Nonclinical Safety Assessment

Nonclinical Safety Assessment

A Guide to International Pharmaceutical Regulations

Edited by

WILLIAM J. BROCK
Brock Scientific Consulting, Montgomery Village, USA

KENNETH L. HASTINGS
Sanofi, Bethesda, USA

KATHY M. McGOWN
FoxKiser, USA

WILEY
A John Wiley & Sons, Ltd., Publication

This edition first published 2013

Registered office
John Wiley & Sons Ltd, The Atrium, Southern Gate, Chichester, West Sussex, PO19 8SQ, United Kingdom

For details of our global editorial offices, for customer services and for information about how to apply for permission to reuse the copyright material in this book please see our website at www.wiley.com.

Library of Congress Cataloging-in-Publication Data

Nonclinical safety assessment : a guide to international pharmaceutical regulations / edited by William J. Brock, Kenneth L. Hastings and Kathy M. McGown.
p. ; cm.
Includes index.
ISBN 978-0-470-74591-5 (cloth)
1. Drug development–International cooperation. 2. Drugs–Toxicology–International cooperation. I. Brock, William J. II. Hastings, Kenneth L. III. McGown, Kathy M.
[DNLM: 1. Drug Evaluation, Preclinical–standards. 2. Drug Approval–methods. 3. Drug Toxicity–prevention & control. 4. International Cooperation. 5. Legislation, Drug. 6. Toxicity Tests–standards. QV 771]
RM301.25.N64 2013
615.1'901–dc23 2012037888

A catalogue record for this book is available from the British Library.

ISBN: 9780470745915

Set in 10/12pt, Times-Roman by Thomson Digital, Noida, India.

Contents

List of Contributors

Shana Azri-Meehan, Forest Research Institute, Jersey City, USA

Matthew S. Bogdanffy, Boehringer Ingelheim Pharmaceuticals, Ridgefield, USA

William J. Brock, Brock Scientific Consulting, Montgomery Village, USA

Leigh Ann Burns-Naas, Gilead Sciences Inc., Foster City, USA

Cristiana Leslie Corrêa, Planitox, Campinas, Brazil

Luc M. De Schaepdrijver, Johnson & Johnson, Belgium

Jamie L. Doran, Intrinsik Health Sciences Inc., Mississauga, Canada

Christopher E. Ellis, CDER, Office of New Drugs, FDA, Silver Spring, USA

Fariza Feraoun, Laboratoires SERB, France

Malik Feraoun, Clinique Feraoun, France

Paul Donald Forbes, Toxarus Inc., Malvern, USA

Douglas Francis, DF Pre-clinical Services Pty Ltd., Hughes ACT, Australia

Lijie Fu, SNLB, China

Osamu Fueki, Pharamaceuticals and Medical Devices Agency, Japan

Hanan Ghantous, CDER, Office of New Drugs, FDA, Silver Spring, USA

Mark T. Goldberg, PlantForm Corporation and Karamella Consulting Inc., Guelph, Canada

Martin D. Green, DVRPA/OVRR/CBER/FDA, WOC2, Rockville, MD, USA

Melanie T. Hartsough, Biologics Consulting Group Inc., Derwood, USA

Kenneth L. Hastings, Sanofi, Bethesda, USA

Robert V. House, DynPort Vaccine Company LLC, Frederick, USA

Mark E. Hurtt, Pfizer, Groton, USA

Louise Latriano, ToxPharm Consulting LLC, Scotch Plains, USA

Kathy M. McGown, FoxKiser, USA

Kazuichi Nakamura, Shionogi & Co. Ltd., Global Regulatory Affairs Department, Japan

S. Natesan, Advinus Therapeutics Limited, India

Robert E. Osterberg, Osterberg Pharm-Tox Consulting, Rockville, USA

Marc J. Pallardy, School of Pharmacy and INSERM, University Paris-Sud, Chatenay, Malabry, France

Robert M. Parker, Huntingdon Life Sciences, East Millstone, USA

James A. Popp, Stratoxon, Lancaster, USA

Mark W. Powley, CDER, Office of New Drugs, FDA, Silver Spring, USA

K.S. Rao, Rao Toxicology Foundation (RTF), Sanjayanagar, India

Christopher P. Sambuco, Downingtown, USA

Giuliana Selmi, Planitox, Campinas, Brazil

Melissa S. Tassinari, CDER, Office of New Drugs, FDA, Silver Spring, USA

Jan-Willem van der Laan, FTBB, Medicines Evaluation Board, The Netherlands

Qingli Wang, Center for Drug Evaluation, SFDA, China

Adam Woolley, ForthTox Ltd., UK

Raymond G. York, RG York & Associates LLC, Manlius, USA

Flávio Ailton Duque Zambrone, Planitox, Campinas, Brazil

Preface

This book, *Nonclinical Safety Assessment: A Guide to International Pharmaceutical Regulations*, was conceived as an update to the Alder and Zbinden text on international nonclinical testing regulations. This out-of-print text was published in 1988 prior to ICH but, at the time, represented a reasonably complete description of the testing requirements for pharmaceuticals. Since that time, the pharmaceutical industry has seen the implementation of ICH, development of new guidance and guidelines from FDA and the EU (CHMP), a new regulatory process in China and other regions, implementation of FDAMA, and so on. It is hoped that this book provides a practical description of nonclinical drug development regulations in the major market regions although we do recognize that this is not a static but a dynamic process that continues to evolve almost on a daily or weekly basis. Although we attempted to capture the state-of-the-art in regulatory toxicology development, we also recognize that certain aspects will change even during the publishing process. Not all regions are covered in this edition of the book. However, with the evolution of ICH, it is likely that all pharmaceutical regions will adopt the ICH concept with minimal alternatives in the testing strategy.

Regardless, the objective of this text is to provide a guide for those involved in nonclinical drug development. As you will see from the layout of the book, the initial section discusses the legislative and regulations for different regions. This is followed by specific chapters on the conduct, interpretation and regulatory considerations of nonclinical studies. The final section of the book describes biotechnology-derived products, vaccines, and so on and the nonclinical challenges and solutions for the clinical development of these sometimes difficult therapeutics.

This text is intended for those actively involved in the clinical development of a pharmaceutical product, whether as a toxicologist, pharmacologist, clinician, project manager, and other functional responsibilities. The approaches and methodologies described throughout this book provide a useful and scientifically valid means to drug approval.

We hope you find this a very useful resource.

The Editors
December 2012

Part I

International Regulations and Nonclinical Studies for Pharmaceuticals

1

Introduction

The Drug Development Process and the Pharmaceutical Market

Kathy M. McGown[1] *and William J. Brock*[2]
[1]*FoxKiser, USA*
[2]*Brock Scientific Consulting, Montgomery Village, USA*

The world market for drugs is large and growing. At the end of 2011, global sales of pharmaceuticals topped $950 billion. The United States (US), Canada, European Union 5 (EU5[1]) and Japan account for almost 85% of pharmaceutical sales (IMS, 2012a) with the balance of the market spread across the rest of the world (ROW). With the consolidation of major corporations and the emergence of small worldwide pharmaceutical enterprises, the face of the pharmaceutical industry continues to evolve. Within this changing global landscape, individual countries and regions continue to have unique regulations and guidances that drug companies must follow for product approval in those regions. Although the larger markets are often the first that are targeted for regulatory submission and approval, this does not mean that an applicant should minimize the regulatory requirements of other areas, in particular those of the "Pharmerging" markets such as India, South America and China. These markets are expected to expand significantly over the next five years and potentially outpace the growth in the more traditional geographic regions. Approvals in those regions can be rigorous and time consuming. However, a basic premise of the

[1] United Kingdom, Spain, Germany, France and Italy.

Nonclinical Safety Assessment: A Guide to International Pharmaceutical Regulations, First Edition.
Edited by William J. Brock, Kenneth L. Hastings and Kathy M. McGown.

industry continues to be that the first to market captures a major portion of the sales while the successive entries in a drug class fight to develop a market presence and maintain market share. Therefore, regardless of the geographic region and the associated challenges, drug development and nonclinical programmes must always integrate this "first to market" view as part of their regulatory strategy.

In this era of evolution, development and marketing has become fiercely competitive. The industry spends millions of dollars on developing new drugs although it is well known that the chance of any single candidate reaching the marketplace is extremely low. Overall, it has been estimated that for every 5000–10 000 candidate drugs, on average only one successfully reaches the consumer market (DiMasi, 2001; PhRMA, 2012), and the probability of that new drug entering the market is highly dependent on the therapeutic class (Adams and Brantner, 2006; Kaitin and DiMasi, 2011). Therefore, industry proceeds with some caution as it pursues development and branches into new classes of drugs or biologics. Companies will often invest a great deal of capital into rapid screening technology to better eliminate those compounds that show limited promise. With the advent of the various "omics" technologies and emphasis on the development of biomarkers of disease, the hope is that these technologies will allow for the targeting of specific disease endpoints and therefore a more selected market segment. Indeed, the development of pharmacogenomics has led to the possibility, as yet unrealized, of personalized medicine and the development of drugs and treatments for targeted subpopulations. Regardless of these advances, early stage drug candidates will still drop out of the development process for a variety of reasons, though most often these will be related to toxicity discovered during the preclinical phase or within the early clinical programme. Later stage development dropouts are most often due to lack of efficacy in the target population although economics plays an increasingly larger role in the choice to discontinue developing a drug or biologic candidate. This later scenario is common with small pharmaceutical enterprises that are dependent on venture firms and other sources of external funding to continue to fuel their development activities.

Efficacy, societal concern for safety and global leveraging of regulatory requirements are driving forces in the processes for drug development. In these processes, drug development strategies and the associated nonclinical safety assessment must consider certain "facts". First, the cost of developing drugs and biologics is extremely high, with investments increasing sharply with each stage of development (DiMasi *et al.*, 2003). Second, as stated earlier, most products will fail during development. While the true success rate for drug development is certainly greater than the often stated 1-in-5000 or more, it is clear that only 3–5% of those products that enter initial clinical evaluations become marketed drugs. With this in mind, many companies choose to undertake only those safety and screening studies "required" to start clinical studies. Larger companies often take a broader, more conservative investigative approach in order to ensure clinical safety and to address anticipated requirements across regions. The downside to this latter approach is that a large number of resources are devoted to a more comprehensive nonclinical programme when later stage clinical success of the candidate is not assured. Over time, several priorities in the nonclinical programmes have developed. First, "kill the losers" as early as possible and, second, minimize the time spent in developing a potentially unsuccessful drug. These principles have produced a spectrum of strategies in the nonclinical safety assessment of drugs, best illustrated by looking at the two extremes.

Strategy A: *Do Only What You Must.* Financial limitations, particularly in small companies, drive the nonclinical and clinical planning. At later stages of development the candidate therapeutic will be licensed to, or a partnership developed with, a larger company. Therefore, the focus is to undertake only the minimum technical and regulatory steps necessary to get a molecule to that critical partnering point in development.

Strategy Z: *Minimize the Risk of Subsequent Failure.* Development proceeds through a series of well-defined and carefully considered milestone decision points. Studies and technical tasks are not often limited to the minimum needed for early development but are often augmented by additional study components. Many of the additional components are short-term toxicity screens or studies which are inexpensive and could be repeated later in the development process. Exactly what these "extra" components include will vary from company to company, and frequently reflect past experiences.

Clearly, most nonclinical programmes fall somewhere in between. Regardless of the strategy chosen, the studies performed to meet regulatory nonclinical safety assessment requirements can be thought of as belonging to three major categories:

- Those necessary to support the successful filing of an Investigational New Drug (IND) application, a Clinical Trial Authorization or equivalent, and to ensure subject safety in the subsequent first in human clinical studies.
- Those required to support the continued long-term clinical development of a drug, up to and including Phase 3 studies. These often include the longer subchronic and speciality studies.
- Those studies required to support a marketing approval application. These nonclinical studies typically include carcinogenicity studies and reproductive toxicity studies. In some cases, the timing of these studies could extend into the post-approval phase of the product lifecycle.

Exactly which study fits into what category is somewhat fluid, and this is heavily influenced by the therapeutic indication, the mechanism of action and the targeted treatment population.

In this book, we examine the international regulations for nonclinical drug development and how the safety of human pharmaceutical products is evaluated around the globe. Clearly, the guidance and regulations established by the US Food and Drug Administration (FDA) over the decades have played a critical role and have provided a baseline or framework for many of the regulations established worldwide. More recently the International Conference on Harmonization (ICH) has emerged as an essential process to consolidate guidance and regulations across the US, Europe and Japan. Although most countries have adopted the concepts of ICH, and many others are expected do so, there still remain country-specific requirements that are necessary for approval. The authors included within this book represent dozens of years of experience in the area of national and international nonclinical drug development. Therefore, we hope to provide a practical, if not comprehensive, assessment of the regulations required for nonclinical toxicology studies around the globe.

1.1 The Global Pharmaceutical Market

The pharmaceutical industry and all of its components operate as part of a global market. This globalization can be seen in all areas, including research, nonclinical and clinical evaluation and production of finished commercial products. Well-known examples of this exist in the sectors of chemical intermediates, active pharmaceutical ingredients (APIs) and in the manufacture of generic drugs. Over the last few decades, these industry segments have made major geographic shifts, with the chemical manufacturing of intermediates and APIs relocating almost entirely from the "West" to India and Asia. Whereas 20 or 30 years ago, Research and Development (R&D) and manufacturing of pharmaceutical products originated in the intended market region, it is now not uncommon to find bulk and finish production occurring in one part of the world for marketing and distribution in an entirely different geographical region.

Over the last 20 years, as the pharmaceutical market has seen robust growth and globalization, the overall cost of health care has been increasing at an alarming rating. Despite widespread public perception, the cost of pharmaceuticals, at least in the US, has not been the driving force behind this spending increase. According to the latest data from Centers for Medicare and Medicaid services (CMS, 2012), pharmaceutical expenditure in the US accounted for only 10% of total healthcare spending in 2010, versus 8.8% in 2000. Regardless of expenditure source, the end result has been heightened media and legislative scrutiny with, in some countries, the healthcare debates taking on a political "life-of-its-own" and the research-based pharmaceutical industry coming under fire as an easy target. It is expected and hoped that healthcare costs will begin to stabilize over time. The effect of currently proposed or future legislative reforms on the pharmaceutical industry is unknown but there is expectation that whatever "fixes" are put in place will result in some negative impact on the industry. With the high cost of pharmaceutical development and outside pressure on the industry, companies will continue to make efforts to control and improve development methods and optimize their expenditures. As part of this trend, there has been an increase in partnering, in-licensing of drug candidates, mergers and acquisitions, and the creation of fully integrated pharmaceutical networks or FIPnets (Kaitin and DiMasi, 2011). The industry has seen larger companies acquiring smaller competitors for R&D expertise, intellectual property, pipelines or marketed portfolio such as Sanofi's acquisition of Genzyme or Takeda's acquisition of Nycomed. There have been several major consolidations, including Pfizer's acquisition of Wyeth and Merck's merger with Schering Plough. As companies continue to examine cost-cutting initiatives, options of mergers and acquisitions and a variety of other "value adding" measures, the overall trend in the pharmaceutical industry appears to be that of consolidation and shrinkage.

In 2011, worldwide sales of drugs were $956 billion, an increase of 5.1% over 2010, with branded drugs accounting for nearly two-thirds of pharmaceutical spending. This branded share is projected to decline, however, to as low as 50% by 2016 as many of the large market products continue to come off-patent (IMS, 2012a; 2012b). The US still accounts for the largest share of the global pharmaceutical market with about $320 billion in annual sales, a slight gain of approximately 3.6% over 2010 (IMS, 2012c). For the same time period, sales in Europe remained relatively flat while Japan saw modest growth of 5.6%. The Pharmerging markets, which include China, Brazil, India and Russia,

Table 1.1 *Top 10 global pharmaceuticals by sales, 2011.*

Rank	Medicine	Company	Primary medical use	2011 sales (USD, billion)	Percent growth vs. 2010
1	Lipitor	Pfizer	Cholesterol	12.5	−3.3
2	Plavix/ Iscover	Bristol-Myers Squibb, Sanofi	Thrombotic events	9.3	3.7
3	Advair/ Seretide	GlaxoSmithKline	Asthma	8.7	0.04
4	Crestor	AstraZeneca	Cholesterol	8.0	14.4
5	Nexium	AstraZeneca	Gastrointestinal disorders	7.9	−6.2
6	Seroquel	AstraZeneca, Astellas Pharmaceuticals	Schizophrenia	7.6	9.5
7	Humira	Abbott	Rheumatoid arthritis	7.3	17.8
8	Enbrel	Amgen, Pfizer	Rheumatoid arthritis	6.8	6.7
9	Remicade	Johnson & Johnson, Merck, Tanabe	Rheumatoid arthritis	6.8	8.4
10	Abilify	Otsuka	Schizophrenia	6.3	14.3

(IMS, 2012d).

outpaced the more developed markets with a 29% gain in pharmaceutical spending in 2011. This growth was largely attributable to increased spending on generic drugs; however, these emerging markets are expected to continue to expand rapidly and could account for as much as 30% of global spending by 2016 (IMS, 2011; 2012a).

The global top 10 branded pharmaceuticals for 2011, which accounted for approximately 8.5% of the total worldwide sales, are presented in Table 1.1.

This list will see dramatic changes over the next few years due to patent expirations and the potential for new competition from biosimilars. Overall, the therapeutic areas that have seen the greatest development have been those encompassing large populations and chronic diseases, resulting in the model of the billion dollar "blockbuster" drug.

The concentration of total sales for a limited number of pharmaceuticals is thought to have distorted, at least for a time, the therapeutic research direction of new drug development. Now, with many of the blockbusters losing patent protection, development is moving away from that paradigm to one of focused therapeutics and specific patient populations. While precise international costs are not available, US pharmaceutical R&D spending is currently estimated to be at least $50–65 billion, based on an estimated 3500 pharmaceutical companies in the US (PhRMA, 2011; 2012). It is expected that there are similar numbers of companies and levels of R&D spending in Europe, and significant value coming from other parts of the world such as China, Australia, India, and Israel. While most of the public focuses on the largest companies, such as those in Table 1.2, the vast majority of companies are mid-sized, small and startups. Significantly, the innovations leading to new molecular entitiess (NME) and biologics appear to be arising primarily from these smaller organizations, with the larger companies licensing these new therapies or purchasing the technology outright.

Table 1.2 *Top 15 global pharmaceutical companies by sales, 2011.*

Rank	Pharmaceutical company	2011 sales (USD, million)	Percent change vs. 2010
1	Pfizer	56 427	−0.7
2	Novartis	51 632	10.1
3	Merck & Co	40 119	6.9
4	Sanofi	39 478	2.4
5	AstraZeneca	36 974	2.9
6	Roche	34 869	5.7
7	GlaxoSmithKline	34 491	1.3
8	Johnson & Johnson	27 664	0.0
9	Abbott	25 871	6.6
10	Teva	23 872	−2.5
11	Lilly	23 716	7.3
12	Takeda	17 767	6.1
13	Bristol-Myers Squibb	16 446	9.7
14	Bayer	16 390	4.3
15	Amgen	16 323	4.6

(IMS, 2012e; IMS, 2012f).

Over the last several years, focused development in targeted therapeutic areas has been the mainstay of many companies. The therapeutic areas that have received the greatest interest over the past decade are shown in Table 1.3. As suggested by this information, the trend has been to pursue therapies for the treatment of chronic diseases, particularly those that affect the ageing population. At the same time, several older or discarded drugs have been repurposed for new uses, such as thalidomide for multiple myeloma, doxepine hydrochloride for insomnia, or the combination of dextromethorphan and quinidine for psuedobulabar affect, and some very old drugs, such as digoxin, continue to be in use. In

Table 1.3 *Top global therapeutic classes by sales, 2011.*

Rank	Therapeutic class	2011 sales (USD, billion)	Percent growth vs. 2010
1	Oncologics	62.2	5.5
2	Respiratory agents	39.4	7.3
3	Antidiabetics	39.2	11.4
4	Lipid regulators	38.7	3.7
5	Antipsychotics	28.4	9.4
6	Angiotensin II Antagonists	27.4	−0.7
5	Anti-ulcerants	26.9	−6.4
8	Autoimmune Agents	24.4	14.1
9	Antidepressants	20.4	−1.5
10	HIV Antivirals	17.4	9.5
11	Platelet Aggregation Inhibitors	16.4	4.1
12	Anti-Epileptics	14.1	10.1
13	Vitamins & Minerals	13.9	6.1
14	Vaccines	13.4	13.0
15	Narcotic Analgesics	12.3	0.7

(IMS, 2012a).

the last 10–15 years, new drug classes have emerged that have grown significantly in terms of expenditures and have shown major therapeutic advances by either reducing disease burden (statins) or unacceptable side effects (atypical antipsychotics) (Dickson and Gagnon, 2004).

A major factor to consider in the development of new therapeutic entities is cost, which can present significant hurdles to the smaller, innovative companies. DiMasi *et al.* (2003) examined the development costs of 68 pharmaceuticals based on a survey from 10 drug companies. The estimated average development cost per new drug was $802 million (in 2000 dollars). Dickson and Gagnon (2004) further demonstrated that the cost of development to approval has increased over time from 1979 to 2003 and, more recently, that cost has been revised upwards to $1 billion or more (Adams and Brantner, 2010). Furthermore, the average time to approval has increased. While the time from discovery to approval in the 1960s was estimated to be about eight years, in the current decade that timeline has increased to 12–14 years (Dickson and Gagnon, 2004; PhRMA, 2012). Although the costs and timing to approval represent primarily "big pharma", the drug development process in smaller enterprises is estimated to be about the same. Active drug development in the small companies is critical for their survival but many of the small companies have limited (one or two) NMEs in their pipeline. Hence, all of their energy and resources are developed to the success of that single entity, at least through early clinical studies. At that point, in order to have the financial resources necessary to continue their programmes, the smaller companies must often look for partnering opportunities.

In the US, the National Institutes of Health (NIH) helps to support the development of pharmaceuticals with funding to academic institutions or nonprofit groups and, more recently, through small business innovation and research (SBIR) grants. Although not completely certain, the costs from discovery through early development of these drugs are anticipated to be the same as those developed in larger industrial laboratories. However, the number of approved drugs that originate through this means is small. For example, it was found that of the 47 approved drugs that reached $500 million in US sales in 1999, only four originated either directly or indirectly through governmental support (DiMasi *et al.*, 2003).

1.2 Looking to the Future

Crommelin *et al.* (2010) provide interesting scenarios and predictions of the pharmaceutical industry during the next decade. Some of the predictions are somewhat disturbing but certainly could reflect the changing environment in the industry. The authors suggest that large target population breakthroughs (blockbuster drugs) will not be delivered into the market. They see drugs for smaller populations, such as orphan diseases, and believe that society will need to spend considerable resources in order to fill the pharmacological "toolbox". Furthermore, the authors believe that advances in delivery technology will blur the distinctions between drugs and devices. Indeed, it is expected that such an increase in combination drug/device products will be seen in the next decade. They further indicate that the major pharmaceutical companies will continue to dominate but only to the extent that they have the resources and expertise for development, and with this shift, Chinese and Indian pharmaceutical companies will slowly enter the group of leading innovative firms. That scenario has already been seen with the accession of Teva Pharmaceuticals, which entered into the international generics market in the 1990s but is now one of the top 10 pharmaceutical companies in the world.

Another complicating factor in considering the pharmaceutical market sector is the sheer diversity of products involved. In the next decade, the number of biotechnology-derived products will continue to expand, particularly in the fields of oncology and immunologic therapies. Small molecules will continue to dominate for some time as NMEs, second, third or fourth generation molecules, line extensions and generics, although biotechnology products will constitute a growing percentage of INDs and, just as important, a larger proportion of total pharmaceutical sales. The challenges of early stage development and assessing the safety of these biologic and biotechnology-derived substances are very different. Although there continues to be an increasing trend towards final drug (biologic) approval, there have also been increases in approval time. The reasons are diverse, some ascribing it to implementation of risk evaluation and mitigation strategies (REMS) but others believe it is only the reasonable rationale to ensure the appropriate time to adequately review increasingly complex products for difficult-to-target conditions (Hughes, 2010).

In summary, the pharmaceutical market will continue see growth although the double digit increases of the 1990s and 2000s are not expected. The era of the "blockbuster" drug is over with the pharmaceutical companies now challenged to go forward with more focused development and to work towards the concept of "personalized" medicine. Continued worldwide regulatory pressures for safe and effective drugs will force drug companies to consider how resources are devoted to the "pipeline" of new molecular entities and biologics. Indeed, there is an expectation by some that eventually the increase in biotechnology-derived therapies will outpace the small molecule in the coming decades.

1.3 Legal and Regulatory Considerations in Drug Development

In the US, the laws that are applicable to the approval of a drug product are the Federal Food and Drug Cosmetic Act (FFDCA) and its various amendments. For each amendment to the FFDCA that is passed, the FDA must develop regulations in order to implement the legislative revisions. Those regulations pass through an administrative rulemaking process that is documented in the Federal Register and the final regulations are then "codified" and published in the Code of Federal Regulations (CFR). For drug and medical devices, as well as foods, cosmetics and dietary supplements, the FDA regulations are contained in Title 21. Those regulations specific to human drugs can be found in Subchapter D (Parts 300–399) while regulations for Vaccines and Biologics are in Subchapter F (Parts 600–680) and Medical Devices are found in Subchapter H (Parts 800–898). For human drugs the definition of a new drug can be found in 21 CFR Subchapter D, Part 310.3(g):

> "A new drug substance means any substance that when used in the manufacture, processing, or packing of a drug, causes that drug to be a new drug but does not include intermediates used in the synthesis of such substance."

The regulations then proceed to define what constitutes an NME, a generic drug and drug combination products. For toxicologists, the most relevant sections of the FDA regulations are 21 CFR Subchapter D, Parts 312 and 314 and Subchapter F, Part 601. These sections describe the Investigational New Drug Application (IND), the New Drug Application (NDA) and Biological License Application (BLA), respectively. Those processes and applications will be described in later chapters in this book. The major focus for a toxicologist working in the pharmaceutical industry is on preparing the toxicology "packages" to support these applications and overseeing the nonclinical studies necessary to support clinical studies. In a nutshell, the law requires solid scientific evidence of safety and efficacy before a new drug or medical device will be permitted in clinical trials or placed into the market.

In the European Union, the process for regulatory drug approval or authorization is somewhat similar. For new biological or high-technology products, orphan drugs, products for HIV/AIDS, cancer, diabetes, neurodegenerative diseases, autoimmune and other immune dysfunctions and viral diseases, the approval pathway is "centralized" through the European Medicine Agency (EMA). A marketing authorization application (MAA) is prepared according to standard format (CTD) and submitted to the Medicines Bureau of EMA. Those applications are then reviewed by the Committee for Medicinal Products for Human Use (CHMP) and registration authorizations decisions for the EU are made. Drugs are reviewed as either Part A or Part B drugs, with Part A drugs having the more formidable process review since these are biotechnology-derived products. Part B drugs, are the usual small molecule drug products as new molecular entities (NME), new formulations or for new indications. Other new active substances might be accepted for consideration under the centralized procedure when it can be shown that the product constitutes a significant therapeutic, scientific or technical innovation. There are several other pathways available for those drug products that fall outside the scope of the EU centralized process. These include the decentralized process for simultaneous authorization in sponsor-selected countries, the mutual recognition procedure, or the national process for product authorization within a single country.

The approval process in Japan is likewise similar to that of the EU and the United States. The Pharmaceuticals and Medical Devices Agency (PMDA) is an independent administrative organization charged with the review of new drug and medical device products. Within this organization, there are different branches, each having responsibility for the review of drugs or medical devices. The regulations of the PMDA do not include the "quasi-drug" category. Quasi-drugs are products ranging from deodorants, hair dyes, hair growers and depilatories, medicated cosmetics (notably whitening agents) and medicated toothpaste to sanitary napkins and over-the-counter health drinks. The quasi-drugs are reviewed within the Japanese authority but outside the regulatory structure for human pharmaceuticals and medical devices.

The legal and regulatory processes briefly described here represent those countries or regions that participate in the ICH process. Other countries and regions have their own processes that must be considered when gaining regulatory approval of a drug. These are discussed further in the appropriate chapters of this book.

1.4 The Drug Development Process – General Considerations

Prior to entry into the drug development process, a large amount of resources and brainpower goes into "discovery" – the research that leads to optimal selection of a substance that shows greater promise than others for ultimate approval and marketing. The discovery process has seen radical changes over the last 5–10 years as research continues to make strides in identifying biomarkers of disease (Amur *et al.*, 2008; Krishna *et al.*, 2008; Tesch *et al.*, 2010). Biomarkers for breast cancers, leukaemia, prostate cancer and diabetes have led to the development and validation of *in vitro* models that are used to determine early efficacy of potential new drugs. *In vivo* animal models of diseases have also furthered the development of specific, targeted therapies. In addition to these animal- and cell-based models, a great effort has been devoted in recent years to *in silico* models and the development of bioinformatic databases which have further reduced the time and resources in the discovery process (Ekins *et al.*, 2007; Muster *et al.*, 2008; Pauli *et al.*, 2008; Hutter, 2009). Using all of these resources, a lead compound and backups are selected for further development.

The drug development process then follows a logical and somewhat general pathway to first-in-human trials although, depending on the product, some companies might choose to take a more customized approach for entry into early human exposure. For the general case approach to nonclinical safety assessment, there are a few fundamental assumptions about the drug under development. The first assumption is that the primary intended route of therapeutic administration is oral, as is indeed the case for the vast majority of both existing and new drugs. Most aspects of nonclinical safety assessment depend on the route of administration, but the use of other routes (e.g., intravenous, topical), will influence what is done for nonclinical safety assessment. A second assumption relates to the frequency of drug administration and the dosage form. Most often, the drug is administered once daily (QD) although there continues to be the development of drugs for twice daily (BID) or three-times daily (TID) as well as weekly or monthly administration; this latter is more common for development of biologics and anticancer therapies. Extended release formulations present their own set of challenges in terms of optimum pharmacokinetics and the evaluation of off-target effects. Dosage forms commonly used include liquids, tablets, and capsules although other delivery means, such as inhalants, topical patches, depots and implants are not infrequent and will need to be considered in the nonclinical programme.

The nonclinical studies required to initiate clinical studies of pharmaceuticals in humans are variously labelled as first-in-human or "FIH enabling" or, in the United States, "IND enabling" studies. For many drug candidates, it may comprise the only regulatory nonclinical safety work that will ever be done, since progression into further development will be based primarily on the successful outcome of these early clinical studies.

The nonclinical studies needed for opening an IND or CTA are to be performed in compliance with Good Laboratory Practice regulations (GLP). Prior to initiating studies, certain preparatory steps must be performed in order to successfully achieve such compliance:

1. Sufficiently pure drug substances must be produced and characterized. It is extremely important that the purity of the drug substance used in the nonclinical studies be no greater than what is intended to be used in the clinical programme in order that the

impurities become "qualified" as the studies progress. Use of a higher purity in nonclinical studies will generally result in a regulatory agency "Clinical Hold" on the clinical trial programme until data are developed to demonstrate the safety of the drug substance relative to potential impurities. In addition, the stability of both the drug substance (API) and drug product (API with included excipients) under appropriate storage conditions and in the anticipated animal dosing formulation must be demonstrated.

2. The GLP-compliant analytical and bioanalytical methods must be developed and validated to verify the purity of the drug substance, concentrations of the drug in dosing solutions as well as detecting the drug substance and metabolite(s) in blood or other matrices. The development and validation of these methods is almost always a rate-limiting step in the nonclinical programme, so it is advisable to complete the method developments prior to initiating the pivotal toxicology studies. Furthermore, the bioanalytical methods must be developed for the selected test species (rodent and nonrodent) that is to be used in the nonclinical studies, and in the concentration range anticipated. Therefore, early analytical development could be critical to the timing and outcome of a competitive nonclinical programme.

With the preparatory work in place, the nonclinical studies can commence. The details of specific study designs are described elsewhere in this book; however, the study designs are generally compliant with those outlined in the OECD guidelines and other internationally recognized testing protocols (for example, the FDA Red Book).

The results of early pharmacology studies, as well as initial pharmacokinetic studies conducted to examine the efficacy and bioavailability of the drug, can often serve to establish dose levels for early dose rangefinding toxicity studies. Acute toxicity studies are not required for entry into the clinical trial although some variation of these studies is usually conducted to help with the setting of dose levels for repeat dose toxicity studies (ICH M3R2). In the absence of such data, a dose escalation study can be undertaken, and is generally advisable for initial studies to be conducted in both rodents and nonrodents.

The IND (CTA)-enabling studies consist of repeat-dose toxicity studies in both a rodent and a nonrodent species. These studies will need to be at *minimum* two weeks in duration followed by a recovery phase. In recent years, the study duration has trended towards four weeks followed by recovery in order to adequately fulfill regulatory requirements. The rat is the typical rodent species, with the dog often used as the nonrodent species. However, the nonhuman primate (NHP) is typical for biotechnology-derived products since this animal model is immunologically competent and similar to humans when compared to other nonrodent species (ICH S6R1). For topical drugs, the minipig is becoming the more acceptable nonrodent species, replacing the rabbit and dog. In all of these studies, blood samples will need to be collected for toxicokinetics.

In the US, it is possible to undertake a single-dose clinical study based on single-dose toxicity studies in rodents and nonrodents. However, these nonclinical studies will need to be "gold-plated". That is, the studies will need to include all parameters typically included in well-designed repeat-dose toxicity studies. Other than the usual in-life measures, the studies will need to include clinical pathology, gross and microscopic pathology, ophthalmology and, for nonrodents, electrocardiogram evaluations. A single-dose nonclinical study to support a single-dose clinical study would be appropriate if the clinical therapy itself is only a single administration, for example, some antivirals. Otherwise, it would be most cost- and time-effective to undertake the repeat-dose studies to support the single-dose clinical study.

Some pharmaceutical companies often prefer to conduct 90-day in addition to 4-week studies as the IND-enabling toxicity studies, and this could be related to experience with previous drug candidates as well as the intended duration of multiple-dose clinical studies. Although this represents a conservative approach to drug development, doing a 90-day study further assures the safety of the drug candidates going forward into early clinical trials. The downside is that there is a large expenditure associated with these studies with no assurance that the clinical candidate will progress far enough in development to justify the cost.

For the IND-enabling programme, genotoxicity studies also are needed. According to ICH guidance (ICH S2 and ICH M3R2), an *in vitro* mutagenicity study and an *in vitro* chromosomal aberration study are generally needed for the IND or CTA. If either of these studies are "positive", then the *in vivo* chromosomal aberration study will be needed along with an evaluation of the weight of evidence approach for genotoxicity. If the *in vivo* study is also positive, it is likely that the drug would be abandoned. Furthermore, the regulatory authority could request that the sponsor undertake other genotoxicity studies, for example, COMET assay, UDS, and so on (see Chapter 14). Similar to the repeat-dose studies described above, some companies will undertake all three initial studies prior to submission of the IND. This decision is often based on prior experience with a similar drug or could represent company policy. Exceptions to the requirement to conduct genotoxicity studies are made for certain drug classes, such as oncologics, and also for certain biologics.

Finally, the core battery of safety pharmacology studies will be necessary (ICH S7). The core battery consists of an evaluation of the central nervous system (CNS) and respiratory systems in the rat and an evaluation of the cardiovascular system (CVS) in the dog. Over the last few years, a combined study of CVS and respiratory system in the dog or nonhuman primates (NHP) has become more common as this tends to reduce the timeline for development (Lindgren *et al.*, 2008; Pugsley *et al.*, 2008). Further, this study design has been found to be acceptable to the regulatory authorities. Development and validation of this combined study in other species, such as the minipig, also has been reported (Authier *et al.*, 2008; 2009; 2011).

The discussion above reflects the general approach of the IND-enabling programme for small molecules. For biotechnology-derived substances, the development approach is more complex and often is done on a "case-by-case" basis depending on the product and the intended application. Most often for biotechnology-derived substances, single-dose studies in the appropriate animal model, usually the NHP, and the rat are undertaken to determine dose levels and species to be used in subsequent repeat-dose studies. For these latter studies, the duration of dosing may only be four weeks although durations of up to six months have been conducted. The dose regimen usually consists of administering the drug 1–3 times/week. Evaluation of the blood levels of biotechnology-derived substances as well as blood levels of neutralizing antibodies is necessary. The development of biologic products is further described in Chapter 18.

The IND or CTA can usually be submitted with the toxicology studies described above. In some cases, an early fertility and embryofetal study (Segment I) and an embryofetal developmental toxicity study (Segment II) are conducted depending on the class of drugs being examined as well as whether toxicity signals are identified in the repeat-dose studies. As described above, some companies may undertake these studies as a matter of established routine in their drug development process. This might seem more than required but could be a reflection of the culture of the company.

Overall, the drug development process described in this introduction represents a general "best" case. It is not uncommon that issues arise during the development process that cause delays for the conduct of additional studies. One must remember that, by design, a biologically-active compound is being intentionally administered to animals and it is expected that some unknown and potentially adverse responses will occur. It is how those responses are managed, how they experimentally translate to risks in humans, and the amount of resources available to the company to evaluate the responses and the risks that will ultimately determine whether this drug proceeds to further development.

References

Adams, C. and Brantner, V.V. (2010) Spending on new drug development. *Health Econ.*, **19**, 130–141.

Adams, C.P. and Brantner, V.V. (2006) Estimating the cost of new drug development. Is it really $802 million? *Health Affair.*, **25**, 420–428.

Amur, S., Frueh, F.W., Lasko, L.J., and Huang, S.M. (2008) Integration and use of biomarkers in drug development, regulation and clinical practice: A US regulatory perspective. *Biomark. Med.*, **2**, 305–311.

Authier, S., Gervais, J., Fournier, S., Gauvin, D., Maghezzi, S., and Troncy, E. (2011) Cardiovascular and respiratory safety pharmacology in Gottingen minipigs: Pharmacological characterization. *J. Pharmacol. Toxicol. Methods*, **64**, 53–59.

Authier, S., Legaspi, M., Gauvin, D., and Troncy, E. (2009) Respiratory safety pharmacology: Positive control drug responses in Sprague-Dawley rats, beagle dogs and cynomolgus monkeys. *Reg. Toxicol. Pharmacol.*, **55**, 229–235.

Authier, S., Legaspi, M., Gauvin, D., Chaurand, F., Fournier, S., and Troncy, E. (2008) Validation of respiratory safety pharmacology models: Conscious and anesthetized beagle dogs. *J. Pharmacol. Toxicol. Methods*, **57**, 52–60.

CMS (2012) National Health Expenditure Data, Historical. www.cms.gov.

Crommelin, D., Stolk, P., Besancon, L., Shah, V., Midha, K., and Leufkens, H. (2010) Pharmaceutical sciences in 2020. *Nat. Rev. Drug Discov.*, **9**, 99–100.

Dickson, M. and Gagnon, J.P. (2004) The cost of new drug discovery and development. *Disc. Med.*, **4**, 172–179.

DiMasi, J.A. (2001) Risks in new drug development. Approval success rates for investigational drugs. *Clin. Pharm. Therap.*, **69**, 297–307.

DiMasi, J.A., Hansen, R.W., and Grabowshi, H.G. (2003) The price of innovation: New estimates of drug development costs. *J. Health Econ.*, **22**, 151–185.

Ekins, S., Mestres, J., and Testa, B. (2007) In silico pharmacology for drug discovery: Applications to targets and beyond. *Br. J. Pharmacol.*, **152**, 21–37.

Hughes, B. (2010) 2009 FDA drug approvals. *Nat. Rev. Drug Discov.*, **9**, 89–92.

Hutter, M.C. (2009) In silico prediction of drug properties. *Curr. Med. Chem.*, **16**, 199–202.

IMS (2011) *The Global Use of Medicines: Outlook Through 2015*, IMS Institute for Healthcare Informatics, May 2011.

IMS (2012a) IMS Forecasts & Reports. The Global Use of Medicines: Outlook Through 2016. http://www.imshealth.com/portal/site/ims/.

IMS (2012b) Top-Line Market Data. Global Pharmaceutical Market Size & Growth by Region, 2011–2016. http://www.imshealth.com/portal/site/ims/.

IMS (2012c) Top-Line Market Data. U.S. Spending Information. http://www.imshealth.com/portal/site/ims/.

IMS (2012d) Top-Line Market Data. Top 20 Global Products, 2011. http://www.imshealth.com/portal/site/ims/.

IMS (2012e) Top-Line Market Data. Top 20 Global Corporations, 2011. http://www.imshealth.com/portal/site/ims/.

IMS (2012f) Top-Line Market Data. Top 20 Global Corporations, 2010. http://www.imshealth.com/portal/site/ims/.

IMS (2012g) Top-Line Market Data. Top 20 Global Therapeutic Classes, 2011. http://www.imshealth.com/portal/site/ims/.

Kaitin, K.I. and DiMasi, J.A. (2011) Pharmaceutical innovations in the 21st century: New drug approvals in the first decade, 2000–2009. *Clin. Pharmacol. Therap.*, **89**, 183–188.

Krishna, R., Herman, G., and Wagner, J.A. (2008) Accelerating drug development using biomarkers: A case study with sitagliptin, a novel DPP4 inhibitor for type 2 diabetes. *Amer. Assoc. Pharmaceut. Sci. J.*, **10**, 401–409.

Lindgren, S., Bass, A.S., Briscoe, R., Bruce, K., Fredrichs, G.S., Kallman, M.J., Margaf, C., Patmore, L., and Pugsley, M.K. (2008) Benchmarking safety pharmacology regulatory packages and best practice. *J. Pharmacol. Toxicol. Methods*, **58**, 99–109.

Muster, W., Breidenbach, A., Fischer, H., Kirchner, S., Muller, L., and Pahler, A. (2008) Computational toxicology in drug development. *Drug Disc. Today*, **137**, 303–310.

Pauli, I., Timmers, L.F., Caceres, R.A., Soares, M.B., and de Azevedo, W.F., Jr. (2008) In silico and in vitro: Identifying new drugs. *Curr. Drug Targets*, **9**, 1054–1061.

Pharmaceutical Research and Manufacturers of America (PhRMA) (2011) 2011 Pharmaceutical Industry Profile. http://www.phrma.org/.

Pharmaceutical Research and Manufacturers of America (PhRMA) (2012) 2012 Pharmaceutical Industry Profile. http://www.phrma.org/.

Pugsley, M.K., Authier, S., and Curtis, M.J. (2008) Principles of safety pharmacology. *Br. J. Pharmacol.*, **154**, 1382–1399.

Tesch, G., Amur, S., Schousboe, J.T., Siegel, J.N., Lasko,L.J., and Bai, J.P. (2010) Success achieved and challenges ahead in translating biomarkers in clinical applications. *Amer. Assoc. Pharmaceut. Sci. J.*, **12**, 243–253.

Websites

European Medicines Agency (EMA). www.ema.eu.int

Food and Drug Administration, Center for Drug Research. www.fda.gov/cder.

International Conference on Harmonization. www.ich.org.

Japan Pharmaceutical Manufacturer Association (JPMA). www.jpma.or.jp/english.

2

ICH: History and Nonclinical Guidances

Jan-Willem van der Laan[1] *and Kenneth L. Hastings*[2]
[1]*FTBB, Medicines Evaluation Board, The Netherlands*
[2]*Sanofi, Bethesda, USA*

2.1 Introduction

The International Conference on Harmonization of Technical Requirements for Registration of Pharmaceuticals for Human Use, commonly referred to as ICH, began in 1988 when a delegation of the European Commission (EC; now the European Union, EU) and the European pharmaceutical industry visited Japan to discuss issues in drug development common to both. During this visit, differences were identified in the technical requirements for registration of pharmaceuticals for human use. Although legitimate differences of opinion on the scientific basis of requirements were acknowledged and discussed, there was recognition that these issues could be resolved. The EC and Japan committed to resolving these issues with the understanding that success would result in significant public health and economic benefits.

It is important to understand that these differences in pharmaceutical development and registration requirements were the result of national laws. Differences in these laws were often the result of public health issues unique to specific countries and regions. For example, many birth defects due to thalidomide (although first reported in Australia) occurred in Europe, where it was first marketed (McBride, 1977). Thus, requirements for establishing the safety of drugs that would be used in women during pregnancy were especially important to the EU. However, in discussions between the EU and Japan, it became apparent that the *scientific* basis of requirements for pharmaceutical development applied to all parties. It was this understanding that made ICH possible.

Nonclinical Safety Assessment: A Guide to International Pharmaceutical Regulations, First Edition.
Edited by William J. Brock, Kenneth L. Hastings and Kathy M. McGown.

In 1989, at the World Health Organization (WHO) International Conference of Drug Regulatory Authorities (ICDRA), specific planning for harmonization of pharmaceutical regulations began. Delegates from this meeting subsequently met with the International Federation of Pharmaceutical Manufacturing Authorities (IFPMA) and proposed a formal initiative involving industry and health regulatory authorities in three regions/countries (Europe, Japan, and the United States) to produce harmonized requirements. It was during these discussions that ICH was conceived.

The first formal meeting of ICH was hosted in Brussels, Belgium in April 1990, by the European Federation of Pharmaceutical Industry Associations (EFPIA). This was a planning meeting to reach agreement on the structure and remit of the ICH. The ICH Steering Committee (SC) was formed, consisting of representatives from six parties (informally referred to as the "Six Pack"; Table 2.1).

In addition to representatives of the Six Pack countries, observers attended from other interested organizations (the European Free Trade Association, EFTA), national regulatory authorities (Sweden, Canada, Australia), and WHO. Sweden represented other authorities (Norway, Switzerland) who would participate in negotiations.[1] At subsequent meetings in Tokyo and Washington, the ICH SC began establishing expert working groups (EWGs) for specific topics.

At the October 1990 ICH SC meeting in Tokyo, an official statement was released expressing commitment to increased international harmonization to ensure that safe and effective medicines would be developed and registered in the most efficient and cost-effective manner. This would become recognized as the principal remit of ICH. In 1991, the First International Conference on Harmonization (ICH) convened in Brussels, with more than 1000 participants. The full list of official conferences is given in Table 2.2.

Presentations given at four conferences were recorded precisely and published in books (D'Arcy and Harron, 1992, 1994, 1996, 1998). Presentations given at subsequent conferences are available via the internet (www.ich.org).

Table 2.1 *ICH Six Pack.*

Regulatory agencies	Industrial associations
1. European Union (including European Medicines Agency and CHMP)	4. European Federation of Pharmaceutical Industry Associations (EFPIA)
2. US Food and Drug Administration	5. Pharmaceutical Research and Manufacturers Association (PhRMA)
3. Japanese Ministry of Health Labour & Welfare (now including PMDA)	6. Japanese Pharmaceutical Manufacturers Association (JPMA)

Secretariat: International Federation of Pharmaceutical Manufacturers Association (IFPMA).

[1] The European Community at that time consisted of 12 member states. Austria, Finland and Sweden joined the EU in 1995, just preceding the establishment of the European Agency for Evaluation of Medicines (EMA – now the European Medicines Agency, EMA) in January 1995.

Table 2.2 *International conferences on harmonization.*

	Year	Place
ICH 1	1991	Brussels
ICH 2	1993	Orlando
ICH 3	1995	Yokohama
ICH 4	1997	Brussels
ICH 5	2000	San Diego
ICH 6	2003	Osaka

2.2 Organization of the ICH

The ICH is not a regulatory authority. ICH Guidelines (or, in the US, Guidances), when promulgated, convey no *legal* authority. These guidelines/guidances are submitted to the appropriate national (or regional) regulatory authorities for official adoption and publication. The ICH working process is illustrated in Figure 2.1.

The process of formulating ICH guidelines is discussed in detail below, but the experiences of the first Expert Working Groups (EWGs) are illustrative. The ICH SC established four categories of guidelines, denoted alpha-numerically: safety (S), efficacy (E), quality (Q), and combined topics (M). Nonclinical topics are covered under safety (S). These were the first ICH safety topics:

1. Toxicity Testing Programme
2. Reproductive Toxicology
3. Biotechnology.

The extent of the process became apparent when discussions began on Topic 1: the Toxicity Testing Programme. It became clear that several issues could be dealt with best

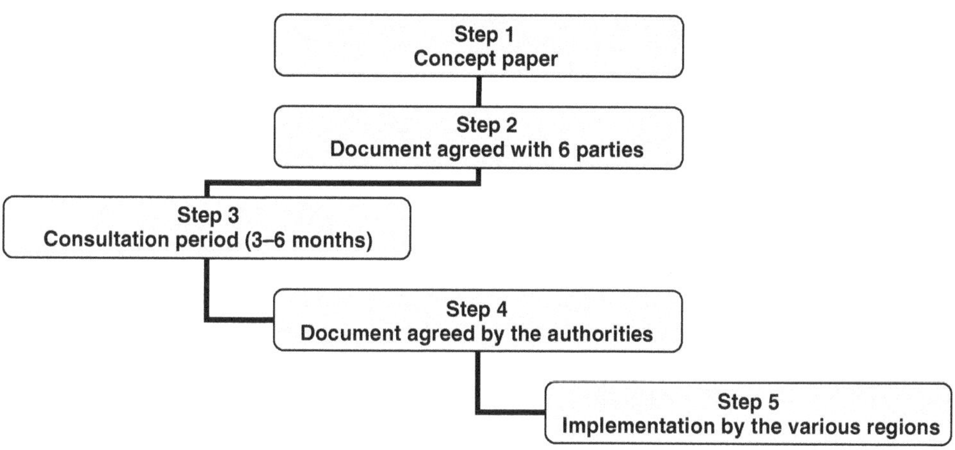

Figure 2.1 *The ICH process.*

as separate topics. Thus, carcinogenicity testing (to become S1) and duration of chronic repeated-dose toxicity studies (to become S4), were assigned to separate EWGs.

One issue was resolved at this conference: the usefulness of mean lethal dose (LD_{50}) determinations in drug development. The decision was taken that LD_{50} added little value to safety assessment and would no longer be used in any of the ICH regions. The parties agreed that a well-designed, single-dose acute toxicity study using increasing doses and detailed descriptions of observed effects would be adequately informative.

A specific issue recognized early by the SC was the need for accurate translation, especially of precisely-defined technical terms. This need became clear with harmonization of the requirements for single-dose acute toxicity tests. An important consideration in recommending elimination of the LD_{50} test was concern over animal welfare. It was difficult to support the utility of a study which used death as an experimental end-point. It soon became clear that an agreement could be reached by recommending a study design in which doses were chosen to demonstrate the *no observable effect level* (NOEL), and particularly the *no observable adverse effect level* (NOAEL). This solution revealed an anticipated problem: "NOAEL" was incorrectly translated from Japanese into English. "Mu Sayo Ryo" means "*no effect dose*" in English, and "Mu Dokusei Ryo" means "*no toxic effect dose*". The problem in interpretation was "effect" in NOEL, which was translated as "toxic". In an attempt to avoid confusion, the Japanese added a third term, "Mu Eikyo Ryo", meaning a dose without any biological effect, which in fact caused even more confusion. The key was to provide precise translations of "adverse effect" and "pharmacologic effect". Harmonization at this point was accomplished by correct and *precise* translation.

A second issue addressed early in ICH discussions was significant differences between Japan and other parties in conduct of reproductive toxicology studies. In Japan, the primary evaluation of reproductive hazard was done on an administrative level without specific toxicological knowledge. A key aspect of study design in Europe and the US was that exposure to the test article, when using pregnant rats and/or rabbits, was a standard period (from gestational days 5 to 16), but this could differ for various authorities (e.g., from gestational days 6 to 18). Japan was especially strict in expecting that exposure would be during the day 5 to day 16 period of gestation. At times, studies had to be repeated because the Japanese requirements were not met. This issue was resolved and it has now been agreed that small differences in dosing intervals will not lead to a request for a new study.

2.3 The ICH Process

As of this writing, ten safety (nonclinical) ICH Guidelines have been published and accepted by the three regions (these documents are listed in Table 2.3). The contents of these documents are discussed in detail in other chapters. Here, a brief description of the ICH process is given.

The first step in producing an ICH guideline is identification of an issue in drug development being addressed by regulatory authorities using discordant approaches. Usually, an informal working group (IWG) is formed to determine whether harmonization of approaches to a given issue is possible and needed. It is important to emphasize that

Table 2.3 *ICH Safety Guidelines.*

ICH Guideline number	Guideline topic
S1	Carcinogenicity testing (3 guidelines)
S2	Genotoxicity testing (2 guidelines, Revision 2011)
S3	Toxicokinetics (2 guidelines)
S4	Duration chronic studies
S5	Reproductive toxicity (2 guidelines)
S6	Preclinical testing of biotech-derived proteins (Addendum 2011)
S7	Safety pharmacology (2 guidelines)
S8	Immunotoxicity
S9	Testing of anticancer drugs
S10	Photosafety (in progress)
	Multidisciplinary
M3	Timing of nonclinical studies (Revision 2009)
M4	Common Technical Dossier
M7	Genotoxic impurities (in progress)

available *scientific* data are key to this process. One of the most important tasks of the IWG is to survey relevant information and determine whether additional data are needed. Often it is found that sufficient data exist to support useful discussion, but these need to be assembled in a useful format. If the IWG determines that a harmonized approach can be recommended and would likely be adopted, a request is made to the ICH SC that an EWG be formed.

When an EWG is formed, each of the Six Pack nominates members (usually two from each party). In addition, other health authorities and trade groups could nominate representatives. For example, Canada and Switzerland usually nominate representatives, officially designated as "observers". In practice, all members of an EWG are equal partners in discussions. The task of the EWG is to write a concept paper, which is the blueprint for negotiations. This concept paper, when presented to the SC, constitutes Step 1 in the ICH process.

When consensus has been achieved in the EWG and a draft guideline is written, this constitutes Step 2. Really, the Step 2 document is the finalized product of Step 1. Step 3 is circulation of the document for consultation and review outside of the EWG. This is a very important step in the ICH process. In this process, the work product of the EWG is critically assessed by those potentially affected by the document. Often, this process involves meetings sponsored by organizations such as the Drug Information Association, professional societies such as the Society of Toxicology, and public meetings sponsored by regulatory agencies such as the US FDA. It is not unusual for outside parties to be critical of the document for various reasons. Most important are issues related to gaps in available knowledge, often identified by relevant experts outside of the EWG. In fact, critiques by outside experts can result in significant changes in the document and delays in accepting a proposed guideline. Thus, it is important that a Step 2 document, when made available for comment outside of ICH, be written as clearly as possible, vetted appropriately by regulatory scientists not involved in the EWG but affected by the guideline, and supported by quality data.

When the Step 2 guideline is judged acceptable by the ICH parties, the EWG begins Step 4, writing the final guidance. Usually this involves clarification of issues raised during the review of the Step 2 document. If there are major objections to the Step 2 document from any of the Six Pack, it will likely be sent back to the EWG for more extensive changes – possibly involving collection and consideration of other data. However, once the recommendation has been made by the three Six Pack regulatory authorities to accept the guideline, the SC begins final consideration. It is unusual for the SC to not accept a properly vetted Step 4 document. The purpose of the SC signing the Step 4 document, referred to as Step 5, is to *recommend* acceptance by the three regulatory authorities in the Six Pack. Usually, this is done without further modifications to the guideline. However, there are examples of "regional differences" being acknowledged in the final guideline (see discussion on ICH M3 below).

Finally, it should be remembered that each region in the Six Pack tends to view the guidelines somewhat differently. US FDA uses the term "guidance", implying that the document does not mandate approaches but establishes best practices which can be altered if there is a compelling rationale. As a general rule, however, ICH guidelines are used with very few exceptions. Europe and Japan tend to view ICH guidelines more strictly.

Another important concept used by ICH is called "maintenance". ICH recognized that any guidance is likely to need updating consistent with advances in science and practical experience. Thus, three processes can be used to address needed changes in the guidelines. The first is called a question-and-answer document. This is designed to address specific (and usually rather minor) issues. The second is called an addendum, and this is a more extensive process, often involving the formation of a new EWG. This approach is designed to deal with significant *new* issues without the need for rewriting the existing guideline (a recent example is the addendum to ICH S6). Finally, maintenance can involve a complete revision of an existing guideline. This has been done recently with revisions of ICH S2 and ICH M3.

2.4 Animal Welfare and Alternative Methods

ICH recognizes the importance of animals in drug development and is sensitive to potential animal welfare issues. Thus, emphasis is placed on the 3Rs (reduction, refinement, and replacement of animals) when evaluating ICH guidelines.

Humane and rational use of live animals to test the safety of new pharmaceuticals was on the ICH agenda from the very beginning. A fundamental fact accepted by ICH was that safety of a new pharmaceutical could not be demonstrated without using animals. Harmonization was explicitly meant to reduce redundant animal studies due to regional differences in requirements.

The following are achievements within the framework of ICH with respect to the 3Rs:

- A better definition of what is needed from acute toxicity studies. Initially, this led to fewer redundant studies. ICH M3(R2) includes a provision that acute toxicity studies might not be needed since most useful acute toxicity information can be obtained in repeated-dose toxicity studies (ICH, 2009).
- A more flexible interpretation of the appropriate interval of exposure in embryo–foetal toxicity tests, which reduced the redundancy in this type of study.

- Reduction of the chronic rat study requirements (only one study of 6 months' duration.) The requirement for a 12-month study in rats was dropped because products to be administered chronically in humans would be evaluated in 2-year rodent carcinogenicity bioassays.
- Refinement (better welfare conditions of animals) can be found in the guideline on dose selection for rodent carcinogenicity bioassays (ICH S1C). The maximum *acceptable* dose is no longer only the maximum tolerated dose (MTD), that is, associated with some toxicity, but can be based also on other criteria, such as a 25-fold AUC exposure as compared with the intended human exposure at therapeutic levels.

Some guidelines appear to *increase* the number of animals used in drug development. For example, in order to comply with ICH S3 (Guideline on Toxicokinetics) extra animals might be needed for determination of systemic exposure to the test article. However, the value added by evaluating systemic exposure in nonclinical studies justifies this exception and other end-points could be included to maximize the usefulness of additional animals.

2.5 ICH M3

The contents of ICH Safety (S) topic guidelines are discussed in relevant sections of this book. However, ICH M3 deserves special consideration: this document outlines the entire nonclinical programme to enable drug development and marketing authorization. The original M3 document (1997) primarily dealt with timing of nonclinical toxicology studies with respect to concurrent clinical trial *duration*. Although the 2009 revision (Guidance for Industry: M3(R2) Nonclinical Safety Studies for the Conduct of Human Clinical Trials and Marketing Authorization for Pharmaceuticals) contains substantially the same information, it is greatly expanded. First, several issues were not resolved in the original document. For example, consensus was not achieved on the duration of chronic toxicity studies in nonrodents. There was also lack of consensus on the timing of reproductive toxicity studies with respect to the stage of drug development. Lack of consensus resulted in "regional differences" being written into the guideline. Second, the need for and timing of special toxicology studies were not addressed in the original guidance. Finally, certain study designs to enable first-in-human clinical trials – the exploratory IND concept – were not included in the 1997 guidance.

A complete revision of M3 was needed, therefore, and the essentials are presented here. The first accomplishment was harmonization of the length of toxicity studies to support clinical trials and marketing authorization for drugs intended for chronic use. The original ICH M3 document stated that either 9- or 12-month repeat-dose toxicity studies in nonrodents would be needed, depending on the region. According to ICH M3(R2), a 9-month repeat-dose toxicity study in nonrodents is acceptable to support both clinical trials and marketing authorization for drugs to be used chronically. In addition, ICH M3(R2) harmonizes the length of both rodent and nonrodent toxicity studies needed to support clinical trials and marketing authorization for drugs used for shorter durations.

Another issue not resolved in the original ICH M3 was high-dose selection for general toxicology studies. At the time of writing the original guideline, the issue of high-dose selection was deferred to the individual regulatory authorities. This resulted in conflicting expectations, lack of a harmonized approach, and needless repetition of some nonclinical studies. ICH M3(R2) includes two new criteria for selecting the high-dose: large exposure multiples in animals compared to clinical exposure to the test article (with 50 times accepted as sufficient in absence of other traditional indicators such as maximum tolerated dose, MTD), and "limit dose" (usually 1 g/kg/day).

ICH M3(R2) contains a section on selection of first-in-human dose based on nonclinical studies. Although the guideline refers to regional guidances (published by FDA and EMA), these are not in conflict, so there are no "regional differences". This also illustrates an important point when considering an ICH guideline: if there is no lack of harmony between the Six Pack regions on a specific issue, no further guidance is needed.

Perhaps the most significant section of ICH M3(R2) concerns nonclinical studies needed to enable exploratory clinical trials. Five approaches are given in the document: two to support "microdose" studies, and three for limited clinical trials using doses anticipated to produce pharmacologic activity. There are two key points: exploratory clinical trials are intended for early selection of candidate compounds based on relatively limited nonclinical data, and once a candidate compound is selected, standard enabling nonclinical studies would be needed. Thus, for the selected candidate, it is possible that *more* nonclinical data would be generated during development. However, for candidate compounds *not* selected, fewer nonclinical studies would be expected. Thus, the positive effect is anticipated to be less animal use overall (Ledwith and DeGeorge, 2011).

Timing of nonclinical embryo–foetal development studies relative to clinical trials is harmonized in ICH M3(R2). Before including women of childbearing potential (WOCBP) in clinical trials, both Europe and Japan expected reproductive toxicity studies to have been conducted. In the US, reproductive toxicity studies were expected prior to Phase 3 clinical trials. ICH M3(R2) allows for including WOCBP in short-term clinical trials without completion of reproductive toxicity studies if proper precautions are taken. In addition, results of dose range-finding embryo–foetal development studies (in two species) can also be used to enable clinical trials enrolling WOCBP.

ICH M3(R2) recommends juvenile animal studies to enable clinical trials in paediatric subjects on a case-by-case basis. Where juvenile animal studies are needed, rodents are preferred. Finally, the guideline emphasizes that many special toxicity studies (immunotoxicity, phototoxicity, abuse potential) should be conducted on an as-needed, case-by-case basis. Some safety issues, such as phototoxicity, can be assessed in clinical trials without the need for special animal studies. ICH M3(R2) provides clear recommendations on what would be needed for combination drug products. In particular, emphasis is placed on knowledge acquired in real-world use of drug combinations and that this information can be more useful than animal studies.

2.6 New Initiatives and Topics

ICH recognizes that there are topics that have not been addressed in the guidelines. In addition, some existing guidelines are in need of maintenance. Some issues have been addressed by other health authorities and might not need ICH guidance. For example, WHO has published guidance on nonclinical development of vaccines: this has been accepted as adequate by the Six Pack (WHO, 2003). Computational toxicology (e.g., quantitative structure-activity relationship, QSAR) is an important tool for some guidances currently being developed (e.g., genotoxic impurities; ICH M7). Although the Organization for Economic Cooperation and Development (OECD) has ceded responsibility for drug approval standards to ICH, computational toxicology standards are being considered by OECD that could be used by the EWG for M7.

ICH M4 – known as the Common Technical Dossier (or Document) – is an administrative rather than a scientific guideline. There are several outstanding issues, many identified by the pharmaceutical industry. For example, rearranging all the studies from one system (e.g., US FDA) to another (e.g., EMA) is an enormous task, including renumbering the studies and rewriting the cross-references. This task could take as much as three months with no purpose other than making the same material available in another part of the world. Lack of harmonization in ICH M4 includes placing acute toxicity studies with pharmacodynamic study reports in one section of the CTD (Part F). In Module 2, the summaries and overviews are now included as a separate part. In Module 2.4, the company should provide a nonclinical overview, which should be a critical description and discussion of the entire nonclinical dossier, describing the strategy chosen to provide proof-of-concept evidence and to support the safety of the active substance. In Module 2.6, the company is requested to give summary descriptions of all nonclinical studies provided in the dossier without any critical analysis of the data. It is clear from the description that the nonclinical overview in Module 2.4, is in fact the European Expert Report, whereas the nonclinical summaries in Module 2.6, are the same as the Factual Summaries from FDA requirements. This is an example of regional differences persisting in an ICH guideline. These technical issues should be addressed in the future.

Nonclinical scientific issues that may need to be addressed by ICH include photosafety and adjuvant safety. An ICH IWG is currently at work on photosafety, and one is likely to begin work soon on adjuvant safety. Finally, the issue of genotoxic impurities is being considered as a combined quality and safety issue. This document, ICH M7, is currently at Step 1 and is under discussion.

References

D'Arcy, P.F. and Harron, D.W.G. (1992) Proceedings of the First International Conference on Harmonisation, Brussels 1991. Queen's University Belfast, p. 590.

D'Arcy, P.F. and Harron, D.W.G. (1994) Proceedings of the Second International Conference on Harmonisation, Orlando 1993. Queen's University Belfast, p. 590.

D'Arcy, P.F. and Harron, D.W.G. (1996) Proceedings of the Third International Conference on Harmonisation, Yokohama 1995. Queen's University Belfast, p. 590.

D'Arcy, P.F. and Harron, D.W.G. (1998) Proceedings of the Fourth International Conference on Harmonisation, Brussels 1997. Queen's University Belfast, p. 590.

International Conference on Harmonisation (2009) ICH Guideline M3(R2), Guidance on Nonclinical Safety Studies for the Conduct of Human Clinical Trials and Marketing Authorization for Pharmaceuticals, June.

Ledwith, B.J. and DeGeorge, J.J. (2011) Changes to ICH Guideline M3: New and revised guidance on nonclinical safety studies to support human clinical trials and marketing authorization. *Clin. Pharmacol. Therapeut.*, **89**, 295–299.

McBride, W.G. (1977) Thalidomide embryopathy. *Teratology*, **16**, 79–82.

World Health Organization (2003) WHO Guidelines on Nonclinical Evaluation of Vaccines, WHO/BS/03, 1969, 21 November.

3

Food and Drug Administration: Nonclinical Program and Pharmaceutical Approval

William J. Brock[1] *and Kenneth L. Hastings*[2]
[1]*Brock Scientific Consulting, Montgomery Village, USA*
[2]*Sanofi, Bethesda, USA*

The fascination of drug discovery and development for toxicologists is that drugs are intended to have a biological function. Therefore, toxicologists and pharmacologists should have some understanding of the mechanism of action of the drug. Furthermore, drug development often allows the toxicologist to be somewhat flexible in developing the toxicology programme that enables clinical trials and marketing applications. Much of the following discussion relates to small molecules although in some cases the same concepts can be applied to biotechnology-derived products such as monoclonal antibodies.

3.1 Legislative Authority of the FDA

The history of health product legislation in the US largely involves the passage of bills in the US Congress, generally in response to public demand. In 1902, Congress passed the Biologics Act in response to a tragedy in St. Louis where ten children died after being given contaminated diphtheria antitoxin. However, Congressional enactment of the Pure Food and Drug Act in 1906 had more to do with tainted and adulterated food than with the regulation of drugs. When Harvey Wiley, chief of the Bureau of Chemistry, Department

---

Nonclinical Safety Assessment: A Guide to International Pharmaceutical Regulations, First Edition.
Edited by William J. Brock, Kenneth L. Hastings and Kathy M. McGown.

of Agriculture and the driving force in the enactment of this early law, did his pioneering work (beginning in 1904) on the effects of various food preservatives on health, he did so using only human subjects with no prior experiments in animals. Legislation in place in 1906 consisted strictly of a labelling law prohibiting the sale of processed food or drugs that were misbranded. No approval process was involved and enforcement relied on post-marketing surveillance and prosecution. Efficacy was not a consideration until 1911 when the Sherley Amendment outlawed fraudulent therapeutic claims.

Current regulations in the US are largely shaped by a law passed in 1938. The pharmacology revolution was in its infancy, primarily due to the development of antibiotics in the 1930s and 1940s. Medical and pharmacy practices were not as we know them now, as few drugs required a physician's prescription. Medicines, called patent preparations, were often marketed with fraudulent claims. For example, Radithor (a solution of radium) was marketed in the 1930s for treatment of 160 diseases. In 1933, Walter G. Campbell (an FDA official who would become commissioner in 1940) delivered a memo to Rexford Tugwell, Undersecretary in the Department of Agriculture, concerning an insecticide (lead arsenite) used on fruits. Tugwell had apparently questioned why this chemical was not banned. At that time, the FDA did not have regulatory power to ban marketed products such as insecticides.

The 1906 law was designed to control blatantly misbranded and/or adulterated foods and drugs. Safety and efficacy were assumed so long as the product was not misbranded; pre-marketing review of a drug was an unknown practice. Amendments to the 1906 law to control bogus therapeutic claims and dangerous preparations were not effective. Paul Dunbar of the FDA suggested to Campbell that an entirely new law was needed. A committee of FDA professionals and outside academic consultants drafted a new law, which no one in Congress was willing to sponsor. However, in 1938 Senator Royal Copeland of New York was convinced to sponsor what we now know as the Federal Food, Drug, and Cosmetic Act (the FD&C Act).

As is so often true in these legislative debates, a tragedy empowered advocates of the proposed FD&C Act. In 1937, the Elixir of Sulfanilamide incident occurred, which remains one of the nation's worst drug tragedies. The Massengil Company was not one of the industry giants. The company's chief chemist was simply trying to develop a product and, in fact, did so in a manner consistent with practices of the time. There was a perceived need for a liquid form of sulfanilamide, but it was difficult to dissolve. The chemist used diethylene glycol. No toxicity tests were performed on the finished product, although the product did pass through the "control lab" where it was checked for appearance, fragrance, and consistency.

The first reports of human toxicity occurred in late 1937 when the American Medical Association (AMA) requested information from the FDA because of six deaths that might have been attributable to the elixir. When samples of the elixir were tested by the AMA, diethylene glycol was found and determined to be the toxic agent. The AMA issued a warning to the public about the elixir in October 1937. In the meantime, the FDA had become aware of the deaths and launched an investigation. By the end of October 1937, at least 73 people had died and another 20 deaths were linked to the elixir. The Agency eventually recovered and accounted for 99.2% of the elixir produced.

Because of this disaster, a new legislative bill was introduced which stated that manufacturers seeking to market new drugs would be required to supply records of testing, lists of components, descriptions of each manufacturing process, and sample labels. Drugs would require certification by the FDA before sale was permitted. In January 1938, debate started on the Wheeler-Lea Bill, which would ensure that all controls over drug advertising would remain in the Federal Trade Commission (FTC). Despite strong opposition by the FDA, the Wheeler-Lea Bill was signed into law in March 1938.

Before passage of the 1938 FD&C Act, drugs could be marketed if the label did not state false or misleading information regarding strength and purity. Efficacy claims included in the label were not regulated. Drugs marketed before the passage of the Act were considered to be effective if the manufacturer did not change claims in the label and there was no evidence that the drug was not safe (referred to as pre-38 drugs). If there was a change in the drug label (e.g., based on new evidence of efficacy for a pre-38 drug), the FDA considered this to be a "new drug" and the manufacturer was required to prove that the drug was safe for its intended use.

The 1938 FD&C Act changed the pharmaceutical industry from a traditional consumer product manufacturer to one in which purchases were controlled by a third party (that is, the physician). In 1929, ethical pharmaceuticals (prescription drugs) comprised only 32% of all medicines while by 1969 this was up to 83% (Temin, 1980). In 1961, Senator Estes Kefauver proposed legislation to amend the FDC Act to increase FDA oversight of the drug industry. Included in the amendment was a provision that new drugs had to be not only "safe", but also "efficacious". There was little support for the amendment at the time.

As in 1938, a tragic incident would influence the legislative process. An anti-anxiety drug marketed in Europe, thalidomide, was prescribed and used by many women for pregnancy-related depression. At about the same time in Europe, there was an apparent increased incidence of phocomelia, a birth defect marked by imperfect development of arms and legs. In 1961, thalidomide was determined to be the causative teratogen and was taken off the market in Europe. The William S. Merrill Company had applied for a New Drug Application (NDA) for thalidomide in the US in 1960. It was never approved because the FDA examiner, Dr Frances Kelsey, had returned the application for lack of sufficient information. Eventually, the company withdrew the application. The newspaper accounts of the thalidomide tragedy created public support for the bill, and it was signed into law in October 1962. It was demonstrated after the fact that thalidomide was teratogenic in the rabbit. Because of this episode, there exists the current practice that human pharmaceuticals are tested for teratogenicity in two species, one generally being the rabbit.

The 1962 Amendment to the FDA Act made three major changes in the new drug approval process. First, and perhaps most important, the 1962 Amendment introduced the concept of effectiveness into the approval process. A New Drug Application (NDA) had to contain evidence that the drug was not only safe, but also effective. The new law required that companies submit to the FDA a request to allow clinical testing under an Investigational New Drug application (IND). No response from the FDA was deemed to be acceptance.

The second major change under the 1962 Amendment was the establishment of a premarket approval system. Under the 1938 law, an NDA would take effect automatically if the FDA did not respond. For example, the only reason thalidomide was not approved was because Dr Kelsey returned the application to the sponsor with a request for more information. In contrast, the 1962 Amendment required affirmative FDA action before a drug could be marketed. Under the 1962 Amendment, the FDA was empowered to withdraw NDA approval and remove a drug from the market for a variety of reasons, including evidence that the product was unsafe or that the sponsor had misrepresented or not reported relevant data.

The third major change expanded the FDA's authority over the clinical testing of new drugs. Thus, substantial evidence consisting of adequate and well-controlled investigations, including clinical investigations by a qualified expert, was required. In setting standards for clinical evidence, the FDA became highly influential in clinical trial design (Merrill, 1994). The FDA was initially quite unprepared for this new level of responsibility. It was not until 1973 that audited regulations on the determination of safety and effectiveness were put in place. While there have been several procedural changes, for example, the 1985 Investigational New Drug (IND) revision, and the 1988 IND procedures for life-threatening disease treatment, there have actually been no major changes in the law from 1992 with Prescription Drug Users Fee Act (PDUFA) and 1997 with the FDA Modernization Act (FDAMA) and subsequent modifications.

The 1962 legislation also applied retroactively to all drugs approved as safe from 1938 to 1962 (referred to as pre-62 drugs). These pre-62 drugs were permitted to remain on the market while evidence of their effectiveness was reviewed. The Drug Efficacy Study Implementation (DESI) programme was established in which the FDA would review the effectiveness of drugs approved between 1938 and 1962. If the DESI review indicated a lack of substantial evidence of a drug's effectiveness, the FDA would publish a Notice of Opportunity for a Hearing (NOOH) in the Federal Register concerning the proposal to withdraw approval of the drug. The manufacturer of the drug had the opportunity to request a hearing and provide the FDA with documentation of effectiveness before a final determination is made. Drugs for which a NOOH has been published are referred to as less-than-effective (LTE) drugs. The FDA continues to use the DESI programme to review pre-1962 drugs, for example, some opiates.

In response to resource constraints resulting in unacceptable drug review delays, Congress passed the 1992 PDUFA. Under the terms of this act, companies would pay a fee to the Agency to defray costs associated with NDA review. These fees would provide the FDA with resources needed to decrease application review time. In return, companies were guaranteed a more rapid review time. By all accounts, PDUFA has been successful. In 1992 (the year PDUFA was passed), 26 NDAs were approved, requiring on average 29.9 months for data review; while in 1996, 53 new drug (or biological) products were approved, each requiring an average of 17.8 months of review time.

The mid 1990s saw the re-inventing government initiatives (RIGO) which issued a report entitled *Reinventing Regulation of Drugs and Medical Devices.* Two bills were introduced in the mid-1990s that provided the essential outline of what would become FDAMA (Pilot and Waldmann, 1998). The Food and Drug Administration Modernization Act (FDAMA) was signed into law in November 1997. The FDA has identified various tasks, regulations and guidance necessary for the implementation of FDAMA. Various guidance documents were issued that are of interest to toxicologists:

- Renewal of PDUFA for another 5 years
- Fast track for break-through products
- Change in the way biological products are regulated, that is, elimination of the Establishment and Product licences, both replaced with a Biological Licence Application (BLA)

- Change in the way antibiotics are developed and regulated
- Incentives for the development of paediatric claims
- Companies will be permitted to disseminate information about approved uses for their products (direct to consumer advertising)
- FDAMA requires that the FDA establish a clinical trials database for drugs used to treat serious and life-threatening diseases, other than AIDS and cancers (databases for these diseases have already been established).

3.2 Nonclinical Drug Development and the FDA

The FDA regulations require that the "safety and efficacy" of a drug be demonstrated prior to marketing approval. For the toxicologist, the design and conduct of nonclinical studies to demonstrate the safety of the drug prior to entry into a clinical trial is of prime importance. The early drug development toxicology programme should be designed to identify a safe first-in-human (FIH) dose, and key toxicity signals and end-points that would prove useful for safety monitoring in Phase 1 clinical studies. The Investigational New Drug (IND) will include the data tables and narrative of the toxicology, pharmacokinetic and pharmacology studies completed and the justification of the dose level(s) selected for the Phase 1 trial. With all of the data developed to initiate a clinical trial, the toxicologist is provided an opportunity to take a "holistic" view of the data.

The nonclinical studies needed to initiate clinical studies are called "IND enabling" or "FIH enabling". Nonclinical toxicology studies needed to initiate a clinical study should be conducted in compliance with Good Laboratory Practice (GLP) regulations.

In preparation for the IND-enabling studies, there are a variety of items that must be addressed in advance of drug administration to the first animal in the first study.

- Characterization of the drug substance. The purity of the drug substance used in the clinical studies should not be of lesser purity than used in nonclinical studies. A good rule of thumb is that the purity of the drug substance used in nonclinical studies should approximate 95–99% with the clinical supply being >99%.
- Development and validation of a GLP-compliant analytical method. These studies are necessary to verify the purity of the drug substance, and measure the drug substance in dose formulations.
- Development and validation of a GLP-compliant bioanalytical method. Although detection of drug metabolites might not be needed in early nonclinical studies, development of methods could be valuable in determination of metabolic differences between animals and humans, especially with respect to potential unique human metabolites.
- Stability of the drug substance under sponsor-specified storage conditions and in the anticipated animal dosing formulation over the expected duration of the study. For example, if the study is 28 days in duration, the stability of the drug substance should cover this duration plus any time required for shipping, storage, protocol preparation, and so on.

Table 3.1 *Content of a standard Investigational New Drug Application.*

IND Section Number	Section Description
1.	IND cover sheets (form FDA-1571)
2.	Table of contents
3.	Introductory statement and general (clinical) investigation plan
4.	Reserved
5.	Clinical investigator's brochure
6.	Proposed clinical protocol(s)
7.	Chemistry, manufacturing, and control information
8.	Pharmacology and toxicology information
9.	Previous human experience with the investigational drug
10.	Additional information
11.	Other relevant information

The principle responsibility of the toxicologist is to design, conduct and interpret non-clinical studies to support each phase of clinical investigation. The FDA issued guidance for industry on the content and format of the IND in 1987 and 1995, prior to promulgation of Good Guidance Practices in 1997 (FDA 1987; 1995). As of this time, these guidances are still in force.

For the toxicologist, the most important stipulation in the 1995 Guidance is that the sponsor is allowed to submit draft, unaudited reports with the IND. If unaudited reports are submitted, the sponsor must finalize the reports within 120 days of submission of the IND. If the integrated summary in the IND was based on unaudited draft reports, then the sponsor will need to submit to the Agency an update of the summary identifying any differences between the unaudited report and audited, final report.

The content of the IND is shown in Table 3.1 (21CFR Part 312.23). Many of the sections identified are self-explanatory although a few notable exceptions are discussed below.

The IND cover sheet, FDA Form 1571, tends to be self-explanatory but this form needs to be included with each submission made to the Agency as it allows the FDA to quickly notice what is being submitted. There are several different "types" of INDs with the most common being the commercial IND. Other INDs consist of Investigator IND, Emergency IND, Treatment IND and the Screening IND. These are described more thoroughly by Mathieu (2005).

Section 8, for the toxicologist and pharmacologist, represents the major section of the IND. This section is discussed in greater detail below.

Section 9 would contain any clinical information that has been generated for the drug substance. This would occur, of course, if the drug was in clinical development in other regions prior to submission of the IND in the US.

Sections 10 and 11 allow the sponsor to provide to the FDA any other information considered to be relevant to the "approval" of the IND. These sections can describe the use of radiolabelled drugs in the clinical trial and a description of the safety of the radiation-absorbed dose, drug dependency, paediatric studies and an assessment for the use of the drug in paediatric populations, and so on. Overall, these sections permit the Sponsor to tell the Agency about special circumstances that potentially impact the approval of the IND.

With the advent of the International Conference on Harmonization (ICH; see Chapter 2), sponsors can use the Common Technical Document (CTD) format as it allows the IND to be rapidly converted to a New Drug Application (NDA) if the drug product proceeds to this stage of development (ICH, 2002). Although the CTD format is not consistent with the IND format described above, this has become the acceptable format for submission to the FDA.

The CTD is organized into five modules:

- Module 1, Administrative Information and Prescribing Information: This module contains documents specific to each region; for example, application forms or the proposed label for use in the region. The content and format of this module can be modified to be consistent with the needs of the FDA.
- Module 2, Common Technical Document Summaries: For the IND, Module 2 contains the bulk of the nonclinical information provided in tabular and narrative form. It should begin with a general introduction to the pharmaceutical, including its pharmacologic class, mode of action, and proposed clinical use.
- Module 3, Quality: Information on the drug product physiochemical properties, drug formulation information, and so on
- Module 4, Nonclinical Study Reports: The nonclinical study reports are to be provided in this section.
- Module 5, Clinical Study Reports: If clinical data are available, the study reports and related information are to be included in this section.

The Good Laboratories Practice (GLP) regulation (21CFR Part 58) was codified in 1978 in response to poor practices by a few laboratories involved in the conduct of preclinical safety studies (Baldeshwiler, 2003). Since that time, many regions have developed GLP regulations. Overall, the regulatory context of those regulations are similar to that of the FDA GLPs although some differences do exist (Swidersky, 2007; Nakashima, 2008; Ertz and Preu, 2008; Huntsinger, 2008). Toxicology studies submitted to FDA to support clinical trials should be conducted according to GLPs. Efficacy pharmacology and pharmacokinetic studies usually are not conducted according to GLPs.

During the last 10 years, the FDA has encouraged sponsors to meet with the respective FDA division prior to undertaking many of the pharmacology and toxicology studies and before submission of the IND. Generally, industry has reacted positively to pre-IND meetings. In preparation for a pre-IND meeting, the sponsor should submit to the Agency a briefing package containing all available pharmacology and toxicology data as well as any Chemistry and Manufacturing Control (CMC) information pertinent to the drug formulation intended for the Phase 1 trial (FDA, 2009).

Tabular summaries of the pharmacology and toxicology data and an overall narrative are critical to ensure that the sponsor conveys to the Agency the potential toxicity and pharmacological activity of the drug substance. Although the format of tabular summaries is not specified in the IND guidance, it is best to use the format described in the Common Technical Document (CTD).

For the briefing package and pre-IND meeting, specific questions to the Agency should be developed about the nonclinical or clinical programme. The intent of these questions is to gain concurrence with the FDA about the nonclinical studies the sponsor intends to undertake as well as questions related to CMC and the clinical programme. An outline of the pivotal protocols with specific endpoints to be measured should be considered particularly where these toxicity endpoints would be important for specific pharmaceutical categories. The sponsor should keep in mind that the FDA has access to large databases that could include drugs of similar structure and pharmacology to the sponsor's test article. Therefore, the sponsor should carefully consider the Agency's opinion and advice regarding the development of the drug.

3.3 Nonclinical Testing: General Conditions and Considerations

For the discussion below, there are fundamental assumptions about the drug under development. The first assumption is that the intended route of therapeutic administration is oral, as this is the case for most drugs. Another assumption is that the drug is intended to be administered once daily.

The next major assumption is that the ICH process has been quite effective. As late as the early 1990s, significant differences existed in requirements between the current ICH parties (Alder and Zbinden, 1988). Many ICH parties either had no written guidelines or had not promulgated acceptable practices. The sole written guidance in the US was a document authored by Edward Goldenthal (Goldenthal, 1968).

IND-enabling studies typically support single- and repeat-dose clinical studies less than two weeks in duration. Toxicology studies for longer clinical trials should be of the same duration (ICH, 2004). The repeat-dose toxicity studies for the IND should be conducted in rodent and nonrodent species although there are exceptions, for example, biological products (see Chapter 18). Additionally, developmental and reproductive toxicity studies are usually needed to include women of child-bearing potential in clinical trials (Chapter 15). Rodent carcinogenicity studies (if required) and the final parts of the reproductive toxicity package are usually conducted prior to NDA submission (Chapters 13 and 15).

For intravenous drug products, nonclinical tests for haemolysis, intravenous/extravascular irritation and protein precipitation are often needed. Immunogenicity and sensitization might be needed for dermal products. Similarly, route-specific irritation assays (eye, skin, muscle, mucosal, etc.) would be needed. The nonclinical development of oncologic products will differ from that of the general case described above. For these products, dosing will mirror at a minimum the clinical dosing regimen (DeGeorge *et al.*, 1998; ICH, 2010).

3.4 Toxicity Testing: Small Molecules and Traditional Pharmaceuticals

Most often, the regulatory development and approval of drugs proceeds in a somewhat fixed and orderly way. The 1938 FDC Act required safety assessment, but no consistent guidelines were available. Testing guidelines were first proposed in 1949 and published in the *Food, Drug and Cosmetic Law Journal* that year (Burns, 1983). Following several revisions, these guidelines were issued as *The Appraisal Handbook* in 1959. While never formally called a guideline, it set the standard for preclinical toxicity test design for several years. The current basic guidelines for testing required for safety assessment in support of the phases of clinical development of drugs were first outlined by Goldenthal (1968) and later incorporated into a 1971 FDA publication entitled *FDA Introduction to Total Drug Quality*.

In the 1970s and more so in the 1980s, other testing guidelines were prepared and were used as a basis for the design of toxicity studies for nonclinical studies. In 1982, the FDA's Bureau of Foods published the guidelines on *Toxicological Principles for the Safety Assessment of Direct Food Additives and Color Additives Used in Food*, that is, the FDA Red Book. Although theses guidelines were specifically directed towards the safety evaluation of food additives, they describe how the FDA incorporates information about expected human exposure and chemical structure-activity relationships for food and colour additives used in food. These guidelines were at times referenced as a basis for testing of new pharmaceuticals. Starting in the early 1980s, the Organization of Economic Cooperation and Development (OECD) began to release testing guidelines that have often been used as a basis for the design of preclinical studies. Concurrent with the OECD guidelines, the FDA began to formalize the guidance documents that described the need for certain end-points, group size, and so on as well as specific studies necessary for drug approval. Furthermore, Japanese guidelines made available from the Ministry of Health, Labor and Welfare (MHLW) also specified the requirements for testing for new molecular entities (Chapter 9).

3.5 Toxicity Testing of Pharmaceuticals – The General Approach

As noted previously, testing of pharmaceuticals usually proceeds in a rather fixed and orderly way. For entry into early clinical trials, testing will be needed to support those trials, and the duration of the repeat-dose studies generally will need to mirror the duration of the clinical trial (Table 3.2).

As the duration of the clinical study increases, the duration of the nonclinical study also will need to be longer. It is possible to initiate a single-dose clinical study for some pharmaceuticals by providing to the Agency a single-dose toxicity study in two species. These studies must include clinical pathology and histopathology as well as be fully GLP-compliant. The FDA prefers, however, a short-term repeat-dose study, for example, 7-day. The dosage level and group size are critical to study designs. Table 3.3 presents general guidance on the number of animals to be used in systemic toxicity studies.

The number of animals in each group shown in Table 3.3 is the minimum based on OECD guidelines. Indeed, for 4-week studies, 10 rats/sex/group is often used and this number of rats is encouraged for 2-week studies. Likewise, the number of nonrodents, for example, dogs, generally has been 3/sex/group for 2- and 4-week studies although the Agency has recommended increasing this number for the treatment phase of the study. Furthermore, additional rodents are often needed in studies for the collection of blood samples for toxicokinetic determinations or other specific endpoints.

In these studies, end-points would include body weights, clinical observations, haematology and clinical chemical parameters, and, at necropsy, organ weights and histopathology. Also, ophthalmological examinations should be conducted in pivotal studies.

Table 3.2 *General guidelines for animal toxicity studies in early development.*

Route of administration	Duration of clinical trial	Animal study duration	Special studies
Oral or parenteral	Several days up to 2 week	2 species; 2 week	For parenteral administered drugs; compatibility with blood where applicable
	Up to 4 week	2 species; up to 4 week	
	Up to 3 months	2 species; up to 3 months	
Inhalation (general anesthetics)		4 species; 5 days (3 h/day)	
Dermal	Single application	2 species; single 24-h exposure followed by 2-week observation	Sensitization
	Single or short-term application	2 species; 4 week (intact and abraded skin)	
Ophthalmic	Single application		Eye irritation tests with graded doses
	Multiple application	1 species; 3 week daily applications, as in clinical use	
		1 species; duration commensurate with period of drug administration	
Vaginal or rectal	Single application	2 species; duration and number of applications determined by proposed use	Local and systematic toxicity after vaginal or rectal application in 2 species
	Multiple application		

Furthermore, for drugs directed to the CNS, for example, antipsychotics, special staining of neural structures should be incorporated into the study (Schmued *et al.*, 1999; Schmued and Hopkins, 2000; Bolon *et al.*, 2006). In the last 10 years there has been increased use of electrocardiograms (ECG) in nonrodent species during the conduct of pivotal repeat dose studies and this has become the standard for biotechnology-derived drugs (Gauvin *et al.*, 2006). Although this continues to be debated in the toxicology community, these end-points have become so common that it is advisable to continue to include them. Furthermore, there has been discussion about including genotoxicity measures, for example, micronucleus formation, in subchronic studies based on guidance from ICH (see Chapter 14). Also, the FDA (and ICH) has encouraged sponsors to include additional animals to examine the reversibility of adverse

Table 3.3 Numbers of animals per sose group.

Study duration (per sex)	Rodents (per sex)	Nonrodents (per sex)
2–4 week	5–10	3
13 week	20	4
26 week	30	4
Chronic	50	4

effects. Indeed, including a recovery phase has become the standard in most pivotal toxicology programmes.

3.6 First-in-Human Dosing: Results from Nonclinical Studies

Initiation of the first-in-human (FIH) clinical study is the beginning of a long road to drug approval. With the completion of the toxicology and pharmacology studies, the toxicologist is often charged with recommending and, more importantly, justifying the FIH dose. Manipulation of the toxicology data to achieve the FIH is not overly complicated. However, it is assurance that the dose will not harm clinical subjects and the justification of that dose can be very much of a concern. Although the details of determining the FIH are well beyond the scope of this chapter, there have been a number of reviews published on this topic (Sharma and McNeill, 2009; Mager *et al.*, 2009; Tibbitts *et al.*, 2010).

Two approaches have been adopted for determining the FIH dose for most therapeutics. The first has been described in FDA guidance (FDA, 2005). In general, the No Observed Adverse Effect Level (NOAEL) determined in pivotal nonclinical studies is identified in the most sensitive and relevant species. The NOAEL is then adjusted with allometric scaling factors or on the basis of pharmacokinetics to determine the human equivalent dose (HED). The HED is further reduced by appropriate safety factors according to the particular toxicological characteristics of the molecule and the design of the clinical trials. The safety factor applied is usually a factor of 10. However, the safety factor used will clearly depend on the results of the nonclinical studies, the therapeutic indication and the design of the clinical trial.

The second approach is the Minimal Anticipated Biological Effect Level (MABEL), and was described in a EU guidance (CHMP, 2007). With consideration of the FIH dose using MABEL, both toxicological and pharmacodynamic data are used. The MABEL is expected to result in a dose that leads to a minimal pharmacological effect. As with the HED, safety factors can be applied to determine the FIH dose.

Oncologic products represent a special case for determining the FIH dose (ICH S9). For these products, it is not necessary to identify a NOAEL. The FIH dose for small molecules is set at 1/10th the Severely Toxic Dose in 10% of the animals (STD 10) for rodents or for nonrodent 1/6th the Highest Non-Severely Toxic Dose (HNSTD). The HNSTD is defined as the highest dose level that does not produce evidence of lethality, life-threatening toxicities or irreversible findings.

References

Alder, S. and Zbinden, G. (1988) *National and International Drug Safety Guidelines*, MTC Verlag, Zollikon, Switzerland.

Baldeshwiler, A.M. (2003) History of FDA good laboratory practices. *Qual. Assur. J.*, **7**, 157–161.

Bolon, B., Garman, R., Jensen, K. *et al.* (2006) A "Best Practice" approach to neuropathic assessment in developmental neurotoxicity testing – for today. *Toxicol. Pathol.*, **34**, 296–313.

Burns, J. (1983) Overview of safety regulations governing food, drug and cosmetics, in *The United States in Safety and Evaluation and Regulation of Chemicals 3: Interface between Law and Science* (ed. F. Homberger), Karger, New York.

Committee for Medicinal Products for Human Use (CHMP) (2007) Guideline on requirements for first-in-man clinical trials for potential high-risk medicinal products www.ema.europa.eu.

DeGeorge, J., Ahn, C., Andrews, P. *et al.* (1998) Regulatory considerations for the preclinical development of anticancer drugs. *Cancer Chemother. Pharmacol.*, **41**, 173–185.

Ertz, K. and Preu, M. (2008) International GLP: A critical reflection on the harmonized global GLP standard from a test facility viewpoint. *Ann. First Super Sanita.*, **44**, 390–394.

Food and Drug Administration (2009) Formal meeting between the FDA and sponsors or applicants www.fda.gov.

Food and Drug Administration (2005) Estimating the maximum safe starting dose in initial clinical trials for therapeutics in adult healthy volunteers www.fda.gov.

Food and Drug Administration (1987) Guideline for the format and content of the nonclinical pharmacology/toxicology section of an application www.fda.gov.

Food and Drug Administration (1995) Guidance for Industry: Content and format of Investigational New Drug Applications (INDs) for Phase 1 studies of drugs, including well-characterized, therapeutic, biotechnology-derived products www.fda.gov.

Gauvin, D.V., Tilley, L.P., Smith, F.W.K., and Baird, T.J. (2006) Electrocardiogram, hemodynamics, and core body temperature of the freely moving laboratory beagle dog by remote telemetry. *J. Pharmacol. Toxicol. Methods*, **53**, 128–139.

Goldenthal, E. (1968) Current view on safety evaluation of drugs. FDA Papers, May 13–18.

Huntsinger, D.W. (2008) OECD and US GLP applications. *Ann. First Super Sanita.*, **44**, 403–406.

International Conference on Harmonization (ICH) (2010) S9 nonclinical evaluation for anticancer pharmaceuticals www.ich.org.

International Conference on Harmonization (ICH) (2004) Guidance on nonclinical safety studies for the conduct of human clinical trials and marketing authorization for pharmaceuticals, M3(R2) www.ich.org.

International Conference on Harmonization (ICH) (2002) The Common Technical Document (CTD) www.ich.org.

Mager, D.E., Woo, S., and Jusko, W.J. (2009) Scaling pharmacodynamics from in vitro and preclinical animal studies to humans. *Drug Metab. Pharmacokinet.*, **24**, 16–24.

Mathieu, M. (2005) *New Drug Development: A Regulatory Overview*, 7th edn, Parexel, Waltham, MA.

Merrill, R.A. (1994) Regulation of drugs and devices: An evolution. *Health Aff.*, **13**, 47–69.

Nakashima, N. (2008) National GLP programmes and implication of regulatory authorities for pharmaceuticals, pesticides and other chemicals. *Ann. First Super Sanita.*, **44**, 363–368.

Pilot, L.R. and Waldmann, D.R. (1998) Food and Drug Administration Modernization Act of 1997: Medical device provisions, *Food Drug Law J.* **53**, 267–295.

Schmued, L., Slikker, W., Clausing, P., and Bowyer, J. (1999) d-Fenfluramine produces neuronal degeneration in localized regions of the cortex, thalamus and cerebellum of the rat. *Toxicol. Sci.*, **48**, 100–106.

Schmued, L.C. and Hopkins, K.J. (2000) Fluoro-Jade B: A high affinity fluorescent marker for the localization of neuronal degeneration. *Brain Res.*, **874**, 123–130.
Sharma, V. and McNeill, J.H. (2009) To scale or not to scale: The principles of dose extrapolation. *Br. J. Pharmacol.*, **157**, 907–921.
Swidersky, P. (2007) Quality assurance and good lab practice. Contract Pharma May, 2007 www.contractpharma.com.
Temin, P. (1980) Regulation and the choice of prescription drugs. *Amer. Econ. Rev.*, **70**, 301–305.
Tibbitts, J., Cavagnaro, J.A., Haller, C.A. *et al.* (2010) Practical approaches to dose selection for first-in-human clinical trials with novel biopharmaceuticals. *Reg. Toxicol. Pharmacol.*, **58**, 243–251.

4

Nonclinical Pharmaceutical Development in MERCOSUR and Brazil

Cristiana Leslie Corrêa, Giuliana Selmi, and Flávio Ailton Duque Zambrone
Planitox, Campinas, Brazil

4.1 Introduction

In South America, the inclusion of nonclinical studies in the safety assessment of pharmaceuticals is an essential requirement when registering products. Although there are some differences amongst the countries and regions, mainly concerning the details of requirements, priority is given for pharmacological, pharmacokinetic and toxicological investigations.

In this chapter, details of nonclinical studies required for registering drugs in Brazil will be presented, as well as the pertinent legislation in the Southern Common Market (MERCOSUR), which is aimed at the harmonization of such matters amongst the associated countries (Argentina, Brazil, Paraguay, Uruguay and Venezuela). Due to the fact that MERCOSUR tends to be a common market in all South America, the requisites presented here could become a reference to all regions.

4.2 MERCOSUR

MERCOSUR, the Southern Common Market, is made up of five countries: Brazil, Argentina, Paraguay, Uruguay and Venezuela. Its aim is to guarantee a better integration amongst the countries, broadening the domestic market and promoting economic

Nonclinical Safety Assessment: A Guide to International Pharmaceutical Regulations, First Edition.
Edited by William J. Brock, Kenneth L. Hastings and Kathy M. McGown.

development. Several initiatives have been implemented, such as free trade, movement of goods, people and currency, the prospect of increased political and commercial integration, coordination of macroeconomic policies and the harmonization of legislation in the concerned areas.

In March 1991, the countries involved signed the Treaty of Asunción, with a view to creating the Southern Common Market – MERCOSUR. In December 1994, at the Presidential Summit at Ouro Preto, an Additional Protocol to the Treaty of Asunción was approved – the Ouro Preto Protocol – which established the institutional structure of MERCOSUR and gave it an international legal authority. Ouro Preto marked the conclusion of the transition period and the adoption of the basic instruments of the common commercial policy which characterizes the Customs Union. The Party States resolved to start a new phase in order to achieve a single market which would generate greater economic growth in their countries by taking advantage of specialization in production, economies of scale, commercial cooperation and the greater negotiating power of the bloc with other blocs or countries (MERCOSUL, 2010).

Amongst the legislations established by MERCOSUR related to drug registration is the 129/1996 Act, which refers to the technical regulations for undertaking clinical trials, specifically those studies carried out in humans for pharmacoclinic and/or therapeutic purposes. According to this Act, it is understood that pharmacoclinic studies are those that aim at the efficacy and/or safety of a pharmaceuticals (MERCOSUL/GMC, 1996).

Such resolution brings specifications related to the following nonclinical studies: pharmacodynamics (therapeutic effect, mechanism of action, interactions); pharmacokinetics (absorption, distribution, biotransformation, elimination); acute toxicity; repeated- dose toxicity; effects on fertility; studies on embryotoxicity (mainly teratogenicity); perinatal and postnatal toxicity; mutagenic activity; oncogenic/carcinogenic potential; local irritation studies; skin sensitization studies; and other studies necessary to characterize the drug product (MERCOSUL/GMC, 1996). The main characteristics to be observed while carrying out a nonclinical study cited by the research legislation involving humans in MERCOSUR are listed below (MERCOSUL/GMC, 1996):

- **Pharmacodynamics:** These studies must evaluate all the main organs and systems in order to determine not only the anticipated therapeutic effect, but also to reveal other possible effects, both therapeutic and adverse. They must be carried out on cardiovascular, respiratory, nervous, neuromuscular, urinary, endocrine and digestive systems. Pharmacodynamic effects related to the proposed indications must be demonstrated to include, for example, dose-response effects and time-related effects. It is mandatory to perform studies that enable the assessment of possible pharmacodynamic interactions and the mechanisms of action of the active moiety that comprises the drug.
- **Pharmacokinetics:** The pharmacokinetic studies must be carried out to assess the systemic exposure of the product, enabling the establishment of the absorption characteristics as absorption rate and Cmax, the tissue distribution, biotransformation, the rate of clearance and the elimination route. The studies to be carried out include single-dose pharmacokinetic studies, repeated-dose pharmacokinetics studies, distribution studies in normal and pregnant animals and biotransformation, excretion and pharmacokinetic interactions.
- **Acute toxicity:** These studies must be carried out in at least three animal species, one of which must be a nonrodent. The age, group and number of animals by gender, administration period, dosage and pathological evaluations are not specified within the

legislation. In the nonclinical study, a minimum of two routes of administration is recommended, one by the clinically relevant route of administration and the other must be a route which assures systemic exposure. During the conduct of the nonclinical study, the animals must be examined for clinical signs and duration of toxic effects, dose-response relationships and reversibility, possible cause of any mortalities, biochemical and haematologic parameters; clinical and pathological observations and an estimation of the maximum tolerated dose. Also, requirements indicate that differences in toxicity be explored between the intended clinical route of administration and by another route of administration. For example, if the clinical route of administration is oral, a second route of administration, for example, intraperitoneal, must be included and the differences in toxicity observed between the two routes highlighted.

- **Repeated dose toxicity:** These studies must use a minimum of two animal species, one of which must be a nonrodent, and the route of administration must be the recommended one for the proposed therapeutic use. The administration time must be from 12 to 24 weeks, according to the nature of the product, the proposed therapeutic use and the animal species being used. A minimum of three doses is recommended. The highest dose must produce toxic effects and the lowest dose must be related to the proposed therapeutic dose, taking into consideration the sensitivity of the species used in the study, that is, identification of a no-observed adverse effect level (NOAEL). The following observations must be made and include clinical signs of toxicity, dose-response relationship and its reversibility, the differences related to gender and species, morbidity and mortality, biochemical haematologic parameters, nutritional parameters (weight evolution, water consumption, etc.), clinical and pathological observations and target organs. The gender, group and number of animals per dose, age and the pathological evaluations are not specified by the legislation.
- **Chronic toxicity (in repeated doses):** The studies on chronic toxicity must have a minimum of two animal species, one of which must be a nonrodent and the route of administration must be related to the one recommended for the proposed therapeutic use. It is recommended that the administration period must not be less than 24 weeks in the rodent species. A minimum of three doses is required: the highest dose must produce a verifiable toxic effect; the lowest dose must be related to the proposed therapeutic dose, taking into consideration the sensitivity of the species used in the study. The following observations must include clinical signs of toxicity, dose-response relationship and its reversibility, as well as the differences related to gender of the species, morbidity and mortality, biochemical and haematologic parameters, nutritional parameters (weight evolution, water consumption, etc.), clinical and pathological observations, the NOAEL) (non-toxic dose), toxic dose and targeted organs. The gender, group and number of animals per dose, age and pathological evaluations are not specified by the legislation. Concerning the duration of administration, the toxicological studies must follow the determinations listed below:

    - When the administration period of the drug in humans is either a single dose or of limited duration (less than two weeks), the proposed administration period for animals in the nonclinical studies must be at least two weeks.
    - When the administration period of the drug in humans is up to four weeks, the administration period for animals in the nonclinical studies must be from three to 26 weeks.

- When the administration period of the drug in human is of more than four weeks, the administration period for animals in the nonclinical studies must be of 26 weeks at a minimum, not including the carcinogenicity studies.

- **Embryotoxicity studies (mainly teratogenicity), perinatal and postnatal toxicity:** The embryotoxicity studies must be conducted in a minimum of two species, one of which must be a nonrodent species. Each study should include at least three doses. The number of groups and number of animals per group, age, route and duration of administration have not been specified in the legislation.
- **Mutagenicity and carcinogenicity:** The mutagenic activity as well as the carcinogenic potential must be established for drug products administered for long durations. For *in vitro* mutagenicity studies, these are to be done with and without metabolic activation.

When necessary, according to the nature of the product, other studies might be required, for instance, studies on local irritability and skin sensitization.

In general, the guidelines given by MERCOSUR for the conduct of nonclinical studies are similar to those of the international recommendations, for example, ICH. The only description that is not according to international guidelines is related to an embryotoxicity study, where it is mentioned that the highest dose must not show toxicity. Generally, the highest dose, even in a teratology study, should produce some evidence of toxicity. Probably, the legislators may have made a mistake in the description.

There is no reference advising for following international guidelines, but the text of the legislation broadly describes the studies consistent with international guidelines. However, importance is given to scientific judgement and a case-by-case analysis in order to achieve the purpose of assessing the safety of the drug in the population. The legislation considers that the nonclinical and clinical studies must be planned and designed in a sound scientific and ethical manner, suitable for the development of new drugs.

4.3 Brazil

4.3.1 Brazilian Regulatory Aspects

In Brazil, the registration of products under the Sanitary Surveillance: Drugs, Food, Cosmetics, Sanitizers and other materials related to Health (such as medical devices, dental instruments, etc.) is the responsibility of the Brazilian National Regulatory Agency (ANVISA – Agência Nacional de Vigilância Sanitária). The Agency is managed by a Collegiate Board of Directors and is comprised of five members, one of whom is the chairman. Since its establishment in 1999, the medication area has been overseen by the chairman of this Board. This area is organized under the General Office Of Drugs (GGMED), which currently is divided into four offices, two units and a nucleus (Table 4.1) which have equal standing under the general management (Nishioka, 2006; ANVISA, 2009).

All ANVISA's regulations are subordinate to the legislation. The legal basis applied to drug registration is established by Law 6360, 23 September 1976 and Decree 79094, 5 January 1977 (ANVISA, 1976; 1977). Both the laws and regulations have been

Table 4.1 *General Office of Drugs (GGMED) from Agencia Nacional de Vigilância Sanitária (ANVISA).*

Division	Abbreviation	Attributions related to the registering
Office of New Drugs, Research and Clinical Trials	GEPEC	Registration of new drugs (synthetic and natural products). It evaluates post-registration alterations that comprise, amongst others, the change or insertion of a new manufacturing site, the changes of excipients, labelling and packaging alterations, the development of new pharmaceutical forms, new concentrations, new therapeutic indications, broadening of indications, text alterations in the leaflet. The assessment of the application for registration of new associations or combinations in the fixed dose of the active principle, which have or not already been registered is also an attribution of GEPEC
Office of Generic Drugs	GEMEG	Generic drug registration
Office of Biosimilar Drugs	GEMES	Biosimilar drug registration
Office of no drug, specific, Herbal drug and homoeopathic	GMEFH	Specific, herbal drug, homoeopathic drug registration and control of drugs with registration exemption
Unit of Biologic Products and Hemotherapic	UPBIH	Biological products registration, including vaccines
Unit of Controlled Products	UPROC	Does not conduct registrations
Nucleus of Information Quality Management in Drugs	NUQUIM	Does not conduct registrations

modified over time, and the main existing regulations from ANVISA about drug registration are described in Table 4.2. The regulations are applicable according to the kind of drug, the definitions and/or classifications of which are found in Table 4.3.

Besides ANVISA, the National Health Council (CNS – Conselho Nacional de Saúde), an organization that belongs to the Health Ministry, also presents regulations that are applicable to the registration of drugs (Resolution 251 of 7 August 1997). Amongst other

Table 4.2 *ANVISA regulations for the registration of pharmaceuticals.*

Drug type	ANVISA regulation	Date of enactment
New (synthetic and semi-synthetic)	RDC No 136 (ANVISA, 2003c)	05/29/2003
Generic	RDC No. 16 (ANVISA, 2007b)	03/02/2007
Biosimilar	RDC No. 17 (ANVISA, 2007c)	03/02/2007
Biologic	RDC No. 315 (ANVISA, 2005)	10/26/2005
	RDC No. 323 (ANVISA, 2003d)	11/10/2003
Herbal drug	RDC No. 14 (ANVISA, 2010)	03/31/2010
Homoeopathic	RDC No. 26 (ANVISA, 2007d)	03/30/2007
Specific	RDC No. 132 (ANVISA, 2003a)	05/29/2003
Already registered drug suitability	RDC No. 134 (ANVISA, 2003b)	05/29/2003

Table 4.3 *Classification and/or definitions used by ANVISA for drug registration.*

Drug type	Classification and/or definition
New (synthetic or semi-synthetic)	Pharmaceutical product, technically obtained or elaborated, with prophylactic aim, curative, palliative or for diagnoses. It is a finished pharmaceutical product that has a synthetic or semi-synthetic active principle, which is usually associated to adjuvant component.
Generic	Drugs that are chemically identical to a brand-name or innovative drug, which are to be interchangeable, usually manufactured either after a patent has expired, or if there are no sole rights by a drug company, once the generic drug meets the same standards for effectiveness, safety and quality and it is designated by the Brazilian Common Denomination (DCB – Denominação Comum Brasileira), or in its absence, by the International Common Denomination (DCI – Denominação Comum Internacional).
Similar	It has the same active principles, it shows the same concentration, pharmaceutical form, administration route, dosage, and therapeutic indication, and that is equivalent to the brand name drug in the Federal Organization responsible for the sanitary surveillance, differing only in some characteristics as size, shape, expiring date, packaging, labelling, excipients and vehicle, having to be identified by a commercial name or brand.
Biologic	Biological drugs are the ones that contain molecules with known biological activity, already registered in Brazil, and which have already passed through all the manufacturing stages. They are vaccines; serums; immunologic substances; hemoderivatives; biomedicines (drugs obtained either from biologic fluids or animal origin tissues and/or drugs obtained by biotechnological procedures); monoclonal antibodies (mAbs); drugs that have microorganisms which are live, tenuous or dead; probiotics; allergenic. A probiotic drug which has live or inactive microorganisms in order to prevent or treat human diseases through interaction with microbiotics or with an intestine epithelial or with immune cells associated or by other mechanisms of action
Herbal drug	Drugs made from medicinal plants. They are made exclusively using derivatives from herbal drugs (extract, tincture, oil, wax, exudate, juice, and others). The medicinal plant or parts thereof, after harvesting, stabilization and drying, whole, scratched, crushed or pulverized, are not to be registered as herbal drug
Homoeopathic	Drug streamlined prepared from substances that are subject to crunches or successive dilutions followed by succussion, or other form of rhythmic agitation, with preventive and curative purpose to be administered according to homoeopathic therapy, or anthroposophic homotoxicological
Specific	The category of specific drug registration is made up by: A: The parenteral solutions of high and low volume, parenteral or not, like: water for injection, glucose solutions, sodium chloride, other electrolytic compositions or sugars; B: Opoterapics – specific drugs prepared from glands, organs, tissues or secretion of animals (for example, propolis); C: Drugs that are mainly from vitamins and/or minerals and/or amino acids, isolated or associated with each other, with at least one of the components above the nutritional limits established by the specific legislation.

duties, it follows up on the development process and the scientific and technological incorporation in the health area in the country. Resolution 251 approves guidelines for research involving human beings as well as research with new active substances, drugs, vaccines and diagnostic tests. It also includes the nonclinical trials necessary for those investigations (ANVISA, 1997).

The evaluation of a registration dossier in Brazil is usually divided into three parts: pharmaceutical properties (or formulation studies); efficacy and safety analysis. The pharmaceutical analysis (type of drug, properties) is carried out by ANVISA's technicians, generally pharmacists. Requests to *ad hoc* consultants for advice are rare. The same does not apply, however, for the safety and efficacy assessment, developed through nonclinical and clinical studies. For historical reasons that preceded the creation of ANVISA, such assessments have traditionally depended on a review by recognized expert consultants, organized into technical councils. The role of ANVISA's technicians in these assessments has always been, and still is, limited, and the Agency continues to rely on outside aid, even though the manner of addressing requests for technical opinion and decision-making has been modified since mid-2003. These changes aim at making the analysis more efficient and decision-making processes more transparent. One of these changes was made in order to improve the efficiency of the analysis process by running the pharmacological analysis and the efficacy and safety analysis in parallel, given that the first is performed internally, and the second is performed by consultants. It is noteworthy that ANVISA is required to be efficient due to deadlines which are legally defined for issuing technical opinions, that is, approval.

Efficacy and safety assessments of new drugs are conducted almost exclusively by consultants contracted either directly or through medical associations. The consultants are selected from amongst their affiliates who have knowledge and experience in the area and do not have conflicts of interest with the issues or technical opinions about the products. Assessments of applications for registration of new drugs are sent to two consultants, while a single consultant is usually engaged for the assessment of supplements and post-registration changes. The overall experience with the assessments by *ad hoc* consultants has shown that the technical opinions are, with few exceptions, very detailed, and clearly point out the reasons for the given recommendations. The transparency of the criteria used for decision-making has been much higher with the current model (ANVISA, 2009).

It is noteworthy that, in recent years, ANVISA has adopted a more independent position on the subject of its internal consultant's opinions and that of other international regulatory agencies. In the case of new molecules, ANVISA requests technical opinions from at least two consultants, and it is not rare that these technical opinions are not in full agreement – indeed, they are occasionally quite divergent. Thus, it should be emphasized that ANVISA has the final approval responsibility. Although the Agency, in most cases, approves the technical opinions of its consultants, allowing or rejecting the petition or making "requirements" (requests for clarification or additional evidence) in accordance with them, this is not always the case. Some of the reasons for the occurrence of disparities between ANVISA and its consultants include: (a) differing technical opinion between different consultants; (b) consultant's recommendations that are in disagreement with recognized regulatory criteria adopted by the Agency, for example, a consultant's support to apply for a registration on the basis of preliminary or incomplete clinical investigation; (c) recommendations which do not have legal support, for example, approval of registration based on the fact that the drug has already been registered in another regulatory agency; (d) ANVISA's disagreement with the recommendations of a consultant. When the Agency has a differing opinion from that of the consultants, the differences are documented in the process. Whether approving the recommendations of the consultants or not, ANVISA explicitly states in its analysis the reasons for the decision, therefore contributing to the transparency of the process.

It is essential that ANVISA has the technical ability to make decisions, and that the reasons for the decision-making are made clear in its analysis. Although ANVISA is aware of and habitually uses, the assessments made by other regulatory agencies, it does not necessarily approve decisions taken by these regulatory agencies (Nishioka, 2006).

4.3.2 Nonclinical Studies Required for Drug Registration

The main regulations in effect in Brazil for drug registration require the conduct of nonclinical studies. The National Health Council Resolution, No. 251, 7 August 1997, ANVISA Resolutions No. 90, March 2004 and No. 323, 10 November 2003 are also included in the following discussion of nonclinical studies (ANVISA, 1997; 2003d; 2004).

Based on the national legislation currently in effect, the registration of new drugs (synthetic and natural products) requires the submission of the following nonclinical studies: pharmacodynamics, pharmacokinetics, acute toxicity, subchronic toxicity, chronic toxicity, reproductive and developmental toxicity, mutagenic activity and oncogenic potential (ANVISA, 2003c). In the case of biologic products, including probiotics, the registration must include the pharmacodynamic, subchronic toxicity, chronic toxicity, reproductive toxicity, mutagenic activity and oncogenic potential. The pharmacokinetic study is required only for biologics, whereas for blood products, only the submission of the pharmacodynamics study is required (ANVISA, 2003d; 2005). According to this legislation, there is no indication of a specific methodology for conducting nonclinical studies for these classes of drugs in the guidelines although international or other regional guidelines, for example, OECD, EPA, and so on, are referenced.

For homoeopathic products, when the substance is not on the Table of Powers for Registration and Streamlined Drug Notification (Tabela de Potências para Registro e Notificação de Medicamentos Dinamizados), the manufacturer is responsible for establishing and proving the safety of use in the intended concentration, by means of toxicology studies, both clinical and nonclinical, suitable for the profile of the substance. This Table of Powers contains a list of homoeopathic substances (n $\approx$ 1867 substances) with a description of the minimum and maximum streamlining per product for production and commercialization. Any other specification that does not meet the power band presented must be researched, as described above. However, the legislation does not establish which studies are to be presented, or the methodology to be followed when conducting these studies (ANVISA, 2007a; 2007d).

The only drug class for which the regulation cites the requirements for nonclinical studies and specifies the minimum requirements to be followed throughout the conduct of such studies is herbal drugs. The nonclinical studies required for this type of drug are pharmacology, acute toxicity, repeated-dose toxicity, and special studies (genotoxicity), the latter being necessary only when there are indications of continuous or prolonged use of the drug in humans (ANVISA, 2004; 2010b).

Table 4.4 *Criteria for acute toxicity studies, according to Resolution for Herbal Drugs.*

Criteria	Characteristics
Species	A mammal species (avoiding animals with particular genetic characteristics)
Gender	Males and females
Groups and number of animals per test (control and healthy groups)	A minimum of 6 males and 6 females per dose
Age	Adults
Route of administration	Same route as proposed for the product
Dosage	Sufficient for observation of possible adverse effects and estimated 50% lethal dose (dose which kills 50% of test animals). If there is no observable adverse effect, use the maximum dose possible
Observations	Signs of toxicity including onset time, progression and reversibility of these symptoms should be recorded. The greatest number of parameters should be noted, such as loss of mobility, respiration rate, piloerection, diarrhoea, salivation, altered muscle tone, hypnosis, convulsions, hyperexcitability of the central nervous system, abdominal contortions, number of dead animals along with the possible causes of the deaths and respective histopathological tests
Observation period	Postdose at 0, 15, 30 and 60 min and every 4 h, and then daily thereafter for 14 d after administration. This period can be extended depending on the observed signs of toxicity. Body weight change and food intake must be observed starting at 24 hr postdose. At the end of the observation period, all surviving animals should be sacrificed and autopsied. If changes are seen in the autopsies, histological examination of the involved organs should be performed
Pathological tests	Not specified

The conduct of nonclinical studies for herbal drugs must follow, as a minimum, the "Guide For Pre-Clinical Toxicity Studies of Herbal Drugs", which is specified by Resolution No 90 March 2004 (ANVISA, 2004). The criteria established by the guideline for each nonclinical study, including acute and repeated dose toxicity tests, are described in Tables 4.4 and 4.5. For genotoxicity, a bacterial reverse mutation assay (with and without metabolic action), or an *in vitro* evaluation of damage to chromosomes of mammalian cells or mouse lymphoma assay and an *in vivo* evaluation of chromosome damage in rodent hematopoietic cells (micronucleus test) must be carried out.

For herbal drugs used topically, in addition to acute toxicity and repeated-dose toxicity, and when genotoxicity is indicated, dermal sensitization, skin irritation and eye irritation should be performed. There is no reference of a methodology to be followed although the studies should conform to acceptable toxicological study designs.

In addition, ANVISA has a system of simplified registration for herbal drugs. In cases where the product is included in the latest publication of the "List of Simplified

Table 4.5 *Criteria for repeated dose toxicity studies, according to Resolution for Herbal Drugs.*

Criteria	Characteristics	
Animal species	A minimum of two mammalian species: one rodent and one nonrodent (no specie specified) The breeds should be defined in order to avoid animals with particular genetic characteristics	
Gender	Males and females	
Groups and number of animals per test	Rodents: a minimum of 10 males and 10 females per dose Nonrodents: a minimum of 3 males and 3 females per dose for study to include a control group with the formulation vehicle	
Age	Adult	
Route of administration	Same route proposed for the drug product	
Administration period	Period of use proposed for therapeutic use of the product:	Minimum duration of the repeated dose study:
	30 d of use per year	4 week
	Over 30 d of use per year	12 week
Dosage	A minimum of three doses: – dose which produces therapeutic effect (the lowest dose) – the highest dose which produces a detectable adverse effect, limited by the dose volume – intermediate dose, such as the geometric average between the highest and lowest dose	
Observations	Behavioural changes, body weight changes (weekly), complete haematology, biochemical blood analyses (sodium, potassium, gamma-glutamyl transferase, aminotransferase, alkaline phosphatase, urea, creatinine, uric acid, cholesterol, triglycerides, glucose, total protein and bilirubin)	
Pathological tests	– Macroscopic tests: in all animals at all dose levels – Histopathological tests: mandatory in animals treated with the highest dose. The material removed from the animals should be kept in a state of conservation for up to five years In the absence of histopathological changes in animals treated with the highest dose and of macroscopic changes at the lower doses, it may be unnecessary to carry out histopathological evaluation for the low and intermediate doses It is recommended that macroscopic and microscopic analysis is carried out on the following organs: liver, kidney, lung, heart, oesophagus and stomach, intestines, sexual organs, pancreas, adrenal gland	

Registration of Herbal Drugs", (Lista de registro simplificado de fitoterápicos – Instrução Normativa No. 5, 2008) there is no need to validate the therapeutic indications and safety of use. In this situation, the specifications stated in the legislation must be fully complied with, such as part of the plant used, indications and usage, therapeutic actions, dosage (mode of administration and preparation), route of administration, and precautions. Other pharmaceutical formulations with the same route of administration could be developed, provided the calculations of dose equivalence between the extract forms and the proposed pharmaceutical formulations are presented. It must be shown that the amount of active ingredient and its bioavailability in both products are similar. The "List of Simplified Registration of Herbal Drugs" is periodically updated and published by ANVISA.

For all classes of drugs, there is no legal requirement that studies should be conducted in Brazil. Therefore the monitoring of the development and guidance of the studies by ANVISA are not necessary.

To supply the absence of specific legislation, in March 2010 ANVISA, through the Management of Safety and Efficiency Assessment (Gerência de Avaliação de Segurança e Eficácia), published a guidance for carrying out nonclinical safety studies during the development of drugs. This was based on documents from recognized agencies which oversee the safety of drugs (FDA – Food and Drug Administration; EMA – European Drugs Agency) and institutions with an interest in the area (ICH – International Conference on Harmonization; OECD – Organization for Economic Cooperation and Development; NCI – National Cancer Institute; WHO – World Health Organization), with a view to increased harmonization with international regulations. The guide is also intended to rationalize nonclinical studies, avoiding duplications and the unnecessary use of animals without compromising the possibility of obtaining reliable information on the safety of the drug tested. Any deviation from the guidelines must always be justified.

The studies covered in the guideline include single dose toxicity (acute), repeated dose toxicity, reproductive toxicity, genotoxicity, local tolerance, carcinogenicity, studies for assessing pharmacological efficacy and toxicokinetics. For all of these, information is included on the objective of the study, animal model to be used, means of administration, dosage, and observation period. In addition, the guideline describes situations where nonclinical studies are necessary to construct a rational set of evidence to form the basis for planning clinical trials (ANVISA, 2010a). The guideline can be accessed through the ANVISA website (www.anvisa.gov.br). On receiving the reports, ANVISA thoroughly evaluates the design and methodology used in conducting these studies and might request clarification on specific points of the studies.

In addition to the specific legislations mentioned above, Resolution No. 251 of the National Health Council, concerning research involving humans, also describes the need for information prior to conducting clinical studies. A detailed presentation of nonclinical information necessary to justify the clinical stage of the project is requested, including a report of experimental studies (materials and methods, animals, laboratory tests, data on the pharmacodynamics, safety margin, therapeutic margin, pharmacokinetic and toxicology). Additionally, the nonclinical results must be accompanied by a discussion of the relevance of the findings in relation to the expected therapeutic effects and possible undesirable effects in humans. The nonclinical toxicology studies required are similar to those described above and include acute toxicity, repeated-dose toxicity and chronic toxicity. In addition, toxicity studies should also include an analysis of the effects on fertility, embryo–foetal development, mutagenic activity, oncogenic potential (carcinogenic) and other studies, according to the nature of the drug and therapeutic use in humans (ANVISA, 1997). A description of the studies is included in Table 4.6.

4.3.3 Comparison with Other Agencies and Harmonization Institutes

The methodologies for conducting nonclinical studies for drugs in Brazil presented in the guidance for conducting nonclinical safety studies during the development of drugs

Table 4.6 *Principle characteristics for the conduct of toxicological studies, according to Resolution No 251 (1997).*

Criteria	Characterístics	
Species	Minimum of 3 animal species, one of which must be a non-rodent mammal.	
Gender	Males and females	
Groups and number of animals per test (control and healthy groups)	Not specified.	
Age	Not specified.	
Route of administration	Acute toxicity:	Two routes of administration: – one route must be related to that recommended for the proposed therapeutic use – and the other must be a route which assures the drug absorption
	Subchronic toxicity:	Same route proposed for the product
	Chronic toxicity:	Same route proposed for the product
Administration period	Subchronic toxicity:	Minimum of 24 week
	Chronic toxicity:	Minimum of 24 week
Dosage	Not specified	
Observations	Not specified	
Pathological tests	Not specified	

(Resolution of the National Health Council, No. 251, 7 August 1997 and Resolution No. ANVISA, 9 March 2004), were compared with methods described in international protocols of some agencies and institutions such as the FDA (Food and Drug Administration), EMA (European Drugs Agency), ICH (International Conference on Harmonisation), OECD (Organization for Economic Cooperation and Development) and WHO (World Health Organization).

For acute toxicity studies, differences occur that are related to the number of species and the recommended routes of administration. ANVISA Resolution No. 90, March 2004 states that the study should be conducted with a mammalian species and the preferred route of administration is the route proposed for the therapeutic use of the product in humans. In Resolution No. 251/1997 of the National Health Council, it is not clear regarding the number of species to be used, but two routes of administration are recommended, one which ensures systemic exposure to the drug; the other route of administration must be the clinically relevant route. Guidance for conducting nonclinical safety studies during the development of drugs describes the use of a minimum of two species, one of which must be a nonrodent mammal; recommends two routes of administration (clinically relevant route for use in humans and intravenous route); dosage; observation period and parameters to be evaluated very similar to international protocols (ANVISA, 1997; 2004b; 2010a). The requirements cited in Resolution No. 90, March 2004 differ from the international protocols which uniformly indicate the use of two animal species and two routes of administration (ANVISA, 2004).

For repeated dose studies, international protocols are generally in agreement for the conduct of these studies, as to the number of species to be used and recommended route of administration. However, Resolution No. 251/1997 of the National Health Council does not describe the number of species to be used (only in a general manner) and mentions that the experimental schedule must have a minimum of 24 weeks of administration for repeated doses, whether or not it is a subchronic or chronic study (ANVISA, 1997; 2004).

Although Resolution No. 251/1997 of the National Health Council requests the submission of genotoxicity studies, only Resolution No. 90/2004 refers to the criteria to be followed when conducting these studies; these are, in general, in agreement with international protocols and guidance. A detailed description of genotoxicity tests can be found in the guidance for conducting nonclinical safety studies during the development of drugs, that is in agreement with international protocols and guidance (ANVISA, 2010a).

There is no national legislation establishing how reproductive toxicity and carcinogenicity studies should be conducted, nor is there any request for the submission of these studies for herbal drugs. However, the new guidance for conducting nonclinical safety studies during the development of drugs describes methodologies proposed for those tests, in accordance with international protocols and guidance.

The same situation is observed in studies on pharmacodynamics, pharmacokinetics, dermal irritation, eye irritation and dermal sensitization, where there is no reference in the national legislation concerning the criteria to be followed when conducting such studies. Only the guidance for conducting nonclinical safety studies during the development of drugs gives the recommendation to carry out these studies according to international harmonization (ANVISA, 2010a).

In general, the legislation is open to incorporate a design recommended by sponsors as long as it is shown that the safety assessment programme is scientifically valid and that, in the development of new drugs, critical assessment of the programme should be allowed and will be conducted on a case-by-case basis. Moreover, the new guidance for conducting nonclinical safety studies during the development of drugs was published with the aim of supplying the absence of specific legislation indicating the nonclinical tests to be applied, with their methodology, for evaluating the safety of drugs when they are registered.

4.3.4 Regional Reality of Drug Registration – Final Comments

Overall, it is noted that the nonclinical tests applied in the registration of drugs in Brazil are not widely evaluated and debated by the national industry, by Brazilian researchers, or by the regulation institute, since analyses and interpretations are entrusted to *ad hoc* consultants. There is no regulation that prohibits or restricts the registration of substances which have adverse findings in nonclinical toxicology studies. Accordingly, it appears that the interpretation of toxicological data will be of fundamental importance in this context and it will depend upon the analyses and scientific judgement made by the outsourced consultants, using the weight of evidence approach. The evolving technical ability of regulators, as well as the careful selection of expert consultants, brings efficiency and good results in this system of assessment of nonclinical studies.

It is emphasized that the quality of information, as well as reviews from scientific consultants, will have a key role in the final assessment of the process. The consultants, chosen directly by ANVISA or indicated by medical societies consulted by the Agency for that purpose, are, in general, specialists – university professors and/or researchers of recognized expertise, Brazilian in the great majority of cases – who must not have conflicts of interest which could potentially interfere with their evaluation of the drug.

In general, Brazilian legislation related to drug registration does not establish criteria for conducting nonclinical studies, nor does it determine that the conduct must based on existing international protocols. It should be noted that it is intended, based on the new guidance published by ANVISA (Guidance for conducting nonclinical safety studies during the development of drugs), that nonclinical safety studies needed for the development of new drugs should be coordinated and scientifically valid, and it is expected that they will provide reliable data to support the subsequent clinical research. The preparation of this guidance was based on documents from recognized agencies that oversee the safety of drugs (FEDA, EMA) and institutions with an interest in the area (ICH, OECD, NCI, WHO), to ensure that Brazilian requirements will present greater harmonization with international regulations.

With respect to MERCOSUR, Brazilian legislation still prevails for the registration of new drugs in Brazil, while MERCOSUR legislation is no more than a possible point of interaction between the member countries. Since MERCOSUR legislation addresses the question of nonclinical tests in broad and general terms, there are no conflicts in discussions which would exclude the possibility of future harmonization between the countries. Brazil has taken a great step forward in harmonization with the publication of the guidance, since it is adopting methodologies proposed by international organizations and institutions which are recognized in this area.

References

Agência Nacional de Vigilância Sanitária/Brasil (ANVISA) (1976) Lei n° 6360, de 23 de setembro de 1976. Dispõe sobre a vigilância sanitária a que ficam sujeitos os medicamentos, as drogas, os insumos farmacêuticos e correlatos, cosméticos, saneantes e outros produtos, e dá outras providências. Diário Oficial [da] União; Poder Executivo, Brasília, DF, Sept 24, 1976.

Agência Nacional de Vigilância Sanitária/Brasil (ANVISA) (1977) Decreto n° 79094, de 05 de janeiro de 1977. Regulamenta a Lei no 6.360, de 23 de setembro de 1976, que submete a sistema de vigilância sanitária os medicamentos, insumos farmacêuticos, drogas, correlatos, cosméticos, produtos de higiene, saneantes e outros. Diário Oficial [da] União; Poder Executivo, Brasília, DF, Jan 07, 1977.

Agência Nacional de Vigilância Sanitária/Brasil (ANVISA) (2003a) Resolução RDC n° 132, de 29 de maio de 2003. Dispõe sobre o registro de medicamentos específicos. Diário Oficial [da] União; Poder Executivo, Brasília, DF, Jun 02, 2003a.

Agência Nacional de Vigilância Sanitária/Brasil (ANVISA) (2003b) Resolução RDC n° 134, de 29 de maio de 2003. Dispõe sobre a adequação dos medicamentos já registrados. Diário Oficial [da] União; Poder Executivo, Brasília, DF, Jun 02, 2003b.

Agência Nacional de Vigilância Sanitária/Brasil (ANVISA) (2003c) Resolução RDC n° 136, de 29 de maio de 2003. Dispõe sobre o registro de medicamento novo. Diário Oficial [da] União; Poder Executivo, Brasília, DF, Jun 02, 2003c.

Agência Nacional de Vigilância Sanitária/Brasil (ANVISA) (2003d) Resolução RDC n° 323, de 10 de novembro de 2003. Aprova Regulamento técnico de registro, alteração e revalidação de registro dos medicamentos probióticos, conforme Regulamento Técnico anexo a esta Resolução. Diário Oficial [da] União; Poder Executivo, Brasília, DF, Nov 12, 2003d.

Agência Nacional de Vigilância Sanitária/Brasil (ANVISA) (2004) Resolução RE n° 90, de 16 de março de 2004. Determina a publicação da "Guia para a realização de estudos de toxicidade pré-clínica de fitoterápicos". Diário Oficial [da] União; Poder Executivo, Brasília, DF, Mar 18, 2004.

Agência Nacional de Vigilância Sanitária/Brasil (ANVISA) (2005) Resolução RDC n° 315, de 26 de outubro de 2005. Dispõe sobre o Regulamento Técnico de Registro, Alterações Pós-Registro e Revalidação de Registro dos Produtos Biológicos Terminados. Diário Oficial [da] União; Poder Executivo, Brasília, DF, Oct 31, 2005.

Agência Nacional de Vigilância Sanitária/Brasil (ANVISA) (2007a) Instrução Normativa n° 5, de 11 de maio de 2007. Dispõe sobre os limites de potência para registro e notificação de medicamentos dinamizados. Diário Oficial [da] União; Poder Executivo, Brasília, DF, Apr13, 2007a.

Agência Nacional de Vigilância Sanitária/Brasil (ANVISA) (2007b) Resolução RDC n° 16, de 02 de março de 2007. Aprova o Regulamento Técnico para Medicamentos Genéricos. Diário Oficial [da] União; Poder Executivo, Brasília, DF, Mar 05, 2007b.

Agência Nacional de Vigilância Sanitária/Brasil (ANVISA) (2007c) Resolução RDC n° 17, de 02 de março de 2007. Dispõe sobre o registro de Medicamento Similar e dá outras providências. Diário Oficial [da] União; Poder Executivo, Brasília, DF, Mar 05, 2007c.

Agência Nacional de Vigilância Sanitária/Brasil (ANVISA) (2007d) Resolução RDC n° 26, de 30 de março de 2007. Dispõe sobre o registro de medicamentos dinamizados industrializados homeopáticos, antroposóficos e anti-homotóxicos. **Diário Oficial [da] União**; Poder Executivo, Brasília, DF, Apr 02, 2007d.

Agência Nacional De Vigilância Sanitária/Brasil (ANVISA) (2009) **Site oficial**: Medicamentos. Web site http://www.anvisa.gov.br/medicamentos/index.htm. Accessed Ago 27, 2009.

Agência Nacional De Vigilância Sanitária/Brasil (ANVISA) (2010a) Guia para a condução de estudos não clínicos de segurança necessários ao desenvolvimento de medicamentos. Brasília, Brasil: Gerência de Avaliação de Segurança e Eficácia, 2010. Web site http://portal.anvisa.gov.br/wps/portal/anvisa/home/medicamentos. Accessed Sept 27, 2010a.

Agência Nacional de Vigilância Sanitária/Brasil (ANVISA) (2010b) Resolução RDC n° 14, de 31 de março de 2010. Dispõe sobre o registro de medicamentos fitoterápicos. Diário Oficial [da] União; Poder Executivo, Brasília, DF, Apr 05, 2010.

Brasil (1997) Resolução CNS n° 251, de 07 de agosto de 1997. Aprova normas de pesquisa envolvendo seres humanos para a área temática de pesquisa com novos fármacos, medicamentos, vacinas e testes diagnósticos. Diário Oficial [da] União, Poder executivo, Brasília, DF, Sept 23, 1997.

MERCOSUL (2010) **Site oficial**: A respeito do MERCOSUL. Web site http://www.mercosur.int. Accessed 21 October 2010.

MERCOSUL/GMC (1996) Resolução n° 129, de 13 de dezembro de 1996. Regulamento Técnico sobre a Verificação de Boas Práticas de Pesquisa Clínica. Diário Oficial [da] União, Poder executivo, Brasília, DF, Dec 14, 1996.

Nishioka, A.S. (2006) Como é feito o registro de medicamentos novos no Brasil. *Prática Hospitalar.*, **45**, 13–17.

5

Nonclinical Safety Assessment: Canada

Jamie L. Doran[1] *and Mark T. Goldberg*[2]
[1]*Intrinsik Health Sciences Inc., Mississauga, Canada*
[2]*PlantForm Corporation and Karamella Consulting Inc., Guelph, Canada*

5.1 Introduction

Canada has a population of about 33.5 million. As a market for global pharmaceuticals, it represents about 2.5% of sales with a total of about US$17 billion annually. This ranks as the sixth largest geographic market. Although it is geographically and politically close to the United States, Canada is a sovereign nation and has its own approach to regulating pharmaceuticals. For example, Canada offers 20 years of patent life protection along with eight years of clinical data exclusivity to innovators.

Health Canada* is the regulatory body of the federal government that approves drug products under the authority of the Food and Drug Act. This act authorizes Health Canada to regulate the safety, efficacy and quality of medications. Health Canada is divided into different agencies and branches which regulate different products and activities.

Canada offers Scientific Research and Experimental Development (SRED) tax credits to innovators. Although changes to this programme have been announced, a great deal of preclinical research has been conducted in Canada as a result of the SRED tax credit. Provinces offer additional SRED incentives such that a Canadian company conducting research in Canada can receive a cash refund for 20–35% of their research costs. Consequently, most of the major pharmaceutical and biotechnology companies currently have

* http://www.hc-sc.gc.ca/dhp-mps/index-eng.php.

Nonclinical Safety Assessment: A Guide to International Pharmaceutical Regulations, First Edition.
Edited by William J. Brock, Kenneth L. Hastings and Kathy M. McGown.

or formerly had research facilities in Canada. For example, most of the preclinical research on Lipitor®, the best selling drug in pharmaceutical history, was conducted in Canada by Warner Lambert Parke Davis, before this firm was acquired.

5.2 Organization of Health Canada

Several branches and agencies report into the Minister of Health and form the basis for Health Canada's organizational structure. The Health Products and Food Branch (HPFB) of Health Canada regulates prescription drugs, over-the-counter (OTC) medications, natural health products, medical devices, food, and veterinary drugs. Foods do not require premarket approval, but all other products do, including dietary supplements, which are called natural health products (NHP) in Canada. Within the HPFB there are six directorates, including:

- Biologics and Genetic Therapies Directorate
- Therapeutic Products Directorate
- Natural Health Products Directorate
- Food Directorate
- Veterinary Drugs Directorate and Marketed Health Products Directorate
- Health Products and Food Branch Inspectorate.

The Directorates responsible for nonclinical safety assessments of new drugs are discussed below.

5.2.1 Therapeutic Products Directorate

Pharmaceuticals (and not biological drugs) and medical devices in Canada are regulated by the Therapeutic Products Directorate (TPD). The TPD consists of 12 offices and bureaux, as depicted in Figure 5.1.

TPD conducts a premarket review of a product's safety, efficacy and quality, as well as a determination of the risks associated with a product's use, relative to its benefits. Preclinical studies are required prior to clinical trial authorization. The preclinical study requirements are discussed in more detail in Section 5.4.

Once preclinical studies have been completed, the sponsor submits a Clinical Trial Application, along with a protocol, investigator's brochure and Ethics Review Board approval. Within 30 days, Health Canada will indicate whether or not the trial can proceed. Health Canada will not approve a clinical trial; rather, they will issue a letter of non-objection, indicating that they are not opposed to the sponsor conducting the clinical trial. Procedures for Clinical Trial Applications in Canada are described in greater detail in Section 5.5.

Once clinical trials have been conducted, the sponsor files a New Drug Submission (NDS). This contains all of the typical information about the product, including preclinical and clinical studies, details on production, chemistry and manufacturing, packaging and labelling, indications, side-effects, and so on. For generic drugs, an Abbreviated New Drug Submission (ANDS) can be filed. This application should show bioequivalency, as well as production, packaging and labelling information. Consequently, it is a much smaller application than an NDS. Review of an NDS can take 300 days while an ANDS review can take 180 days.

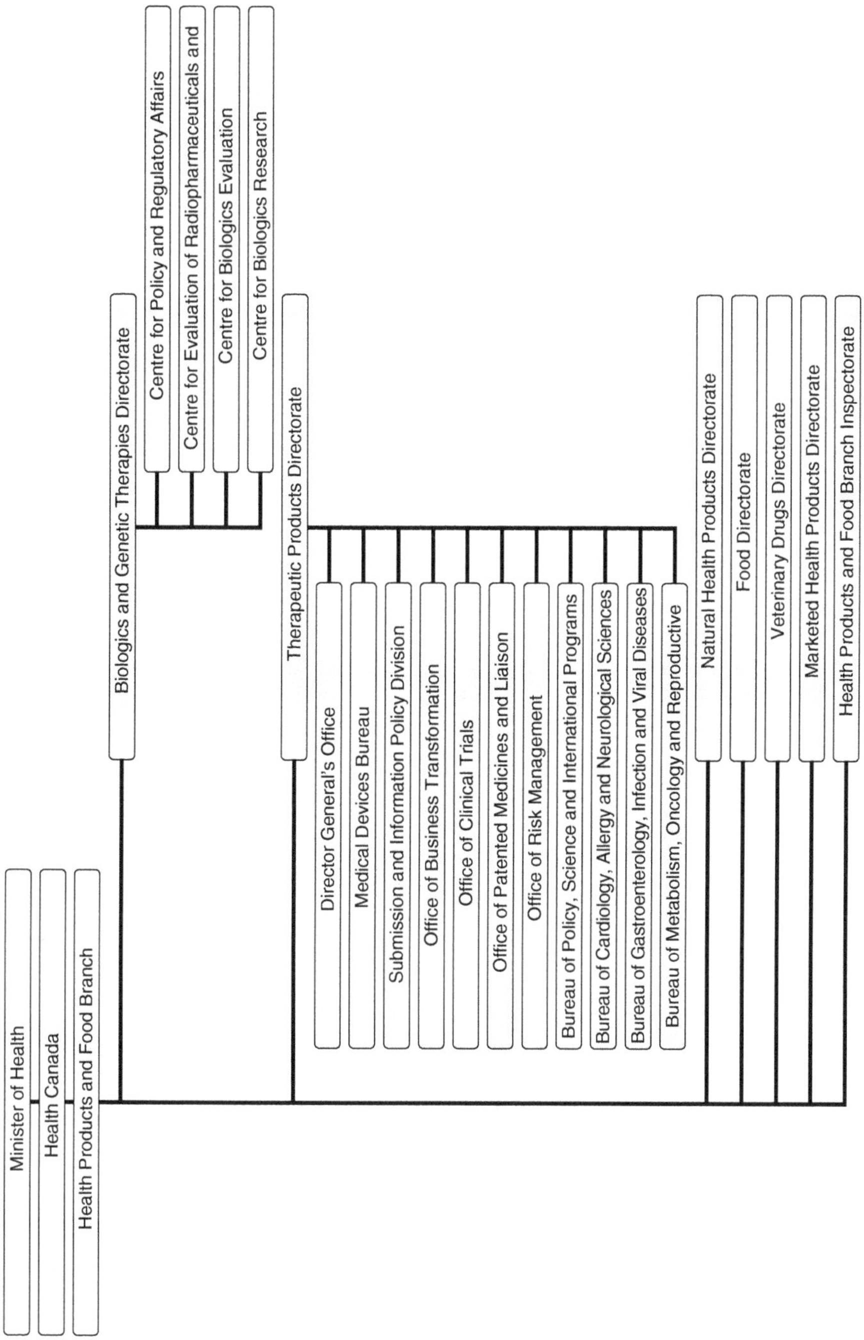

Figure 5.1 *Health Canada Organization.*

Once the product has been approved by Health Canada, a Drug Identification Number (DIN) is issued.

5.2.2 Biologics and Genetic Therapies Directorate

Biological drugs and radiopharmaceuticals are regulated by the Biologics and Genetic Therapies Directorate (BGTD). Products regulated by the BGTD include, but are not limited to, blood and blood products, vaccines, antibodies, gene therapy products, organs and xenografts. In essence, the BGTD is responsible for enforcing the Regulations that govern the directives for drugs described in Schedules C and D of the Food and Drugs Act. The BGTD is organized into four centres and four offices, as depicted in Figure 5.1.

5.2.3 Natural Health Products Directorate

NHPs in Canada are similar to Dietary Supplements in the United States and include vitamins and minerals, herbal remedies, homoeopathic medicines, traditional medicines such as traditional Chinese medicines, probiotics, and other products like amino acids and essential fatty acids. They deserve special mention because, in Canada, these products all require *premarket* approval. NHPs must make a health-related claim, which could include a structure/function claim, and they must be manufactured using Good Manufacturing Practices (GMP). NHPs in Canada are regulated by the Natural Health Products Directorate of Health Canada. Generally, the more compelling the scientific evidence is for a claim, the stronger the claim that will be accepted. Depending on the claim, a sponsor might wish to conduct a clinical trial on an NHP. The clinical trial must follow the guidelines for conducting clinical trials in Canada, as outlined for therapeutic products (see Section 5.5).

Once a NHP has been approved for sale in Canada, Health Canada will issue a unique identifier for the product, called a Natural Product Number or NPN. For homoeopathic products, this could be a Drug Identification Number for Homoeopathic Medicines (DIN-HM).

5.3 The Regulatory Framework for Drug Approval in Canada

Health Canada is the department of the federal government responsible for assisting Canadians in maintaining and improving their health. The Minister of Health, as leader of this department, is responsible to Parliament for administering various Acts and Regulations, including the Food and Drug Act and its corresponding regulations, the Food and Drug Regulations.

5.3.1 The Food and Drugs Act

The Food and Drugs Act is applicable to all food, drugs, cosmetics and therapeutic devices sold in Canada. For the purpose of this Act, the following definitions apply:

Food: Any article manufactured, sold or represented for use as food or drink for human beings, chewing gum and any ingredient that may be mixed with food for any purpose.

Drug: Any substance or mixture of substances manufactured, sold or represented for use in (a) diagnosis, treatment, mitigation or prevention of disease, disorder or abnormal physical state, or its symptoms, in human beings or animals; (b) restoring, correcting or modifying organic functions in human beings or animals; or (c) disinfection in premises in which food is manufactured, prepared or kept.

Cosmetic: Any substance or mixture of substances manufactured, sold or represented for use in cleansing, improving or altering the complexion, skin, hair or teeth, and including deodorants and perfumes.

Device: Any article, instrument, apparatus or contrivance, including any component, part or accessory thereof, manufactured, sold or represented for use in (a) the diagnosis, treatment, mitigation or prevention of a disease, disorder or abnormal physical state, or its symptoms, in human beings or animals; (b) restoring, correcting or modifying a body function or the body structure of human beings or animals; (c) the diagnosis of pregnancy in human beings or animals; or (d) the care of human beings or animals during pregnancy and at and after birth of the offspring, including care of the offspring. A contraceptive device is included but does not include a drug.

The Act is divided into two parts and has four completed Schedules (i.e., annexes or attachments). Part I of the Act describes the general governing aspects of the sale and advertisement under which a food, drug, cosmetic or device can be sold. This Part restricts the sale and advertisement to the general public of any food, drug, cosmetic or device that claims treatment, prevention of cure of diseases listed in Schedule A of the Act. This Schedule includes disorders such as cancer, depression, glaucoma, obesity, and sexually transmitted disease. For drugs, Schedule B lists recognized international standards that can be used to develop and approve a drug; these include the United States Pharmacopoeia and the National Formulary.

Drugs regulated as biologics or radiopharmaceuticals (i.e., those regulated by the Biologics and Genetic Therapies Directorate) are listed in Schedule C (radiopharmaceuticals) and Schedule D (biologics) of the Act. The Act states that the drugs listed in these Schedules may not be sold unless the Minister of Health has indicated that the drug manufacturing premises and the processes for manufacture of the drug are suitable to ensure the safe use of the drug.

Administration and enforcement issues are addressed in Part II of the Act. This Part includes provisions for inspection of manufacturing premises, and seizure and/or forfeiture of Food and Drug Act products. The Act provides for the ability of the regulatory body to establish regulations for purposes of enforcing the Act. The main regulations in enforcement under this act include the Food and Drug Regulations, the Medical Device Regulations and the Natural Health Product Regulations. The Food and Drug Regulations are most relevant to the focus of this chapter and thus are discussed below.

5.3.2 The Food and Drug Regulations

The purpose of the Food and Drug Regulations (Regulations) is to enforce the provisions under the Food and Drug Act for products classified as "food" and "drug". The Regulations consist of seven parts; Parts A through J (see Figure 5.2a). Part A contains primarily administrative information but also provides rules for labelling, importation, regulatory definitions, language requirements and packaging. Part B of the Regulations addresses food products and thus will not be discussed in detail.

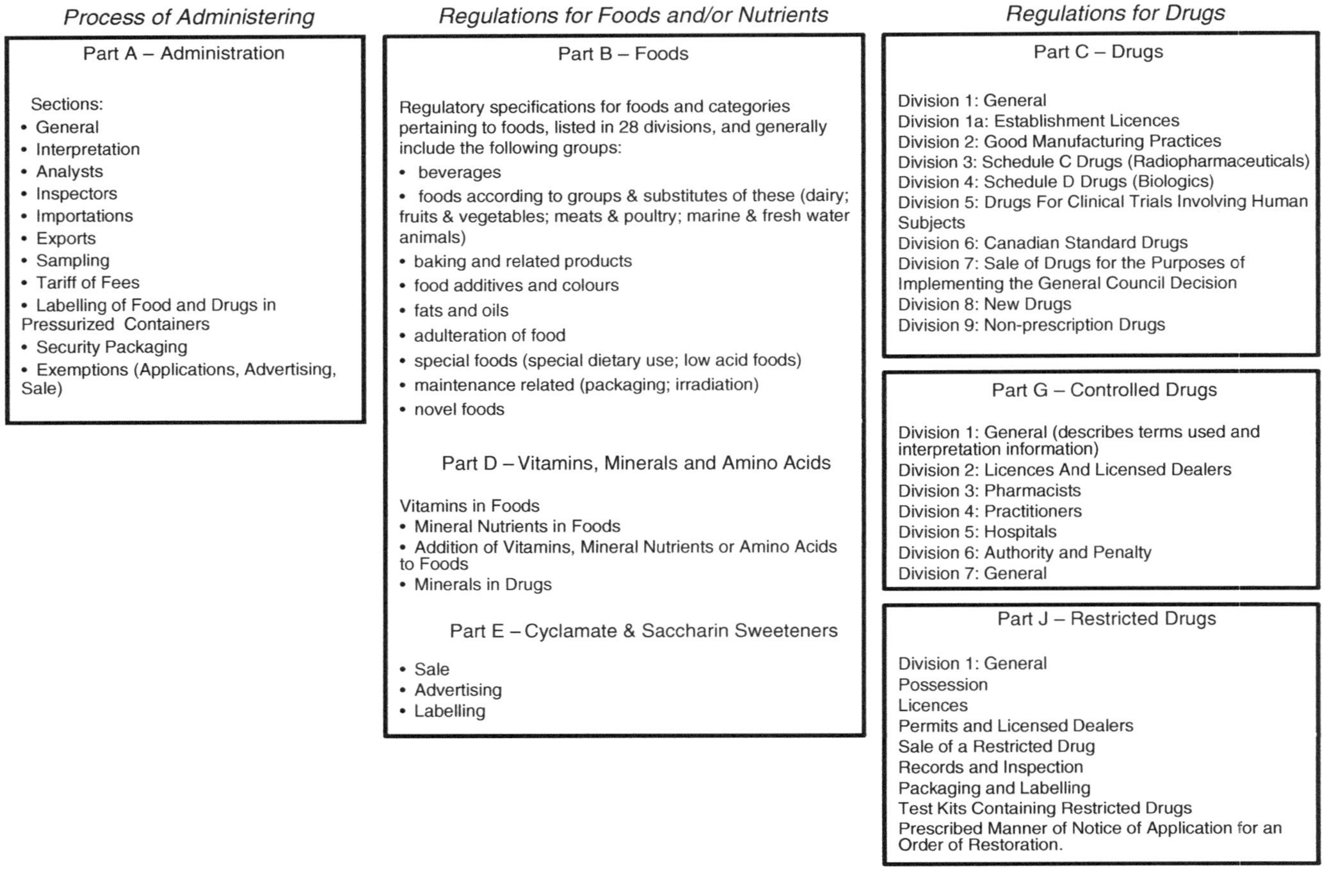

(a)

Figure 5.2 *Food and Drug Regulations in Canada. (a) Breakdown of Parts A–J. (b) Breakdown of Part C – Drugs.*

Divisions 1, 1a, and 2

Paragraphs within Division 1:

- General
- Assignment and Cancellation of Drug Identification Numbers
- Tablet Disintegration Times
- Adverse Drug Reaction Reporting
- Limits of Drug Dosage
- Cautionary Statements and Child Resistant Packaging
- Miscellaneous *(Restrictions and exceptions)*
- Colouring Agents
- Schedule F Drugs [list of medicinal ingredients]
- Recalls
- Limits of Variability
- Mercuric Chloride Tablets
- Synthetic Sweeteners [repealed]
- Aminopyrine and Dipyrone
- Coated Potassium Salts
- Antibiotics
- Chloramphenicol
- Veterinary Drugs
- Contraceptive Drugs

Paragraphs within Division 1a (*Establishment Licences*):

- Application
- Prohibition
- Application for Establishment Licence
- Issuance
- Refusal to Issue
- Terms and Conditions
- Notification
- Suspension
- Designation

Paragraphs within Division 2 (*Good Manufacturing Practices*):

- Sales
- Premises
- Equipment
- Personnel
- Sanitation
- Raw Material Testing
- Finished Product Testing
- Records
- Samples
- Stability
- Sterile Products
- Medical Gases

Divisions 3, 4 and 5

Division 3 (*Schedule C Drugs, Radiopharmaceuticals*):

Regulatory specifications for radiopharmaceutical drugs, which are defined as: 'a drug that exhibits spontaneous disintegration of unstable nuclei with the emission of nuclear particles or photons.'

Paragraphs within Division 4 (*Schedule D Drugs, Biologics*):
Regulatory specifications biological drugs, which are drugs that are made from living organisms.

Division 4 contains information for the following groups:

- Vaccines and Bacteriophage
- Toxins, Toxoids and Antitoxins, Antisera
- Preparations from Human Sources (including plasma)
- Insulin related paragraphs (preparations; injections; different types; labelling)
- Globin Insulin with Zinc
- Anterior Pituitary Extracts

Paragraphs within Division 5 (*Drugs For Clinical Trials Involving Human Subjects*):

- Application
- Prohibition
- General
- Application for Authorization
- Authorization
- Notification
- Amendment
- Additional Information and Samples
- Sponsor's Obligations
- Suspension and Cancellation

Divisions 6, 7, 8 and 9

Drugs listed in Division 6 (*Canadian Standard Drugs*):

Canadian Standard Drugs are drugs that have official standards, such as for: purity, quality and other physical and identity related parameters. These drugs include the following groups:

- Conjugated Estrogens
- Digotoxin
- Digoxin
- Esterified Estrogens
- Gelatin
- Thyroid

Division 7 (*Sale of Drugs for the Purposes of Implementing the General Council Decision*) Breakdown:

- Application
- Application for Authorization
- Authorization
- Notice to Commissioner of Patents
- Marking and Labelling
- Records
- Notice to Minister

Division 8 (*New Drugs*) Breakdown:

Regulatory specifications for New Drugs, which are defined as: 'a drug that contains or consists of a substance, whether as an active or inactive ingredient, carrier, coating, excipient, menstruumor other component, that has not been sold as a drug in Canada for sufficient time and in sufficient quantity to establish in Canada the safety and effectiveness of that substance for use as a drug.'

- New Drugs (including New Drug submissions)
- Sale of New Drug for Emergency Treatment
- Sale of Medicated Feeds
- Experimental Studies

Division 9 (*Non-prescription Drugs*):

- New Drugs
- Analgesics
- Acetaminophen
- Salicylates

(b)

Figure 5.2 (Continued)

Part C addresses regulations concerning drugs and consists of ten divisions (see Figure 5.2b). Division 1 includes (but is not limited to) statements on proper names that must be used in place of chemical names and/or synonyms for a drug, describes the drug identification numbers assignment and cancellation process, requirements for adverse drug reaction and recall reporting, as well as variation limits on finished products. Division 1A provides regulations on the application and maintenance of an establishment license for the manufacture of drugs.

Division 2 of Part C outlines the principles of Good Manufacturing Practice (GMP) for Canada. Division 3 describes the regulations specific to drugs listed under Schedule C of the Act (radiopharmaceuticals). Division 4 describes regulations specific to drugs listed under Schedule D of the Act, which includes biological drugs. There are variations in requirements, such as Health Canada testing requirements prior to the sale of a Schedule D drug, divergent labelling requirements and divergent definitions (such as date of manufacture and date of issue) that are described in this Division and thus diverge biologics regulations from those regulating other drugs.

Division 5 of Part C of the Regulations outlines the processes for applications to perform clinical trials in Canada. These are described in detail in the section on Clinical Trial Applications. Division 6 provides definitions of specific drugs, which have exceptional definition rules in comparison to those described by other jurisdictions. Definitions for drugs such as conjugated oestrogen, digitoxin and thyroid are described in this section. Division 7 outlines the authority and restrictions on the sale of drugs in Canada. Division 8 outlines the requirements for approval of new drugs, including the New Drug Submission (NDS) process, the generic drug approval process and sale of new drugs for emergency treatment. Division 9 outlines the specific requirements for the sale and labelling of analgesics, acetaminophen- and salicylate-containing drugs.

The remaining parts of the Regulations include Part D, Vitamin, Minerals and Amino Acids; Part E, Cyclamate and Saccharin Sweeteners; Part G, Controlled Drugs, Part J, Restricted Drugs. Four Schedules are attached to the Regulations; these schedules address primarily food-related issues.

5.4 Nonclinical Assessment in Canada

5.4.1 Canada and the International Conference on Harmonization

5.4.1.1 The Role of Canada in the International Conference on Harmonization

The International Conference on Harmonization of Technical Requirements for Registration of Pharmaceuticals for Human Use (ICH) was formed in 1990 with the goal of achieving harmonization in the guidelines and requirements for new drug registration. The regulatory authorities of Europe, Japan and the United States are the active participants forming this group. Since its initiation, observers from non-ICH countries and regions have been appointed to act as links between the ICH and the non-ICH regions. Canada is one of these observers and is represented by Health Canada.

As an observer, Canada takes part in ICH Steering Committee and ICH Global Cooperation Group meetings. The ICH Steering Committee sets ICH policies and procedures, topics for harmonization and monitors initiatives. The Committee meets a minimum of two times per year. Canada nominates participants to attend the Committee meetings; these participants do not have voting authority.

The ICG Global Cooperation Group is a subcommittee of the Steering Committee and was formed in response to interested parties beyond the three ICH regions. The objectives of the ICH Global Cooperation Group include: reduction of regional differences in technical requirements for new drugs; promotion of safe, effective and high quality drugs from an international perspective; and promotion of the practice of clinical trials to meet high international standards. Canada forms part of the ICH Global Cooperation Group.

5.4.1.2 ICH Guidance Documents: Adoption Process

In accordance with Step 2 of the ICH process for harmonization of guidelines, Health Canada releases draft guidance documents for stakeholder consultation and comment. These comments are forwarded to the appropriate ICH working group for consideration.

In the past, delays for formal adoption were experienced, causing issues for Canadian drug development programmes seeking authorization in international countries and vice versa. These delays also caused uncertainty in the industry with respect to the acceptance status of the ICH guidance document. Health Canada now strives to adopt ICH guidance documents once administrative steps for adoption have been completed, thus accelerating the formal adoption period and effective date. Once ICH guidance documents are adopted, they become official Health Canada guidance.

5.4.1.3 Adopted ICH Guidance

The majority of ICH guidance documents related to nonclinical safety ("Safety" guidance) have been adopted by Health Canada (see Chapter 2 for listing of documents).

The following ICH guidance documents have not been adopted by Health Canada at the time of this publication:

ICH S8 – Immunotoxicity studies for human pharmaceuticals
ICH S9 – Nonclinical evaluation of anticancer pharmaceuticals

According to a contact with Health Canada, the Government encourages stakeholder use of these documents as they anticipate approving them shortly (e-mail, 2010).

ICH M3 (R2) (Guidance on nonclinical safety studies for the conduct of human clinical trials and marketing authorization for pharmaceuticals) is still under consideration by Health Canada. According to our contact in the Government, many comments were received during the regional regulatory consultation and this has caused delays in approving the document (e-mail, 2010).

Although these three documents have not been formally approved by the Government, the majority of companies filing a CTA or NDS follow the general guidelines provided in these document. Therefore, there is little difference in the development path of anticancer therapeutics in Canada versus the United States or Europe; immunotoxicity studies are conducted under the general guidelines provided in ICH S8 and Health Canada generally accepts or advises to conduct nonclinical studies of duration indicated in ICH M3 (R2) (depending on the type of therapeutic and indication). Canadian or foreign pharmaceutical organizations rarely focus clinical trials or market authorization solely in Canada given the small market and thus drug development plans often follow the internationally-accepted guidelines of the ICH.

5.4.2 Good Laboratory Practices in Canada

5.4.2.1 History and Background

The principles of Good Laboratory Practices (GLP) are intended to promote the quality and validity of test data. As a member country in the Organization for Economic Cooperation and Development (OECD), Canada is required to adhere to the Decisions and Recommendations set out by the OECD on various aspects of GLP as it relates to chemical testing. In 1981, an OECD Council Act relating to the Mutual Acceptance of Data (MAD) was adopted. This Act states that all OECD member countries will accept safety data developed in another member country for the purposes of assessing the safety of a product. Further to this Act, an additional Act was adopted in 1989 that was intended to put provisions in place to assure that these data were being developed in compliance with the OECD Principles of GLP. This act states that any member country carrying out the testing of a chemical (in relation to protecting health and the environment) must establish national compliance monitoring procedures, designate an authority to execute and monitor these activities and require a declaration of GLP compliance by testing facilities' management.

In August 2009, the UK GLP monitoring authority for the Medicines and Healthcare Products Regulatory Agency published a statement on their opinion of test data garnered from test sites in Canada (GLP, 2009). At that time, Environment Canada (EC) was responsible for GLP monitoring of testing of industrial chemicals and the Standards Council of Canada (SCC) was responsible for GLP monitoring of testing of agrochemicals (i.e., pesticides). Health Canada had responsibility for monitoring the compliance of pharmaceutical product testing; however, this agency had not previously established a monitoring programme in accordance with the 1989 OECD Act that mandates this activity. Therefore, the UK monitoring authority stressed in their statement that key members of a testing study team (Study Director, Principle Investigator, and Quality Assurance) verify the GLP compliance status of any Canadian facility contracted to perform GLP testing of a pharmaceutical product.

In June 2009, Health Canada partnered with the SCC to enable the SCC to act as Canada's monitoring authority for GLP compliance of testing facilities involved in the testing of pharmaceutical, biologic and radiopharmaceutical products. A draft guidance document on the adherence to Good Laboratory Practices was issued for public consultation in August 2009. The final version was adopted in February 2010 and became effective in April 2010 (GD, 2010). Testing facilities were expected to be assessed and compliant within one year from this date. This policy guidance has been reviewed and accepted by the OECD.

5.4.2.2 Guidance Document Overview and Highlights

The Health Canada Guidance Document, "Non-Clinical Laboratory Study Data Supporting Drug Product Applications and Submissions: Adherence to Good Laboratory Practices", sets policies stating that when data from a nonclinical study are included in drug product submissions (such as Clinical Trial Applications (CTAs), Drug Identification Number (DIN) applications, and New Drug Submissions (NDSs)), a GLP compliance statement must be provided; that non-GLP studies must be justified; that assessment and compliance documentation must be provided by a GLP monitoring authority; and that all nonclinical study documentation supporting an approved drug product be archived for a minimum of 10 years after the first date of sale. Health Canada intends tp proceed with mandatory GLP requirements when the Food and Drugs Act is revised and amended.

5.4.2.3 *Applicability*

The guidance document applies to all nonclinical data relating to pharmaceutical (including disinfectants), radiopharmaceutical and biologic drugs for human use. The guidance document does not apply to nonclinical data supporting veterinary drugs, natural health products, medical devices (including some combination products), food additives or cosmetics. It is Health Canada's intention and legal obligation to implement mandatory GLP monitoring of studies for veterinary drugs, food and feed additives and medical devices. There is currently no intention to set guidelines for cosmetics, due to the lack of regulated premarket safety data requirements or for natural health products, due to their exemption from OECD GLPs. Non-prescription drugs (also known as Over-the-Counter or OTCs) are not exempt from this policy.

Some nonclinical studies, such as primary pharmacology studies conducted during the discovery phase of development and certain safety pharmacology and pharmacodynamic studies conducted outside of the core battery of studies are not required to be GLP-compliant. Bioanalytical studies supporting human bioequivalence studies are not subject to GLP requirements; rather, they are required to comply with Good Clinical Practices (GCP). Health Canada has indicated that GLP requirements for clinical studies involving products could be waived unless novel nonclinical data are required to support the planned trial.

5.4.2.4 *Recognition*

Health Canada will require OECD or equivalent recognition of domestic or foreign facilities conducting nonclinical studies for all nonclinical data covered under the scope of the guidance document. All nonclinical study reports must include a management declaration indicating that the study was conducted in accordance with GLP principles. Available evidence indicating the facility's GLP compliance status should be included in the section of CTD Module 1.2.5 – Compliance and Site Information (within CTA and NDS submissions).

5.4.3 Case Studies and Summary Basis of Decision

5.4.3.1 *Summary Basis of Decision*

The Summary Basis of Decision (SBD) procedure was implemented in response to Canadians' growing concern regarding the transparency of the approval process for market authorizations of pharmaceuticals in Canada. Prior to the pilot SBD projects in 2004, Canadians were forced to gather detailed information on the basis of market authorizations from similar documents published internationally. Similar to the European Public Assessment Reports, the SBD document contains Health Canada's considerations on the safety, efficacy and quality (chemistry, manufacturing and controls) of a new drug and thus provides the basis for Health Canada's decision to grant market authorization for a new drug. The process is being phased in, initiating with new active drug substances and certain medical devices. A Notice of Decision forms part of the SBD and is often published prior to the SBD. The Notice of Decision is a short (one page) summary of the authorization and a general overview of the drug or device.

SBDs for drug products regulated by the Therapeutic Product Directorate are available at: http://www.hc-sc.gc.ca/dhp-mps/prodpharma/update-miseajour/index-eng.php.

SBDs for drug products regulated by the Biologics and Genetic Therapies Directorate are available on the above website or: http://www.hc-sc.gc.ca/dhp-mps/brgtherap/update-miseajour/index-eng.php.

The SBD contains detailed technical information on the scientific and regulatory basis for decision, which includes quality basis (drug substance and drug product), facilities and equipment for manufacture, evaluation of adventitious agents, nonclinical basis (pharmacodynamics, pharmacokinetics, toxicology), clinical basis (efficacy, safety), the benefit/risk assessment and recommendation as well as an overview of the submission milestones and dates.

5.4.3.2 *Case Studies (Examples of Summary Basis for Decision of Approved Drugs in Canada)*

Presented below are four case examples of approved drug products in Canada, with interesting nonclinical basis of decision.

5.4.3.3 *^{Pr}Besivance™ (Besifloxacin, 06% w/v, suspension); Baush & Lomb Inc.*

Besivance™ was approved by the US FDA in May 2009 and in Canada in October 2009. It is indicated for the treatment of patients one year of age and older with bacterial conjunctivitis caused by specific aerobic gram-positive and gram-negative bacteria.

In vitro activities of the active ingredient were satisfactory; sensitivity assays were not required due to topical ophthalmic nature of the suspension. *In vitro* studies also revealed a low propensity for resistance. Primary pharmacodynamic studies are not generally required for antibacterial agents and thus were not evaluated for this product. Adverse effects were observed on safety pharmacology studies following systemic administration of the drug (prolongation of the QT interval and reduced creatinine clearance). However, given the topical ocular application of this drug and low systemic availability following repeat dosing in animals and humans, these risks were considered negligible.

Typical ADME (Adsorption, Distribution, Metabolism and Excretion) studies were conducted in rats, rabbits and monkeys. Rapid absorption and distribution were observed with topical ocular application of the drug product, although low systemic exposure was also observed following ocular administration.

Toxicity studies were conducted in rats and dogs and local tolerance studies were conducted in rats, dogs and guinea pigs. Single and repeat toxicity studies suggested a wide safety margin for the drug. The drug was mutagenic in some bacterial strains and positive in the *in vivo* mouse micronucleus assay at levels much higher than those expected following topical ocular administration. Due to short-term use of the product and the low systemic exposure following topical ocular administration, Health Canada decided that market authorization should not be prevented in light of these findings. Carcinogenicity studies were not conducted due to the short-term use and low systemic availability of the drug.

Peri- and post-natal development studies as well as embryo-foetal development studies demonstrated that the drug is foetal-toxic. These effects were observed at plasma levels much higher than those that would occur following topical administration.

Local tolerance studies did not provide any basis for concern with regard to the topical ocular administration of the product.

Despite the concerns with respect to genotoxicity and foetal-toxicity, Health Canada based the positive nonclinical safety assessment on the fact that Besivance™ has minimal systemic exposure when administered topically to the eye, suggesting that the risks to the treated patients are minimal. This submission was filed in November 2008 and authorized in October 2009.

5.4.3.4 ^{Pr}Abilify (Aripiprazole, 2 mg, 5 mg, 10 mg, 15 mg, 20 mg, and 30 mg tablets); Bristol-Myers Squibb Canada*

Abilify was first approved by the US FDA in November 2002, the EMA in June 2004 and in Canada in July 2009. It is indicated for schizophrenia and bipolar disorder and is administered orally.

Nonclinical studies were not reviewed for the Abilify drug submission based on the fact that the drug had been marketed internationally (US and Europe) for approximately seven years at the time of submission (an estimated cumulative human exposure to the drug was over 4 million patients). The FDA and EMA approval reports were consulted to confirm the proposed text for the Product Monograph. No nonclinical safety concerns were identified by Health Canada during the agency's review of these FDA and EMA documents.

5.4.3.5 ^{Pr}Ongylza™ (Saxagliptin Hydrochloride, 5 mg, Tablet); Bristol-Myers Squibb Canada

Ongylza™ was approved in the United States in July 2009, Europe in October 2009 and in Canada in September 2009. It is classified as an oral antihyperglycemic agent and is indicated for type 2 diabetes patients in combination with metformin or a sulfonylurea.

A comprehensive nonclinical investigational programme was conducted to establish the nonclinical safety profile of Ongylza. *In vivo* and *in vitro* pharmacology studies were conducted to establish the potent efficacy for the drug product. No adverse effects were noted in safety pharmacology studies conducted in rats and dogs. In pharmacokinetic studies (conducted in rats, dogs and monkeys), the major observation was that the drug appears to be metabolized via the cytochrome P450 (CYP) 3A4/3A5 pathway; therefore Health Canada suggested that co-administration with drugs that inhibit or induce CYP3A4/5 should be carefully evaluated.

A full battery of toxicology studies was performed in mice, rats, rabbits and monkeys. This included single and repeat toxicity studies, genotoxicity, carcinogenicity, reproduction and development, and local tolerance studies. There were minimal observations in these studies; however, the use of the drug has been limited in pregnant and lactating women.

Where appropriate, the nonclinical data for Ongylza™ were also compared to other drugs in the same class. Following a review of these data and those generated for Ongylza, Health Canada found that there were no major safety issues identified in the nonclinical safety studies evaluating Ongylza™. The submission was filed in July 2008 and authorized in September 2009.

5.4.3.6 Arepanrix™ H1N1 (AS03-Adjuvanted H1N1 Pandemic Influenza Vaccine) GlaxoSmithKline Biologicals

Arepanrix was approved on an interim basis by Health Canada in October 2009 in response to a request by the Public Health Agency of Canada, further to the anticipation of an influenza A H1N1 pandemic. Due to the expedited nature of this authorization, prototype ("mock") and reference vaccines were used in the safety and efficacy evaluation of the H1N1 vaccine. These prototypes and references primarily included Arepanrix H5N1 and Pandemrix H5N1 for the purposes of the nonclinical evaluation as the major distinction between these vaccines and the H1N1 vaccine was the different strains of influenza used in the manufacture of the vaccine.

Immunogenicity studies were conducted with naïve female mice using Arepanrix H1N1 and Pandemrix H1N1. Similar studies were performed in ferrets using Arepanrix H5N1. All studies indicated an increased immune response following administration. Secondary pharmacodynamics and drug interactions were not examined in nonclinical studies for this vaccine.

A repeat-dose toxicity study was conducted in rabbits with an AS03-adjuvanted A/H3N2 influenza antigen or the adjuvant alone. Genotoxicity and carcinogenicity studies were not performed with this vaccine. Historical genotoxicity studies conducted with an influenza antigen control and the adjuvant were reviewed in this evaluation.

Reproductive and development studies were not performed with Arepanrix H1N1; two studies were conducted with the Arepanrix H5N1 and Pandemrix H5N1. Some adverse effects were noted in both studies; however, the findings were not consistent for both studies. Therefore, the reviewer was unable to ascertain the toxicological significance of these findings.

Local tolerance, single dose toxicity tests were performed in rabbits with a model vaccine (A/H3N2 antigen). No adverse effects were observed on this study and local dermal reactions were considered minimal and not related to the test treatment.

Overall, Health Canada concluded that the toxicity studies conducted with the model strains and strain variants were representative of Arepanrix H1N1 and thus could be used as surrogate data for the nonclinical evaluation of the vaccine. Further, the evaluators concluded that from a nonclinical perspective, the vaccines were well-tolerated and efficacious in stimulating an immune response. The first part of the rolling new drug submission was filed in August 2009 and the interim order for authorization was issued in October 2009.

5.5 Clinical Trial Applications

5.5.1 History and Regulations

Provisions under the Food & Drug Regulations governing the use of drugs in clinical trials were initially developed in the early 1960s. These Regulations described the requirements for an Investigational New Drug Submission (IND), which was required to be submitted prior to distribution and/or sale of a new drug for use in clinical trials. There are several provisions in the current Regulations that define the requirements applicable to the sale and use of new or approved drugs in clinical trials. However, in the 1980s a working group was formed to provide recommendations on the Canadian drug submission review process, including the review time for approval of INDs, which was not defined. In 1987, the Regulations were amended to include a 60-day default review time for IND approval, to allow for more timely access to new drugs and to encourage new research in Canada.

Following recognition of the need to harmonize clinical trial practice with international regulatory guidelines such as Good Clinical Practices (GCPs), the Regulations were amended to include Division 5, Drugs for Clinical Trials Involving Human Subjects. Coming into effect in 2001, this new regulation introduced the Clinical Trial Application (CTA), which replaced the previously required IND for approval of clinical trials. Other features included the incorporation of a 30-day review period, defined sponsor responsibilities with respect to documentation, record keeping (25 years in Canada) and GCPs, defined investigator responsibilities and qualifications, and provided expanded authorities to the Minister. All CTAs are required to be signed by the Senior Medical Officer or Scientific Officer, who represents the sponsor and is responsible for providing an attestation with respect to the CTA at the time of filing.

As a consequence to this amendment, the following guidance and policy documents are no longer valid: Conduct of Clinical Investigations (1989), Preparation of Investigational New Drug Submissions (1991), Clinical Trials Review and Approval Policy (1997).

5.5.2 Clinical Trial Application Overview

Clinical Trial Applications (CTA) are required for Phase I–III clinical studies for any new drug. A CTA is also required for approved products being studied on a clinical trial outside the parameters of clinical use defined in the approved Notice of Compliance (NOC) or Drug Identification Number (DIN) application. Phase 4 studies do not require a CTA. A CTA must be filed and approved prior to the commencement of the trial. The target review period for Phase 1 Healthy Volunteer or Bioequivalence studies is seven days, with the exemption of applications involving specific types of therapies (gene therapies, for example). For all other studies, Health Canada is required under the Regulations to review the CTA and within 30 days of receipt notify the sponsor the approval or notice of deficiency.

The CTA is first subject to a screening phase to ensure that all components are present. Once screening is complete, the CTA is processed for review and an acknowledgement letter is sent to the sponsor. Upon completion of the review, the CTA is either approved (a No Objection Letter is issued) or rejected (a Not Satisfactory Notice is issued).

The majority of applications filed to Health Canada are to the Therapeutic Products Directorate (TPD) (ADSP-I, 2007). In 2007, 2021 CTAs were filed; 86% of these applications were filed to the TPD and the remaining were filed to the Biologics and Genetics Therapies Directorate (BGTD) (ADSP-I, 2007; ADSP-II, 2007). In the TPD, these applications were primarily for Phase 1 Bioequivalence studies (54%), with Phase 2 and Phase 3 studies being the second most common type of study. In the BGTD, the applications were primarily for Phase 2 and Phase 3 studies. In the same year, 931 and 393 CTA amendments (CTA-A) were filed to the TPD and BGTD, respectively. Over the past three years, the influx of applications and amendments has remained relatively steady. The statistics on CTAs and CTA-As filed to the Natural Health Products have not been published.

5.5.3 Pre-Submission Meetings and Consultations

Open communication with regulators is pivotal to the drug approval process. At minimum, sponsors are encouraged to request a pre-CTA consultation meeting with the appropriate Directorate prior to submitting a CTA. Sponsors also have this option, to hold a meeting with the Directorate prior to submission of an NDS or related submission (supplement to an NDS, abbreviated NDS). Health Canada specifies the particular usefulness of this meeting for applications involving new active ingredients, novel therapies and/or first-time submission sponsors (GCTS, 2003). We have observed that Regulatory Officers at Health Canada are open to informal discussion or questions further in advance of the pre-CTA consultation phase, to assist with issues such as drug classifications, high-level preclinical study design and navigating regulatory documents and forms. These initial consultations allow the sponsor to establish a relationship with the regulatory authorities early on in the development of their new drug.

Pre-CTA meetings must be requested in writing to the appropriate Directorate. The sponsor must provide four potential dates and times for the meeting; the earliest date should be no less than one month after the formal request for a meeting. The sponsor is required to submit a pre-CTA information package 30 days prior to the meeting date. The information package contains summarized information related to the available nonclinical and clinical data, global clinical development plans and regulatory status, a detailed synopsis of the proposed clinical trial, and detailed summary of the chemistry, manufacturing and controls (GCTS, 2003). The sponsor is responsible for preparing minutes of the pre-CTA meeting within 14 days after the meeting date.

5.5.4 CTA Content and Format

In 2003, Health Canada formally endorsed ICH guideline M4 (The Common Technical Document) for submission of information to the appropriate Directorate. The scope of the CTD guidelines does not extend to the clinical development stage; however, Health Canada has maintained the modular format of the CTD for consistency of documentation in subsequent stages of the drug authorization process (GCTS, 2003).

Section C.05.005 of Division 5 of the Regulations specifies the required information and documentation to be submitted with the CTA. The CTA is composed of three modules:

Module 1: Administrative/Clinical Information This module should include information such as the Drug Submission Application Form (HC/SC 3011), the Investigator's Brochure, the Protocol Safety and Efficacy Assessment Template – Clinical Trial Application (PSEAT-CTA) for pharmaceuticals, the Submission Rationale/Summary of Drug Product for biological/radiopharmaceuticals, clinical information (protocol, for example) and other administrative information.

Module 2: Common Technical Document Summaries This module contains only Quality (Chemistry, Manufacturing, Controls) Information for the purposes of a CTA. The Quality Overall Summary is presented using templates provided by Health Canada. There are specific templates depending on the type of product (pharmaceutical versus biologic) and phase of development.

Module 3: Quality This module contains the body of the required data presented in Module 2.

All modules and supporting documentation are to be submitted in hard copy to the appropriate Directorate. Specific sections of the CTA are required to be submitted in electronic format on a CD-ROM; investigator's brochure, PSEAT-CTA, and study protocol, in addition to the hard copy. Applications for combination products (medical device plus a drug or pharmaceutical plus a biological/radiopharmaceutical drug) must be submitted in duplicate. CTAs for Comparative Bioavailability Trials are formatted slightly differently than the typical CTA; information pertaining to these applications can be found on the Health Canada website.

5.5.5 Nonclinical Aspects of the CTA/CTA-A Process

Unlike the US FDA Investigational New Drug application (IND), full nonclinical study reports are not requested by Health Canada in a CTA. Rather, summaries are provided in the Investigator's Brochure and the PSEAT-CTA (pharmaceuticals) or Submission Rationale (biologics). Full nonclinical study reports are submitted with the New Drug Submission (NDS). CTAs are updated annually through the submission of an updated Investigator's Brochure; updated nonclinical information is provided in this document.

5.5.6 CTA-A Content and Format

Division 5 of the Regulations defines provisions for defining a CTA amendment (CTA-A) and when an amendment needs to be approved by the governing authority or simply notified post-change. CTA-As are classified into two categories: Clinical and Quality. Significant changes in either of these categories require authorization by Health Canada and thus CTA-As of this nature are subject to the 30-day review period. Other minor or urgent changes (i.e., when the safety of the clinical trial subject is in jeopardy) can be made without prior approval within 15 days of implementing the change under the notification process.

Significant clinical changes include changes to the protocol that affect the disposition of a clinical trial subject, affect evaluation of the efficacy or safety of the drug, alter the risk to the health of a subject; or extend the duration of the clinical trial. Significant quality changes include, but are not limited to: the use of new ingredients during manufacture; identification of a new impurity or degradation product; removal of control tests; test method limits relaxed; or altered stability information. For biologics and radiopharmaceuticals, some changes might be considered outside the scope of a CTA-A and could be reclassified as a CTA by the Directorate. These changes include, but are not limited to: altering facility for any stage of production; changes in expression systems; changes to the purification process; and significant changes to release specifications.

The main components of an amendment include a copy of the revised protocol, a copy of the recently-approved protocol, a description of the proposed changes including substantiation for each change. The format of the CTA-A is similar to that of the CTA; only Module 1 is submitted for a clinical CTA-A unless there are quality amendments as well. All CTA-As should include the Drug Submission Application Form (HC/SC 3011). As with the CTA, in addition to the hard copy the components noted above need to be submitted electronically. For changes to the Quality section, an electronic copy of the Quality Overall Summary is required as well.

5.5.7 CTA and CTA-A Review Process

When a CTA or CTA-A is received, Health Canada issues an acknowledgement letter that initiates the default 30-day review period. A control number is assigned to all CTAs and CTA-As; these numbers are used to track applications and amendments. The CTA or

CTA-A is screened and deficiencies are addressed by a Request of Clarification (Clarifax) or Screening Rejection Letter. All Clarifax's should be responded to within two calendar days. If a timely response is not received for a Clarifax or if there are significant deficiencies in the application, a Not Satisfactory Notice (NSN) will be issued. A No Objection Letter (NOL) is issued to the sponsor when no deficiencies have been identified or all deficiencies have been addressed (GI, 2009).

5.6 Special Regulatory Considerations

5.6.1 Generic Drugs

Due to the universal health care system and management of drug costs in Canada, the Canadian generic drug industry is thriving. Manufacturers of generic drugs are required to provide equivalency to Canadian reference product from a quality (chemistry and control) perspective as well as clinically via the conduct of bioequivalent studies. A Canadian reference product is defined as a drug that has been authorized for sale and is marketed in Canada by the innovator company. If this drug is no longer available for sale in Canada, a similar drug suitable for bioequivalency purposes might be deemed acceptable by the Government. Part C of the Food and Drug Regulations includes provisions for a generic manufacturer to file an Abbreviated New Drug Submission (ANDS).

5.6.2 Subsequent Entry Biologics in Canada

In March 2010, Canada released its official guidance document, Guidance for Sponsors: Information and Submission Requirements for Subsequent Entry Biologics (SEB), to assist sponsors in satisfying the requirements under the Food and Drugs Act and Regulations for the authorization of sale of SEBs in Canada (GS, 2010). The release of this document follows regulatory initiatives begun in 2005 which included the release of a draft guidance in 2008 and an extensive open consultation process. This process included face-to-face meetings to provide a forum for in-depth discussion of the issues with key stakeholders worldwide.

Health Canada defines an SEB as "A biologic drug that enters the market subsequent to a version previously authorized in Canada and with demonstrated similarity to a reference biologic drug". In Europe, these types of products are referred to as "biosimilars" or "similar biological medicinal products", and in the United States they are "follow-on protein products" or "follow-on biologics". The term SEB was used by Health Canada in order to distinguish the SEB regulatory approval process from that which is followed for chemical generic drugs. The concepts and existing principles within the Food and Drugs Act and Regulations will govern the regulation of SEBs. The Biologics and Genetic Therapies Directorate (BGTD) will provide oversight over and regulate the approval of SEBs. SEBs are further subject to existing concepts and principles within the Patented Medicines (Notice of Compliance) Regulations, C.08.004.1 of the Food and Drug Regulations, the Patent Act, and their accompanying guidance documents.

5.6.2.1 Reference Biologic Drug

Given the definition of an SEB (a biologic drug that enters the market subsequent to a version previously authorized in Canada and with demonstrated similarity to a reference biologic drug), the term Reference Biologic Drug (RBD) must be adequately defined in order to assist the sponsor with conforming to the Health Canada guidance. Health Canada defines an RBD as "a biologic drug authorized on the basis of a complete quality, nonclinical and clinical data package, to which an SEB is compared in studies to demonstrate similarity".

Health Canada provides guidance on the choice of a RBD, including:

- The RBD should be authorized for sale and marketed in Canada;
- The same RBD should be used throughout comparability studies and SEB product development;
- The RBD should have the same dosage form, strength and route of administration as that planned for the SEB;
- The RBD should have sufficient safety and efficacy data accumulated to allow for adequate comparison to the SEB.

As with most new drug submissions and applications, the sponsor is encouraged to dialogue with the Directorate early on in the process. However, when choosing an RBD for development of an SEB, particularly if the RBD is non-Canadian, Health Canada specifically encourages early discussions to confirm the suitability of the product.

5.6.2.2 Non-Canadian Reference Biologic Drug

The sponsor is required to name a biological drug authorized for sale and marketed in Canada to which the SEB will be subsequent. This product should be used for the comparability programme. However, a sponsor can use a non-Canadian reference drug, subject to the following:

- The sponsor must demonstrate that the non-Canadian reference drug is a suitable surrogate for the Canadian version;
- The non-Canadian reference drug must be marketed by the same innovator company or corporate entity as the Canadian RBD;
- The non-Canadian drug must be from a region that has an established relationship with Health Canada (a Mutual Recognition Agreement country, for example);
- The non-Canadian drug should be marketed in a region that adopts ICH guidelines and has pre- and post-marketing regulations comparable to those of Canada

5.6.2.3 Nonclinical Information and Submission Requirements

A full chemistry and manufacturing package, as well as side-by-side characterization studies to the RBD to establish similarity, are required for all SEB drug submissions. During comparability exercises where physical/chemical or biological assays are considered inadequate, data from nonclinical studies might be used to demonstrate that the higher order of the SEB is comparable to that of the RBD. However, nonclinical data should not be relied upon heavily, as this could be indicative that consideration of the drug as an SEB is inappropriate. In addition, where the SEB exhibits impurities different from the RBD, nonclinical studies could be used to help confirm that the safety or the efficacy of the SEB is not adversely impacted by the impurity.

From a nonclinical perspective, the requirements for testing might be reduced if similarity to the RBD is demonstrated in the comparability exercises included in the quality package. As with any new drug, specific nonclinical requirements could differ depending on clinical parameters relating to the specific class of drug and the applied indications. The same RBD that was used in the comparability exercise should be used in any nonclinical studies required. Further, the SEB used in the nonclinical testing should be that for which approval is sought; any quality changes to the SEB during nonclinical or clinical development could require bridging studies depending on the effect these changes have on the product.

Some nonclinical studies are required by the Health Canada guidance and should be conducted prior to the initiation of any clinical studies. These include both *in vitro* and *in vivo* studies and should be comparative in nature and designed to detect differences between the SEB and RBD. *In vitro* studies include receptor binding studies or cell-based assays when appropriate and *in vivo* studies include animal pharmacodynamic studies relevant to the clinical indication, at least one repeat-dose toxicity study, and other relevant safety observations that can be made during the toxicity study. The duration of the toxicity study should be sufficiently long so as to detect differences in toxicity or immune response between the SEB and RBD and should also include toxicokinetic studies. Results of the repeat-dose toxicological studies could warrant further studies (such as safety pharmacology or reproduction studies) that would otherwise not generally be required for an SEB submission.

The nonclinical studies discussed above should be conducted following the principles recommended by ICH S6 (Preclinical Safety Evaluation of Biotechnology-Derived Pharmaceuticals). These general principles state that nonclinical safety studies involving biological drugs are primarily used to define the pharmacological and toxicological effects prior to and throughout clinical development. The selection of the most suitable animal species, age, physiological state, manner of delivery (including dose, route of administration and regimen), and stability of the test article under the conditions of use, must all be considered when conducting nonclinical safety testing. The further considerations provided in ICH S6 regarding exposure assessment and specific types of studies, such as immunotoxicity, genotoxicity and carcinogenicity studies, should be reviewed during development of the SEB.

5.6.2.4 Case Study: Omnitrope™: The First SEB Approval in Canada

In April 2009, Health Canada authorized the first SEB for market in Canada, Omnitrope™ (Somatropin, Sandoz Canada Inc.). Omnitrope™ is indicated for long-term treatment of Growth Hormone Deficiency in children and long-term replacement therapy of Adult Growth Hormone Deficiency in adults. Interestingly, approval of this SEB occurred prior to release of the final guidance document on the information and submission requirements for SEB authorization.

Following evaluation of quality information on the SEB and RBD, a reduced clinical package was accepted for the new drug submission. The RBD was Genotropin®, which was authorized for sale in Canada in 1998 but was never actually marketed in Canada. Pharmacodynamic studies demonstrated comparable efficacy to the RBD. Pharmacokinetic studies were not conducted due to the similar responses of the RBD and the SEB in efficacy studies and the fact that both drugs could stimulate an immune response in foreign species. Single-dose toxicity studies were not conducted. One repeated-dose toxicity study was conducted in rats. The RBD was not used as a comparator in the repeated-dose study. Health Canada had no safety concerns following review of the results of these studies; adverse effects observed in females were deemed related to the pharmacodynamic action of the drug. Genotoxicity, carcinogenicity and reproductive/developmental toxicity studies were not conducted. Local tolerance studies were conducted with Omnitrope^{TM} and the RBD in rabbits. Some adverse effects were noted and thus Health Canada has recommended that the injection site be rotated on a daily basis.

From a nonclinical perspective, Health Canada deemed the comparability exercises and the nonclinical safety profile sufficient to support the use of the Omnitrope^{TM} for the indications described above. The first submission for Omnitrope^{TM} was filed in April 2007; a notice of deficiency was issued in March 2008 for this submission. A response was filed in June 2008 and the SEB was authorized for market in April 2009.

5.6.3 Orphan Drugs in Canada

Several jurisdictions have adopted Orphan Drug policies or acts to enable patients with rare diseases greater access to innovative drugs, as well as encouraging pharmaceutical/ biotechnology companies to focus research and development in emerging, rare diseases with small markets. At this time, no such policy has been implemented in Canada; however, the federal Government announced in October 2012 that a new regulatory framework is being developed for the authorization of orphan drugs in Canada. During development of the new approach, Health Canada has suggested that there are provisions in place to assist Canadians with access to innovative drugs and stimulate research in this area. These provisions include the Priority Review Policy, the Notice of Compliance with Conditions Policy and the Special Access Program as well as tax incentives and reduced fees.

5.6.3.1 Priority Review Policy

The Priority Review Policy was implemented to "fast-track" the approval of new drug submissions intended for treating serious, life-threatening or severely debilitating diseases or conditions for which there is evidence that the drug provides effective treatment, prevention or diagnosis or a significant increase in efficacy (or significant decrease in risk) such that the overall risk/benefit profile is improved over existing therapies. The Guidance for Industry: Priority Review of Drug Submissions provides a basic guidance on the criteria for qualifying for a Priority Review (GI, 2006). Discretion on the part of Health Canada is exercised when defining a condition as serious, life-threatening or severely debilitating, although some examples and guidance are provided in the document. Substantial evidence is required for clinical effectiveness, in the form of at least two adequate and well-controlled clinical trials; this need for evidence is flexible based on the therapy and indication. Health Canada highly encourages pre-submission meetings prior to filing a request for Priority Review status. The request for Priority Review must be submitted prior to the filing of a drug submission. If the application is approved, the screening of the drug submission is reduced to 25 days and 180 days for the full submission review.

5.6.3.2 Notice of Compliance with Conditions

If a drug has a favourable risk/benefit profile and promising clinical evidence that it can provide benefits (in the form of treatment, diagnosis or prevention) to patients suffering from severely debilitating, life-threatening or serious disease, a Notice of Compliance with conditions (NOC/c) may be granted (GD, 2006). The sponsor must also prove that the drug is of high quality. Prior to approval, the sponsor must outline in a Letter of Undertaking the confirmatory clinical studies that will be conducted to confirm the clinical benefit of the drug. Further in this letter, the sponsor must outline and agree to an expanded post-marketing surveillance programme. The product monograph must clearly define the conditions under which the drug has been authorized and, prior to approval, the sponsor must prepare educational material outlining the use and authority of the product.

5.6.3.3 Special Access Programme

In accordance with Sections C.08.010 and C.08.011 of the Food and Drug Act, Health Canada can authorize the sale of a specific quantity of an unauthorized drug for use in the emergency treatment of a patient under the care of a practitioner. The request must be received from the practitioner and each request is considered by the Special Access Programme (SAP) on a case-by-case basis (GDIP, 2008). This programme is specifically intended for emergency use of a drug for serious or life-threatening conditions where no suitable therapy is available or conventional therapies have failed. The results of using the unauthorized drug in the emergency situation must be provided to the manufacturer of the drug.

References

E-mail correspondence with Nick Orphanos (2010) International Programs Division, Bureau of Policy, Science, and International Programs, Therapeutic Products Directorate, Health Products and Food Branch, Health Canada on 31 August 2010 at 10:02 AM EST.

Good Laboratory Practice: Use of Test Sites in Canada (2009) UK Good Laboratory Practice Monitoring Authority, Medicines and Healthcare Products Regulatory Agency, August 2009.

Guidance Document (2010) *Nonclinical Laboratory Study Data Supporting Drug Product Applications and Submissions: Adherence to Good Laboratory Practice*, Health Products and Food Branch, Health Canada, Ottawa, Ontario, April 2010.

Annual Drug Submission Performance – Part I (2007) Ottawa, Ontario: Therapeutics Product Directorate, Health Products and Food Branch, Health Canada, 2007.

Annual Drug Submission Performance – Part II (2007) Ottawa, Ontario: Biologics and Genetic Therapies Directorate, Health Products and Food Branch, Health Canada, 2007.

Guidance for Clinical Trial Sponsors: Clinical Trial Applications (2003) Ottawa, Ontario: Health Products and Food Branch, Health Canada, June 2003.

Guidance for Industry: Management of Drug Submissions (2009) Ottawa, Ontario: Health Products and Food Branch, Health Canada, September 2009.

Guidance for Sponsors: Information and Submission Requirements for Subsequent Entry Biologics (SEBs) (2010) Ottawa, Ontario: Health Products and Food Branch, Health Canada, March 2010.

Guidance for Industry: Priority Review for Drug Submissions (2006) Ottawa, Ontario: Health Products and Food Branch, Health Canada, March 2006.

Guidance Document: Notice of Compliance with conditions (NOC/c) (2006) Ottawa, Ontario: Health Products and Food Branch, Health Canada, March 2006.

Guidance Document for Industry and Practitioners: Special Access Programme for Drugs (2008) Health Products and Food Branch, Health Canada, January 2008.

6

European Pharmaceutical Regulation – Nonclinical Testing Requirements

Adam Woolley[1] *and Jan Willem van der Laan*[2]
[1]*ForthTox Ltd., UK*
[2]*FTBB, Medicines Evaluation Board, The Netherlands*

6.1 Introduction

Broadly, the goal of pharmaceutical development and regulation can be seen from two apparently diametrically opposed viewpoints: those of the pharmaceutical industry and the regulatory authorities in countries across the world. From the point of view of the pharmaceutical industry, the objective is to bring drugs to the market and to sell them at a profit so that the next drug can be developed. The role of the regulator is to ensure that the drugs for which they receive applications for clinical trials or marketing are effective and safe. The two camps have tended to view each other with suspicion; however, this is counterproductive as both are supportive of the common goal of bringing drugs to market for the benefit of patients. In Europe, as in other jurisdictions, drug development should be seen as a collaborative effort between industry and regulators; communication can ensure a smooth development path and, eventually, successful application to market the product.

The process of nonclinical development of pharmaceuticals is evolving continuously and, for the most part, becoming increasingly complex and more expensive. It is fair to say that if penicillin had been subject to the current testing requirements it would not have been brought to market so quickly and many more patient lives would have been lost as a result. This does not mean that flexibility and pragmatism have no role in the current climate; it might be possible to fast-track some developments if there is a critical

Nonclinical Safety Assessment: A Guide to International Pharmaceutical Regulations, First Edition.
Edited by William J. Brock, Kenneth L. Hastings and Kathy M. McGown.

unmet medical need for the product. Another example is the approach to biopharmaceutical drugs which, in some cases, can be brought to market with a more pragmatic approach to nonclinical testing (see Chapter 18) than that used for more conventional products.

Nonclinical development of pharmaceuticals has had a number of wake-up calls in recent history, which have had huge influences on the nonclinical testing process. Without reiterating the whole history of the field over the last 50 years, some seminal events stand out which have changed the course of nonclinical testing. The first and most important event was the thalidomide disaster in the 1960s. This demonstrated unequivocally that the testing paradigm used up to that point was deficient and, inevitably, there was a new emphasis on reproductive toxicology as a result, especially for developmental effects. This led to the extensive use of the rabbit in developmental studies. Another milestone was the inception of Good Laboratory Practices (GLP) in the late 1970s and the resultant huge increase in the quality of nonclinical testing – for example, the requirement for standard toxicity protocols such as those related to chronic toxicity and carcinogenicity. Testing practices and requirements have also been influenced by further adverse events in patients, such as cardiac toxicity shown by non-cardiovascular drugs such as cisapride and terfenadine.

Pressures on testing are also seen through initiatives such as the 3Rs of Russell and Burch, which seek to reduce, refine and replace the use of animals in medical research. The danger here is that, while this is a worthwhile objective, it is possible to be overwhelmed by the pressure to use fewer animals and to lose sight of the intention of nonclinical testing which is to develop safer drugs for humans through the rational support of clinical trials used in the various phases of clinical development. This becomes more difficult if the group sizes in animal studies are reduced to such an extent that normal variation in the endpoints investigated overwhelms the detection of differences from controls that could be clinically significant.

Pharmaceutical development in Europe is made more complex relative to other jurisdictions or markets such as the USA or Japan by specifically European factors. In Europe, while there is one overall regulatory authority, the European Medicines Agency (EMA) based in London in the UK, there are 27 independent countries, 23 official languages and more than 60 minority languages, ranging from Basque in Spain to Kashubian in Poland and Irish Gaelic. The power of the harmonization, which was felt in Europe in the late 1980s facilitated the DG-Enterprise of the European Commission to take the initiative in starting the process of International Harmonization (ICH) in 1989.

Fortunately for the pharmaceutical industry, the challenge of such diversity has been smoothed in recent years by the processes of the International Conference on Harmonization (ICH or, in full, the International Conference on Harmonization of Technical Requirements for Registration of Pharmaceuticals for Human Use). There are, however, sufficient variations from this theme to justify writing a separate chapter on nonclinical development in Europe.

Another regional factor to consider is that, although practically all the countries in Europe are members of the Organization for Economic Cooperation and Development, not all are members of the European Union (EU); although there are more than 40 countries in Europe, only 27 are members of the EU (although Norway, Iceland and Liechtenstein are active observers). Some others (and EU members) are members of other trade cooperatives such as the Council for Europe (the majority of countries in this continent) or the European Free Trade Association (EFTA). This consists of Iceland, Liechtenstein, Norway and Switzerland (which represents EFTA as an observer in ICH). All these countries have close ties with each other and the European Commission of the EU, based in Brussels, Belgium.

The broad concept of nonclinical development is the same in Europe as in other parts of the world – the extent of nonclinical testing required increases as the duration of clinical trials increases. Broadly, the process is driven by the provisions of ICH although there are some exceptions, which are explored below. This chapter reviews the development of first-to-market drugs, without exploring the complexities of generic drug development or marketing applications.

6.1.1 Definitions

Before embarking on a description of pharmaceutical development in any jurisdiction, it is essential to define what is covered by the text that follows and, hence, perhaps to indicate what is not covered.

The definition is given in the relevant EU directive (Directive 2001/83/EC(EU, 2008a). This definition of a medicinal product is given in two parts or limbs:

- Any substance or combination of substances presented as having properties for treating or preventing disease in human beings;
- Any substance or combination of substances which may be used in or administered to human beings either with a view to restoring, correcting or modifying physiological functions by exerting a pharmacological, immunological or metabolic action, or to making a medical diagnosis.

It is pointed out in this document that medicinal products might be covered by both limbs of this definition but that the European Court of Justice has confirmed that falling under either limb is enough to classify a product as a medicinal product. Occasionally there is uncertainty about whether a product falls under the regulations for medicinal products or for medical devices; the MHRA (Medicines and Healthcare products Regulatory Agency) has a Borderline Section that can give advice when needed. The MHRA document (MHRA, 2008) makes the point that full harmonization of European Community legislation has not yet been fully achieved. On this basis, a product classified as a medicine in some countries might be classified as a food in some others. However, the judgements of the European Court of Justice hold sway eventually, as every member state has to follow them rather than insist on its own legislation.

In the USA, the definition is set by the US Code; the following is a description from the Food Drug and Cosmetic Act (Chapter 3, Definitions Sec. 201 g [21 USC 321].

> (1) The term "drug" means (A) articles recognized in the official United States Pharmacopoeia, official Homoeopathic Pharmacopoeia of the United States, or official National Formulary, or any supplement to any of them; and (B) articles intended for use in the diagnosis, cure, mitigation, treatment, or prevention of disease in man or other animals; and (C) articles (other than food) intended to affect the structure or any function of the body of man or other animals; and (D) articles intended for use as a component of any article specified in clause (A), (B), or (C). A food or dietary supplement for which a claim, subject to sections 403(r)(1)(B) and 403(r)(3) or sections 403(r)(1)(B) and 403(r)(5)(D), is made in accordance with

> the requirements of section 403(r) is not a drug solely because the label or the labeling contains such a claim. A food, dietary ingredient, or dietary supplement for which a truthful and not misleading statement is made in accordance with section 403(r)(6) is not a drug under clause (C) solely because the label or the labeling contains such a statement.

There are, of course, differences between the USA and the EU about what is classified as a drug; for instance, in the USA sunscreen products are classified as over-the-counter (OTC) or non-prescription drugs but are classified as cosmetics in the EU. As indicated above, there are careful distinctions to be drawn between drugs and food supplements.

6.2 Regulation of Medicinal Products in the European Union

6.2.1 Overview

As suggested above, there are essentially (and simplistically) two blocks of countries in Europe: those that are EU Member States and those that are not. However, the margins between these two apparently distinct blocks become blurred on closer examination. For example, Switzerland is not an EU Member State but has close ties with the EU to the extent that its requirements and expectations for nonclinical testing are very similar to those of the EU. Employees of SwissMedic, the Swiss Agency for Therapeutic Products, are representatives of the European Free Trade Association (EFTA) in the current ICH processes, and these countries follow ICH guidelines in their assessment procedures. Likewise, in answer to a survey of European nonclinical requirements (see below for more details), no specific requirements outside those of EU states were identified for Norway. On this basis, much of the following discussion is based on EU expectations and regulatory process.

In essence, there are two approaches to pharmaceutical regulation in the EU:

- the centralized (or Community) authorization procedure;
- national procedures and mutual recognition/decentralized procedure.

It should be noted at the outset that certain types of product have to be registered by the centralized procedure; these include biological and orphan medicinal products.

6.2.2 Role of the European Medicines Agency in the Regulation of Medicines

The primary role of the EMA is to assess applications for the marketing of medicinal products in the EU; these assessments are based on quality, safety and efficacy. Of course, it does this for applications made via the central route but also serves as an arbitrator in cases of dispute when mutual recognition procedures break down. EMA opinions (essentially recommendations) are produced for all products assessed in the centralized procedure and these are passed to the European Commission who takes the final decision on grant, refusal, revocation or suspension of marketing.

With particular relevance to the current chapter, the EMA is also responsible for designation of orphan medicinal products and assessing paediatric investigation plans for products intended for use in children. They also draft regulatory and scientific guidance documents in a broadly analogous manner to the FDA relating to the nonclinical development of new drugs. Importantly, from the point of view of companies wishing to develop a new drug but are uncertain what developmental approach they should take to better ensure success, the EMA offers scientific advice and comment on proposals for nonclinical evaluation of products.

6.2.3 Scientific Structure of the EMA

The scientific work of the EMA is driven by six scientific committees:

- Committee for Medicinal Products for Human Use (CHMP)
- Committee for Medicinal Products for Veterinary Use (CVMP)
- Committee for Orphan Medicinal Products (COMP)
- Committee on Herbal Medicinal Products (HMPC)
- Paediatric Committee (PDCO)
- Committee on Advanced Therapies (CAT)

From the point of view of this discussion, the most important of these are the CHMP, the PDCO and the CAT, which are discussed in more detail below. Of the others, the COMP does not give advice on the marketing of products, only on their status as orphan drugs, giving companies the opportunity to receive protocol assistance for nonclinical and clinical studies. The CVMP is not discussed in this chapter and the HMPC has a restricted brief which covers herbal products, with plant-derived products of a nature that is often weakly defined with respect to chemical composition.

The following comments are summarized from the EMA website, having regard to the objectives of the current chapter.

6.2.3.1 Committee for Medicinal Products for Human Use (CHMP)

This is the pivotal committee for the approval of medicinal products for human use as well as for any questions that relate to them, either before or after marketing.

The CHMP plays a vital role in the marketing procedures for medicines in the European Union. Amongst a wide range of activities, its responsibilities relevant to nonclinical development include:

- Initial assessment of products submitted under the centralized procedure.
- Authorizing post-authorization activities, such as modifications (e.g., new formulations) or extensions to the existing marketing authorization.
- It acts as an arbitrator when there are disputes between member states arising out of the mutual recognition and/or decentralized procedures and acts in referral cases from other sources, for instance where there is concern about protection of public health.
- Playing a key role in EU-wide pharmacovigilance as it monitors adverse drug reaction reports. It can make recommendations to the European Commission about changes to a product's marketing status. Such activities could lead to additional nonclinical study, such as specific mechanistic work.
- Publishing a European Public Assessment Report for every product authorized via the central procedure; this includes a summary of product characteristics (SPC) which includes some nonclinical information. These are available publically via the EMA website.

One of the other most useful functions of the EMA/CHMP is to provide scientific advice to companies, who can present nonclinical development proposals for comment. The Scientific Advice procedure is designed to speed up the development of medicines for the benefit of patients. For potential orphan drugs, a special form of advice is available as protocol assistance. The Scientific Advice procedure is intended to aid companies when there is insufficient detail in EU guidelines or other regulatory documents, or when the company wants to deviate considerably from the guidelines. As companies can request scientific advice at any stage of development, the nonclinical part of the development phase could also benefit from this procedure, as it might ensure that appropriate tests and designs are being used, preventing delays during the evaluation phase of the marketing authorization application.

Scientific advice from the EMA is not legally binding, neither on the side of the sponsor nor on the side of the authorities, as new data and new insights could be raised during further development.

It is not in the scope of the Scientific Advice procedure to provide any kind of pre-assessment, although it is current practice of many companies to include such a general question in their Scientific Advice application.

Another function to be aware of are the activities of the special working parties on Efficacy (EWP), Safety (SWP), Quality (QWP) and Biologicals (BWP) in preparation of scientific and regulatory guidelines for nonclinical development, together with cooperation with international partners such as those involved in ICH.

These working parties are in practice the sparring partners of the other parties in the ICH.

6.2.3.2 Paediatric Committee (PDCO)

The Paediatric Committee does not authorize medicinal products; this remains firmly a responsibility of the CHMP. However, it is likely to be consulted by the CHMP for its opinion on the safety of a paediatric medicinal product, as defined by the nonclinical programme, if the data have been generated according to a previously agreed paediatric investigation plan.

The chief responsibility of the PDCO is to assess paediatric investigation plans, including assessing applications for full or partial waiver and applications for deferral of paediatric investigation.

The PDCO is also responsible, if requested by the CHMP, for assessing data that result from paediatric investigation plans and providing opinions on the quality, safety or efficacy of any medicinal product to be used in children.

6.2.3.3 Committee for Advanced Therapies (CAT)

The process of evaluating the safety of small molecules has been well established over several decades and has become ever more refined (and complex) with increasing knowledge and experience. This applies to a somewhat lesser extent to biological products such as monoclonal antibodies, but it is fair to say that a body of experience is building with these substances as more and more of them enter clinical development and, eventually, marketing and post-marketing pharmacovigilance. However, the emergence of new therapeutic strategies and technologies has required a re-evaluation of the existing paradigms for safety evaluation and this has been recognized by the establishment of the Committee for Advanced Therapies (CAT).

These include products that use or take advantage of regenerative medicine or more personal therapeutic initiatives and the development of nanomedicines. Examples of such products include those based on gene therapy, cell therapy (potential use of stem cells) and tissues for tissue engineering. Such products or strategies hold out the prospect of revolutionary treatment for disease or injury, including skin in burns, and in diseases that affect many of the population such as neurodegeneration (dementia) and cancer.

The regulation on advanced therapies (Regulation (EC) 1394/2007; EU,) was designed to provide a more homogenous approach to the evaluation of such therapies. The CAT was established under this regulation. One of the aspects of these products that is recognized by the regulation is that they could be a combination of, for example, cells and polymer frameworks or metal implants. It is clear that such products do not lie completely within the normal or traditional guidelines for nonclinical evaluation of "traditional" pharmaceuticals or of medical devices and might well contain elements relevant to both. This is likely to present a significant challenge in terms of nonclinical development and safety evaluation.

Another emerging aspect of advanced therapies is the prospect of using genetic information from individual patients to inform the strategy for their treatment – the area of pharmacogenomics. It is clear that these new strategies will require a re-evaluation of the current standards for nonclinical development and a more targeted approach to safety evaluation is likely to become necessary. This is likely to include the evaluation of the safety of a new or existing drug in experimental models relevant to the target patient population and also of its safety if it is used outside this group.

6.2.4 Regulatory Process in the EU

Although much of the process of and requirements for nonclinical development within the EU are similar to those in other jurisdictions such as the USA, it is worth outlining the basic principles of pharmaceutical regulation in Europe.

There are two basic procedures: central via the EMA based in London, UK or decentralized via the individual authorities of the member states. The latter has to be subdivided, however, in a so-called decentralized and a mutual recognition (MR) procedure. Although apparently similar, in fact the decentralized procedure is different from that for mutual recognition because of the momentum of the formal decision. The MR procedure is based upon the decision of one member state, which is to be "mutually" recognized by others with only small margins for change. The decentralized procedure is led by one country, but the decision is taken after having the input from all the contributing member states, which could be less than all European countries in that round.

Use of the centralized procedure is obligatory for biological products (including genetic engineering products), orphan drugs and those intended for treatment of HIV/AIDS, autoimmune diseases and other immune dysfunctions, cancer, diabetes and neurodegenerative disorders. This procedure has the advantage that it provides a marketing authorization that is immediately valid in all 27 member states as well as in Iceland, Liechtenstein and Norway. This process is described in Annex I of Regulation (EC) No 726/2004.

The centralized procedure works through the appointment of a member (or alternate) of the CHMP (the rapporteur) with a second member of another state to act as co-rapporteur. This has the advantage that there are two independent views on the full dossier which, from a quality (ISO9002) point of view, contributes to the independence of the decisions.

Rapporteurs and co-rapporteurs are appointed through a process which is influenced mainly by factors such as specific expertise for the therapeutic area and (sometimes) work load. Some countries are more often selected as rapporteurs than others; these are mostly in northern and western Europe; less extensive contributions are made by some of the smaller countries and less by those in eastern and south-eastern Europe. Although the workload is not evenly distributed amongst the member states this does not seem to be the cause for complaint amongst applicants, who see much benefit in having an expert assessment team to work with.

Broadly, the process consists of the circulation of a list of new requests through CHMP members and members express their interest in the products, where appropriate offering themselves as rapporteur or co-rapporteur. These pairs are chosen for all three areas in the application: Quality, Safety and Efficacy; the choice is made by the Chair and/or vice-Chair of the CHMP after a preselection by the EMA. Particular attention is paid to areas of expertise of the country teams although the fair distribution of workload is also taken into account. Rapporteurs are allowed to choose assessment teams (where needed) from amongst the list of experts of the EMA network, irrespective of their nationality.

The documentation required for a marketing authorization application has undergone worldwide harmonization in the so-called electronic Common Technical Dossier (eCTD). The specific requirements for Europe are summarized in the Notice to Applicants 2B (EU, 2008b).

An important document from a European point of view is the Nonclinical Overview (CTD 2.4) which in fact is the successor of the previous European Expert Report. The Overview should be a critical assessment that considers and reflects the testing strategy of the company when developing the product at hand. It should contain reflections and considerations regarding the choice of species, and the weight-of-evidence that the risk-benefit of the product is sufficient for marketing.

6.3 Nonclinical Testing in the Support of Clinical Trials

The EMA plays a limited role in the authorization of clinical trials, which is achieved through national authorities and local ethics committees. This procedure started in 2004 in most countries, although the UK and Sweden were far ahead in this respect.

There is a Clinical Trial Facilitatory Group (CTFG) which has the mandate to smooth the implementation of the directive (there is no permanent position associated with this), but it is possible that it might get a greater role after review of the Clinical Trial Directive in the future. In the Netherlands the nonclinical assessment is done by the 25 individual Medical Ethical Evaluation Committees (METC) instead of a single national office (as in most of other countries). The Central Committee for Human Research (CCMO) should only be involved for special products (vaccines, gene therapy, and advanced therapy) and specific populations (e.g., children).

The data requirements before initiating a clinical trial in Europe are broadly similar to those of the ICH, although it is possible that the competent authorities of individual member states could have specific requirements or that the authorizing ethics committee(s) might request additional studies. In each case, the need for such studies should be assessed by consultation with the relevant authority and ethics committee before any application to run a trial is made.

Formal requirements in the EU are slightly different from the US requirements, as in Europe the dossier is called the Investigational Medicinal Product Dossier (IMPD).

> The IMPD includes summaries of information related to the quality, manufacture and control of the Investigational Medicinal Product, data from non-clinical studies and from its clinical use. An overall risk-benefit assessment, critical analyses of the non-clinical and clinical data in relation to the potential risks and benefits of the proposed study have to be part of the IMPD.
>
> (Citation from the website: www.impd.eu).

This IMPD includes also a nonclinical part (often incorporated in the Investigator's Brochure, describing the discovery and developmental phase of a new product).

6.3.1 Role of Individual Country Regulatory Agencies/Authorities

The EU has expanded significantly in recent years, there now being 27 member states. Despite this expansion, the new states have not had significant impact on the processes of pharmaceutical development in the EU, although Hungary has well-established toxicological processes and knowledge.

One of the authors (J-W van der Laan) carried out a survey of national authorities in Europe by means of a questionnaire. Replies were received from 19 authorities, including two non-member states – Norway and Switzerland. The questions were:

1. Can you identify any specific study or trial that is required by your country that is not contained in European or ICH guidelines?
2. Do you know of any that is required (or just not required) by other countries in Europe
3. Is there any national documentation (in English or national language) that supports these national standpoints?
4. Are there specific nonclinical issues that your own authority or country require to be covered before clinical trials?
5. What are the requests for biotechnology-derived products?
6. Is there any request for *in vitro* testing, for example, for monoclonal antibodies?
7. Any other additions?

In addition, two historical questions were asked about the start date of nonclinical evaluation and whether there had been any changes as a result of specific medical disasters such as thalidomide or TGN1412 or simply as a result of joining the EU.

The following responses were received:

1. **Can you identify any specific study or trial that is required by your country, that is not contained in European or ICH guidelines?**
   The majority of replies were negative. Italy identified the potential for specific requirements for studies conducted before Phase I clinical trials with new radiopharmaceuticals or with advanced therapy medicinal products. Romania also identified radiopharmaceuticals but also indicated that trials with engineered tissues would require specific studies to be conducted before Phase 1 trials.
2. **Do you know of any specific study or trial that is required (or just not required) by other countries in Europe?**

The answer to this question was universally negative, that is, no other studies are required.

3. **Is there any national documentation (in English or national language) that supports these national standpoints?**
The majority of answers to this question were negative. The German authority provided a link to a website that indicated broad adherence to ICH guidelines.
The French authority indicated that their nonclinical requirements before Phase 1 clinical trials were different in some respects but did not provide additional reference.
The Italian authority indicated that they have, since 2004, specific guidelines on cellular therapy and gene therapy, in Italian (available at http://www.iss.it/binary/publ/publi/0478.1106653420.pdf).
The Danish authority indicated that they deviate from ICH M3 in respect of safe contraception as they do not accept sexual abstinence due to low compliance, especially in longer studies. This could be expected to have some impact on the type and extent of reproductive toxicity studies that are required before the three classic clinical trial phases.
4. **Are there specific nonclinical issues that your own authority or country requires to be covered before clinical trials?**
Most of the responses to this were negative, with reference to ICH guidelines. The Spanish authority indicated that sometimes there were insufficient nonclinical data for clinical trials covering two phases (for example I/II or II/III), particularly with anticancer drugs. The UK has procedural requirements for handling trials with higher risk compounds; these are discussed below.
5. **What are the requests for biotechnology-derived products?**
Most responses to this question referred to the use of ICH or EMA/CHMP guidelines. The Swiss authority indicated that these were handled on a case-by-case basis taking into account the indication and sufficient safety factors due to possible interspecies differences in biological activities, with an indicated preference for calculations based on the Minimum Anticipated Biological Effect Level (MABEL).
While the Italian authority indicated adherence to ICH S6 it also pointed to a case-by-case approach to justify the lack of data in particular areas or the presentation of different data than those requested by the ICH guideline.
The Danish authority also referred to ICH S6 and said that the case-by-case evaluation was based on the characteristics of the molecule, including size or similarity to known products.
The UK MHRA referred to the answer of the previous question.
6. **Is there any request for *in vitro* testing, for example, for monoclonal antibodies?**
Of the 19 responses received, 14 indicated that there were no specific guidelines outside ICH S6. Most of the six other responses emphasized, directly or indirectly, the importance of a case-by-case approach. Switzerland indicated that tissue cross reactivity and pharmacodynamic investigations (e.g., receptor binding, specificity of binding) would be required while Italy said that *in vitro* tests were not routine. In contrast, the Hungarian authority said that two types of *in vitro* tests could be requested: receptor binding and cell-based studies.
Austria indicated a case-by-case approach while suggesting that *in vitro* tests could be a substantial part of a nonclinical test programme. However, this depends on the

nature of the product (monoclonal antibody or other biologic) and the target. For the latter, targeting of a blood group-associated antigen might be associated with tests for coagulation to ensure compatibility with human serum and that ADCC/CDC for special blood groups might be requested. This is consistent with ICH S6 and the extent of testing depends on the package as a whole.

The Danish agency suggested the need to show the comparability of target affinity in animals and humans or to establish no observed binding. Functional potency could be investigated *in vitro* using human cells or cells transfected with the human receptor. They also emphasized the importance of tissue cross-reactivity studies.

7. **Any other additions?**
   Although most responses to this were negative, Italy and Romania indicated that critical calculation of the first-in-man dose for biotechnology derived products was not based on the NOEL. While the Hungarian response was also negative, they emphasized that the nonclinical part of clinical trial applications is assessed according to international legislation. Their assessor should request the necessary nonclinical studies based on the characteristics of the active substance, on the type and phase of the intended clinical study and on the target population.

In addition to the above specific questions, two historical questions were asked:

- When was the start of the nonclinical evaluation (sometimes by a ministerial department or by an agency for medicines)?
- Were there any changes in relation to specific disasters, for example, thalidomide, TGN1412? Or just to fulfil European regulation by joining the EU?

Unsurprisingly, given the breadth of the European Union and the cumulative history of countries joining, there was a broad band of answers to the first of these questions. The progenitor of the current UK MHRA, with those of Italy, Spain and Sweden, started assessment of data for clinical trials in the 1970s. Other member states, which joined more recently, started formal procedures in the years following 2000. In between these extremes was a range of dates in the 1980s and 1990s for the start of formal procedures.

The response to disasters such as the TGN1412 clinical trial has usually been robust. Not surprisingly, as the disaster occurred in the UK after approval of the protocol by the MHRA, the UK instituted a set of procedures for high-risk compounds and the EMA published a draft guideline: Guideline on Requirements for First-In-Man Clinical Trials for Potential High-Risk Medicinal Products. Although TGN1412 has been the most recent high profile case, others have occurred, such as Letigen, which was removed from the market in Denmark in 2002.

The following discussion looks at the nonclinical approach to high-risk products, as described in the EMA CHMP guideline.

6.3.2 Risk Mitigation in Nonclinical Development of Medicinal Products

Following the incident with TGN1412 in 2006, there was a brief vogue for referring to "high-risk medicinal products" which were defined as those for which there are concerns for serious adverse reaction in first-in-human clinical trials. A guideline on this was published in March 2007, this was fully superseded by the final "risk mitigation" guideline published in July of the same year. These originated in part as a response to the TGN1412 affair in which serious adverse reactions were seen in human volunteers on first treatment with this substance. The risk mitigation guideline acknowledges that there are risks with all medicinal products and that in some cases additional data might be required or that a different approach to the clinical trials is necessary (in which case there may also be changes to the intended non-clinical programme).

The EMA guideline on "Strategies to Identify and Mitigate Risks for First-in-human Clinical Trials with Investigational Medicinal Products" (CHMP, 2007) was produced to assist companies sponsoring clinical trials to make the transition from nonclinical to early clinical development. One of the authors (JWvdL) was highly involved in the production of this guideline which sets out to identify factors that influence risk for new investigational medicinal products and, together with consideration of aspects of quality and clinical testing strategies, considers nonclinical requirements for first-in-human clinical trials. This essential document gives strategies for mitigating and managing risk, including the calculation of the initial dose to be used in humans. At this point, it is worth noting that risk is inversely proportional to knowledge; the lower the level of understanding, the greater the inherent risk – a relationship tragically underlined by the TGN1412 trial but also by previous episodes such as thalidomide, benoxaprofen, terbinafine and cispapride. Broadly, the more innovative a product is, the more likely it is that understanding will be lower and – potentially – could be based on false premises or unproven hypotheses.

One of the first caveats given is the warning that nonclinical studies might not predict safety issues in humans because, for example, the target is more specific to humans, although other aspects could interfere with nonclinical predictivity, such as physiology. However, it is accepted that toxicologists have to use the results of nonclinical tests, in combination with other knowledge, to predict the likely effects of new medicinal products on humans.

One of the first steps in this process is to assess risk factors that are relevant to the compound under investigation and the human population to be exposed in first-in-human studies. Although this guideline refers specifically to prediction of "severe adverse reactions", this process should be undergone for all substances before every trial, irrespective of whether the compound is considered to be of high risk. Factors to consider include the mode of action of the substance (pharmacological as well as toxicological), the nature of the target (particular pharmacological receptors or proteins) and the relevance of any available animal model.

This guideline has been reviewed in detail by Milton and Horvath (2009) who point out that it has a number of potential weaknesses, not least that it was conceived initially with biologicals in mind but has been expanded subsequently to cover new chemical (small molecule) entities. The major drawback of this approach is that the risk assessment paradigm for biologicals has been based on receptor dynamics as opposed to that for small molecules for which distribution and metabolism are often critical, coupled with what could be called classical biochemical mechanisms of toxicity. The guideline does not give priority to distribution and metabolism. It is usually assumed that biologicals distribute poorly through the body and that metabolism follows the usual pathways of protein catabolism. Of course, for small molecules these are important processes to consider and *in vitro* metabolism studies play a significant part in choice of second species. For biologicals, the choice of second species is dependent on factors such as receptor specificity, cross-species reactivity and homology.

Although the guideline title refers specifically to mitigation of risk in first-in-human clinical trials, such mitigation is to a large extent the result of consideration of nonclinical aspects of the test compound's activity – be it pharmacological or toxicological. On this basis, it is appropriate to consider it here in some detail.

6.3.2.1 Mode of Action

It is quite common that the mechanism or mode of action of a small molecule is not fully understood at the time of first-in-human trials. Theoretically, this should be less of a problem with biologicals, which have been more specifically designed for the target. Novelty of mode of action is not necessarily an added risk factor; what is critical is the extent of understanding of the action and how that can affect the organism to which the substance will be administered. Comparison of action between laboratory test systems – *in vivo* or *in vitro* – is a critical part of the risk assessment. The following aspects of any mechanism of action should be considered:

- Nature and intensity, including extent and potency, any amplification, duration of effect and its reversibility at the target site;
- Nature and extent of effects at non-target receptors or tissues;
- Slope of the dose response curve and its shape, particularly if it is U-shaped or bell-shaped.

The guidance suggests that the following modes of action might require special attention:

- Action at a target which is connected to multiple signalling pathways;
- A biological cascade or cytokine release including those resulting in amplification of an effect that is not sufficiently controlled by physiological feedback mechanisms.

As part of this process it is important to consider any previous exposure of humans to substances with similar modes of action. Evidence from animal models (including transgenic rodents) could be useful to assess the risk of serious, pharmacologically-mediated toxicity. It is also appropriate to consider any novelty in the molecular structure which might lead to enhanced interaction with receptors when compared with any previous molecule or, in some cases, to the parent compound.

6.3.2.2 The Nature of the Target

The nature of the target itself is likely to impact on the risks associated with first-in-human trials and in future studies. One of the points made by Milton and Horvath (2009) is that even if the initial dose of TGN1412 had been reduced, expression of the serious effects could well have been delayed until the point when the toxic dose was reached. While it is clear that the molecular structure of the target should be known, it is equally important to assess the distribution of the target in normal and abnormal tissues, its specificity for cell type, including its presence (or absence) in normal or diseased tissue. In addition, the biological function of the human target should be considered and compared with that in the test systems used in the nonclinical programme. Polymorphisms in structure – both in animals and humans – and their potential impact should be considered.

6.3.2.3 Relevance of Animal Species and Models

In the absence of data relating to the effects of a novel compound in man, the experiments and tests conducted before first-in-human studies assume critical importance in terms of risk assessment and, as a consequence, in risk mitigation. These include the establishment of a credible database on the factors considered above.

It is critical to understand any differences that might exist between humans and the test system that is considered to be the most relevant for the safety evaluation. Factors to be considered include structural homology, distribution, signal transduction pathways and the nature of pharmacological effects expressed at the target. It is also important to assess and understand any difference in physiological function between the animal and human forms of the target. Perceived lack of relevance to humans increases the risks for first-in-human studies.

While there will always be discussion about the utility of animal models in medical research, their use is a pragmatic recognition that they represent a major tool for the evaluation of the pharmacology and toxicology of novel medicinal products. However, it should be remembered that, while they are essential to the development of new drugs, they are fallible; like all tools, misuse is likely to produce undesirable results. Even if the results of nonclinical experiment are relevant, lack of understanding of their significance might lead to their misapplication and faulty interpretation. Desire to see an effect could lead to its "observation" and to the ignoring of relevant counter-evidence. This is sometimes exemplified by attempts to use statistics as an Aristotelian lever to demonstrate that a marginal difference is statistically significant in a direction favourable to the continuation of the project.

There are increasingly well-understood differences between animal models and humans; between *in vivo* models and *in vitro* (bear in mind that human *in vitro* might not relate to human *in vivo*). Although animals and humans might possess the same pharmacological target or receptor, this does not mean that the response to activation or antagonism will be the same in both species. Receptor binding or affinity for the target could be different, as could be the distribution of the target in the cell or in the various tissues; different routes of distribution or metabolism (especially for small molecular entities) might mean that receptor occupancy is of lower duration in humans than in animals or vice versa. Even if an animal or test system is relevant to humans, differences in presentation – formulation or route of administration – could make the results in tests irrelevant.

Where it has been shown that there are relevant differences between the species, it is possible that the response in test systems might be less valuable for predicting the human response. Although similarity of response in, for example, rats and dogs might give some confidence that humans would respond similarly, this assumption should be carefully assessed. A more cautious approach is needed where a difference between the two species chosen for the toxicology programme has been demonstrated: which is relevant to man and why?

One of the features of modern pharmaceutical development is the increasing specificity of action of many new medicinal products, especially biologicals such as antibodies. For such products, animals might not reproduce the pharmacological effect that is intended for humans and might not indicate any relevant toxicity. This could be due to differences in receptor expression and binding, pharmacokinetics or pharmacodynamics.

In assessing and mitigating the risk in first-in-human clinical trials, the EMA guideline advocates a weight-of-evidence approach involving the integration of information from *in vivo*, *ex vivo* and *in vitro* studies. Although it points out that high human specificity of a medicinal product could complicate the nonclinical evaluation of risk, the guideline suggests that this does not necessarily imply increased risk. The guideline indicates that demonstration of relevance of an animal model (or models) could include comparison with humans for:

- Target expression, distribution and primary structure although, as suggested above, comparable structural homology should not be taken to imply similarity of effect.
- Pharmacodynamics, including binding to any receptor and comparison of functional consequences, including any cell signalling.
- Assessment and comparison of any additional functional domains in animals, for instance the Fc receptor system for monoclonal antibodies.
- Absorption, distribution, metabolism and elimination.
- Tissue cross-reactivity studies, where relevant.

The relevance of the chosen animal models should be documented and justified in detail. For the majority of small molecules, the two default species are the rat and the dog. The use of the rat is a matter of tradition and its deficiencies and advantages in the context of individual molecules should be understood as far as possible when interpreting the studies that result. While testing in the rat is almost obligatory for small molecules, its use for more human-specific biologicals is likely to be inappropriate. This could well hold for the dog as well, driving the increasing use of appropriate nonhuman primates for the assessment of biologicals. In the absence of a clearly relevant test species, the use of homologous proteins or transgenic animals expressing the human target may be the only viable route.

In common with ICH guidelines, the European paradigm for pharmaceutical development is that, wherever possible, two species should be used for the toxicology programme. This does not necessarily include the nonrodent species used in reproductive toxicity testing, the rabbit and, increasingly, the minipig (Van der Laan et al, 2010). Having said that, the minipig offers a credible alternative to the beagle dog for toxicity evaluation, giving the advantage that the general and reproductive studies can be conducted in the same species. For ethical reasons, the use of nonhuman primates in Europe has increasingly to be justified based on human relevance and the absence of suitable alternatives.

6.3.2.4 Pharmacodynamic, Safety Pharmacology and Pharmacokinetics

The relevance of the animal model selected should be supported by pharmacodynamic studies of mode of action and biology of the target. The studies undertaken should assess primary and secondary pharmacodynamics and should include target interactions; where possible or appropriate, these should be linked to functional response, for example receptor binding and occupancy and duration of effect and dose response. This should result in a dose-response curve for the pharmacological effect, which could identify a threshold for effect; the identification of abnormally-shaped curves (U- or bell-shaped) is cited as a priority. Although the intention is to identify effects that might be present at low doses, it should be remembered that this might not mitigate the risk of such effects being seen as doses are increased. However, it should be remembered that even if the TGN1412 trial had been started at a lower dose, it is still possible that the adverse events would have been expressed at higher doses in subsequent volunteers.

The EMA guideline points out that, although it is not mandatory that these studies should be compliant with Good Laboratory Practices (GLP), they should be of high quality and consistent with the principles of GLP.

Safety pharmacology studies from the standard core battery should be conducted before first-in-human clinical trials. As with the main ICH guideline on safety pharmacology, it is stated that additional studies should be carried out on a case-by-case basis. In deference to the TGN1412 episode, there is a clause indicating special attention to the immune system when the product is intended to target immune function.

As far as pharmacokinetics are concerned, it is axiomatic that these should be defined in all species used for the nonclinical studies before first-in-human studies, as detailed in ICH guidelines. The guideline says that exposures should also be characterized at pharmacodynamic doses in the relevant animal models, especially when pharmacodynamic effects could contribute to safety concerns. However, it does not offer any suggestions as to how this should be achieved. As implied above, knowledge of the target could indicate that the pharmacodynamics in animals are expressed at different plasma or target tissue concentrations than in humans or that there are other differences, for instance due to different receptor affinity, response or tissue distribution. Although Milton and Horvath (2009) indicate that there is little mention in the guideline of distribution and metabolism – which are seen as especially relevant to small molecules – the guideline mentions that, in general, determination of the NOAEL is the basic approach and adjustment should be done.

6.3.2.5 Toxicology

In common with similar guidelines, the EMA document states that the toxicology programme should use relevant species and include toxicokinetics. In addition, if there are factors that could influence risk, the inclusion of additional endpoints (by implication, nonroutine parameters or measurements) should be considered on a case-by-case basis. In common with other points in this document, this is easy to write but more difficult to put into effect. Whilst knowledge of a product might indicate that there are specific areas of risk that should be investigated in the animals used for the toxicity studies, actually identifying and validating a new endpoint or parameter could pose insuperable challenges. Additional complexity is added when the comparable significance of the endpoint in animals is compared with that in humans; differential expression of the parameter adds another layer of uncertainty to the interpretation mix.

While the guideline says that toxicity studies in nonrelevant species are discouraged as they might encourage misinterpretation, it is important to recognize that some expressions of toxicity are irrelevant to humans, even if the species is, in other respects, human relevant. The guideline indicates that the use of homologous proteins or transgenic animals might be useful; the caveats given above about this approach remain relevant. Even if a species is considered to be relevant, the immunogenicity of human proteins in animals should be considered; repeat dosing beyond a certain point could become uninformative. However, although antibodies could be raised to an injected protein, the question as to whether they are neutralizing antibodies or not might need to be answered.

A number of products developed recently have targeted proteins present in human disease that are not present in healthy humans or laboratory animals. In these cases, use of animal models of the disease might be useful but should be justified. One of the challenges here is to identify a relevant model of the human disease and to show that a response seen in the animal can be sensibly extrapolated to human patients.

When considering the nonclinical aspects of a pharmaceutical development from the European point of view, it is worth considering a possible difference between the US

FDA and the EMA. The FDA guidelines are generally interpreted as spelling out requirements while the EMA prefers to elicit thought in the construction of a nonclinical programme; it is for this reason that the title of the risk mitigation guideline includes the word "strategies". Although thought is encouraged in non-clinical planning, it should be remembered that all aspects of a programme should be justifiable in scientific terms.

6.3.2.6 Estimation of the First Dose in Humans

The EMA guideline acknowledges the widespread use of the No Observed Adverse Effect Level (NOAEL) in the derivation of a first-in-human starting dose but promotes the use of a newer concept – the Minimal Anticipated Biological Effect Level or MABEL.

In common with the FDA guidance on first-in-human dose selection (FDA, 2005), the EMA refers to the use of the NOAEL in the selection of safe starting doses. The selection should be based on the NOAEL in the most sensitive and relevant animal species and that this should be adjusted with allometric factors. In contrast to the FDA guidance, the EMA document places more emphasis on the use of pharmacokinetic and pharmacodynamic data in the assessment. As with the FDA, the use of safety factors is indicated for adjustment of the final dose, although these are not discussed as extensively as in the FDA guidance. It should be noted that the NOAEL approach was used in calculating the first dose for the TGN1412 trial; Milton and Horvath (2009) suggest that the safety factor used (160-fold) was derived from the dose after it had been set. This tends to exemplify the somewhat *ad hoc* use of safety factors and the lack of rigour in their choice. The use of the NOAEL in this case also highlights the disadvantages of this approach, as the NOAEL for a toxic effect might not be extrapolatable to humans due to the types of difference reviewed above.

Where risk factors have been identified in respect of target or mode of action, the MABEL approach is recommended. This is the dose that is the "anticipated dose level leading to a minimal biological effect level in humans". Factors to be taken into account when using MABEL include any expected or known differences in sensitivity between humans and animals. The term "minimal" is not defined and, although Milton and Horvath (2009) criticize this in their paper, it should be acknowledged that this cannot be defined in any general sense as the criteria for decision will be different for every compound assessed. As with other systems of dose calculation, the use of safety factors is envisaged, albeit without discussion. The EMA guideline states:

> The calculation of MABEL should utilise all *in vitro* and *in vivo* information available from pharmacokinetic/pharmacodynamic (PK/PD) data such as:
>
> - target binding and receptor occupancy studies *in vitro* in target cells from human and the relevant animal species;
> - concentration-response curves *in vitro* in target cells from human and the relevant animal species and dose/exposure-response *in vivo* in the relevant animal species.
> - exposures at pharmacological doses in the relevant animal species.
>
> Wherever possible, the above data should be integrated in a PK/PD modelling approach for the determination of the MABEL.

Any safety factor used should take into account risks associated with: the novelty of the compound (although it is earlier stated that this is not necessarily a risk *per se*); mode of action; potency; species specificity; and the shape of the dose-response curve.

Impenetrably, the guideline also adds an implied factor to take account of the uncertainty inherent in the calculation of the MABEL. The use of any safety factors needs to be justified; clearly, deciding a dose and then calculating the resulting safety factor is not acceptable.

Although the guideline indicates that the NOAEL approach is the current default method for first-in-human dose selection, it recommends that MABEL should be used in parallel and that any differences in dose estimation be investigated and, if appropriate, the lower dose used. Although use of the NOAEL is discussed, it is our opinion that the use of MABEL, including its inherent uncertainties, should become the preferred method for selection of first-in-human doses for the majority of compound classes, including small molecules.

6.4 Overview

While the nonclinical development of medicinal products in Europe is driven in large part by ICH guidelines, there are procedural differences in the approach of member states to the authorization of clinical trials and, in some cases, in the studies that might be required to support such applications. The recent EMA guideline on risk mitigation (EMA 2007) gives extensive guidance on risk assessment and species choice for toxicity studies and, crucially, in selection of the first-in-human dose. While the NOAEL is acknowledged as an acceptable approach for dose selection for first-in-human studies, it is our opinion that the MABEL should become more important in the future and, ultimately, be the preferred method for all medicinal products.

References

CHMP (2007) EMA/CHMP/SWP/28367/07 Guideline on strategies to identify and mitigate risks for first-in-human clinical trails with investigational medicinal products.

EU (2007) Parliament of the Council of 13 November 2007 on advanced therapy medicinal products and amending Directive 2001/83/ECand Regulation (EC) No 726/2004. http://eur-lex.europa.eu/LexUriServ/LexUriServ.do?uri=OJ:L:2007:324:0121:0137:en:PDF

EU (2008a) Directive 2001/83/EC Of The European Parliament and of the Council of 6 November 2001 on the Community code relating to medicinal products for human use (consolidated version dated December 2008).

EU (2008b) Notice to Applicants 2B http://ec.europa.eu/health/files/eudralex/vol-2/b/update_200805/ctd_05-2008_en.pdf

FDA (2005) Guidance for Industry: Estimating the Maximum Safe Starting Dose in Initial Clinical Trials for Therapeutics in Adult Healthy Volunteers. U.S. Department of Health and Human Services, Food and Drug Administration, Center for Drug Evaluation and Research.

Milton, M.N. and Horvath, C.J. (2009) The EMA guideline on first-in-human clinical trials and its impact on pharmaceutical development. *Toxicol. Pathol.*, **37**, 363–371.

Van der Laan, J,W., Brightwell, J., McAnulty, P., Ratky, J. and Stark, C. (2010) Regulatory acceptability of the minipig in the development of pharmaceuticals, chemicals and other products. *J. Pharmacol. Toxicol. Methods*, **62**, 184–195.

Useful Websites

EMA: http://www.ema.europa.eu/ema/Heads of Medicines Agency
http://www.ema.europa.eu/
Heads of Medicines Agency: http://www.hma.eu/http://www.hma.eu/uploads/media/Assessment_in_MS_public_dec_08__2_B.pdf

Main agencies

MHRA: http://www.mhra.gov.uk/index.htm
Netherlands CBG: http://www.cbg-meb.nl
NetherlandsCCMO: http://www.ccmo.nl
BfArm: http://www.bfarm.de/EN/Home/homepage__node.html
Swedish MPA: http://www.lakemedelsverket.se/Tpl/StartPage_395.aspx
French Afssaps: http://afssaps.sante.fr/
Hungary (National Institute of Pharmacy): www.ogyi.hu/

7
South Africa

Fariza Feraoun[1] *and Malik Feraoun*[2]
[1]*Laboratoires SERB, France*
[2]*Clinique Feraoun, France*

7.1 Introduction

South Africa is often called "A World in One Country" because of the contrast in its technologically advanced cities, its natural beauty and the many cultures that make up the South African nation.

Over the last 40 years, South Africa has developed a medicines regulatory authority with internationally recognized standing. Over the past 15 years, it has been transformed in order to improve its performance and regulatory processes. It is the role of the Department of Health to ensure that all South Africans have access to good quality healthcare. There are more than 20 000 medicines approved by the South African regulatory authority: the Medicines Control Council (MCC). The medicine registration is a long and complex process by which the Medicines Regulatory Authority (MRA) approves the use of medicines based on evidence of their quality, safety and efficacy. The aim of this process is to promote and protect the public health.

Medicines regulations integrate several activities that are carried out by the MRA during the pre- and post-approval periods. These include the regulation of nonclinical, clinical, pharmaceutical and analytical processes and the evaluation of data submitted to ensure compliance with the standards of Good Manufacturing Practices (GMP), Good Laboratory Practices (GLP) and Good Clinical Practices (GCP).

There are different stages to drug development including nonclinical, clinical and post-marketing phase IV-trials. The "critical path" of the research and development process starts when candidate products are selected for development, involving nonclinical and

Nonclinical Safety Assessment: A Guide to International Pharmaceutical Regulations, First Edition.
Edited by William J. Brock, Kenneth L. Hastings and Kathy M. McGown.

clinical studies. The nonclinical and clinical data gathered during these stages are then submitted for assessment by the MCC in order to have the approval of the medicine. This is what we will present in this chapter.

7.2 Country Information

7.2.1 Description

The Republic of South Africa is a country located at the southernmost region of the continent of Africa. The South African coast borders both the Atlantic and Indian Oceans. To the north of South Africa lie Namibia, Botswana and Zimbabwe, to the east are Mozambique and Swaziland, while the Kingdom of Lesotho is an independent enclave surrounded by South African territory. The location of South Africa has had a great influence on its climate and on several aspects of development. Due to a varied topography and oceanic influence, there is a considerable variation in climate from the extreme desert of the southern Namib in the farthest northwest to the subtropical climate in the east along the Mozambique border and the Indian Ocean.

7.2.2 Economy

According to the United Nation classification, South Africa is a middle-income country with an abundant supply of resources, and well-developed financial, legal, communications, energy and transport sectors. A modern infrastructure supports an efficient distribution of goods to major urban centres throughout the entire region. South Africa has a large agricultural sector and is an exporter of farming products.

7.2.3 Country Organization

South Africa consists of nine provinces. The administrative capital is Pretoria, the legislative capital is Cape Town and the judicial capital is Bloemfontein.

South Africa has a bicameral parliament: the National Council of Provinces and the National Assembly.

7.2.4 The Rainbow Nation

Eleven official languages are recognized in the constitution. South Africa is a nation of more than 49 million people of diverse origins, cultures, languages and religions, hence the name "Rainbow Nation".

7.2.5 Health and Medicines

Basic healthcare is a fundamental right. One of the goals of the government is therefore to provide healthcare that is affordable and accessible. In South Africa, parallel private and public healthcare systems exist. The health system consists of a wide public sector and a smaller but fast-growing private sector. Healthcare varies from the most basic primary healthcare, freely offered by the state, to highly specialized health services available in the private sector for those who can afford it.

The public system serves about 80% of the population, but is chronically underfunded and understaffed. The wealthiest 20% of the population uses the private system and are far better served as most resources are concentrated in the private health sector. The state contributes approximately 40% of all expenditure on health. The drug expenditure per person varies widely between the sectors. Public health consumes around 11% of the government's total budget, which is allocated and spent by the nine provinces. How these resources are allocated, and the standard of healthcare delivered, varies from province to province. The Medicines Regulatory Authority is charged with ensuring the safety, quality and effectiveness of all medicines sold in South Africa.

7.3 The Regulatory Aspects

7.3.1 The Registration of Medicines: Introduction and Scope

The Department of Health is committed to providing quality healthcare to all South Africans. The Medicines Control Council (MCC) is the statutory body charged with evaluating all medicines through a registration process before granting to some of them the marketing authorization for South Africa.

7.3.2 The Legal Framework

Legislation requires that the MCC shall register every medicine before it can be marketed. An application for registration of a medicine must be submitted for evaluation and approval prior to being marketed. It is a legal requirement that data submitted for evaluation should substantiate all claims and meet technical requirements of quality, safety and efficacy of the product for the purposes for which it is intended.

The Medicines and Related Substances Control Act No. 101 of 1965 (the "Act"), as amended, and its Regulations, is the principal act governing the manufacture, registration, distribution and marketing of drugs in South Africa. The Act requires that all medicines registered in the Republic of South Africa are of acceptable quality, efficacy and safety. The regulatory authority applies standards laid down by the Act. It is appointed by the Minister of Health.

The applicants must also comply with the MCC guidelines and application forms that are available from the office of the Registrar of Medicines and the MCC website. Also throughout the registration procedures, applicants must comply with the Committee recommendations and the MCC resolutions to the applications.

The South African guidelines shall be read in conjunction with the Act and its Regulations. They outline the format, the information and the data requirements for preparation and submission of an application for registration of medicines. We will develop these requirements further.

The guidelines are meant to guide the applicant in meeting the requirements of the Act. They are intended to provide recommendations and to assist applicants in the preparation of documentation for the registration of medicines. Whenever there is doubt, applicants are advised to consult the MCC for confirmation and clarification before completing and submitting the application form.

Guidelines represent the MCC's current thinking on safety, quality and efficacy of medicines. However, MCC reserves the right to request any additional information to establish the safety, quality and efficacy of a medicine in keeping with the knowledge current at the time of evaluation. Guidelines are constantly evolving as a result of scientific developments and harmonization of the requirements of regional and international regulatory authorities. The MCC regularly updates the guidelines to reflect current thinking and keep its technical requirements and evaluation policies in line with the "best international medicines regulatory practice".

It is acknowledged, however, that in some instances scientific developments may dictate alternative approaches. When a deviation from a guideline is decided on, a detailed justification for the deviation and a scientific and technical justification for the alternative approach should be included in the expert report submitted with the application.

7.3.3 Role, Structure and Organization of the MCC

7.3.3.1 Role

The Medicines Control Council (MCC) was established to oversee the regulation of medicines in South Africa. Its main purpose is to safeguard and protect the public through ensuring that all medicines that are manufactured, packed, distributed and marketed in South Africa are safe, therapeutically effective and consistently meet acceptable standards of quality. The MCC, in considering whether a medicine is suitable for use for its intended purpose, assesses its relative risk against the benefits. Another role of the MCC is to prepare guidelines to assist the industry in complying with the requirements from the Act.

7.3.3.2 Structure and Organization of the MCC

The MCC operates through expert council committees manned by external specialists from various institutions around the country to carry out the assessment. These MCC members are appointed by the Minister of Health for a 5-year period that can be renewed once. The role of these experts is to evaluate data sets submitted by the pharmaceutical industry for purposes of registration. As they are drawn from various academic institutions (mainly medical and pharmacy schools), from industry and government, they have to declare commercial interests related to the pharmaceutical industry and to remove themselves from any discussion or decision-making related to these interests.

Several technical committees with about 150 members evaluate volumes of data submitted by pharmaceutical companies for registration purposes. Since the MCC is a legal entity, it can face civil litigation. This could have an impact on the decision-making process, since individuals can become cautious in making decisions for fear of being sued.

These committees include the complementary medicines committee, analytical committee, clinical committee, pharmaceutical/bioavailability committee, scheduling committee, African traditional medicines committee, veterinary clinical committee, biological committee, clinical trials committee and pharmacovigilance committee.

The skills of the MCC and its committees are written into law. A Regulation of the Act stipulates that the MCC shall include experts in pediatrics, internal medicine, public health, clinical pharmacology, pharmaceutical chemistry, toxicology and drug safety, biotechnology, pharmaceutics, virology and microbiology. Also included are persons with knowledge of the study of adverse drug reactions, complementary medicines, and law. In addition, a person with specialized knowledge in veterinary clinical pharmacology, and a veterinarian designated by the Minister of Agriculture also make up the MCC.

The Cluster Medicines Regulatory Affairs is headed by the Registrar of Medicines. The office of the Registrar provides administrative and technical support to the MCC and its activities. The Registrar is also an executive secretary to the MCC. The Registrar's office is a Chief Directorate – MRA within the Department of Health.

There are four Directorates which are largely responsible for coordination and execution of different activities: Operations and Administration; Inspectorate and Law Enforcement; Clinical Evaluation and Trials; and Medicine Evaluation and Research. The staff complement of MRA includes doctors, pharmacists, veterinarians, other scientists and administrative staff.

7.3.4 The Regulatory Procedures

There are three types of regulatory evaluation procedures.

7.3.4.1 Routine Review Process

The Routine Review Process is the normal process, with the regular evaluation timelines observed and the full application data package.

7.3.4.2 Abbreviated Medicine Review Process

The Abbreviated Medicine Review Process (AMRP) shortens the evaluation time of pharmaceutical products that are registered in a country with which the MCC aligns itself, if the evaluation reports of this Health Authority are available. The MCC aligns itself with a regulatory authority which is:

- a member of the International Conference on Harmonization of Technical Requirements for Registration of Pharmaceuticals for Human use (ICH), i.e., United States of America (FDA), European Union (EMA and National Regulatory Authorities), and Japan (MHLW);
- an ICH observer, i.e., Switzerland (Swissmedic) and Canada (Health Canada);
- a regulatory authority associated with an ICH regulatory authority member through a legally binding mutual recognition agreement, i.e., Australia (TGA), Norway, Iceland and Liechtenstein;
- a member of the PIC/S (Pharmaceutical Inspection Cooperation Scheme) for quality matters relating to GMP. This process applies to new chemical entity (NCE) products approved within the last three years of the licence.

The AMRP is an abbreviated evaluation process and not an abbreviated application; therefore, it requires a full submission according to the standard format, with the following additional documents:

- certificate of approval of registration of the medicine by this Health Authority;
- expert reviewers' reports on chemical–pharmaceutical, pharmaco–toxicological and clinical documentation;
- relevant correspondence both negative and positive (e.g., queries, non-acceptance of certain claims/statements) between the applicant and the registering Authority;

- written confirmations that the data submitted and the formulation applied for to the MCC are identical to that approved by the registering Authority; and that the proposed package insert is based on the package insert and the complete dossier of the licensing country;
- a letter authorizing the MCC to contact the relevant Authority for an evaluator's or assessor's report.

The raw data of experimental and clinical studies should be excluded from the application.

7.3.4.3 Expedited Review Process/Fast-Track Review Process

Under certain circumstances, the MCC can accelerate the registration process for specific medicines that have important therapeutic benefit and which are required urgently to deal with key health problems. In such cases, an accelerated review system is applied: the Expedited Review Process, also named the Fast-track Review Process.

The applicant should submit an Expedited Review Request to the Minister of Health with a copy to the Registrar of Medicines before submitting the full application. Products that will be considered for expedited review are either medicines that appear on the Essential Drugs List (EDL) or medicines containing new chemical entities that are considered essential for national health but do not appear on the EDL.

The following should be submitted with the application:

- Expert report; a package insert (where the product has been approved);
- Summary Basis for the Registration Application (SBRA) and, depending on the medicines, either a declaration by the applicant that this medicine appears on the EDL or, in the case of a NCE considered essential for national health, a written notification to that effect from the Minister.

The process when an applicant applies for a Fast-track Review Process is as follows:

- The applicant shall be notified by the Registrar within 30 days of the date of receipt of the application whether or not this application is to be subjected to the Expedited Registration Process.
- The MCC might request any information with respect to the application under consideration and such information shall be furnished by the applicant within a period indicated by the MCC, failing which the MCC may reject the application.
- The MCC shall, within nine months from the date of receipt of the application by the Registrar, make a decision with regard to the application and inform the applicant of such decision.

7.3.5 The Registration Requirements for Preparation of the Application Package

The process of getting a new drug on the market for a pharmaceutical company starts with preliminary research. Pharmaceutical companies spend a large portion of their budgets on research and development. Nonclinical and clinical trials are undertaken to determine the safety and efficacy of drugs. Animal tests are carried out to determine the toxicity of the drug. Human tests are used to determine the efficacy and the levels and rates of absorption, distribution around the body, metabolism and excretion.

In order to apply for registration of a drug in South Africa, the applicant shall first reside and do business in South Africa. He shall submit the application dossier following a specific format (South African CTD format), with a completed screening form, a proposed label for use on the medicine, a sample, a copy of the manufacturing licence and a current GMP certificate from the regulatory authority of the medicine's country of origin, a site master file, and all data from nonclinical and clinical studies. The application procedure is very elaborate, involving strict compliance with the administrative, scientific and technical information requirements.

Previously, there was a specific South African format for the applications for registration of a medicine, referred to as the Medicine Registration Form 1 (MRF1; 6.01 Dec03 v1 from December 2003), which was made up of five parts. It was similar to the Common Technical Document elaborated by the International Conference on Harmonization (ICH). The main differences were that the Modules were called Parts and the bioavailability and bioequivalence studies were addressed in Part 2A instead of Module 5. The requirements for registration used to be quite similar to those of the European Union.

In June 2010, the MCC announced its intention to implement the South African Common Technical Document (ZA CTD) format as a replacement for the previous MRF1 format. From 1 June 2011, submissions of new product applications for registration in ZA CTD format are mandatory. The applicants shall submit to the MCC dossiers for the registration of medicines following the new South African format. The format and organization of the Summaries, Quality, Nonclinical, and Clinical Modules (Modules 2 to 5, respectively), are described in the European Notice to Applicants: Medicinal products for Human Use [Volume 2B: Presentation and format of the dossier CTD (July 2003)].

The CTD guidelines, together with the South African Regulatory Guidelines (SARG), provide detailed information about the contents of an application. These guidelines apply to applications to register medicines and all related variations. Applicants should not modify the overall organization of the CTD.

The documents outlining the format and data requirements for preparation and submission of an application for registration of medicines are the General Information Guideline (2.01 Jul12 v8 from August 2012), the Guidance for the Submission of the South African CTD/eCTD-General & Module 1 (2.24 Guidance General Module 1 Jul12 v5 from August 2012) and the South African Common Technical Document (ZA CTD Jul v5 from August 2012).

Some information is also presented in the Pharmaceutical and Analytical CTD/eCTD Guideline (2.25 PA CTD Jun11 v3 from June 2011), in the Pharmaceutical and Analytical guideline (2.02 PA Jun11 v6 from June 2011) and in the Package Inserts for Human Medicines Guideline (2.16 PI for human medicines Aug09 v3 from October 2009).

The South African Common Technical Document contains the South African Module 1 which is region specific and the CTD Modules 2, 3, 4 and 5.

7.3.5.1 Module 1 Administrative Information and Prescribing Information

Relevant administrative documentation should be submitted in Module 1 of the CTD dossier.

This Module contains the Letter of Application, the Comprehensive table of contents, the Application Form (Module 1.2.1) with the relevant Annexes to the application form, the South African labelling and packaging and the Information about the experts for Quality, Nonclinical and Clinical Modules (resume and declaration signed by the experts).

It also contains the specific requirements for different types of applications, the environmental risk assessment, the Good Manufacturing Practice information, the details of compliance with screening outcomes, the individual patient data-statement of availability, the foreign regulatory status, the bioequivalence trial information, the pediatric development program and the risk management plan.

The Application Form to use for the application for registration of a medicine is available on the MCC website (Module 1.2.1 Mar11 v3 from March 2011). Once completed, it is included in Module 1.

In cases concerning well-known active pharmaceutical ingredients, the MCC may grant exemption from the submission of the information about the nonclinical and clinical experts (1.4.2 and 1.4.3).

7.3.5.2 Module 2 CTD Summaries

Module 2 contains the Quality Overall Summary, Nonclinical Overview, Clinical Overview, Non-clinical Written and Tabulated summaries, and the Clinical Summary. We will present further the nonclinical documentation that needs to be included in this Module.

7.3.5.3 Module 3 Quality

Module 3 contains all information about the Active Pharmaceutical Ingredient and the Pharmaceutical Product.

7.3.5.4 Module 4 Nonclinical Study Reports

Module 4 of the dossier contains the nonclinical (pharmaco-toxicological) data relevant to the application. It contains the table of contents of Module 4, the study reports and the literature references.

In cases concerning well-known active pharmaceutical ingredients, the MCC may grant exemption from the submission of nonclinical study reports in Module 4.

7.3.5.5 Module 5 Clinical Study Reports

The Module contains the table of contents of Module 5, the tabular listing of all clinical studies, the clinical study reports and the literature references.

In the next paragraphs, we present the documents and data needed for the application package with the different steps of submission.

7.3.5.6 Requirements for an Application

The procedure for submitting an application for the registration of a medicine has several steps. This is linked to the review process which begins by the administrative checking of the package, followed by the scientific review of the data and documents submitted.

7.3.5.6.1 Foreign Registration Information

The applicant shall furnish the list of all countries in which the application has been registered, and the status of that registration. It shall indicate the status of the application: approvals with indications, deferrals, withdrawals and rejections. As previously explained, the MCC aligns itself with the regulatory authorities of the following countries and region: USA, European Union, all European Union countries, Japan, Switzerland,

Canada, Australia, Norway, Iceland, Liechtenstein. For quality matters relating to GMP, the MCC also aligns itself with any member of the PIC/S.

If the medicine has already been registered in any of these countries, the administrative documentation shall be provided (copy of registration certificate; approved package insert; conditions of registration; confirmation of similarity of package). For rejections or withdrawals relating to safety matters the details for each case should be provided. If not registered and/or applied for registration in the country of origin, the reason should be given.

7.3.5.6.2 Manufacturing Requirements

Only medicines manufactured, packed and quality controlled at sites compliant with the current principles of GMP as prescribed by the MCC are considered for registration. The Act requires that overseas manufacturers of medicine supplied to South Africa should comply with the same or equivalent manufacturing standards as expected of South African manufacturers. Evidence in relation to compliance with GMP of the overseas manufacturer is required for applications for registration of imported medicines. When acceptable evidence of GMP compliance is not available, overseas manufacturers are inspected by the GMP Inspectorate to assess manufacturing standards before registration of the medicine is approved.

7.3.5.7 Steps of Submission

7.3.5.7.1 Pre-Screening Step

On receipt at the MCC, all applications for registration are subject to the pre-screening step. In the previous submissions, the applicants had to complete and include the pre-screening checklist, which was Attachment A of the previous version of the general information guideline and the Application for registration of a medicine screening form entitled MRF2 for dossiers in MRF format (form available on MCC website MRF2; 6.02 Jun07 v3 from June 2007).

From 1 July 2010, the pre-screening step has become the first part of administrative screening, and technical screening is carried out by the evaluator before evaluation commences. If the applicant does not comply with the pre-screening requirements the application is returned as "incomplete". If the pre-screening step is successful, a screening number for the application, an acknowledgement receipt and the required pre-screening fee are sent to the applicant. Once completed, the screening step can take place.

7.3.5.7.2 Screening Step

In the previous submissions, the screening submission package contained a covering letter, the completed pre-screening checklist, the completed screening form MRF2, a complete application for registration dossier (MRF1) and several other administrative documents.

Now, when submitting a dossier in South Africa, the screening submission package contains a covering letter, the completed screening template for new applications for registration (6.15 screening template SA Jun11 v5_1) from March 2012, the complete application for registration dossier in ZA CTD format and several other administrative documents. The screening template is to be used on receipt of an application for registration of a medicinal product submitted to the South African Regulatory Authority. Usually a separate application for each pharmaceutical form is required.

If the applicant screening package does not comply with the screening requirements, the screening status "hold" or "return as incomplete" is communicated to the applicant with reasons and time frames for submitting outstanding information or for collecting the application. In case of contest, a decision is taken at the next MCC meeting.

If the applicant screening package complies with the screening requirements, the screening status "accepted" is communicated to the applicant together with the required application fee, the number of copies of the different parts of the MRF1 and the application number. Once the screening step is successfully completed, the full submission can take place. This date is regarded as the date of submission of the application for registration.

At this stage, what is checked is the presence of the data required, not the actual scientific content of these data. Justification for the omission of data is required. The role of the pre-screening and screening steps is to check whether all the data required have been included but these steps do not involve evaluation of the data or evaluation of the motivation for omission of data. These evaluations will need to be carried out by the reviewers during the scientific review phase.

7.3.5.7.3 Full Submission Step

Several sets are then prepared and sent to several expert committees. Their contents depend on the committee. In the previous format, the clinical set contained the complete Part 1: Administrative information which consisted of the administrative particulars; the table of contents; the labelling; and the foreign registration information. It also contained Part 2B: Summary basis for registration application, or Part 2D: Preclinical expert report and Part 2E: Clinical expert report. The other parts that were included in the clinical set were Part 3B: Formulation and the complete Parts 4 and 5: Preclinical and Clinical studies, respectively.

For the ZA CTD format, the clinical set contains: the Letter of Application (1.0); the comprehensive table of contents (1.1); the Application Form (1.2.1); South African labelling and packaging (1.3); information about the experts (1.4); details of compliance with screening outcomes (1.8); and the foreign regulatory status (1.10). It also contains the nonclinical and clinical overviews (2.4 and 2.5), the nonclinical written and tabulated summaries (2.6), the clinical summary (2.7), the description and composition of the pharmaceutical product (3.2.p.1) and the nonclinical and clinical study reports (Modules 4 and 5, respectively).

7.3.6 The Registration Process: Several Steps of Review

7.3.6.1 Evaluation of the Application Dossier by MCC Reviewers and Outcome

Once the copies of the application are given to members of the relevant expert committees, the scientific evaluation takes place. In parallel, a copy of the registration dossier, the site master file and sample are given to the Inspectorate, who will organize an inspection of the applicant. The registration of the medicine depends on the Inspectorate's recommendation to the MCC. If the inspection reveals errors or omissions, the medicine will not be registered. The Inspectorate evaluates the applicant's facilities according to GMP in order to ensure the quality of the medicine. The Inspectorate may also conduct different types of inspections, including those related to GCP.

After assessing the large amounts of data from the application and writing the corresponding expert reports, the expert committees have to compile these reports for the MCC. These expert reports also follow strict procedures. The committee members give their evaluation reports to the chair of their committees. The peer review of the evaluation of the application takes place at the committee meetings. Discussions and clarifications are obtained from the evaluators if needed.

The recommendations are submitted to the MCC for a resolution that is sent to the applicant. If the application receives a positive recommendation, the product is registered and a certificate is provided to the sponsor. If questions have been raised by the reviewers, the applicant is given a 3-month period to respond to the pharmaceutical recommendation and a 6-month-period to respond to the clinical recommendation.

7.3.6.2 Timelines

There are no official timelines for the evaluation phase carried out by the MCC reviewers. Yet time is a major factor in the pharmaceutical world. A slow registration process has a potentially negative impact on both the pharmaceutical company and the patient. While the pharmaceutical firms' operations are potentially limited until the approval of a medicine, patients who could be treated by this medicine have to wait. Like many other Health Agencies, the MCC suffers from a lack of resources and this is seen by the long timelines observed. Currently, the registration process takes from 18 months up to four years with an average of two years.

7.3.6.3 Specificity of the MCC

A specificity of the MCC is that applicants are not allowed to communicate directly with the evaluators. All queries and issues should be communicated through the secretariat.

7.4 The Nonclinical Safety Assessment

7.4.1 Introduction

The regulations on nonclinical requirements are indicated in the Act and its Regulations; the Clinical guideline (2.09 Clinical Dec03 v1) from December 2003; for the previous format, the medicine registration form MRF1 Part 4; and for the ZA CTD format, the South African Common Technical Document (ZA CTD Jul v5 from August 2012); and the Guidance for the submission of the South African CTD/eCTD – General & Module 1 (2.24 Guidance General Module 1 Jul12 v5 from August 2012). In this section, we describe what needs to be included in the application for a medicine in terms of nonclinical data.

7.4.2 Nonclinical Evaluation

The Clinical Evaluation Unit (CEU) is responsible for the evaluation of both the clinical and the nonclinical data. This CEU is also in charge of the evaluation of clinical aspects of the package inserts and relevant changes to package inserts.

The safety is evaluated through nonclinical studies in animals, animal toxicity, comparative pharmacokinetics and pharmacodynamics studies in animals. The applicant has to include the details of the results of any experiments carried out in animals confirming the safety of the medicine. The nonclinical studies that were in part 4 of the MRF1 form for the previous format are now in the Module 4 of the ZA CTD format. The details of results from tests depend on the state of scientific knowledge at the time when the application is lodged. Any interim and final results of ongoing studies should be submitted as soon as these data become available. Also, an alternative route of administration than used for the registered product or an increased daily dose of unknown inactive pharmaceutical ingredients could result in the need for additional pharmaco-toxicological data.

7.4.3 Content of the Application for Safety Assessment

The nonclinical information, studies and results are in Modules 2 and 4 and some information is also, in some cases, in Module 1.

7.4.3.1 Module 2: Summaries

The nonclinical information presented in Module 2 is the CTD summaries with the nonclinical overview (2.4) and the Nonclinical written and tabulated summaries (2.6).

The Nonclinical written and tabulated summaries (2.6) contain an Introduction (2.6.1), the Pharmacology, Pharmacokinetics and Toxicology written summaries (2.6.2, 2.6.4 and 2.6.6), and the Pharmacology, Pharmacokinetics and Toxicology tabulated summaries (2.6.3, 2.6.5 and 2.6.7).

The Pharmacology written summary (2.6.2) contains a Brief Summary, the primary and secondary pharmacodynamics, the safety pharmacology, the pharmacodynamic medicine interactions, the discussion and conclusions and the tables and figures.

The Pharmacology Tabulated Summary (2.6.3) contains the pharmacology overview, the primary and secondary pharmacodynamics, the safety pharmacology and the pharmacodynamic medicine interactions.

The Pharmacokinetics Written Summary (2.6.4) contains a brief summary, the methods of analysis, the absorption, distribution, metabolism (interspecies comparison), and excretion. It also contains the pharmacokinetic medicine interactions, the other pharmacokinetic studies, the discussion and conclusions and the tables and figures.

The Pharmacokinetics Tabulated Summary (2.6.5) contains the pharmacokinetics overview, the analytical methods and validation reports, the pharmacokinetics data for the absorption after a single dose and for the absorption after repeated doses, the pharmacokinetics data for the organ distribution, for the plasma protein binding, for the study in pregnant or nursing animals, for the other distribution study, and for the metabolism *in vivo* and *in vitro*. it also contains the pharmacokinetics data on possible metabolic pathways, on induction/inhibition of medicine-metabolizing enzymes, on excretion, including excretion into bile, on medicine–medicine interactions and other data.

The Toxicology Written Summary (2.6.6) contains a Brief Summary, the single-dose toxicity, the repeat-dose toxicity (including supportive toxicokinetics evaluations), and the genotoxicity. there is also the carcinogenicity (including supportive toxicokinetics evaluations), the reproductive and developmental toxicity (including range-finding studies and supportive toxicokinetics evaluations), the local tolerance, the other toxicity studies (if available), the discussion and conclusions and the tables and figures.

The Toxicology Tabulated Summary (2.6.7) contains the toxicology overview, the toxicokinetics overview of toxicokinetics studies and toxicokinetics data and the toxicology of active pharmaceutical ingredient. it also contains the single-dose toxicity, the repeat-dose toxicity (non-pivotal and pivotal studies), the genotoxicity: *in vitro* and *in vivo*, and the carcinogenicity. the other sections of the toxicology tabulated summary are the reproductive and developmental toxicity with non-pivotal studies, with fertility and early embryonic development to implantation (pivotal), with effects on embryofoetal development (pivotal) and with effects on pre- and postnatal development including maternal function (pivotal). the last parts of this summary are the studies in juvenile animals, the local tolerance and other toxicity studies.

7.4.3.2 Module 4: Nonclinical Study Reports

The nonclinical information presented in Module 4 are the nonclinical study reports (4.2) with the nonclinical (pharmaco-toxicological) data relevant to the application, the literature references (4.3), and the table of contents of Module 4.

The study reports module (4.2) contain the pharmacology (4.2.1), the pharmacokinetics (4.2.2), and the toxicology (4.2.3) study reports.

The pharmacology study reports module (4.2.1) contain the primary and secondary pharmacodynamics, the safety pharmacology and the pharmacodynamic medicine interactions.

The pharmacokinetics study reports module (4.2.2) contain the analytical methods and validation reports, the absorption, distribution, metabolism, excretion, the pharmacokinetic medicine interactions (non-clinical) and other pharmacokinetic studies.

The toxicology study reports module (4.2.3) contain the single-dose and repeat-dose toxicity, the genotoxicity, the carcinogenicity, the reproductive and developmental toxicity, the local tolerance and other toxicity studies.

The different sections of this Toxicology study reports are the following:

- Single-dose toxicity is in order by species and by route;
- Repeat-dose toxicity is in order by species, by route and by duration. The supportive toxicokinetics evaluations are included in that section;
- Genotoxicity presents the *in vitro* and *in vivo* data, including supportive toxicokinetics evaluations;
- Carcinogenicity is split into the long-term studies (in order by species, including range-finding studies that cannot be appropriately included under repeat-dose toxicity or pharmacokinetics), short- or medium-term studies (including range-finding studies that cannot be appropriately included under repeat-dose toxicity), and 'other' studies. The supportive toxicokinetics evaluations are included in the carcinogenicity section;
- Reproductive and developmental toxicity is split into fertility and early embryonic development, embryo–fetal development, prenatal and postnatal development (including maternal function) and the studies in which the offspring (juvenile animals) are dosed and/or further evaluated. If modified study designs are used, these subheadings should be modified accordingly. The range-finding studies and supportive toxicokinetics evaluations are included in the part on reproductive and developmental toxicity;
- Local tolerance;

- Other toxicity studies (if available), such as antigenicity, immunotoxicity, mechanistic studies (if not included elsewhere), dependence, metabolites, impurities and other.

These studies are listed in Appendix B of the South African Common Technical Document (ZA_CTD_Jul_v5 from August 2012), which is the Nonclinical Tabulated Summaries templates. The MCC advises to refer to the European Commission, NTA, Vol. 2B-CTD, Module 2, edition 2003 for examples of templates.

In the previous format, the applicant had to complete and submit two forms: the MRF1 and the MRF2. The MRF2 form was the application for registration of a medicine screening form, needed for the screening step. In that form, the applicant had to indicate in the "Type of Application" part that he was submitting nonclinical data. Also, in Parts 1C and 1D "Labelling and foreign registration", he had to indicate that nonclinical data were submitted in Part 4.

The MRF1 form was the application for registration dossier. In this form, it was required on Part 1C to furnish the Summary of Product Characteristics (SPC), which was the labelling information for healthcare professionals with regard to the nonclinical safety data. In the MRF1 form, it was required on part 2B to furnish a Summary Basis for Registration Application (SBRA) which was a summary of the core data in support of the clinical safety and efficacy. It was the basis for registration and consisted of an overview of the application.

This was intended to be a very brief and concise document containing the core data, on the basis of which the applicant intended to obtain registration for the product. It was to be presented as a summary only. Hence, no articles or reports were to be incorporated into the SBRA, nor were such papers to be attached to it either, as these belonged with the full submission. It contained only the main safety issues and information on animal and *in vitro* toxicology data with the list of all nonclinical studies carried out.

It was also required in the MRF1 form to present in Part 2D a nonclinical expert report (PCER). The PCER is an independent, objective and encompassing report on all the relevant aspects in the specific field of expertise of the reporter who was familiar/acquainted with the development of the product in light of current scientific knowledge addressing all the nonclinical aspects of the development of the product and of the relevant aspects referred to in the package insert. The ICH guidelines were often followed for the preparation of the PCER.

All issues and properties of the product in the submission had to be clearly identified and critically discussed in the expert report in light of current scientific knowledge. The expert report had to address all the aspects of the package insert. A list of the key references used in compiling the expert report and the curriculum vitae of the expert had to be included.

In cases concerning well-known active pharmaceutical ingredients, or if nonclinical and clinical overviews were submitted, the MCC could grant exemption from the submission of an SBRA, and vice-versa: if an SBRA was submitted, the MCC could grant exemption from the submission of the PCER.

In the South African dossier, the nonclinical information is detailed in Modules 2, 4 and in some cases in the Module 1.

7.4.3.3 Module 1.3.1: Summary of Product Characteristics (SPC), labelling and Package leaflet

The nonclinical information may also be provided in the Module 1.3.1. Usually, the SPC/package insert statements of new chemical entity should be referenced to the clinical data and other references submitted. In case of a well-known entity, the Martindale (the Complete Drug Reference) can be used for the safety information.

In general, the nonclinical safety information is not included in the package insert. However, in some situations, it might be deemed necessary by the MCC to include it in the "Pharmacological action" paragraph, with the Summary of clinical studies, for example, the relevance to pregnancy.

7.4.3.3.1 Paragraph on Pharmacological Action

A summary of clinical studies can be included, if necessary, in the "Pharmacological action" paragraph, which consists of "Pharmacokinetics" and "Pharmacodynamics". The other paragraphs to complete with such data, if relevant, are "Warnings", "Interactions", "Pregnancy and lactation" and "Side effects and special precautions".

7.4.3.3.2 Paragraph on Pregnancy and Lactation

The conclusions from nonclinical toxicity studies, which are of relevance for the assessment of risks associated with exposure during pregnancy, should be included in the "Pregnancy" paragraph. The other parts to complete with such data if relevant are "Women of Childbearing Potential;" "Lactation;" and "Fertility." Cross-reference to "Contraindications" or "Warnings" sections can be given, as appropriate.

7.4.4 The Focus of the Nonclinical Evaluation

The applicant needs to provide the results obtained and conclusions drawn from tests performed nonclinically to demonstrate all aspects of the toxicity of the medicine and to prove the safety of its use, with special reference to:

- acute toxicity;
- subacute toxicity studies;
- chronic toxicity studies;
- subchronic toxicity studies;
- reproduction toxicity (maternal toxicity, teratogenicity, embryotoxicity);
- carcinogenicity studies;
- mutagenicity/oncogenicity studies;
- other tests to substantiate the safety of the medicine (for example, arthropathy, dermal, ocular toxicity);
- pharmacokinetic studies.

The applicant will also provide the methods and experimental results and conclusions from tests performed with reference to the efficacy of the medicine. There will be a special emphasis on the relationship between the tests performed and the purpose for which the medicine is, or will be used or for which it will be propagated, and further, with regard to the dosage and method of administration of the medicine.

7.4.5 Pharmacology Testing

7.4.5.1 Pharmacodynamics

The primary effects of the medicine, with results in different animal species (ED_{50} values, if possible), should be addressed. Comparison of the effects of the product with that of reference products is valuable information. Where relevant, the pharmacology of significant metabolites should be investigated. Other pharmacodynamic effects, especially those that might be of significance for adverse effects of the medicine, should be studied and described. Drug interaction studies, where relevant, should be included.

7.4.5.2 Pharmacokinetics

To assist in the interpretation of toxicological studies, it is important to compare the exposure of the animals used in the toxicity testing with that anticipated in patients given the proposed therapeutic dose regimen. The applicant will provide data which includes C_{max} (after a single dose and at steady state) and AUC. Also, comparative pharmacokinetics data should be included for the parent drug and major metabolite(s), where relevant, in human and all species used in the toxicity, carcinogenicity and reproduction studies. These data should preferably be obtained from the toxicity studies. Other information (for example, $t_{1/2}$ and clearance) could be of value where important differences have been shown between animals and man.

7.4.6 Toxicology Testing

A summary or expert report should be submitted for each animal species studied, with information on the sex of the animals, number of animals, dosage, route of administration, duration of study and toxic manifestations. Important points to consider that pertain to nonclinical toxicity are: the dose-response and the time-response relationships; the species and the target organ specificities: and the reversibility/irreversibility of toxic effects. Medicines that show specific toxicological effects, such as immunotoxicity, hepatotoxicity or neurotoxicity should be investigated further. The points to address in the reproduction studies include: fertility; embryonal toxicity; teratogenicity; and perinatal and postnatal effects. New medicines, which belong to classes that are known to produce a particular toxic effect, should be tested appropriately. The possible mechanism(s) underlying the changes observed in toxicity studies need to be investigated and addressed.

Due to the South African climatic conditions, the phototoxic potential of a medicine, should be considered.

7.5 Conclusion

The medicine registration process in South Africa is an elaborate process by which the regulatory Authority grants the marketing authorization approval for a medicine based on evidence of its quality, safety and efficacy. In this chapter, we have presented the current status of the nonclinical safety assessment. However, this leads to a general reflection about the nonclinical safety studies.

7.5.1 Withdrawals

Recently, several medicines have been withdrawn from the worldwide market due to safety concerns as a result of adverse reactions, and this has raised concerns from a public health perspective. Withdrawals have negative impacts for the reliability of the pharmaceutical industry and for the credibility of the regulatory authorities. These withdrawals have led to the idea that Health Authorities might approve medicines too rapidly and without due consideration of the harmful effects the medicines could have on public health.

7.5.2 Consequences

As a result, some Health Agencies might have become more stringent and less flexible in their requirements for granting marketing authorizations. In recent years, the worldwide pharmaceutical industry has noticed the risk-averse nature of regulatory decision-making. A few companies believe that some Health Agencies are bowing to pressure from the public and refuse to approve some medicines due to their possible rare toxicity or side effects.

7.5.3 New Safety Approach

The traditional model of nonclinical development is currently subject to debate from a public, scientific and regulatory point of view. Some people consider that several tools used for toxicology and human safety testing are too old and fail to predict the specific safety problems. They challenge the current regulatory models for assessing safety of the products. Indeed, they disregard the approach of using animal models and extrapolating safety data to humans and argue strongly against vivisection. They recommend a change in approach from the historical nonclinical studies required, sometimes carried out as a routine but without real added value. Therefore, different models have been proposed to review the nonclinical approach and to increase the development of new studies in order to better adapt the nonclinical world to our needs. Also, it has been shown that, due to genetic factors, the responses to drug could vary among individuals. A possible solution to improve safety could be to consider the interaction of medicines with individuals depending on their genetic constitution.

8

Asia Pacific: China

Lijie Fu[1] *and Qingli Wang*[2]
[1]*SNLB, China*
[2]*Center for Drug Evaluation, SFDA, China*

8.1 Introduction

China's pharmaceutical market has been growing at more than 15% on average since 1978, and continues to grow at nearly 20% annually. In 2010, the total pharmaceutical market size, including the active pharmaceutical ingredient (API), chemical finished product, biological product, Traditional Chinese Medicine (TCM) and medical instruments, was around US$200 billion. According to a report released by IMS Health, the Chinese pharmaceutical market could double by 2013. The sale of prescription drugs will grow to approximately US$40 billion by 2013 (IMS, 2012). The industrial environment in China has been transformed for the better, and pharmaceutical-related regulations have been implemented over the last 10 years. However, companies entering into the Chinese pharmaceutical market will continue to face challenges. Amongst them are the significant regulatory differences between China and other parts of the world. It is crucial for the pharmaceutical industry to understand the regulatory system in order to be competitive.

While creating an open and fair market and promoting a rapid, healthy and sustainable development of the pharmaceutical industry, China has recognized the importance of drug safety by gradually establishing a legal framework which includes state law, regulations and guidelines, and the enhancement and centralization of the authority of the drug regulatory agency and organization. Since the founding of the People's Republic of China, and especially during the past 30 years, China has been continuously improving its drug safety administration organization, drug safety technical supporting system and related laws and regulations to ensure the organizational and legal support of the drug registration

Nonclinical Safety Assessment: A Guide to International Pharmaceutical Regulations, First Edition.
Edited by William J. Brock, Kenneth L. Hastings and Kathy M. McGown.

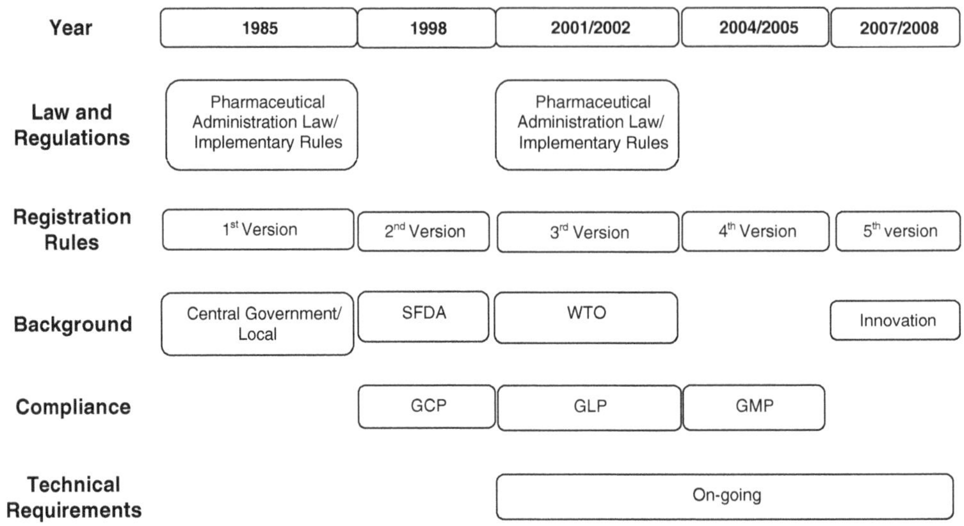

Figure 8.1 History of drug administration and registration in China.

and marketing infrastructure. Based on national conditions and with reference to international experience and focusing on the improvement of drug safety, effectiveness and quality control, China has established an administrative infrastructure covering all areas of research, production, distribution and use of drugs. Since China became a member of the World Trade Organization (WTO) in 2001, the Chinese government has taken, to a certain degree, the necessary steps to standardize the country's pharmaceutical market in order to meet the general requirements of pharmaceutical globalization (China State Council Information Office, 2008).

Compared to the long history of the country, China's regulatory system is in its infancy. The pharmaceutical regulations are still in development and are becoming more streamlined and consistent with international standards and practices (Figure 8.1). However, the Chinese regulatory system remains significantly different from regulatory systems in other countries including the US, Europe and Japan. Its "categorized registration of drugs" makes it more complicated than other countries.

8.2 History of Drug Administration

The earliest regulations on drug registration in China can be traced back to the early 1960s. In 1963, the first regulation, "Rules on Drug Administration", was issued jointly by three Central Government ministries: the Ministries of Health, Chemical Industry and Commerce. This rule defined when a pharmaceutical was a "new product" and laid out procedures for registration, clinical trials and approval of manufacture and marketing of pharmaceuticals. It also established a committee to review and approve applications. In

1965, the Ministries of Health and Chemical Industry issued the "Regulation for Administration of New Pharmaceutical Products". Although this regulation further defined the responsibility with detailed procedures, it had not been consistently enforced since the Cultural Revolution (1966–1978) which occurred shortly after its promulgation.

In 1978, China's State Council promulgated its first "Regulation for Drug Administration of the People's Republic of China" which was issued by the Ministry of Health as the "Rules on New Drug Administration of the People's Republic of China" in 1979. These were comprehensive and systematic regulations and rules that specified definition, classification, preclinical research, clinical trials, identification and analysis, regulatory approval and market entry of new pharmaceuticals. The responsibility for drug registration and approval was divided into two levels. At the national level, the Ministry of Public Health of the Central Government is responsible for products that are "novel", new radioactive substances, controlled substances, birth control drugs, and synthesized traditional Chinese medicines. The responsibilities for other categories including small molecule drugs (primarily generic drugs) are administrated by government agencies at the provincial level. This division of responsibility caused some problems since there were no national standards and guidelines across the whole of China.

In 1984, the Standing Committee of the National People's Congress (NPC) adopted the "Drug Administration Law of the People's Republic of China" (the Drug Law). This new law governed the research, production, marketing and use of drugs. In addition, the law specified the control of production and enforcement against illegal marketing of counterfeit and inferior drugs. The law requires that market entry of pharmaceuticals is subject to regulatory inspection and must be prequalified by regulatory authorities at the provincial level. Production or distribution permits are granted only when enterprises meet the requirements, and then a business license is issued. Only licensed enterprises are allowed to produce or market a drug. By law, applicants for new drug registration must submit a set of technical documents prior to initiation of a clinical trial, which include manufacturing information and pharmacology and toxicology data, and which are then subject to safety evaluation and regulatory approval.

To comply with the Drug Law, in 1985 the Ministry of Health (the national drug authority then), formulated the "Regulations for New Drug Evaluation and Approval". This regulation specifically focused on new drug evaluation and registration and outlined the regulatory procedures and technical requirements for a new drug application. These changes have led to a centralized authority for drug approval. According to the regulation, prior to production of new pharmaceuticals, sponsors must submit nonclinical and clinical data for regulatory review and approval for efficacy and safety and the nonclinical research and clinical trials must follow national standards. Since this regulation laid out regulatory rules on registration for the first time in Chinese history, it is considered the first version of the Provisions for Drug Registration. In 1988 and 1992, the Ministry of Health supplemented the Regulations for New Drug Evaluation and Approval with two special rules which defined and detailed requirements on Traditional Chinese Medicine (TCM) and biological products.

In 1995, China started to explore a more categorized administrative oversight of drugs, biologics and medical products and devices, and the State Drug Administration (SDA) was established as the administrative and regulatory body of the central government of China. The agency was responsible for administrative and technical supervision over the research, production, distribution and use of drugs including TCM raw material, TCM tablets, TCM preparations, chemical drug substances and their preparations, antibiotics, biologics, radioactive pharmaceuticals, serum, vaccines, blood products and diagnostic agents and medical devices. In 1999, China promulgated the Measures for the Categorized Administration of Prescription and OTC Drugs, which resulted in implementing specific regulatory divisions and administration processes for prescription and OTC drugs. Also in 1999, the SDA revised the Regulations for New Drug Evaluation and Approval and promulgated several other regulations, including the Regulations for Import Drugs, Regulations for New Biologics Evaluation and Approval, Regulations for Administration of Generic Drugs, and Regulations for New Drug Protection and Technology Transformation. The *Regulations* for New Drug Evaluation and Approval redefined the definition of a "new drug" as "pharmaceuticals not yet produced/manufactured in China". This regulation has incorporated some of the common regulatory practices seen in other regions, and it was a turning point towards international harmonization. For example, accelerated (expedited) procedures were established for certain categories of pharmaceuticals, such as drugs for cancer, HIV, and new formulas or indications of some TCMs that are protected as national trade secrets.

In 2001, the China significantly revised its drug administrative law, the "Drug Administration Law of the People's Republic of China" (DALPRC, 2001). The revised law unified drug standards, abolished regional standards and provided the legal framework for the drug administration to ensure drug safety. The revised law states that any drug manufacturer, drug distributor, institution for nonclinical safety study, or institution for clinical trials, must comply with good manufacturing practice (GMP), good supply practice (GSP, for pharmaceutical products), good laboratory practice (GLP) or good clinical practice (GCP). Specifically, the new version of the law clearly states that "institutions for nonclinical safety evaluation study and clinical study shall respectively implement GLP and GCP." Failure to comply with the regulations can result in warnings accompanied by instructions to rectify the violations within a specified time limit. If the organization fails to comply, it will be instructed to suspend production, business operations or other work until the violations are rectified.

To enforce the revised law, in 2002 the State Council of China promulgated the "Regulations for the Implementation of the Drug Administration Law of the People's Republic of China" (2002). This regulation once again defined a "new drug" as "pharmaceuticals not yet marketed in China". China implemented "The Implementation Regulations of the Drug Administration Law of the People's Republic of China" (amended in 2002), a policy for the protection of drug data that provides a data exclusivity period of six years.

Following the 2002 revision of the drug law and the regulation for implementation, "Provisions for Drug Registration" was formulated, and the five regulations issued in 1999, including the "Regulations for New Drug Evaluation and Approval", were abolished. Under the new "Provisions for Drug Registration", the scope of a new drug application was defined as an application to apply for registration of a pharmaceutical that had not been marketed. Additionally, changes in formulation and route of administration for marketed pharmaceuticals would also be regulated as "new drug". The regulation authorizes provincial drug authorities to "pre-evaluate" new drug applications and conduct on-site inspections of research institutes and manufacturing sites. Drug samples from the sites are also to be taken by the provincial authority for testing and verification to support registration instead of being submitted by the sponsors, as done previously. The regulation also clearly states that a new drug application must be complete at the time of submission or the application would be returned for resubmission. Additional Administrative Rules of Drug Registration and other policies have been issued since to resolve some issues in the implementation of the "Provisions for Drug Registration".

In 2003, the State Drug Administration (SDA) became the State Food and Drug Administration (SFDA), and China continues to establish the organization of drug authorities under the unified leadership of the central government.

To comply with the Administrative Permission Law of the People's Republic of China, and in response to some of the challenges in carrying out the "Provisions for Drug Registration", a series of regulatory rules and guidance have been included in a revision. The revision further clarified key definitions, standardized regulatory requirements for drug applications, and detailed procedures of submission, review and approval, and emphasized the legal obligations of the regulatory agency.

The revised law defines both the Inspection of Drugs and Legal Liabilities. The law grants SFDA the authority to supervise drug research and development, production and distribution, and use of drugs in medical institutions, and to conduct selective inspection and testing of drug quality. The regulation also specifically addresses fraudulent practices and states that providing any false documents, data or samples to the regulatory agency or obtaining the license by any other fraudulent means will result in a withdrawal or revocation of the drug approval for a period of five years, accompanied by a fine.

The regulation also gives the SFDA and the local organization (local SFDA) authority to supervise and inspect the research and development, production, distribution and use of drugs in accordance with the Drug Administration Law. Clinical trials, manufacturing or importation will be reviewed and approved by the SFDA, and the SFDA can authorize its local SFDA to conduct inspections of research and development sites, to conduct preliminary reviews of the submitted dossier, and to test the pilot samples. The SFDA is also authorized by the regulation to re-evaluate approved drugs. It can request revision of the package insert, suspend production, marketing or use of a drug, or even withdraw the approval. All approvals include a drug approval number, an Import Licence and Pharmaceutical Product Licence that are valid for five years. To continue the production or importation, the applicant has to submit a re-registration application six months prior to the expiry date of the approved license.

For production of a drug admitted by the national standards, an applicant submits technical data and supporting documents to the local SFDA. The local authority should review the application, and provide a review opinion, inspection report and the application dossier to the SFDA of the central government for a full review and notify the applicant within 30 working days of receipt. If all requirements are fulfilled upon review, the national SFDA will issue an approval number. When a drug is produced to an interim standard, an applicant should make a submission for formalization of the standard three months prior to the expiry of the interim standard. The national SFDA should review and approve the interim standard as formal one within 12 months if all requirements are met for formalization. If an applicant does not apply for, or the original interim standard fails to fulfill the requirements for formalization, the agency will withdraw the interim standard and also the approval number for drug production.

8.3 The Provisions for Drug Registration

Chapter 2 of the Provisions (Application for Drug Registration) requires that a domestic applicant shall be legally registered within the territory of China. An application from an overseas applicant for import registration must be done by its branch or entrusted agency within the territory of China.

The Provisions define nonclinical drug studies for registration applications as evaluations of the drug synthetic processes, extraction methods, physical and chemical properties, purity, selection of dosage form, screening of formula, preparation processes, testing methods, quality specifications, stability, nonclinical pharmacology, toxicology and pharmacokinetics. For biological products, it also includes studies on the source, quality specifications, storage conditions, biological characteristics and genetic stability of the starting materials such as bacterial or viral stocks/strains, cell lines, and tissues. All preclinical drug research "shall be in conformity with relevant requirement", and GLP for "nonclinical laboratory studies shall be implemented in the study of safety evaluation".

The Provisions require that the nonclinical studies be conducted according to the relevant technical guidelines issued by the SFDA. Otherwise, supporting data on scientific feasibility of other methods and techniques must be provided in the application. The Provisions also state that the drug research institution shall have adequate staff, equipment and management systems to ensure the "authenticity of all experimental data". Applicants, including those who outsourced all or part of research to other institutions, are responsible for the authenticity of the research data in their application dossier. The SFDA can request the applicant or the drug research institution responsible for testing to repeat the test based on the items, methods and data specified in the application documents, and also to authorize a drug testing institute or another drug research institution to repeat the test or conduct methodological verification.

For data in the application dossier provided by an overseas research institution, the applicant shall attach to the data notarized documents which prove that the research institution is legally registered overseas. The SFDA can send its staff to conduct on-site inspection if needed for the drug review.

Regulatory testing for drug registration is an important step in the approval process in China. This regulatory testing consists of sample testing and verification of specifications. Sample testing refers to the testing of samples conducted by a drug testing institute according to the specifications submitted by an applicant or verified by the SFDA. Verification of specifications refers to the laboratory testing and review conducted by a drug testing institute on the feasibility and scientific basis of the testing methods and the control of the drug quality in the submitted specifications. The National Institutes for Food and Drug Control (NIFDC) or the drug testing institutes of the local SFDA shall take charge of the testing for drug registration. Testing of import drugs, biological products and radioactive pharmaceuticals in support of registration, and that of some categories of new drugs for special review and approval, should be arranged only by the NIFDC.

All institutes engaged in testing for drug registration must be in compliance with the requirements set out by the SFDA GLP, have qualified personnel and adequate equipment, and comply with the quality assurance system and technical requirements of the testing for drug registration.

8.4 The SFDA

The SFDA's major responsibilities in regulating pharmaceuticals are (SFDA, 2010):

1. Formulating policies and programmes in regulating pharmaceuticals, and participating in drafting relevant laws, regulations and normative documents;
2. Administrative and technical supervision of drugs and medical devices, formulating good practices for research, production, distribution and use of drugs, medical devices, and supervision of the implementation of these practices;
3. Registration of drugs and medical devices; drafting national standards for drugs and medical devices, and supervising their implementation; carrying out the Adverse Drug Reaction (ADR) monitoring and adverse event monitoring on medical devices, as well as re-evaluation and elimination; organizing the implementation of a classification system for prescription and nonprescription drugs;
4. Formulating regulations of TCMs and drugs, and supervising their implementation, setting up quality standards, and formulating Good Agricultural Practices (GAP) for Chinese crude drugs and Processing Standards and supervising their implementation, and execution of the national protection system for certain TCMs;
5. Supervising the quality and safety of drugs and medical devices and regulating radioactive pharmaceuticals, narcotics, toxicants and psychotropic drugs, and release quality and safety information of drugs and medical devices;
6. Organizing the investigation and punishment of illegal activities in the research, production, distribution and use of drugs and medical devices;
7. Instructing local authorities on drug administration, emergency response, inspection, and other related works;
8. Carrying out international exchanges and cooperation that relate to pharmaceutical administration and regulation.

The Department of Drug Registration in the agency responsible for drug registration has three divisions in charge of registrations for chemical drugs, biologics, and TCMs respectively, with a division for drug research monitoring and inspection, and one for administrative and coordinate office.

8.5 The SFDA Affiliated Organizations

Sixteen affiliated organizations operate directly under the SFDA, nine of them providing technical and other support to the SFDA (Table 8.1).

The three more prominent centres and NIFDC related to drug approval are described below.

8.5.1 Center for Drug Evaluation (CDE)

This is one of the first regulatory institutions in pharmaceutical evaluation in China. The Center, formerly called the Office of Drug Evaluation and Approval, was established in 1985, one year after the Drug Law was adopted. The CDE is the SFDA's institution that provides technical review and other technical supports for drug registration. The CDE's

Table 8.1 *Affiliated organizations of the SFDA.*

National Institutes for Food and Drug Control
Chinese Pharmacopoeia Commission
Center for Drug Evaluation
Certification Committee for Drugs
National Committee on the Assessment of Protected Traditional Chinese Medicinal Products (Center for Health Food Evaluation)
Center for Drug Re-evaluation (National Center for ADR Monitoring)
Center for Medical Device Evaluation
Information Center
Institute of Executive Development
China Center for Pharmaceutical International Exchange

mission is to support drug registration and administration in its scientific development, standardization and modernization, and to organize and carry out technical reviews of applications for registration of new drugs, generic drugs, and import drugs, according to the national law and regulations in pharmaceuticals administration.

8.5.2 Center for Drug Re-evaluation (CDR)

The primary responsibilities of the CDR are:

1. To provide technical and coordinated support for the SFDA on the implementation of the nation's categorized administration between prescription and OTC drugs, including generating and updating the national "basic drug" list and OTC list;
2. Responsibility for drug re-evaluation as well as review and surveillance of the safety of drugs on the market, and abolishment of unsafe drugs;
3. To provide technical support for the SFDA on the national reporting and monitoring of adverse drug reactions (ADR), and to provide technical guidance to ADR monitoring institutions at the level of provincial, autonomous regions and municipalities;
4. To provide technical support for the SFDA on the national monitoring and re-evaluation system for the adverse event of medical devices, and provide technical guidance to monitoring institutions at the level of provincial, autonomous regions and municipalities.

8.5.3 Certification Committee for Drugs (CCD)

The Certification Committee for Drugs (CCD) was established to prepare standards for GLP, GCP, GAP, GSP and GMP and provisions for their implementation as well as inspection of facilities that conduct studies.

8.5.4 National Institutes for Food and Drug Control (NIFDC)

NIFDC, formally called the National Institute for the Control of Pharmaceuticals and Biological Products (NIFDC), is one of the first institutions established for regulating pharmaceuticals. As an affiliated organization of the SFDA, the NIFDC performs up to 15 "major functions". Designated by the Provisions for Drug Registration, NIFDC's primary role includes conducting sample testing and verification for drug, biological product and radiopharmaceutical registration. It is responsible for the characterization of national reference standards and includes organizing the relevant drug testing institutes of provinces, autonomous regions, and municipalities of SFDA, drug research institutions or drug manufacturers to undertake collaborative assays of the standards. The NIFDC is responsible for the overall technical evaluation of the characterized reference standards with respect to source material selection, preparation methods, testing methods and results, accuracy of value assignment, traceability, stability, filling and packaging conditions and for making decisions on whether or not the candidate materials can be used as "national reference standards" (SFDA, 2007b). The organization also carries out many other functions such as drug safety evaluation, testing method research, development and standardization, conservation of strains of laboratory animals (rodent) and their quality monitoring.

8.6 General Registration Procedures

Drug evaluation and registration in China is governed by different categories, and thus the requirements of regulatory submission depend on the categories applied.

Currently, pharmaceuticals in China are categorized into three types: TCM and botanicals, chemical pharmaceuticals, and biologics. Each of these categories is further classified into "classes". There are nine classes under TCM and botanicals (eight are treated as "new drugs"), six classes of chemicals (five are administrated as "new drugs"), and 15 classes of biologics (14 of which are "new biologics"). Requirements and procedures between an international application and domestic applications are different. In other words, sponsors outside China must follow the requirements and procedures of "import drugs".

As mentioned previously, there are five types of applications for drug registrations in China: new drugs; generic drugs; import drugs and their supplementary applications; and re-registration applications. Application for new drugs refers to application for registration of drugs that have not been marketed within China, and includes changes in dosage form or route of administration, or claims for a new indication for currently marketed drugs. Application for generic drugs refers to registration application for producing the drugs that have an "approved national drug standard" for marketing by the SFDA, whereas the application for biological products must be submitted as the process of new drug application.

8.7 Pharmaceutical Application

Application for new chemical pharmaceuticals refers to an application for the registration of a new chemical entity that has not been marketed within China. It has been classified into six classes and 10 sub-classes (Table 8.2).

The dossiers required in China must contain four parts:

Part 1 General Data and Administrative Documents
Part 2 Chemical, Pharmaceutical and Biological Data
Part 3 Pharmacological and Toxicological Data
Part 4 Clinical Data.

Table 8.2 Classification of NCE by SFDA.

Classification	Sub-classification
Class I: Drug not previously registered in China or other countries	I-1 Synthesized or semi-synthesized active ingredient and its formulation I-2 NME and its formulation which is extracted or fermented from natural products I-3 Optical isomer and its formulation from existing product I-4 New formulation with less components prepared from a marketed drug with more components I-5 New "fixed-dose compounds" (i.e., formulated with multiple components) I-6 New indication of a drug marketed in China that has not been approved domestically or abroad
Class II: New route of administration not previously approved in China or other countries	None
Class III: Drug approved in other countries but not in China	III-1 A drug (and its active ingredients) marketed abroad, and/or a new dosage form of those drugs without change in route of administration III-2 Fixed-dose compounds marketed abroad, and/or a new dosage form of those drugs without change in route of administration III-3 New route of administration of a drug marketed abroad III-4 New indication of approved drugs in other countries and marketed in China
Class IV: Changing the salt form without changing the pharmacological activity of a marketed drug	None
Class V: Changing the dosage form without changing the route of administration	None
Class VI: Drugs currently marketed in China	None

Reproduced from http://eng.sfda.gov.cn/WS03/CL0769/61658.html and http://eng.sfda.gov.cn/WS03/CL0769/61657.html. Copyright (2012) SFDA Last accessed 15/08/2012.

Part 3 of the dossier (Data number 16 to 27, see below) are nonclinical data to support the efficacy and safety of the new drug substance. The contents of this section include:

- Summary of nonclinical pharmacology and toxicology;
- Primary pharmacodynamics;
- Safety pharmacology;
- Single dose toxicity;
- Repeated dose toxicity;

- Local tolerance study, including immunological study, phototoxicity, haemolytic and irritation tests, and other special toxicity;
- Interaction of multiple components in fixed-dose compound on efficacy, toxicity, pharmacokinetics;.
- Genetic toxicity;
- Development and reproductive toxicity;
- Carcinogenicity;
- Preclinical data on drug dependence study;
- Nonclinical pharmacokinetics.

8.8 Import Drug Application

Application for importing chemical pharmaceuticals follows the requirements of domestic application. For an NCE that has not been marketed in China or abroad, it must be in at least in Phase II abroad, and application should submit the same dossiers as Class I, while other NCEs follow the requirements of Class III. The SFDA accepts applications in a CTD format that follows ICH guidelines. The data on specifications and test methods of API, and finished product must be in the format of Chinese Pharmacopoeia.

The application must be in Chinese, but data in other languages can be appended as references.

Although there is no clear distinction between the European (EMA) clinical trial applications (CTA) or the US NDA and the Chinese dossier, the application procedure for importing drugs into China can be divided into two steps clinical trial approval and import drug license (Figure 8.2).

One of the important procedures in Step 1 is to deliver the CMC section of the dossier to NIFDC within two weeks after filing the application with the SFDA Registration Office and obtaining a Notification of Acceptance. With the NIFDC's request, applicants may have to deliver three batches of testing samples to NIFDC for testing and verification. It may take 60–90 working days for the testing in NIFDC, while technical evaluations are conducted by CDE (90 or 80 working days for regular approval). If any deficiencies are found in the dossier, the SFDA may request the sponsor to submit supplemental information within 3–4 months after the request is issued to the sponsor. Following responses, the SFDA may take an additional 30–50 working days to review the supplemental information. The agency might also call for an advisory committee meeting in which the sponsor can make presentations and answer reviewers' questions prior to the CDE submitting the final report of evaluation and recommendation to the SFDA Registration Department and the SFDA Registration Department issuing a clinical trial permit (CTP). All of these processes could be undertaken in parallel with the NIFDC testing.

If there is variation, addition, or cancellation of the items or contents approved in the original application for an imported drug, a supplementary application must be submitted. For the purpose of the supplemental application, a sponsor should assess the implications of the variation for the safety, efficacy and quality of the drug, and conduct corresponding technical studies following relevant guidelines, and submit relevant dossier and

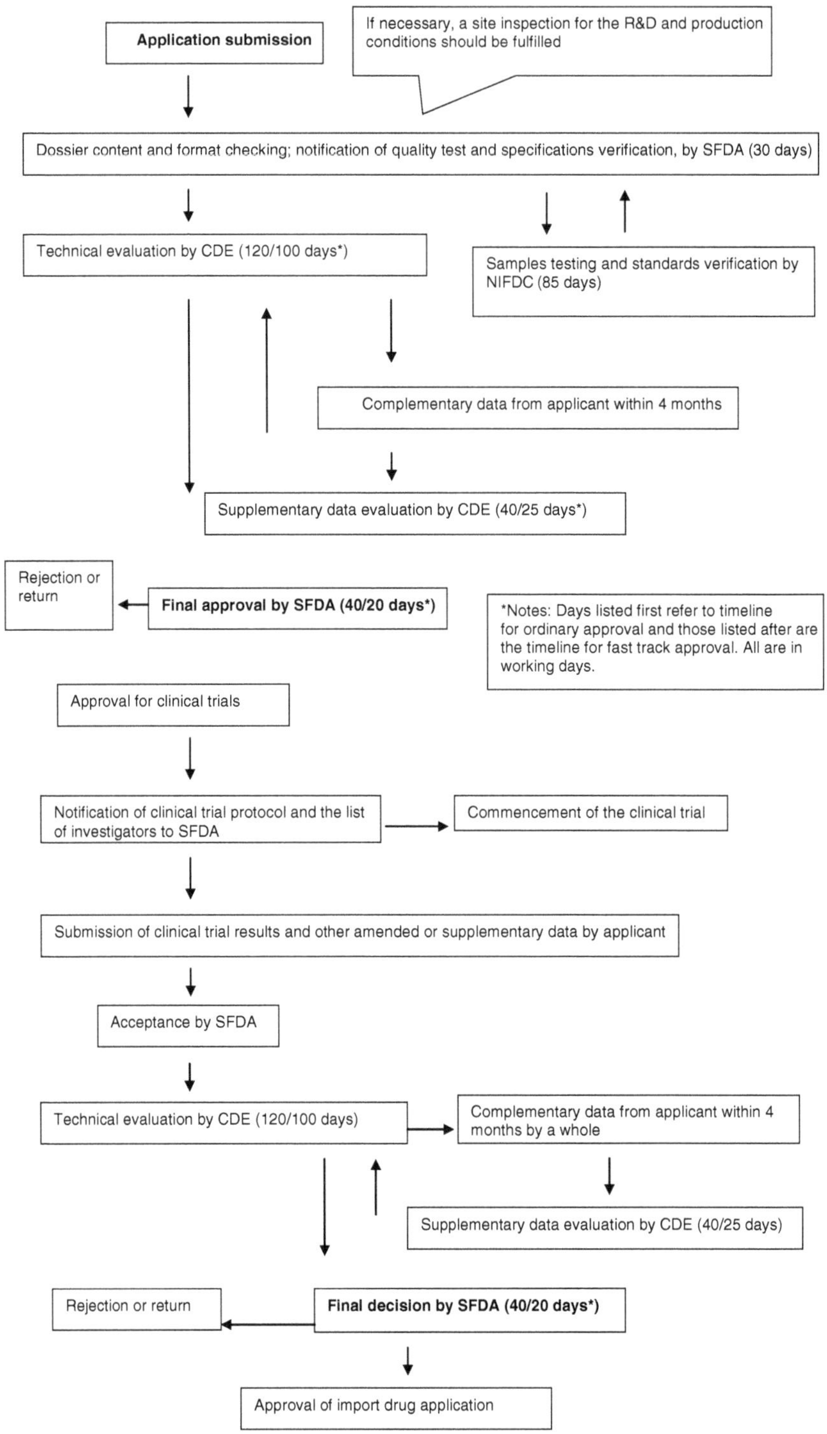

Figure 8.2 *Application and approval procedure for import drugs. Source: http://eng.sfda.gov.cn/WS03/CL0769/61658.html; http://eng.sfda.gov.cn/WS03/CL0769/61657.html).*

explanations to the SFDA, and documents approving the variation issued by regulatory agency of the producing country. The SFDA will conduct the preliminary review of the application dossiers, and issue an acceptance notice of drug registration application if requirements are met, or issue a non-acceptance notice for the drug registration application if requirements are not met. In the case of a non-acceptance notice, the reasons for non-acceptance will be given.

In conclusion, China has made excellent progress on drug registration regulations, including well-defined regulatory guidelines, increased emphasis on innovative medicines and product safety and quality. However, there are still significant challenges, especially to global pharmaceutical companies or sponsors abroad ("international applicant"). Some examples of the challenges are the complicated application and approval process due to categorized registration, and different procedures between domestic and international sponsors.

8.9 Testing Guidelines and Safety Evaluation

According to the Provisions for Drug Registration, the study is conducted according to the relevant technical guidelines issued by the SFDA. Where an applicant conducts the study by adopting other evaluation methods and techniques, the scientific feasibility of alternative methods and techniques must be provided.

Since 2002, the SFDA has begun to issue technical guidelines for testing, submission and technical evaluation. A total of 75 guidelines have been issued by the CDE of SFDA, consisting of 30 for chemical, 13 for TCM, 26 for biologics, and six for technical evaluation. In 2009, the CDE changed its approach to guidelines and began translating and adopting international guidelines with necessary modifications. The first guideline using this approach, Guidelines for Necessity of Carcinogenicity Research of Drugs, was officially issued in May 2010. Twenty SFDA guidelines on toxicological testing and safety evaluation have been issued (Table 8.3). Although the guidelines can be found on the SFDA webpage (www.sfda.gov.cn), they are not available in English.

These regulatory guidelines cover most of the areas in toxicological testing and safety evaluation. When comparing them with ICH and US FDA guidance, however, some guidelines have not yet been issued. Additionally, depending on the time of issuance, differences might exist between the SFDA and international guidelines for the same type of study. Nevertheless, SFDA now accepts studies conducted abroad that follow ICH guidance.

One example of such a difference is in the Guidance for Nonclinical Pharmacokinetic Study of Chemical Drugs. This guidance provides details of dose levels, number of animals, sampling points (at least 9–14 time-points) and parameters that should included, e.g., $t_{1/2}$, Vd, CL, C_{max} and T_{max}, $AUC_{(0-t)}$. The guidance does not require cross-validation of analytical method, and metabolite data are only required if excretion of the parent compound is less than 50% of the administered dose. Another example is the guideline for acute toxicity study of chemical drugs which covers single-dose or repeat-doses within 24 hours. For animal selection, there is a requirement to use both rodent and nonrodent species. Rationale and justification must be provided on a case-by-case basis for not including a nonrodent species. The dose selection should include the range from no

Table 8.3 *SFDA Technical Guidelines on Safety Testing and Evaluation (selected).*

General and Chemical Drugs

- Guidance for Non-clinical Pharmacokinetic Study of Chemical Pharmaceuticals (Issued in 2005)
- Guidance for Acute Toxicology of Chemical Pharmaceuticals
- Guidance for Chronic Toxicology of Chemical Pharmaceuticals
- Guidance for General Pharmacology of Chemical Pharmaceuticals
- Guidance for Irritation, Allergy and Haemolysis Research of Chemical Pharmaceuticals
- Guidance for Summary Format and Content Composed of Chemical Drugs – Summary of Pharmacology and Toxicology Research
- Guidance for Genotoxicity Testing of Pharmaceuticals
- Guidance for Dependency Studies of Pharmaceuticals
- Guidance for Evaluation of Cytotoxic Anti-cancer Pharmaceuticals
- Guidance for Development and Reproductive Toxicity Studies of Pharmaceuticals
- Guidance for Necessity of Carcinogenicity Studies of Pharmaceuticals

Biologics

- Guidance for Preclinical Studies of Preventive DNA Vaccine
- Guidance for Preclinical Safety Studies of Preventive Biologic Products
- Guidance for Preclinical Studies of Preventive Vaccines

TCM and Botanicals

- Guidance for Acute Toxicology of Traditional Chinese Medicines and Botanical Drugs
- Guidance for Chronic Toxicology of Traditional Chinese Medicines and Botanical Drugs
- Guidance for General Pharmacology of Traditional Chinese Medicines and Botanical Drugs
- Guidance for Local Irritation and Haemolysis of Traditional Chinese Medicines and Botanical Drugs
- Guidance for Immunotoxicity (Allergy, Photoallergy) of Traditional Chinese Medicines and Botanical Drugs
  Guidance for Summary Format and Content Compose of Traditional Chinese Medicines and Botanical Drugs – Pharmacology and Toxicology Research

toxicity observed to severe toxicity ("life threatening"). Although it is mentioned that death is not a necessary parameter for a study in nonrodent species, determination of the LD_{50} is still widely used in acute toxicity studies in China.

The recently issued Guideline on Necessity for Carcinogenicity Study of Pharmaceuticals was adopted, with some modifications, from the ICH S1A, Guideline on the Need for Carcinogenicity Study of Pharmaceuticals (ICH, 1995). The guidance applies not only for chemical drugs but can also apply to TCM, pharmaceuticals derived from "natural products" (botanicals), and biological therapeutics. This is one of the few test guidelines in China that applies to all categories of drugs, while most of other, earlier guidelines are specifically for one category of product. It is also the first time that such guidelines encourage interactions between sponsors and the regulatory agency.

Another major change is that this guideline does not include the section of Genotoxicity (4.3) from "Factors to Consider for Carcinogenicity Testing (4.0)". According to the SFDA, the primary reason for not adopting this section is that the background information of the section is not yet fully understood, especially with "unequivocally genotoxic compounds". The CDE made this decision after multiple internal and external discussions including exchanges with former reviewers of US FDA and did not reach an agreement; it plans to revisit this issue in the future.

8.10 GLP Compliance in China

As mentioned previously, the current version of China's Drug Administration Law (the Drug Law, 2001) clearly states that "institutions for nonclinical safety evaluation study and clinical study shall respectively implement GLP for nonclinical laboratory studies and GCP for clinical trial". Any drug manufacturer, drug distributor, institution for nonclinical safety study, or institution for drug clinical trials that does not implement good laboratory practice (GLP) will be given a disciplinary warning and be instructed to rectify their practice within a certain time limit.

The "Good Laboratory Practice (GLP) for Nonclinical Laboratory Studies" (proposed) was promulgated by the State Science and Technology Commission in 1993, and became effective in 1994. In 1999, the predecessor to the SFDA, the Bureau of Drug Administration (SDA) proposed a draft version of nonclinical GLP regulations, which was approved after several years of validation by the government. At the same time, "Inspection of Nonclinical GLP Certification (proposed)" was issued and took effect in 2003 (SFDA, 2003). A supplemental document requires all safety evaluation studies on new drugs to be conducted in GLP-compliant laboratories, otherwise the SFDA will not accept the application. All toxicological data for new drug registrations must be generated in SFDA-certified GLP laboratories. Although these regulations have had a very positive influence on the industry, they also pose challenges to international laboratories which follow US GLPs and have not been certified for Chinese GLP compliance.

In general, SFDA GLP follow the format of the US FDA regulations; therefore, the final Chinese version of the GLP regulations is very similar to that of the US. There are differences between the China and US GLPs although they might not cause potential problems in terms of different testing and compliance requirements. However, there could be some differences in laboratory systems and daily operation of a testing facility (Jia et al., 2007).

A major difference to make note of is that the US does not require laboratories to be "certified" or "accredited" in order to conduct GLP studies. In contrast, laboratories in China must be certified for GLP compliance by the SFDA.

Another important difference to note is in the dates of study initiation and completion. For the SFDA, the dates of protocol and final report approval by test facility management are the study initiation dates and study completion dates. This is in contrast to the US FDA where the study initiation date and completion date are the dates when the protocol and final report are signed by the study director. This reflects the greater weight of responsibility given to the test facility management under SFDA GLP.

While the personnel requirements are similar in general between US FDA and SFDA, the SFDA has specific educational requirements for test facility management. For SFDA, the facility management is required to have an education above the Bachelor degree level in medicine, pharmacology or other related fields and adequate professional qualities and abilities. US FDA only speaks generally about qualifications in the sections covering personnel and does not provide specific educational requirements. There are major differences in management responsibilities under SFDA GLP. Test facility management has the overall responsibility for the establishment, organization and management of the nonclinical test facility. Moreover, SFDA places the responsibility of establishing documentation for the personnel including education, professional trainings and experience with facility management, as well as the administrative functions of creating a master schedule and tracking the progress of the ongoing studies. Under SFDA GLP, management is also required to take the lead in generating and updating standard operating procedures (SOPs) and to ensure that personnel clearly understand the SOPs related to the function they are to perform.

Under the SFDA GLP, the Quality Assurance Unit has additional responsibilities and requirements that include review of the study protocol and periodic inspection of the animal facilities, laboratory instruments and archiving, SOP development and maintenance, and the schedule for audit activities based on the nature and duration of the study. Many of these responsibilities are implied but are not specifically addressed in the FDA GLP. In addition, the SFDA requires that the study director ensures all personnel involved in the study clearly understand their function and the applicable SOPs. It also requires that the study director ensures study data and documentation follow the SOPs and provides suggestions for revising or supplementing procedures in a timely manner.

SFDA GLP requires that the animal facility shall be suitably designed and appropriately equipped. Environmental conditions such as temperature, humidity and air ventilation, lighting and other conditions should be able to be adjusted on an as-needed basis. Animal environments shall meet the national requirements for the grade/class of animals housed. The animal housing facility shall include housing areas for different animal species and test systems. There shall be a separate area for animal quarantine and veterinary treatment. There shall be waste collection and disposal facilities, a sanitization area and a designated area for bio-hazardous material/wastes. For waste disposal, the SFDA GLP consider potential adverse effects that should be avoided or prevented. US FDA GLP also requires that separate laboratory space be provided, as needed, for the performance of the routine and specialized procedures required by nonclinical laboratory studies. This is an area which is not addressed by SFDA.

The GLP Certification process is designed to be an overall evaluation of regulatory compliance by a nonclinical laboratory. The process includes inspection of the organization, personnel, facility and equipment, study conduct and management. To be eligible to apply for the certification, a laboratory needs to operate under GLP for at least one year and complete at least one study in full GLP compliance. The SFDA accept applications for one or more of the following categories:

- Single and multiple dose toxicology study in rodents
- Single and multiple dose toxicology study in nonrodents
- Reproductive and developmental toxicology (Segment I, Segment II, Segment III)
- Genetic toxicology (Ames, micronucleus, chromosome aberration, L5178Y mouse lymphoma test)
- Carcinogenicity study
- Local toxicology study
- Immunogenicity study
- Safety pharmacology study

- Dependency study
- Toxicokinetic study
- Safety evaluation test for radioactive material
- Safety evaluation test for bio-hazardous material
- Other toxicity study

The Certification process could take several months to a year from application to "approval", with multiple steps in between. In short, the applications, usually a package of 130–150 pages in Chinese, are submitted to the SFDA local office for "pre-review" and then transferred to the SFDA Office of Acceptance. The division of Safety Monitoring and Inspection in Drug Registration Department is the regulatory authority for the certification. The Certification Committee for Drugs, authorized by the Safety Monitoring and Inspection Division, is responsible for on-site inspection and technical evaluation.

8.11 Animal Welfare Requirements

Preclinical studies, as well as other types of biomedical research in China, are required to comply with national law, and national and local regulations and guidance ("standards") on laboratory animal care and use, often referred to as animal welfare.

The first regulation specifically for laboratory animal welfare in China was the "Regulation for Laboratory Animals", approved and promulgated by the State Council of China in 1988. This regulation states that animal breeding, production and transportation, and use of animals in biomedical teaching and research are subject to the restrictions of the Regulation, which applies to all institutions and individuals involved in the above activities. It also authorizes the State Science and Technology Commission (SSTC), the predecessor to the Ministry of Science and Technology (MST), as the nation's regulatory and administrative body on laboratory animals. Since then, several regulations, guidance and national standards have been issued by MST, including Guidance for Laboratory Animal Welfare (2006), and some provinces and municipalities have adopted local regulations and/administrative rules as well. All of these are very similar to international standards and practice such as the Guide for the Care and Use of Laboratory Animals (National Research Council, 1996).

The first AAALAC International accredited animal care and use programme in China was fully accredited in February 2006. By February 2012, the number of accredited units had reached 34, and 18 are involved in preclinical research and safety evaluation studies. With this noteworthy progress, China begins to hold a leading position in number of units accredited by AAALAC International in the Asian region, and becomes the fastest growing area in a number of application across the world (AAALAC, 2012).

References

AAALAC International (2012) www.aaalac.org.

China State Council Information Office (2008) White Paper on Drug Safety Administration in China, www.sfda.gov.cn.

Drug Administration Law of the People's Republic of China, 1 December (2001) www.sfda.gov.cn.

ICH (1995) S1A:Guideline on the need for carcinogenicity study of pharmaceuticals. www.ich.org.

IMS (2012) "China Could Be 3rd Largest Pharma Market By 2011" http://www.manufacturing.net/news/2010/03/china-could-be-3rd-largest-pharma-market-by-2011, Manufacturing.net (Advantage Business Media), retrieved 3 January 2012.

Jia, L., Zhu, Y., Wang, Y. *et al.* (2007) Harmonizing Good Laboratory Practice Rules in the US and China. RAJ Pharma Mar, 147–152.

National Research Council (1996) *Guide for the Care and Use of Laboratory Animals*, National Academy Press, Washington, D.C.

Regulations for the Implementation of the Drug Administration Law of the People's Republic of China (2002) www.sfda.gov.cn.

SFDA (2003) Non-clinical GLP regulation, the 2nd order of the SFDA Commissioner, www.sfda.gov.cn.

SFDA (2007a) Administrative Rules on GLP Certification of Non-clinical Research Institutes, SFDA Issue No 214, www.sfda.gov.cn.

SFDA (2007b) Provisions for Drug Registration, www.sfda.gov.cn.

SFDA (2010) Technical Guideline on the Need for Carcinogenicity Studies of Pharmaceuticals, www.sfda.gov.cn.

SFDA (2010) Technical Guideline for Pre-Clinical Research of Preventive Vaccines, www.sfda.gov.cn.

9

Pharmaceutical Regulations for Nonclinical Safety Assessment in Japan

Kazuichi Nakamura[1] *and Osamu Fueki*[*2]
[1]*Shionogi & Co., Ltd., Global Regulatory Affairs Department, Japan*
[2]*Pharmaceuticals and Medical Devices Agency, Japan*

9.1 History of Regulation for Nonclinical Safety Assessment in Japan

In the late 1950s to the early 1960s, the teratogenicity of thalidomide became a socially recognized problem. This tragic event set off active discussions on the need to assess the potential of adverse reactions of drugs. In response to the rise of social awareness and discussion on drug safety, the "Guideline on Nonclinical Assessment of Effects on the Fetus" was notified by the Japanese Ministry of Health and Welfare (now the Ministry of Health, Labor and Welfare; MHLW) in 1963. This was the first guideline dealing with specific toxicity testing in Japan. In 1967, "Basic Policy of Drug Manufacturing Approval" was published to define the documents required for the drug approval application. Acute toxicity, sub-acute toxicity, chronic toxicity, teratogenicity and other special toxicity such as local irritation studies were stipulated in the Policy. Thereafter, principles for the conduct of toxicity studies of combination drugs were notified in 1968, and those for dependence and reproductive toxicity studies followed in 1975.

The Pharmaceutical Affairs Law was first enforced in 1960 and underwent several revisions. In line with the 1980 revision, documents which should be attached to drug approval application were redefined, and then other additional nonclinical studies were included. According to the revision, acute toxicity, sub-acute toxicity, chronic toxicity,

[*] The views expressed in this article are those of the authors and do not necessarily reflect the official views of Pharmaceuticals and Medical Devices Agency.

Nonclinical Safety Assessment: A Guide to International Pharmaceutical Regulations, First Edition.
Edited by William J. Brock, Kenneth L. Hastings and Kathy M. McGown.

reproductive toxicity, dependence, antigenicity, mutagenicity, carcinogenicity and local irritation (tolerance) study reports were to be submitted when considering the classification of new drugs. The Japanese Good Laboratory Practice (GLP) standard for the conduct of nonclinical safety testing was indicated as the MHLW bureau notification and implemented in 1982 to ensure the quality of toxicity studies. The GLP guideline was later published as the MHLW ordinance in 1997 and revised in 2008. Guidelines for acute, sub-chronic and chronic toxicity studies, reproductive toxicity, mutagenicity and carcinogenicity studies were established in 1984 with the Food and Drug Administration (FDA) and European Medicines Agency (EMA) guidelines as the reference. Revised and newly added guidelines including single-dose toxicity, repeated-dose toxicity, reproductive and developmental toxicity, mutagenicity, carcinogenicity, skin sensitization and skin photosensitization studies were published in 1989 (MHLW, 1989).

Because of growing momentum toward marketing of drugs, mutual acceptance of study data and guidelines amongst countries and regions were increasingly demanded. The International Conference on Harmonization of Technical Requirements for Registration of Pharmaceuticals for Human Use (ICH) was organized in 1990 to harmonize technical guidelines and requirements for product registration in order to promote the prompt supply of effective and safe drugs to patients on a global scale. Most of the current Japanese nonclinical safety guidelines are consistent with the ICH safety guidelines (www.ich.org).

9.2 Approval Application of New Drugs in Japan

Documents submitted by the sponsor for drug approval application are reviewed by the PMDA (Pharmaceuticals and Medical Devices Agency) under the auspices of the MHLW. Based on the review by the PMDA, the MHLW approves the marketing of the new drug. The application and review process are illustrated in Figure 9.1. In addition to the review, the PMDA is involved in the post-marketing pharmacovigilance and relief services for adverse health effects of drugs.

9.2.1 Nonclinical Safety Studies Required for Drug Approval

Nonclinical pharmacology, absorption, distribution, metabolism and excretion (ADME) and safety studies required for ethical drug approval are described (MHLW, 2005). Tables 9.1 and 9.2 indicate basic principles of the conduct. Amongst the types

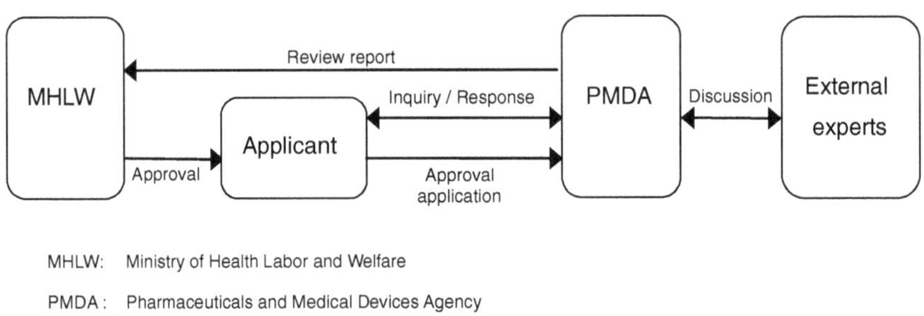

Figure 9.1 Procedures for drug approval application in Japan.

Table 9.1 *Range of nonclinical pharmacology and ADME data required for application for ethical drugs.*

Type of drugs	Pharmacology	Safety pharmacology	Other pharmacology	Absorption	Distribution	Metabolism	Excretion	Biological equivalency	Other metabolism
1. Drugs containing new active ingredients	○	○	□	○	○	○	○	×	□
2. New ethical combination drugs	○	□	□	○	○	○	○	×	□
3. Drugs with a new administration route	○	□	□	○	○	○	○	×	□
4. Drugs with a new indication	○	×	×	□	□	□	□	×	□
5. Drugs in a new dosage form	×	×	×	○	○	○	○	×	□
6. New dosage drugs	○	×	×	○	○	○	○	×	□
7. Biosimilar	○	×	×	□	□	□	□	×	□
8. Drugs supplied in an additional dosage form	×	×	×	×	×	×	×	○	×
9. Similar ethical combination drugs	□	□	×	×	×	×	×	×	×
10. Other drugs	×	×	×	×	×	×	×	○	×

○: required ×: not required □: required on a case-by-case basis.

Table 9.2 *Range of nonclinical and clinical safety data required for application for ethical drugs.*

Type of drugs	Single-dose toxicity	Repeated-dose toxicity	Genotoxicity	Carcinogenicity	Reproductive/developmental toxicity	Local irritation	Other types of toxicity	Clinical data
1. Drugs containing new active ingredients	○	○	○	□	○	□	□	○
2. New ethical combination drugs	○	○	×	×	×	□	×	○
3. Drugs with a new administration route	○	○	×	□	○	□	□	○
4. Drugs with a new indication	×	×	×	×	×	×	×	○
5. Drugs in a new dosage form	×	×	×	×	×	×	×	○
6. New dosage drugs	×	×	×	×	×	×	×	○
7. Biosimilar	□	○	×	×	×	□	□	○
8. Drugs supplied in an additional dosage form	×	×	×	×	×	×	×	×
9. Similar ethical combination drugs	○	□	×	×	×	□	×	○
10. Other drugs	×	×	×	×	×	×	×	×

○: required ×: not required □: required on a case-by-case basis.

of drugs in Table 9.1, biosimilars are currently defined in the MHLW bureau notification (MHLW, 2009).

Some studies may be unnecessary with some rationale provided. For example, if the exposure level of a drug is not increased with a new administration route, long-term repeat-dose toxicity and reproductive and developmental toxicity studies might not be required. On the other hand, some studies need to be added for drugs even with a new indication. If the drug is later planned for chronic indication, longer-term repeated toxicity and carcinogenicity studies may be required. Case-by-case approaches should be taken. Face-to-face consultation meetings with the PMDA are possible at a fee for providing advice on nonclinical study plans and strategies when necessary.

9.3 Current Nonclinical Safety Guidelines Available in Japan

The following nonclinical guidelines are currently available in Japan: genotoxicity studies, carcinogenicity studies, single-dose toxicity studies, repeat-dose toxicity studies, toxicokinetics, repeated-dose tissue distribution studies, reproductive and developmental toxicity studies, safety pharmacology studies including an evaluation of QT prolongation, immunotoxicity studies, microdose studies, nonclinical evaluation of biotechnology-derived pharmaceuticals, nonclinical evaluation for anti-cancer pharmaceuticals, skin sensitization studies, skin photosensitization studies. Most of the guidelines were adapted from the ICH guidelines except those for skin sensitization studies and skin photosensitization studies.

Although several toxicology areas have not yet been covered, Japanese as well as foreign companies consider the guidance documents of other agencies such as the FDA and EMA because most new drugs tend to be simultaneously developed across the world. Some attempts and efforts are made to create new Japanese guidelines on the uncovered toxicity areas.

9.4 Current Trends of Conduct of Nonclinical Safety Evaluation in Japan

9.4.1 Single-Dose Toxicity Studies

While single-dose toxicity studies are not commonly conducted in the USA or the EU, Japanese pharmaceutical companies and the regulatory agency regard these studies as a regulatory requirement. In addition, companies use the information from single-dose toxicity studies to select doses for repeated-dose toxicity studies. Even after the ICH M3 (R2) guideline was published as a Step 5 document in Japan in 2010, there is still a guideline for single-dose toxicity studies, which is very confusing. Some companies might think that single-dose studies are still necessary in Japan. However, the PMDA does not recommend these studies merely to obtain acute toxicity information.

9.4.2 Nonclinical Evaluation of the Potential for QT Interval Prolongation

For nonclinical evaluation of QT interval prolongation, *in vitro* hERG assay and *in vivo* electrocardiography are generally performed. Although an assay for action potential duration (APD) is defined as an *in vitro* follow-up test in the ICH S7B guideline, the assay is sometimes included in Japanese pharmaceutical companies core battery for nonclinical evaluation of QT interval prolongation in because this study is thought to be useful to determine effects on each individual ion channel.

9.4.3 Carcinogenicity Studies

Carcinogenicity studies are conducted according to the ICH S1A, S1B and S1C (R2) guidelines. Japanese pharmaceutical companies are hesitant about conducting a 6-month carcinogenicity study with genetically modified mice including Tg-rasH2 mice, $p53^{(+/-)}$ mice and Tg-Ac mice. The principle reason for not using these transgenic mice is lack of experience in the Japanese companies. The PMDA and MHLW accept the data generated from short-term carcinogenicity studies using genetically modified mice. Benefit and risk balance are considered when positive results are obtained in the carcinogenicity studies.

9.4.4 Safety Evaluation of Drug Metabolites

Since the FDA guidance "Safety Testing of Drug Metabolites" was published in 2008, attention has been drawn to toxicity of drug metabolites in Japan. The FDA guidance for "Safety Testing of Drug Metabolites" states that human metabolites that can raise a safety concern are those formed at greater than 10% of parent drug systemic exposure at steady state. In the ICH M3 (R2) guideline, in contrast, nonclinical characterization of a human metabolite(s) is only warranted when that metabolite(s) is observed at exposures greater than 10% of total drug-related exposure in principle. Although the ICH guideline should supersede the FDA guidance on this point, detailed description in the FDA guidance document is referred to under the circumstances where there is no guideline in Japan.

9.4.5 Phototoxicity Studies

Nonclinical phototoxicity studies are considered to be important for the clinical setting in Japan. The guideline for skin photosensitization studies for prediction of skin chemical photoallergy was published in Japan in 1989. Since then, photosensitization studies have been required for drugs applied to the skin according to the guideline in which several guinea pig models are described. The sensitivity and predictability of the above studies, however, have been under discussion for years. In contrast, there is no guideline for phototoxicity studies in Japan. Many Japanese pharmaceutical companies traditionally conduct *in vivo* phototoxicity studies, particularly using guinea pigs because guinea pig studies are described in the skin photosensitization study guideline. Mouse studies have recently become common. Phototoxicity testing is initiated based on photochemical properties and tissue distribution of compounds. Light absorption of compounds does not necessarily cause phototoxicity, but generation of reactive oxygen species (ROS) is essential for phototoxicity. ROS assay, in which ROS such as superoxide and singlet oxygen generated from photo-irradiated and -excited compounds are determined, is thought to be a useful method to determine additional photochemical properties of drugs directly leading to phototoxicity. As for *in viro* methods, neutral red uptake assay using 3T3 cells is employed. This method, however, often results in false positives. The phototoxicity study is now under discussion as an S10 topic in the ICH.

9.4.6 Skin Sensitization Studies

With relation to local tolerance, sensitization studies are only required for dermal application drugs. The guideline includes several guinea pig models such as the Maximization test and Buhler test. Local lymph node assay, which has not been listed in the guideline, can be accepted by the regulatory agency if the method is well validated in test facilities.

9.4.7 Nonclinical Evaluation of Paediatric Drugs

A guidance for pediatric studies was published in 2012 (MHLW, 2012). One appropriate species (male and female) is usually selected. Age of animals to start dosing is determined considering the corresponding age to human, effects and target organs of drugs and development of organs during dosing. Dosing is terminated at the age when dosing is started in repeat dose toxicity studies in adult animals.

9.4.8 Antigenicity Studies

Due to the genetic polymorphism of immune responses amongst individual humans, humoral immune responses such as anaphylactic reaction, it is difficult to predict these from animal studies. The draft guideline was published by the former Ministry of Health and Welfare (now the MHLW) in 1988, but not finalized because of criticisms about the methodology. Although people might believe that there used to be or even exists the guideline of antigenicity in Japan, there has never been such a guideline. Japanese pharmaceutical companies especially those manufacturing antibiotics, however, have been cautious about the manifestation of life-threatening anaphylaxis in a very small population. Most other drugs other than antibiotics are not tested for antigenicity in Japan.

9.4.9 Safety Evaluation of Chiral Pharmaceuticals

Safety evaluation of chiral pharmaceuticals was discussed at the first ICH meeting in 1991. Thereafter, the FDA published a "Policy statement for the development of new streoisomeric drugs" in 1992, the EEC (at that time) published an "Investigation of chiral active substances (3CC29a)" in 1994, and Health Canada published "Stereochemical issues in chiral drug development" in 2000, respectively. Internal chiral conversion of an enantiomer should be determined to justify the toxicity of the drug for dose selection in first-in-human clinical trials. In addition, the internal converted enantiomer should be considered as a metabolite which is assessed according to the guideline for metabolite toxicity.

9.4.10 Safety Evaluation of Impurities

Safety evaluation of impurities is performed according to the flowchart depicted in the ICH Q3A/Q3B and Q6A guidelines. Unselected enantiomer of chiral drugs and photodegraded compound are also regarded and handled as the impurity.

9.4.11 Other Studies

Assessment of genotoxic impurities has not been required by the Japanese regulatory agency. In future, Japanese pharmaceutical companies will evaluate genotoxic impurities according to the ICH guideline M7, "Assessment and control of DNA reactive (mutagenic) impurities in pharmaceuticals to limit potential carcinogenic risk". A guideline for environmental risk assessment of drugs is now being discussed within the Japanese regulatory agency.

9.5 Safety Assessment of Unapproved Drugs

According to the Japanese White Paper No. 39 published by the Office of Pharmaceutical Industry Research, there is an average lag time of 3.9 years from when major drugs were first marketed elsewhere in the world to when they were marketed in Japan, with 2.4 years between the USA and Japan. Several reasons are mooted for the delay in Japan. Difference in reviewing periods was nominal, but the delay of launching clinical trials was 1.9 years compared with the USA. In addition to insufficient infrastructure for clinical studies and the possible unattractiveness of the Japanese market, there may be overloaded nonclinical assessment for clinical trials or drug application in Japan. Especially for drugs evaluated in the past, additional testing may be required in compliance with current Japanese guidelines. In such cases, sponsors could be excused from doing the studies if justified or specific procedures need to be created to encourage clinical trials or the drug application.

9.6 Necessity of 3Rs (Reduction/Refinement/Replacement) of Animal Studies

Because of growing public interest in animal welfare, the 3Rs – that is,, reduction, refinement and replacement – are considered. Aiming at developing *in vitro* alternative methods for assessing several toxicities, the JaCVAM (Japanese Center for the Validation of Alternative Methods), which corresponds to the ICCVAM (Interagency Coordinating Committee on the Validation of Alternative Methods) in the US and ECVAM (European Center for the Validation of Alternative Methods) in the EU, was founded in 2005 under the auspices of the National Institute of Health Sciences. JaCVAM's policy and mission are to promote the 3Rs in animal experiments for the evaluation of chemical substance safety in Japan and to establish guidelines for new alternative experimental methods through international collaboration (JACVAM, 2012). Applied methods are validated and reviewed by the team at JaCVAM. Validated methods are recommended for regulatory guidance after they are accepted by regulators. *In vitro* alternative assays are being developed for tests for corrosivity test, phototoxicity, skin sensitization, skin irritation, ocular irritation, genotoxicity, skin absorption, acute oral toxicity, as well as endocrine disrupter screening, cell transformation assay and pyrogen screening.

9.7 Attitude of Japanese Pharmaceutical Companies and the Regulatory Agency toward Nonclinical Safety Assessment

Japanese pharmaceutical companies are conservative about safety assessment of drugs. Companies tend to conduct every testing according to the guidelines to avert the risk of delay in drug development due to incompliance with regulatory requirements and possible adverse events occurring in the clinical setting. On the other hand, the regulatory agency unduly requires nonclinical safety studies because it is also concerned that adverse events might occur. Historically, it was in 1997 when consultation with the regulatory agency started. Regulatory communication had not been intense between companies and the agency until then. Opportunities of regulatory communications are not as frequent even now due to the PMDA's limited resources. Therefore, both companies and the agency rely on nonclinical guidelines.

American and European pharmaceutical companies often believe that data review is different between the PMDA and other agencies such as, for example, the FDA and EMA. This difference seems to be related to the strict adherence to testing guidelines in Japan. This stems from a lack of experienced reviewers for nonclinical safety evaluation in the PMDA. The reviewers are not prepared to think about flexible or alternative approaches to nonclinical development. As of 2011, only about 15 reviewers are assigned to nonclinical safety evaluation in the PMDA, amongst which half were young and inexperienced. The PMDA carefully employs researchers who have conducted several nonclinical studies in pharmaceutical companies, because Japanese people are concerned about possible collusion of regulatory agencies with private companies. However, an exchange of personnel between the agency and companies should be encouraged to streamline flexible review.

In addition, we have to consider that Japanese people are very sensitive to safety of drugs as well as foods. Japanese people have been cautious about bovine spongiform encephalopathy, genetically modified foods and residual agricultural pesticides. People carefully watch safety of foods in daily life. As a result, Japanese foods have a good reputation for being safe. There is also public pressure with regards to drug safety. Japanese people subconsciously think that drugs should bring health to people and do not expect adverse effects. The safety awareness of Japanese people forces the agency to not take risk of taking a flexible approach in reviewing data. Zero-risk cannot be applied, especially for drugs. It is important to further assimilate the idea of benefit and risk balance for drugs amongst Japanese people which would create proper safety standard of drugs.

References

Japanese Center for the Validation of Alternative Methods (JACVM) (2012). New Testing Method Assessment, Division of Pharmacology, National Biological Safety Research Center (NBSRC), National Institute of Health Sciences (NIHS).

Ministry of Health, Labour and Welfare (MHLW) (1989). Guidelines for toxicity studies required for application for approval to manufacture or import drugs. Pharmaceutical Affairs Bureau/Evaluation and Registration Division. Notification No. 24, dated 11 Sept. 1989.

Ministry of Health, Labour and Welfare (MHLW) (2005). Application for approval of medicinal products. Pharmaceutical and Food Safety Bureau. Notification No. 0331009, dated 31 March 2005.

Ministry of Health, Labour and Welfare (MHLW) (2009). Guidance on quality, safety and efficacy of biosimilars. Pharmaceutical and Food Safety Bureau. Notification No. 0304007, dated 4 March 2009.

Ministry of Health, Labour and Welfare (MHLW) (2012). Guideline on the Nonclinical Safety Study in Juvenile Animals for Pediatric Drugs. Pharmaceutical and Food Safety Bureau Notification No. 1002–5 dated 2 October 2012.

10

Indian Regulatory Process for Nonclinical Drug Development

K.S. Rao[1] *and S. Natesan*[2]
[1]*Rao Toxicology Foundation (RTF), Sanjayanagar, India*
[2]*Advinus Therapeutics Limited, India*

10.1 Introduction

The Indian pharmaceutical industry has been attracting prime attention from global pharmaceutical companies and not-for-profit organizations for research, development, manufacture and marketing of active pharmaceutical ingredients, intermediates, drug products and medical devices. India's strength is her large scientific pool coupled with the demonstrated capability of her generic pharmaceutical industry, together with the government's support for research, development and intellectual property rights through enactment of policies. India became a signatory to the World Trade Organization's Trade Related Intellectual Property Rights (TRIPS) in 1995, and utilized the transition period of 10 years given to the developing countries to bring national laws in accordance with TRIPS (The Patents (Amendment) Act, 2005). The mandatory compliance with TRIPS, including recognition of product patents, became effective from 1 January 2005 through the enactment of the law for adoption. Such policies sent the right signals to global pharmaceutical companies to see opportunities for drug discovery and development in India.

While several universities and national institutes provide educational, training and research opportunities in basic sciences, there are certain specific institutes and

Nonclinical Safety Assessment: A Guide to International Pharmaceutical Regulations, First Edition.
Edited by William J. Brock, Kenneth L. Hastings and Kathy M. McGown.

departments that primarily focus on the fields of drug research and development, including safety evaluation and toxicity testing. Currently, scientific personnel in the fields of chemistry, biology and veterinary sciences have become the backbone of 24 Good Laboratory Practice (GLP) accredited facilities for safety evaluation and testing of chemicals, pharmaceuticals, veterinary drugs, pesticides, and so on (India GLP, http://indiaglp.gov.in/TestFacilities.html).

The Indian regulatory system for nonclinical safety evaluation, prior to seeking clinical trial approval, is predominantly similar to the requirements of many countries. This chapter provides an overview of Indian requirements and relevant quality systems that are required to be adhered to by organizations involved in drug development, including nonclinical safety evaluation. Finer aspects of nonclinical safety evaluation covering animal toxicology and animal pharmacology studies are covered in detail to enable readers to have a comparative understanding with global practices.

10.2 Drug Development

The drug development process in India is in principle no different from that in other countries. Select Indian pharmaceutical companies, both by themselves and in collaboration with global pharmaceutical companies, have focused their R&D efforts in select therapeutics areas. Also, several contract manufacturing organizations are involved in commercial drug product supply while contract research organizations provide drug development service deliveries to global requirements. All such organizations involved in R&D in pharmaceuticals get their units recognized and adopt the Indian regulatory system as applicable for the different stages as depicted in Figure 10.1.

To promote discovery research and development, the Department of Scientific and Industrial Research (DSIR) in the Ministry of Science and Technology recognizes R&D units under either "in-house R&D" or "commercial R&D", and extends several supports, such as income tax benefits for R&D units, grant-in-aid as well as loans for pharmaceutical and other industries, and collaborative research with national laboratories. In addition, the government of India has established the National GLP Compliance

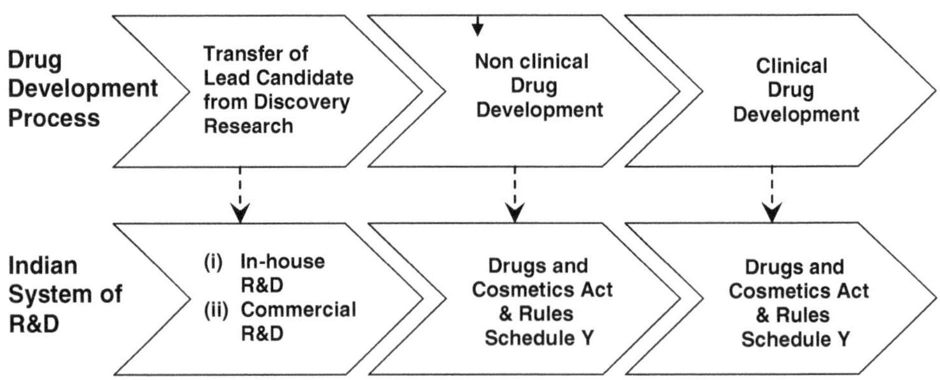

Figure 10.1 *Drug development process – Indian regulatory system.*

Monitoring Authority (http://indiaglp.gov.in/), adopting the OECD quality system of the principles of GLP, for the inspection, monitoring and accreditation of test facilities in India conducting non-clinical and environmental safety studies. India was recently recognized in March 2011 by the OECD Council with the Full Adherence status for Mutual acceptance of Data (MAD), with all of the rights and obligations of member countries of the OECD for GLP. India is a member of the OECD Working Group on GLP and also a member of the OECD Test Guidelines programme.

The Central Drugs Standard Control Organization (CDSCO) is the sole organization under the Ministry of Health and Family Welfare, Government of India, responsible for the regulatory aspects of drugs in India. The various regulatory aspects related to drug testing and approval are covered under the Drugs and Cosmetics Act of 1940 and the ensuing Drugs and Cosmetics Rules of 1945 which is the central legislation that regulates India's drug development and registration process, besides control on commercial manufacture, distribution and sale of drugs and drug products.

The CDSCO functions under the Directorate General of Health Services. Its senior officers include Drugs Controller General of India, Deputy Drugs Controllers, Assistant Drugs Controllers and Technical Officers. The CDSCO headed by the Drugs Controller General of India (DCGI) discharges the functions of the Central Government (similar to the US FDA). The CDSCO is attached to the office of the Directorate General of Health Services in the Central Ministry of Health and Family Welfare. In the context of drug development, the DCGI office is primarily responsible for, but not limited to:

1. Developing standards of drugs, cosmetics, diagnostics and devices
2. Developing regulatory measures, amendments to Acts and Rules
3. Providing permission to manufacture a drug for the purpose of examination, test or analysis (includes manufacture of investigational new drugs)
4. Providing permission to conduct clinical trials, and regulate clinical research in India
5. Regulating market authorization for new drugs
6. Regulating the standards of imported drugs
7. Guidance on technical matters

The Indian system is taking all necessary initiatives to strengthen CDSCO and the office of the DCGI to support new drug discovery and development. The Indian regulatory system also works closely with other regulatory agencies, such as the US Food and Drug Administration (FDA) for strengthening diverse areas of drug development, manufacture and marketing. The US FDA has recently opened an India Office of International Programs at New Delhi and Mumbai in 2008–09.

10.3 Quality Systems

The Drugs and Cosmetics Rules (1945) of the government of India describe Quality Assurance (QA) as a wide-ranging concept concerning all matters that individually or collectively influence the quality of a product. It is the totality of the arrangements made with the object of ensuring that products are of the quality required for their intended use. The system of QA appropriate to the manufacture of pharmaceutical products ensures that pharmaceutical products are designed and developed in a way that takes account of the requirements of Good Manufacturing Practices (GMP) and other associated codes such as those of Good Laboratory Practices (GLP) and Good Clinical Practices (GCP). Essentially, the quality systems are similar to those covered by US FDA (1978), ICH, EMA, WHO, OECD (1997), US EPA (1989a, 1989b), EC Directive (2004), and others (MHW Japan 1997 and MAFF Japan 1999).

Specifically, with respect to nonclinical safety assessment, Schedule Y (2005) of Drugs and Cosmetics Rules, under the general principles for animal toxicology (nonclinical toxicity studies), provides the regulatory requirements and guidelines for toxicity studies, which should comply with GLPs. Key aspects included in Schedule Y (2005) of Drugs and Cosmetics Rules are: (i) such studies should be performed by suitably trained and qualified staff; (ii) employ properly calibrated and standardized equipment of adequate size and capacity; (iii) studies should be done as per written protocols with modifications (if any) verifiable retrospectively; (iv) standard operating procedures (SOPs) should be followed for all managerial and laboratory tasks related to the studies; (v) test substances and test systems (*in vitro* or *in vivo*) should be properly characterized and standardized; (vi) all documents belonging to each study, including its approved protocol, raw data, draft report, final report, and histology slides and paraffin tissue blocks should be preserved for a minimum of five years after marketing of the drug.

The recent amendment in November 2008 to the Drugs and Cosmetics Rules 1945 includes a new Schedule L-1 (2008) which covers the "Good Laboratory Practices and Requirements of Premises and Equipments", primarily for laboratories that support manufacture. Despite such specific emphasis of its applicability, the details of GLP requirements are in alignment with the requirements of Principles of GLP covered in OECD, USFDA, US EPA, etc.

The Schedule Y (2005) of nonclinical safety evaluation also describes application of GLP for the animal studies to be conducted in an accredited laboratory. Where the safety pharmacology studies are part of toxicology studies, these studies should also be conducted in an accredited laboratory.

Thus the quality system needed for nonclinical drug development is similar to international requirements of the Principles of GLP covered in US FDA, US EPA, OECD, and European Council Acts, etc.

10.4 Nonclinical Drug Development – Key Regulatory Requirements

In the process of drug development towards product registration, the clinical development in different phases has been and will continue to be the dominant and critical process that not only requires significantly higher time, efforts and investments than any other process but also helps the drug development company to take decisive actions at the end of each of the successive phases of the clinical development. In view of such importance, a primary requirement as formulated by regulatory agencies has therefore been the nonclinical development, including *in vitro* and *in vivo* studies, all of which provide evidence of safety and support application for approval of clinical studies. Thus, like the regulatory systems in the developed countries, the Indian regulatory system directs the pharmaceutical R&D organizations seeking approval of clinical studies to complete the nonclinical drug development as outlined broadly in Figure 10.2.

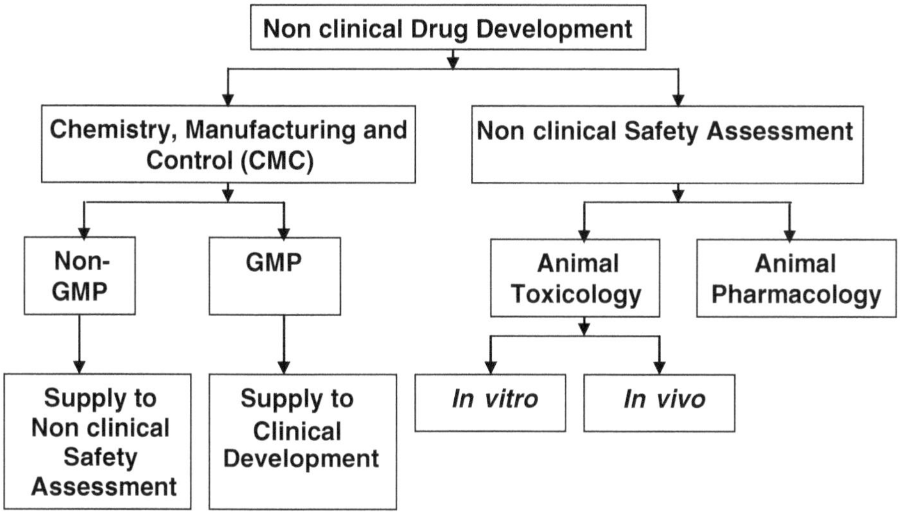

Figure 10.2 *Regulatory requirements of nonclinical drug development.*

While this chapter focuses on nonclinical safety assessment of new chemical entity (NCE) or drug products, it is considered pertinent to have a brief understanding of the test article employed in such assessment. The chemistry, manufacturing and control aspects of production of such test article as well as its characterization including physical, chemical and stability aspects help in the design of studies, both *in vitro* and *in vivo*, of nonclinical safety evaluation. Also, the Schedule Y (2005) of the Indian Drugs and Cosmetics Rules do require such data along with the results of nonclinical safety assessment studies for consideration prior to approval of clinical trials.

10.5 Nonclinical Safety Assessment – Key Approval Requirements

Schedule Y (2005) of the Drugs and Cosmetics Rules provides a detailed requirements of nonclinical safety assessment studies, both *in vitro* and *in vivo*, applicable for seeking approval prior to initiating each of the clinical phases. Additionally, regulations relating to animal welfare demand approval of use of animals prior to undertaking such nonclinical safety evaluation studies on NCEs, drug products, and medical devices. Also, when the test articles happen to be recombinant DNA-based products, then such products require biosafety approval (Figure 10.3) for transport, handling and conduct of studies.

A test facility conducting nonclinical safety assessment studies involving animals to evaluate NCEs, drug products or recombinant DNA-based products needs to comply with the following requirements:

1. The Committee for the Purpose of Control and Supervision of Experiments on Animals (CPCSEA) in the Animal Welfare Division of Ministry of Environment and Forests (see http://moef.gov.in/divisions/awd/awd_overview.html) is responsible for:

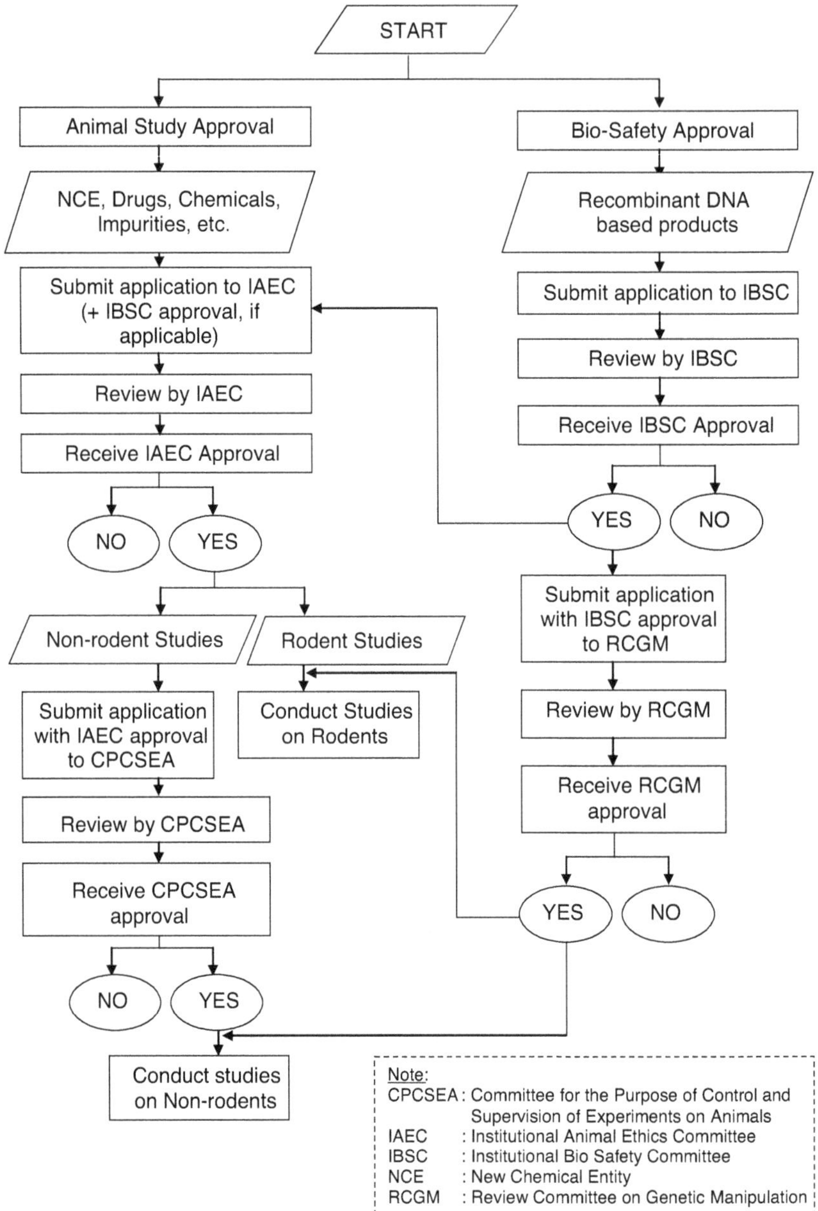

Figure 10.3 *Approval process for nonclinical safety assessment studies involving animals.*

(a) Inspection and approval of animal house facility for breeding and conduct of experiments
(b) Assigning CPCSEA nominees as members to the test facility's Institutional Animal Ethics Committee (IAEC). The IAEC functions are similar to the Institutional Animal Care and Use Program (IACUC)
(c) Review and approval of nonclinical safety studies involving rodents by IAEC

   (d) Review and approval of nonclinical safety studies involving nonrodents, first by IAEC and subsequently by CPCSEA
   (e) Approval of animal import for studies or breeding
   (f) Any other requirements relating to animals and animal products.
2. The Review Committee on Genetic Manipulation (RCGM) in the Department of Biotechnology (DBT) in the Ministry of Science and Technology is responsible for:
   (a) Monitoring safety-related aspects in respect of research projects and activities involving genetically engineered organisms/hazardous microorganisms
   (b) Assigning a DBT nominee to the test facility's Institutional Biosafety Committee (IBSC; see http://dbtbiosafety.nic.in/)
   (c) Review and approval of nonclinical safety studies involving genetically engineered/modified organisms by IBSC.
   (d) Review and approval of import/development, transport and conduct of studies involving genetically engineered/modified organisms by RCGM, based on initial approval by IBSC
   (e) Any other requirements relating to genetically engineered/modified organisms.

A flow chart of approval process for the conduct of nonclinical safety evaluation studies on NCEs, drugs or any other products is given in Figure 10.3. Accordingly, organizations involved in the conduct of such studies need to take a synchronized approach and timely actions by coordinating with all associated parties. Key factors that are frequently considered by test facilities involved in conduct of nonclinical safety studies are:

- Nature of drug substance or drug product as test article.
- Whether such test article is available within the country or to be received from overseas for conduct of studies.
- Required time for delivery of test article, including its related information on characterization, certificate of analysis, material safety data sheet, and so on.
- Required animals: species, numbers, sex, and age, and whether they are locally available, in-house bred or to be imported.
- Required approval from IAEC, IBSC, CPCSEA, and RCGM.
- Sponsor's responsibility in providing documents and approvals as applicable.
- Availability of animal house to receive, quarantine (if applicable), and conduct studies.
- Test protocol requirements to send any animal samples (plasma, tissue, etc.) to overseas laboratories for any specific testing.
- Target time to complete the study and deliver the study report to the sponsor or adhere to the in-house development plan.

10.6 Data Required for Clinical Study Approval

A typical application for permission to undertake clinical trials in humans would need the following information:

1. Chemical and pharmaceutical information
2. Animal pharmacology consisting of:
   (a) Specific pharmacological information
   (b) General pharmacological information

   (c) Pharmacokinetic data related to the absorption, distribution, metabolism and excretion of the test substance.
3. Animal toxicology data include the following:
   (a) General aspects
   (b) Systemic toxicology studies
   (c) Male fertility study
   (d) Female reproduction and developmental toxicity studies
   (e) Local toxicity
   (f) Allergenicity/hypersensitivity
   (g) Genotoxicity
   (h) Carcinogenicity

As the requirements of chemical and pharmaceutical information (often described as CMC by the industry and regulatory authorities) are outside the scope of this chapter, a detailed account of the animal toxicology and animal pharmacology aspects are given in Sections 10.7 and 10.8, respectively.

10.6.1 Animal Toxicity Studies as Mandated by Clinical Phases

The Indian regulatory system requires submission of nonclinical safety assessment data as well as all other applicable data for review and approval for each of the clinical phases. Thus, the nonclinical safety assessments needed prior to seeking approval of each of the clinical phases are summarized in Table 10.1. Briefly, the key objectives of each of the clinical phases are:

- **Phase I Human pharmacology:** Estimation of safety and tolerability (maximum tolerated dose, pharmacodynamics and early measurement of drug activity) with the initial administration of an investigational new drug (IND) into human(s), usually nontherapeutic objectives in healthy volunteers subjects.
- **Phase II Therapeutic exploratory trials:** To evaluate the effectiveness of a drug for a particular indication or indications in patients with the condition under study and to determine the common short-term side-effects and risks associated with the drug. Also, the goal is to determine the dose(s) and regimen for Phase III trials, and evaluation of potential study endpoints.
- **Phase III Therapeutic confirmatory trials:** Demonstration or confirmation of therapeutic benefit(s), safety and effectiveness for use in the intended indication and recipient population, provide an adequate basis for marketing approval, explore the dose-response relationships, and so on.
- **Phase IV Post marketing trials:** For optimizing the drug's use, additional drug–drug interaction(s), dose-response or safety studies and trials designed to support use under the approved indication(s), for example, mortality/morbidity studies, epidemiological studies, and so on.

10.6.2 Animal Toxicity Studies as Mandated by Proposed Route and Duration of Administration

Schedule Y (2005) of the Drugs and Cosmetics Rules also describes the long-term toxicity study requirements, taking into consideration the proposed human route of

Table 10.1 *Non-clinical toxicity testing and safety evaluation data of an IND needed for the conduct of different phases of clinical trials.*

Clinical phase	Requirement of safety assessment studies
I	(a) Single dose toxicity studies (b) Dose ranging studies (c) Repeat-dose systemic toxicity studies of appropriate duration to support the duration of proposed human exposure (d) Male fertility study (e) *In vitro* genotoxicity tests (f) Relevant local toxicity studies with proposed route of clinical application (duration depending on proposed length of clinical exposure) (g) Allergenicity/hypersensitivity tests (when there is a cause for concern or for parenteral drugs, including dermal application) (h) Photo-allergy or dermal phototoxicity test (if the drug or a metabolite is related to an agent causing photosensitivity or the UV absorbance characteristic of the drug)
II	(a) Provide a summary of all the nonclinical safety data (listed above) already submitted while obtaining the permissions for Phase I trial, with appropriate references • In case of an application for directly starting a Phase II trial – complete details of the nonclinical safety data needed for obtaining the permission for Phase I trial, as per the list provided above, must be submitted (b) Repeat-dose systemic toxicity studies of appropriate duration to support the duration of proposed human exposure (c) *In vivo* genotoxicity tests (d) Segment II reproductive/developmental toxicity study (if female patients of child-bearing age are going to be involved)
III	(a) Provide a summary of all the nonclinical safety data (listed above) already submitted while obtaining the permissions for Phase I and II trials, with appropriate references • In case of an application for directly initiating a Phase III trial – complete details of the nonclinical safety data needed for obtaining the permissions for Phase I and II trials, as per the list provided above, must be provided. (b) Repeat-dose systemic toxicity studies of appropriate duration to support the duration of proposed human exposure (c) Reproductive/developmental toxicity studies (d) Segment I (if female patients of child-bearing age are going to be involved) (e) Segment III (for drugs to be given to pregnant or nursing mothers or where there are indications of possible adverse effects on foetal development) (f) Carcinogenicity studies (when there is a cause for concern or when the drug is to be used in humans for more than 6 months)
IV	(a) Provide a summary of all the nonclinical safety data (listed above) already submitted while obtaining the permissions for Phase I, II and III trials, with appropriate references • In case an application is made for initiating the Phase IV trial, complete details of the nonclinical safety data needed for obtaining the permissions for Phase I, II and III trials, as per the list provided above, must be submitted.

Table 10.2 *Systemic toxicity studies required for clinical trials in different phases.*

Route of administration	Duration of proposed human administration	Human clinical trial phase	Long-term toxicity requirements	
			No. of species	Duration
Oral or parenteral or transdermal	Single dose or several doses in one day, up to 1 week	I, II, III	2 species	2 week
	>1 week but up to 2 week	I, II, III	2 species	4 week
	>2 week but up to 4 week	I, II, III	2 species	12 week
	Over 1 month	I, II, III	2 species	24 week
Inhalation (general anaesthetics, aerosols)	Up to 2 week	I, II, III	2 species	1 month (Exposure time 3 h/day, 5 day/week)
	Up to 4 week	I, II, III	2 species	12 week (Exposure time 6 h/day, 5 day/week)
	>14 week	I, II, III	2 species	24 week (Exposure time 6 h/day, 5 day/week)

administration as well as the proposed duration of the administration. Such details and the number of animal species, including the duration of systemic toxicity studies and local toxicity studies, are given in Tables 10.2 and 10.3, respectively.

In addition, certain special toxicity studies (Table 10.4) are mandated by the Indian regulatory system as part of application submission to the DCGI for review and approval of each of the clinical phases.

Animal toxicity data generated in other countries may be accepted in India, and might not be asked to be repeated in India depending upon the quality of data and the accreditations of the laboratory where such data have been generated.

10.7 Animal Toxicology

Animal toxicity studies should comply with GLPs as described in Section 10.3. Toxicokinetic studies (generation of pharmacokinetic data either as an integral component of the conduct of nonclinical toxicity studies or in specially designed studies) should be

Table 10.3 *Local toxicity studies required for clinical trials in different phases.*

Route of administration	Duration of proposed human administration	Human clinical trial phase	Long-term toxicity requirements	
			No. of species	Duration
Dermal Ocular or otic or nasal Vaginal or rectal	Up to 2 week	I, II	1 species	4 week
		III	2 species	4 week
	>2 week	I, II, III	2 species	12 week

Table 10.4 *Special toxicity studies required for clinical trials in different phases.*

Toxicity study	Human clinical trial phase	Specific requirements
Male fertility study	I, II, III in male volunteers/patients	One species
Female reproduction and developmental toxicity studies	II, III involving female patients of child-bearing age	Segment II studies in 2 species
	III involving female patients of child-bearing age	Segment I study
	III for drugs to be given to pregnant or nursing mothers for long periods or where there are indications of possible adverse effects on foetal development.	Segment III study
Allergenicity/ hypersensitivity	I, II, III – when there is a cause of concern or for parenteral drugs (including dermal application)	Guinea pig or mouse
Photo-allergy or dermal phototoxicity	I, II, III – if the drug or a metabolite is related to an agent causing photosensitivity or the nature of action suggests such a potential	Guinea pig
Genotoxicity	I	*In vitro* studies
	II, III	Both *in vitro* and *in vivo*
Carcinogenicity	III (when there is a cause for concern, or when the drug is to be used in humans for more than 6 months)	Rodent species (preferably rat)

conducted to assess the systemic exposure achieved in animals and its relationship to dose level and the time course of the toxicity study. Other objectives of toxicokinetic studies include obtaining data to relate the exposure achieved in toxicity studies to toxicological findings. In addition, these data may contribute to the assessment of the relevance of these findings to clinical safety. Furthermore, these data will help support the choice of species and treatment regimen in nonclinical toxicity studies and to provide information which, in conjunction with the toxicity findings, contributes to the design of subsequent nonclinical toxicity studies.

10.7.1 Systemic Toxicity Studies

10.7.1.1 Single-dose Toxicity Studies

These studies should be carried out in two rodent species (mice and rats) using the same route as intended for humans. In addition, unless the intended route of administration in humans is only intravenous, at least one more route should be used in one of the species to ensure systemic availability of the drug. This route should depend on the nature of the drug. A limit of 2000 mg/kg (or 10 times the normal dose that is intended in humans, whichever is higher) is recommended for oral dosing. At least four doses should be given to develop a dose–response curve. Each group should contain at least five animals of either sex. Animals should be exposed to the test substance in a single bolus or by continuous infusion or several doses within 24 hours. Signs of intoxication, effect on body weight, and gross pathological changes should be reported. It is desirable to include histopathology of grossly affected organs. Animals should be observed for 14 days after the drug administration, and minimum lethal dose (MLD) and maximum tolerated dose (MTD) should be established. If possible, the target organ of toxicity should also be determined. Mortality should be observed for up to seven days after parenteral administration and up to 14 days after oral administration. Symptoms, signs and mode of death should be reported, with appropriate macroscopic and microscopic findings where necessary. The LD_{10} and/or LD_{50} should be reported preferably with 95% confidence limits. If LD_{50} cannot be determined, reasons should be stated.

The dose causing severe toxic manifestations or death should be defined in the case of cytotoxic anticancer agents, and the post-dosing observation period should be up to 14 days. Mice should first be used for determination of MTD. Findings should then be confirmed in rats for establishing the linear relationship between toxicity and body surface area. In the case of nonlinearity, data of the more sensitive species should be used to determine the Phase I starting dose. Where rodents are known to be poor predictors of human toxicity (e.g., antifolates), or where the cytotoxic drug acts by a novel mechanism of action, MTD should be established in nonrodent species.

10.7.1.2 Repeated-dose Systemic Toxicity Studies

10.7.1.2.1 Dose-Ranging Study

Prior to initiating typical repeated-dose toxicity studies, it is desirable to conduct dose-range finding studies on rodents and nonrodents with the objectives of identification of target organ toxicity and establishment of maximum tolerated dose (MTD) for subsequent studies.

Rodents: A study should be performed in one rodent species (preferably rat) by the proposed clinical route of administration. At least four graded doses, including control, should be given, and each dose group as well as the vehicle control should consist of a minimum of five animals of each sex. Animals should be exposed to the test substance daily for at least 10 consecutive days. The highest dose should be the MTD based on the results of the single-dose study. Animals should be observed daily for signs of toxicity (general appearance, activity and behaviour, etc.), and periodically for the body weight and clinical pathology parameters. Gross examination of viscera and microscopic examination of affected organs should be done.

Nonrodents: One male and one female are to be used for ascending Phase MTD study. Dosing should start after initial recording of cage-side and laboratory parameters. The starting dose could be 3–5 times the extrapolated effective dose or MTD (whichever is less), and dose escalation in suitable steps should be done every third day (based on the PK profile of the drug) after drawing the samples for laboratory parameters. The dose should be lowered appropriately when clinical or laboratory evidence of toxicity is observed. Administration of test substance should then continue for at least 10 days at the tolerated dose level, following which samples for laboratory parameters should be taken. Sacrifice, autopsy and microscopic examination of affected tissues should be performed as in the case of rodents.

10.7.1.2.2 Repeated-dose Toxicity Studies

These studies should be carried out in at least two mammalian species, one of which should be a nonrodent. Dose-ranging studies should precede the longer-term toxicity

Table 10.5 *Number of animals required for repeated-dose toxicity studies.*

Group	14–28 days				84–182 days			
	Rodent (rat)		Nonrodent (dog or monkey)		Rodent (rat)		Nonrodent (dog or monkey)	
	Male	Female	Male	Female	Male	Female	Male	Female
Control	6–10	6–10	2–3	2–3	15–30	15–30	4–6	4–6
Low dose	6–10	6–10	2–3	2–3	15–30	15–30	4–6	4–6
Intermediate dose	6–10	6–10	2–3	2–3	15–30	15–30	4–6	4–6
High dose	6–10	6–10	2–3	2–3	15–30	15–30	4–6	4–6

studies. Duration of the final systemic toxicity study will depend on the duration, therapeutic indication and scale of the proposed clinical trial. If a species is known to metabolize the drug in the same way as humans, it should be preferred for toxicity studies.

In repeated-dose toxicity studies, the drug should be administered seven days a week by the route intended for clinical use. The number of animals required for these studies, that is, the minimum number of animals on which data should be available, is shown in Table 10.5.

Wherever applicable, a control group of animals given the vehicle alone should be included, and three other groups should be given graded doses of the drug. The highest dose should produce observable toxicity. The lowest dose should not cause observable toxicity, but should be comparable to the intended therapeutic dose in humans or a multiple of the therapeutic dose. To make allowance for the sensitivity of the species, the intermediate dose should cause some symptoms, but not gross toxicity or death, and should be placed logarithmically between the other two doses. Dose levels are to be scientifically justified.

The parameters to be monitored and recorded in repeat-dose toxicity studies should include behavioural, physiological, biochemical and microscopic observations. In case of parenteral drug administration, the sites of injection should be subjected to gross and microscopic examination. Initial and final electrocardiogram and fundus examination should be carried out in the nonrodent species.

In the case of cytotoxic anticancer agents, dosing and study design should be in accordance with the proposed clinical schedule in terms of days of exposure and number of cycles. Two rodent species can be tested for initiating Phase I trials. A nonrodent species should be added if the drug has a novel mechanism of action, or if permission for Phase II, III or marketing is being sought.

For most compounds, it is expected that single-dose tissue distribution studies with sufficient sensitivity and specificity will provide an adequate assessment of tissue distribution and the potential for accumulation. Thus, repeated-dose tissue distribution studies should not be required uniformly for all compounds and should only be conducted when appropriate data cannot be derived from other sources. Repeated-dose studies may be appropriate under certain circumstances based on the data from single-dose tissue

Table 10.6 *Laboratory parameters to be included in toxicity studies.*

Sl. No.	Category	Parameters
1	Haematological parameters	Haemoglobin, total RBC count, haematocrit, reticulocyte, total WBC count, differential WBC count, platelet count, terminal bone marrow examination, ESR (nonrodents only), general blood picture *Coagulation parameters (Nonrodents only):* bleeding time, coagulation time, prothrombin time, activated partial thromboplastin time
2	Urinalysis parameters	Colour, appearance, specific gravity, 24-hour urinary output, reaction (pH), albumin, sugar, acetone, bile pigments, urobilinogen, occult blood, microscopic examination of urinary sediment
3	Blood biochemical parameters	Glucose, cholesterol, triglycerides, HDL & LDL cholesterol (nonrodents only), LDL, bilirubin, ALT, AST alkaline phosphatase (ALP), GGT (nonrodents only), blood urea nitrogen, creatinine, total proteins, albumin, globulin (calculated values), sodium, potassium, phosphorus, calcium
4	Gross and microscopic pathology	Brain* cerebrum, cerebellum, midbrain, (spinal cord), eye, (middle ear), thyroid, (parathyroid), spleen, thymus, adrenal*, (pancreas), (trachea), lung*, heart*, aorta, oesophagus, stomach, duodenum, jejunum, terminal ileum, colon, (rectum), liver*, kidney*, urinary bladder, epididymis, testis*, ovary, uterus*, skin, mammary gland, mesenteric lymph node and skeletal muscle

* Organs marked with an asterisk should be weighed.
() Organs listed in parenthesis should be examined if indicated by the nature of the drug or observed effects.

distribution studies, toxicity and toxicokinetic studies. The studies might be most appropriate for compounds which have an apparently long half life, incomplete elimination or unanticipated organ toxicity.

The list of various parameters applicable for toxicity studies is given in Table 10.6. Many of the parameters listed in Table 10.6 are similar to those covered in OECD Guidelines for Testing of Chemicals. There are some differences in the parameters and terminology in Schedule Y (2005). However, the Indian Regulatory system would accept studies conducted according to OECD guidelines.

14–28 day repeated-dose toxicity studies: One rodent (6–10/sex/group) and one nonrodent (2–3/sex/group) species are needed. Daily dosing by the proposed clinical route at three dose levels should be done, with the highest dose having observable toxicity, mid-dose between high and low dose, and low dose. The doses should preferably be multiples of the effective dose and free from toxicity. Observation parameters should include cage-side observations, body weight changes, food/water intake, blood biochemistry, haematology, and gross and microscopic studies of all viscera and tissues (Table 10.6).

90-day repeated-dose toxicity studies: One rodent (15–30/sex/group) and one nonrodent (4–6/sex/group) species are needed. Daily dosing by the proposed clinical route at three graded dose levels should be done. In addition to the control, a "high-dose-reversal" (recovery) group and its control group should be also included. Parameters should include signs of intoxication (general appearance, activity and behaviour, etc.), body weight, food intake, blood biochemical parameters, haematological values, urine analysis, organ weights, gross and microscopic study of viscera and tissues. Half the animals in "recovery" groups (high-dose-treated and control) should be sacrificed after 14 days following the end of the dosing phase. The remaining animals should be sacrificed after 28 days of stopping the treatment or after the recovery of signs and/or clinical pathological changes – whichever comes later, and evaluated for the parameters used for the main study.

180-day repeated-dose toxicity studies: One rodent (15–30/sex/group) and one nonrodent (4–6/sex/group) species are needed. At least four groups, including control, should be taken. Daily dosing by the proposed clinical route at three graded dose levels should be done. Parameters should include signs of intoxication, body weight, food intake, blood biochemistry, haematology, urine analysis, organ weights, gross and microscopic examination of organs and tissues.

10.7.2 Male Fertility Study

One rodent species (preferably rat) should be used. Dose selection should be done from the results of the previous 14- or 28-day toxicity study in rats. Three dose groups, the highest one showing minimal toxicity in systemic studies, and a control group should be included. Each group should consist of six adult male animals. Animals should be treated with the test substance by the intended route of clinical use for minimum 28 days and maximum 70 days before they are paired with untreated female animals of proven fertility in a ratio of 1:2 for mating.

Drug treatment of the male animals should continue during pairing. Pairing should be continued until the detection of vaginal plug or 10 days, whichever is earlier. Any pregnant females should be examined for their fertility index after day 13 of gestation. All the male animals should be sacrificed at the end of the study. Weights of each testis and epididymis should be separately recorded. Sperms from one epididymis should be examined for their motility and morphology. The other epididymis and both testes should be examined for their histology.

10.7.3 Female Reproduction and Developmental Toxicity Studies

These studies need to be carried out for all drugs proposed to be studied or used in women of child bearing age. Segment I, II and III studies (see below) are to be performed in albino mice or rats, and the Segment II study should include albino rabbits also as a second test species.

Female fertility study (Segment I): The study should be done in one rodent species (rat preferred). The drug should be administered to both males and females, beginning a sufficient number of days (28 days in males and 14 days in females) before mating. Drug treatment should continue during mating and, subsequently, during the gestation period. Three graded doses should be used, the highest dose (usually the MTD obtained from previous systemic toxicity studies) should not affect the general health of the parent animals. At least 15 males and 15 females should be used per dose group. The control and treated groups should be of similar size. The route of administration should be the same as intended for therapeutic use.

Dams should be allowed to litter and treatment should continue to weaning of pups. Observations on body weight, food intake, clinical signs of intoxication, mating behaviour, progress of gestation/parturition periods, length of gestation, parturition, post-partum health and gross pathology (and histopathology of affected organs) of dams should be recorded. The pups from both treated and control groups should be observed for general signs of intoxication, sex-wise distribution in different treatment groups, body weight, growth parameters, survival, gross examination, and autopsy. Histopathology of affected organs should be done.

Teratogenicity study (Segment II): One rodent (preferably rat) and one nonrodent (rabbit) species are to be used. The drug should be administered throughout the period of organogenesis, using three dose levels as described for Segment I. The highest dose should cause minimum maternal toxicity and the lowest one should be proportional to the proposed dose for clinical use in humans or a multiple of the clinical dose. The route of administration should be the same as intended for human therapeutic use.

The control and the treated groups should consist of at least 20 pregnant rats (or mice) and 12 rabbits in each dose level. All foetuses should be subjected to gross examination, one of the foetuses should be examined for skeletal abnormalities and the other half for visceral abnormalities. Observation parameters should include: (dams) signs of intoxication, effect on body weight, effect on food intake, examination of uterus, ovaries and uterine contents, number of corpora lutea, implantation sites, resorptions (if any); and for the foetuses, the total number, gender, body length, weight and gross/visceral/skeletal abnormalities, if any.

Perinatal study (Segment III): This study is recommended if the drug is to be given to pregnant or nursing mothers for long periods or where there are indications of possible adverse effects on foetal development. One rodent species (preferably rat) is needed. Dosing at levels comparable to multiples of human dose should be done by the intended clinical route. At least four groups (including the control), each consisting of 15 dams should be used. The drug should be administered throughout the last trimester of pregnancy (from day 15 of gestation) and then the dose that causes low foetal loss should be continued throughout lactation and weaning. Dams should then be sacrificed and examined as described below.

One male and one female from each litter of F_1 generation (total 15 males and 15 females in each group) should be selected at weaning and treated with vehicle or test substance (at the dose levels described above) throughout their periods of growth to sexual maturity, pairing, gestation, parturition and lactation. Mating performance and fertility of F_1 generation should thus be evaluated to obtain the F_2 generation whose growth parameters should be monitored till weaning.

Animals should be sacrificed at the end of the study and the observation parameters should include: (dams) body weight, food intake, general signs of intoxication, progress of gestation/parturition periods and gross pathology (if any); and for pups, the clinical signs, sex-wise distribution in dose groups, body weight, growth parameters, gross examination, survival and autopsy (if needed) and, where necessary, histopathology.

10.7.4 Local Tolerance Studies

These studies are required when the clinical dose of the new drug is by routes other than, for example, oral. Those routes of administration would incldue intravenous, topical, subcutaneous, intramuscular, and so on. The drug should be applied to an appropriate site (e.g., skin or vaginal mucous membrane) to determine local effects in a suitable species. Typical study designs for these studies should include three dose levels and untreated and/or vehicle control, preferably use of two species, and increasing group size with increase in duration of treatment. Where dosing is restricted due to anatomical or humane reasons, or the drug concentration cannot be increased beyond a certain level due to the problems of solubility, pH or tonicity, a clear statement to this effect should be given. If the drug is absorbed from the site of application, appropriate systemic toxicity studies will also be required.

Dermal toxicity study: The study should be done in rabbit and/or rat. Daily topical (dermal) application of test substance in its clinical dosage form should be carried out. Test material should be applied on shaved skin covering not less than 10% of the total body surface area. Porous gauze dressing should be used to hold liquid material in place. Formulations with different concentrations (at least three) of the test substance, several-fold higher than the clinical dosage form should be used. Period of application may vary from seven to 90 days depending on the clinical duration of use. Where skin irritation is grossly visible in the initial studies, a recovery group should be included in the subsequent repeated-dose study. Local signs (erythema, oedema/edema and eschar formation) as well as histological examination of sites of application should be used for evaluation of results.

Photo-allergy or dermal phototoxicity: It should be tested by the Armstrong/Harber Test in the guinea pig. This test should be carried out if the drug or a metabolite is related to an agent causing photosensitivity or the nature of action suggests such a potential (e.g., drugs to be used in treatment of leucoderma). Pretest in eight animals should screen four concentrations (patch application for 2 hours ±15 min.) with and without UV exposure (10 J/cm^2). Observations recorded at 24 and 48 hours should be used to ascertain the highest nonirritant dose. The main test should be performed with 10 test animals and five controls. Induction with the dose selected from pretest should use 0.3 ml/patch for 2 hours ±15 min followed by 10 J/cm^2 of UV exposure. This should be repeated on days 0, 2, 4, 7, 9 and 11 of the test. Animals should be challenged with the same concentration of test substance between days 20 to 24 of the test with a similar 2-hour application followed by exposure to 10 J/cm^2 of UV light. Examination and grading of erythema and oedema formation at the challenge sites should be carried out 24 and 48 hours after the challenge. A positive control like musk ambrett or psoralin should be used.

Vaginal toxicity test: The study is to be done in rabbit or dog. The test substance should be applied topically (vaginal mucosa) in the form of pessary, cream or ointment. Six to 10 animals per dose group should be taken. Higher concentrations or several daily applications of the test substance should be given to achieve multiples of the daily human dose. The minimum duration of drug treatment is seven days (more according to clinical use), subject to a maximum of 30 days. Observation parameters should include swelling, closure of introitus and histopathology of vaginal wall.

Rectal tolerance test: For all preparations meant for rectal administration this test can be performed in rabbits or dogs. Six to 10 animals per dose group should be taken. Formulation in volume comparable to human dose (or the maximum possible volume) should be applied once or several times daily, per rectally, to achieve administration of multiples of daily human dose. The minimum duration of application is seven days (more according to clinical use), subject to a maximum of 30 days. Size of suppositories may be smaller, but the drug content should be several-fold higher than the proposed human dose. Observation parameters should include clinical signs (sliding on backside), signs of pain, blood and/or mucus in faeces, condition of anal region/sphincter, gross and (if required) histological examination of rectal mucosa.

Parenteral drugs: For products meant for intravenous or intramuscular or subcutaneous or intradermal injection, the sites of injection in systemic toxicity studies should be specially examined grossly and microscopically. If needed, reversibility of adverse effects can be determined on a case-by-case basis.

Ocular toxicity studies (for products meant for ocular instillation): These studies should be carried out in two species, one of which should be the albino rabbit which has a sufficiently large conjunctival sac. Direct delivery of drug onto the cornea in case of animals having small conjunctival sacs should be ensured. Liquids, ointments, gels or soft contact lenses (saturated with drug) should be used. Initial single dose application should be done to decide the exposure concentrations for repeated-dose studies and the need to include a recovery group. Duration of the final study will depend on the proposed length of human exposure subject to a maximum of 90 days. At least two different concentrations exceeding the human dose should be used for demonstrating the margin of safety. In acute studies, one eye should be used for drug administration and the other kept as control. A separate control group should be included in repeated-dose studies.

Slit-lamp examination should be done to detect the changes in cornea, iris and aqueous humour. Fluorescent dyes (sodium fluorescein, 0.25 to 1.0%) should be used for detecting the defects in surface epithelium of cornea and conjunctiva. Changes in intraocular tension should be monitored by a tonometer. Histological examination of eyes should be done at the end of the study after fixation in Davidson's or Zenker's fluid.

Inhalation toxicity studies: The studies are to be undertaken in one rodent and one non-rodent species using the formulation that is to be eventually proposed to be marketed. Acute, subacute and chronic toxicity studies should be performed according to the intended duration of human exposure. Standard systemic toxicity study designs (described above) should be used. Gases and vapours should be given in whole body exposure chambers; aerosols are to be given by nose-only method. Exposure time and concentrations of test substance (limit dose of 5 mg/L) should be adjusted to ensure exposure at levels comparable to multiples of intended human exposure. Three dose groups and a control (plus vehicle control, if needed) are required. Duration of exposure may vary subject to a maximum of six hours per day and five days a week. Food and water should be withdrawn during the period of exposure to test substance.

Temperature, humidity and flow rate of exposure chamber should be recorded and reported. Evidence of exposure with test substance of particle size of 4 micron (especially for aerosols) with not less than 25% being 1 micron should be provided. Effects on respiratory rate, findings of bronchial lavage fluid examination, histological examination of respiratory passages and lung tissue should be included along with the regular parameters of systemic toxicity studies or assessment of margin of safety.

10.7.5 Allergenicity/Hypersensitivity

Standard tests include guinea pig maximization test (GPMT) and local lymph node assay (LLNA) in mouse. Any one of the two can be done

Guinea pig maximization test: The test is to be performed in two steps: first, determination of maximum nonirritant and minimum irritant doses; and second, the main test. The initial study will also have two components. To determine the intradermal induction dose, four dose levels should be tested by the same route in a batch of four male and four female animals (two of each sex should be given Freund's adjuvant). The minimum irritant dose should be used for induction. Similarly, a topical minimum irritant dose should be determined for challenge. This should be established in two males and two females. A minimum of six male and six female animals per group should be used in the main study. One test and one control group should be used. It is preferable to have one more positive control group. Intradermal induction (day 1) coupled with topical challenge (day 21) should be done. If there is no response, re-challenge should be done 7–30 days after the primary challenge. Erythema and oedema (individual animal scores as well as maximization grading) should be used as evaluation criteria.

Local lymph node assay: Mice used in this test should be of the same sex, either only males or only females. Drug treatment is to be given on ear skin. Three graded doses, the highest being maximum nonirritant dose plus vehicle control should be used. A minimum of six mice per group should be used. Test material should be applied on ear skin on three consecutive days and on day 5, the draining auricular lymph nodes should be dissected out five hours after i.v. ^{3}H-thymidine or bromo-deoxy-uridine (BrdU). Increase in ^{3}H-thymidine or BrdU incorporation should be used as the criterion for evaluation of results.

The Indian Government will recognize and accept either of the above tests for assessing sensitization.

10.7.6 Genotoxicity

In the absence of other data, genotoxic compounds shall be presumed to be trans-species carcinogens, implying a hazard to humans. Genotoxic compounds need not be subjected to long-term carcinogenicity studies although registration of these drugs may be more difficult than drugs that are not genotoxic. However, if such a drug is intended to be administered for chronic illnesses or otherwise over a long period of time, a chronic toxicity study (up to one year) might be necessary to detect early tumorigenic effects.

In vitro and *in vivo* genotoxicity tests are conducted to detect compounds that induce genetic damage directly or indirectly. These tests should enable a hazard identification with respect to damage to DNA.

The following standard test battery is generally expected to be conducted:

(a) A test for gene mutation in bacteria (Ames)
(b) An *in vitro* test with cytogenetic evaluation of chromosomal damage with mammalian cells or an *in vitro* mouse lymphoma assay
(c) An *in vivo* test for chromosomal damage using rodent hematopoietic cells.

Other genotoxicity tests, for example, tests for measurement of DNA adducts, DNA strand breaks, DNA repair or recombination serve as options in addition to the standard battery for further investigation of genotoxicity test results obtained in the standard battery. Only under extreme conditions in which one or more tests comprising the standard battery cannot be employed for technical reasons, alternative validated tests can serve as substitutes provided sufficient scientific justification is provided to support the argument that a given standard battery test is not appropriate.

For cytotoxic anticancer agents, genotoxicity data are not required before Phase I and II trials, but these studies should be completed before applying for Phase III trials.

Ames' Test (reverse mutation assay in Salmonella): S. typhimurium tester strains such as TA98, TA100, TA102, TA1535, TA97 or *Escherichia coli* WP2 *uvrA* or *Escherichia coli* WP2 *uvrA* (pKM101) should be used. *In vitro* exposure (with and without metabolic activation, S9 mix) should be done at a minimum of five log dose levels. "Solvent" and "positive" controls should be used. The positive control could include 9-amino-acridine, 2-nitrofluorine, sodium azide and mitomycin C, respectively, in the Ames' tester strains mentioned above. Each set should consist of at least three replicates. A 2.5-fold (or more) increase in number of revertants in comparison to spontaneous revertants would be considered positive.

***In vitro* cytogenetic assay**: The desired level of toxicity for *in vitro* cytogenetic tests using cell lines should be greater than 50% reduction in cell number or culture confluency. For lymphocyte cultures, an inhibition of mitotic index by greater than 50% is considered sufficient. It should be performed in Chinese hamster ovary (CHO) cells or on human lymphocyte in culture. *In vitro* exposure (with and without metabolic activation, S9 mix) should be done using a minimum of 3 log doses. "Solvent" and "positive" controls should be included. A positive control like cyclophosphamide with metabolic activation and mitomycin C for without metabolic activation should be used to give a reproducible and detectable increase in clastogenic effect over the background which demonstrates the sensitivity of the test system. Each set should consist of at least three replicates. An increased number of aberrations in metaphase chromosomes should be used as the criteria for evaluation.

***In vivo* micronucleus assay**: One rodent species (preferably mouse) is needed. Route of administration of test substance should be the same as intended for humans. Five animals/sex/dose groups should be used. At least three dose levels, plus "solvent" and "positive" controls should be tested. A positive control like mitomycin C or cyclophosphamide should be used. Dosing should be done on days 1 and 2 of study followed by sacrifice of animals six hours after the last injection. Bone marrow from both the femora should be taken out, flushed with foetal bovine serum (20 min.), pelletted and smeared on glass slides. Giemsa-MayGruenwald staining should be done and increased number of micronuclei in polychromatic erythrocytes (minimum 1000) should be used as the evaluation criteria.

***In vivo* cytogenetic assay**: One rodent species (preferably rat) is to be used. The route of administration of test substance should be the same as intended for humans. Five animals/sex/dose groups should be used. At least three dose levels, plus "solvent" and "positive" controls should be tested. The positive control could include cyclophosphamide. Dosing should be done on day 1 followed by intra-peritoneal colchicine administration at 22 hours. Animals should be sacrificed two hours after colchicine administration. Bone marrow from both the femora should be taken out, flushed with hypotonic saline (20 min.), pelletted and resuspended in Carnoy's fluid. Once again, the cells should be pelletted and dropped on clean glass slides with a Pasteur pipette. Giemsa staining should be done and increased number of aberrations in metaphase chromosomes (minimum 100) should be used as the evaluation criteria.

10.7.7 Carcinogenicity

Carcinogenicity studies should be performed for all drugs that are expected to be clinically used for more than six months as well as for drugs used frequently in an intermittent manner in the treatment of chronic or recurrent conditions. Carcinogenicity studies are also to be performed for drugs:

- if there is concern about their carcinogenic potential emanating from a previous demonstration of carcinogenic potential in the product class that is considered relevant to humans; or
- where the structure-activity relationship suggests carcinogenic risk;or
- when there is evidence of pre-neoplastic lesions in repeated-dose toxicity studies; or
- when long-term tissue retention of parent compound or metabolite(s) results in local tissue reactions or other pathophysiological responses.

For pharmaceuticals developed to treat certain serious diseases, the Licensing Authority may allow carcinogenicity testing to be conducted after marketing permission has been granted.

In instances where the life-expectancy of a patient may be short (i.e., less than 2–3 years) as might occur in cancer patients, carcinogenicity studies might not be required. In cases where the therapeutic agent for cancer is generally successful and life is significantly prolonged, there may be later concerns regarding secondary cancers. When such drugs are intended for adjuvant therapy in tumour-free patients or for prolonged use in non-cancer indications, carcinogenicity studies might be needed. Completed rodent carcinogenicity studies are not needed in advance of the conduct of large-scale clinical trials, unless there is special concern for the patient population.

Carcinogenicity studies should be done in a rodent species (preferably rat). Mouse may be employed only with proper scientific justification. The selected strain of animals should not have a very high or very low incidence of spontaneous tumours.

At least three dose levels should be used. The highest dose should not induce mortality and it should not reduce the life span of animals by more than 10% of expected normal. The lowest dose should be comparable to the intended human therapeutic dose or a multiple of the dose, for example, 2.5-fold to make allowance for the sensitivity of the species. The intermediate dose is to be placed logarithmically between the other two doses. An untreated control and (if indicated) a vehicle control group should be included. The drug should be administered seven days a week for a fraction of the life span comparable to the fraction of human life span over which the drug is likely to be used therapeutically. Generally, the period of dosing should be 24 months for rats and 18 months for mice.

Observations should include macroscopic changes observed at autopsy and detailed histopathology of organs and tissues. Additional tests for carcinogenicity (short-term bioassays, neonatal mouse assay or tests employing transgenic animals) could also be carried out depending on their applicability on a case-to-case basis.

Each dose group and concurrent control group not intended to be sacrificed early should contain at least 50 animals of each sex. A high- dose satellite group for evaluation of pathology other than neoplasia should contain 20 animals of each sex while the satellite control group should contain 10 animals of each sex. Observation parameters should include signs of intoxication, effect on body weight, food intake, clinical chemistry parameters, haematology parameters, urine analysis, organ weights, gross pathology and detailed histopathology. Comprehensive descriptions of benign and malignant tumour development, time of their detection, site, dimensions, histological typing, and so on, should be given.

10.8 Animal Pharmacology

10.8.1 General Principles

Specific and general pharmacological studies should be conducted to support use of therapeutics in humans. In the early stages of drug development, enough information may not be available to rationally select the study design for safety assessment. In such a situation, a general approach to safety pharmacology studies can be applied. Safety pharmacology studies are studies that investigate potential undesirable pharmacodynamic effects of a substance on physiological functions in relation to exposure within the therapeutic range or above.

10.8.2 Specific Pharmacological Actions

Specific pharmacological actions are those which demonstrate the therapeutic potential for humans.

The specific studies that should be conducted and their design will be different based on the individual properties and intended uses of the investigational drug. Scientifically-validated methods should be used. The use of new technologies and methodologies in accordance with sound scientific principles should be preferred.

10.8.3 General Pharmacological Actions – Essential Safety Pharmacology

Safety pharmacology studies need to be conducted to investigate the potential undesirable pharmacodynamic effects of a substance on physiological functions in relation to exposure within the therapeutic range and above. These studies should be designed to identify undesirable pharmacodynamic properties of a substance that may have relevance to human safety; to evaluate adverse pharmacodynamic and/or pathophysiological effects observed in toxicology and/or clinical studies; and to investigate the mechanism of the adverse pharmacodynamic effects observed and/or suspected.

The aim of the essential safety pharmacology is to study the effects of the test drug on vital functions. Vital organ systems such as cardiovascular, respiratory and central nervous systems should be studied. Essential safety pharmacology studies may be excluded or supplemented based on scientific rationale. Also, the exclusion of certain test(s) or exploration(s) of certain organs, systems or functions should be scientifically justified.

Cardiovascular system: Effects of the investigational drug should be studied on blood pressure, heart rate, and the electrocardiogram. If possible *in vitro*, *in vivo* and/or *ex vivo* methods including electrophysiology should also be considered.

Central nervous system: Effects of the investigational drug should be studied on motor activity, behavioural changes, coordination, sensory and motor reflex responses and body temperature.

Respiratory system: Effects of the investigational drug on respiratory rate and other functions such as tidal volume and haemoglobin oxygen saturation should be studied.

10.8.4 Follow-up and Supplemental Safety Pharmacology Studies

In addition to the essential safety pharmacological studies, additional supplemental and follow-up safety pharmacology studies might need to be conducted as appropriate. These depend on the pharmacological properties or chemical class of the test substance, and the data generated from safety pharmacology studies, clinical trials, pharmacovigilance, experimental *in vitro* or *in vivo* studies, or from literature reports.

10.8.4.1 Follow-up Studies for Essential Safety Pharmacology

Follow-up studies provide additional information or a better understanding than that provided by the essential safety pharmacology.

Cardiovascular system: These include ventricular contractility, vascular resistance and the effects of chemical mediators, their agonists and antagonists on the cardiovascular system.

Central nervous system: These include behavioural studies, learning and memory, electrophysiology studies, neurochemistry and ligand binding studies.

Respiratory system: These include airway resistance, compliance, pulmonary arterial pressure, blood gases and blood pH.

10.8.4.2 Supplemental Safety Pharmacology Studies

These studies are required to investigate the possible adverse pharmacological effects that are not assessed in the essential safety pharmacological studies and are a cause for concern.

Urinary system: These include urine volume, specific gravity, osmolality, pH, proteins, cytology and blood urea nitrogen, creatinine and plasma proteins estimation.

Autonomic nervous system: These include binding to receptors relevant for the autonomic nervous system, and functional response to agonist or antagonist responses *in vivo* or *in vitro*, and effects of direct stimulation of autonomic nerves and their effects on cardiovascular responses.

Gastrointestinal system: These include studies on gastric secretion, gastric pH measurement, gastric mucosal examination, bile secretion, gastric emptying time *in vivo* and ileocaecal contraction *in vitro*.

Other organ systems: Effects of the investigational drug on organ systems not investigated elsewhere should be assessed when there is a cause for concern. For example, dependency potential, skeletal muscle, immune and endocrine functions may be investigated.

10.8.5 Conditions under which Safety Pharmacology Studies are not Necessary

Safety pharmacology studies are usually not required for locally applied agents, for example, dermal or ocular, in cases when the pharmacology of the investigational drug is well known, and/or when systemic absorption from the site of application is low. Safety pharmacology testing is also not necessary, in the case of a new derivative having similar pharmacokinetics and pharmacodynamics.

10.8.6 Timing of Safety Pharmacology Studies in Relation to Clinical Development

Prior to first administration in humans: The effects of an investigational drug on the vital functions listed in the essential safety pharmacology should be studied prior to first administration in humans. Any follow-up or supplemental studies identified should be conducted if necessary, based on a cause for concern.

During clinical development: Additional investigations may be warranted to clarify observed or suspected adverse effects in animals and humans during clinical development.

Before applying for marketing approval: Follow-up and supplemental safety pharmacology studies should be assessed prior to approval unless not required, in which case this should be justified. Available information from toxicology studies addressing safety pharmacology end-points or information from clinical studies can replace such studies.

10.9 Safety Assessment Requirements: Indian Schedule Y and International Guidelines

The regulatory guidelines adopted for nonclinical safety assessment during drug development are primarily ICH, US FDA, EMA, MHLW (Japan) and OECD. Table 10.7 provides a comparative list of guidelines corresponding to the Schedule Y (2005) requirements of India. Principally, the Indian Schedule Y requirements of safety evaluation are in accordance with the international requirements. The Indian regulatory system also accepts any animal toxicity data generated in other countries.

10.10 Good Laboratory Practice Quality System in India

10.10.1 Indian National Compliance Monitoring Authority (NGCMA)

Considering the need for aligning with the internationally-accepted good laboratory practice (GLP) quality system as adopted by OECD, US FDA, US EPA, etc., the Government of India has established the National GLP Compliance Monitoring Authority (NGCMA) in 2002. The NGCMA has a role in monitoring and accrediting test facilities engaged in the conduct of nonclinical health and environmental safety studies on test items contained in pharmaceuticals, pesticides, cosmetics, veterinary drugs as well as food additives, feed additives, and industrial chemicals. The Indian system has adopted the OECD Principles of GLP (OECD 1997).

Recently, the Drugs and Cosmetics Rules introduced a new Schedule L-1 (2008), entitled, "Good Laboratory Practices and Requirements of Premises and Equipments", primarily applicable for laboratories attached to or supporting pharmaceutical productions.

Table 10.7 Regulatory guidelines applicable for animal toxicity studies.

Indian Schedule Y Guideline	ICH	US FDA	EMA/EU	OECD
1. Animal Toxicology				
1.1 Systemic toxicity study				
1.1.1. Single dose toxicity studies	ICH S3A, S3B, M3 (R2)	Guidance for Industry: Sinlge dose acute toxicity testing for pharmaceuticals, 1996;	CPMP/ICH/384/95, CPMP/ICH/385/95, CPMP/ICH/286/95	OECD 420 (fixed dose), 423 (toxic class method) 425 (up & down procedure)
1.1.2. Repeated dose toxicity studies • Dose Ranging •14-28 day • 90-day • 180-day	ICH S3A, S3B, S4, M3 (R2)	Guidance for Industry M3(R2) Nonclinical safety studies for the conduct of human clinical trials and marketing authorization for pharmaceuticals, 2010.	CPMP/ICH/384/95, CPMP/ICH/385/95, CPMP/ICH/300/95, CPMP/ICH/286/95, CPMP/SWP/1042/99	OECD 407, 408, 409 and 452
1.2 Male Fertility study	ICH S5 (R2)		CPMP/ICH/386/95	—
1.3 Female reproduction and development toxicity studies 1.3.1. Female fertility study (Segment I) 1.3.2. Teratogenicity study (Segment II) 1.3.3 Prenatal study (Segment III)	ICH S5 (R2)		CPMP/ICH/386/95	OECD 414, 415, 416 and 443
1.4 Local tolerance (i) Dermal toxicity (ii) Photo-allergy or dermal phototoxicity (iii) Vaginal toxicity (iv) Rectal tolerance test (v) Parenteral drugs (vi) Ocular toxicity (vii) Inhalation toxicity	ICH S3A, M3(R2)		CPMP/ICH/384/95, CPMP/ICH/286/95, CPMP/SWP/2145/00	OECD 402 & 404 (Acute dermal toxicity & irritation/corrosion), OECD 432, (in vitro 3T3 NRV phototoxicity test), OECD 405 (Acute eye irritation/corrosion), OECD 403 & 436 (Acute), 412 (28/14 Day), 413 (90 Day) - Inhalation

(*continued*)

Table 10.7 (*Continued*).

	ICH	US FDA	EMA/EU	OECD
1.5 Allergenicity / Hypersensitivity (i) Guinea pig maximization test (ii) Local lymph node assay	ICH S8 Not Known		CHMP/ICH/167235/04	OECD 406 OECD 429
1.6 Genotoxicity (i) Ames' test – *in-vitro* exposure (ii) In-vitro cytogenetic assay (iii) In-vivo micronucleus assay (iv) In-vivo cytogenetic assay	ICH S2 (R1), M3(R2), Q3A(R2)		EMA/CHMP/ICH/126642/2008, CPMP/ICH/286/95, CPMP/ICH/142/95	OECD 471, 473, 474 and 475
1.7 Carcinogenicity	ICH S1A, S1B & S1C(R2)		CPMP/ICH/140/95, CPMP/ICH/299/95, CPMP/ICH/383/95, CPMP/SWP/2877/00	OECD 451, 453
2. Animal Pharmacology	ICH S7A, S7B		CPMP/ICH/539/00, CHMP/ICH/423/02	—

References: ICH Guidelines, US FDA 1997, US FDA 2010, EMA, OECD Guidelines for the testing of Chemicals. Also, these references provide exhaustive list of guidelines.

The term GLP applicable for production units in this context is often mistaken for nonclinical regulatory studies performed in compliance with the Principles of GLP, such as OECD (1997) and US FDA (1978). However, the requirements of premises and equipments described in Schedule L-1 (2008) are similar to those needed for nonclinical studies.

10.10.2 Mutual Acceptance of Data (MAD)

Following the establishment of the NGCMA in 2002, India has been a provisional member of the OECD for GLP. As a provisional member, India has been an Observer to the OECD Working Group on GLP and also a member of the OECD Test Guidelines Program. With the experience gained by Indian NGCMA as a provisional member, the OECD Council organized the Mutual Joint Visit (MJV) in 2010 by leading inspectors of OECD member countries along with the inspectors from India. Following the MJV, the OECD Council recognized the Indian GLP system and invited India to be a Full Adherent member to the OECD Council based on the Mutual Acceptance of Data (MAD). India joined as a Full Adherence member in March 2011. Thus, the key implication of India's full adherence status to the MAD system is that nonclinical health and environmental safety data generated in accredited GLP test facilities in India must be accepted by OECD member countries and other adhering countries for the purpose of assessment for the protection of man and environment. Similarly, India would accept all such regulatory data generated from test facilities from OECD member countries.

10.11 Safety Assessment Test Facilities in India

In India, basic research on safety assessment and toxicology is primarily conducted in the national laboratories. In addition, there are contract research laboratories which are accredited to conduct regulatory toxicology studies. Currently, 24 Indian laboratories have been accredited by the Indian National GLP Compliance Monitoring Authority. The Indian GLP compliance monitoring system of inspection of test facilities and accreditation of such facilities when they meet the requirements of OECD Principles of GLP began in 2004 (India GLP: see http://indiaglp.gov.in).

Until the early 1990s, although there were laboratories conducting nonclinical safety assessment studies, there was no contract research laboratory accredited to conduct regulatory toxicology studies as per the Principles of GLP. The first move to develop a test facility for conducting regulatory toxicology studies in accordance with international guidelines (OECD) was initiated by the Rallis Research Centre (earlier name of the authors' Advinus test facility) during the late 1980s. The animal facility was designed and systems and procedures were established, and an initial set of regulatory toxicology studies was conducted to support regulatory submissions on agrochemicals. As there was no GLP compliance monitoring authority/system from the Indian government in those days, the Rallis facility approached other regulatory authorities, such as the European monitoring authority, for inspection and accreditation of the facility. Considering the national laws and systems of individual countries, provision for accreditation of the test facility was available only under the OECD Principles of GLP which has provision to establish Monitoring Authorities and monitor GLP compliance of test facilities. The German GLP Federal Bureau inspected the Rallis test facility in 1992, and provided GLP accreditation certificate to the Rallis test

Table 10.8 *Forms for application for IND/IMPD.*

Regulatory system	Form title	Form No.	Reference
India	Application for grant of permission to import or manufacture a new drug or undertake clinical trial	Form 44	Drugs and Cosmetics Rules, 1945 (as amended vide GSR 780(E), dt. 10.11.2008
US FDA	Investigational New Drug (IND)	Form 1571	http://www.fda.gov/downloads/aboutfda/reportsmanualsforms/forms/ucm083533.pdf
European Commission (applicable for EMA)	Investigational Medicinal Product Dossier (IMPD)	Annex 1 ENTR/F2/BL D(2003) Detailed guidance for the request for authorization of a clinical trial on a medicinal product for human use to the competent authorities, notification of substantial amendments and declaration of the end of the trial April 2003 (also Eudract database)	http://ec.europa.eu/health/files/pharmacos/docs/doc2003/april/cp-guidance-ca_230403_en.pdf

facility that same year. Thus, the Rallis test facility (currently the Advinus) became the first GLP-accredited test facility. Subsequently, other Indian test facilities have been inspected and accredited by OECD member countries.

10.12 Investigational New Drug Application for Undertaking Clinical Trials

The Indian system requires preclinical toxicology data as well as CMC (chemistry manufacturing and control) data and other information similar to the US FDA and EMA practices. A brief summary is given in Table 10.8 for reference.

References

CPCSEA. Committee for the Purpose of Control, Supervision of Experiments on Animals, Animal Welfare Division, Ministry of Environment and Forests, Government of India. http://moef.gov.in/divisions/awd/awd_overview.html.

EC Directive 2004/10/EC of 11 February 2004, Official Journal of the European Union, L 50/44, 20.2.2004, on the harmonisation of laws, regulations and administrative provisions relating to the application of the principles of good laboratory practice and the verification of their applications for tests on chemical substances (codified version).

EMA European Medicines Agency, http://ema.europa.eu/.

IBSC. Institutional Bio-Safety Committee, Department of Biotechnology, Ministry of Science and Technology, Government of India. http://dbtbiosafety.nic.in/

ICH Guidelines International Conference on Harmonization, http://www.ich.org.

India GLP. National Good Laboratory Practice (GLP) Compliance Monitoring Authority, http://indiaglp.gov.in.

MAFF Japan (1999) Notification on the Good Laboratory Practice (GLP) Standards for Agricultural Chemicals, 11-Nousan-No. 6283, 1 October, 1999.

MHW Japan (1997) PAB Notification No. 424, March 27, 1997, Standard of Conduct of Non-Clinical Studies of Drug Safety.

OECD (1997) OECD Principles of good laboratory practice (as revised in 1997): Council Decision [C(97)186/Final] 26th November 1997.

OECD Guidelines for the testing of chemicals, http://www.oecd.org/.

Schedule Y (2005) Requirements and guidelines for permission to import and/or manufacture of new drugs for sale or to undertake clinical trials. Drugs and Cosmetics (IInd Amdt.) Rules, 2005, vide GSR 32(E), dated 20 January 2005, w.e.f. 20 January 2005.

Schedule L-1 (2008) Good Laboratory Practices and requirements of premises and equipments. Drugs and Cosmetics Rules, vide GSR 780(E), dated 10-11-2008, w.e.f. 1-11-2010.

The Drugs and Cosmetics (Amendment) Act (2008) (An Act further to amend the Drugs and Cosmetics Act, 1940), dated 5 December 2008.

The Drugs and Cosmetics Rules (1945) (As amended vide GSR 780(E), dated 10 November 2008, w.e.f. 1 November 2010).

The Patents (Amendment) Act (2005) This Act shall be deemed to have come into force on the 1st day of January, 2005.

US EPA (1989a) 40 CFR Part 160: Good laboratory practice standards – FIFRA and FFDCA (1989 and its subsequent revisions).

US EPA (1989b) 40 CFR Part 792: Good laboratory practice standards – TSCA (1989 and its subsequent revisions).

US FDA (1978) 21 CFR Part 58: Good laboratory practice for nonclincal laboratory studies (1978 and its subsequent amendments).

US FDA (1997) Guidance for Industry M3 Nonclinical Safety Studies for the Conduct of Human Clinical Trials for Pharmaceuticals.

US FDA (2010) M3(R2), Guidance on M3(R2), Nonclinical Safety Studies for the Conduct of Human Clinical Trials and Marketing Authorization for Pharmaceuticals, Federal Register, Vol. 75, No 13, Docket No. FDA/2008/D/0470, p. 3471, 21 January 2010.

11

Asia Pacific: Australia

Douglas Francis
DF Pre-clinical Services Pty Ltd., Hughes ACT, Australia

11.1 Introduction

The Australian pharmaceutical drug industry is in a state of relative infancy in relation to other developed regions of the world such as the United States of America (USA), Japan and Europe. The term "infancy" refers to the relatively low number of innovative pharmaceutical companies that have been established and operate in Australia. The pharmaceutical industry within Australia has grown to a market capitalization greater than AUD200 million. Such companies include CSL, Cochlea and Resmed. The relatively small size of the innovative pharmaceutical industry reflects the small number of clinical and nonclinical support companies in Australia.

Despite the low number of companies that offer clinical and nonclinical support to the pharmaceutical industry, the standard to which they operate is high. All clinical support companies operate within a tightly legislated environment and conduct current good clinical practice (cGCP)-compliant clinical trials, the data from which are accepted for evaluation by all major regulatory agencies such as the Australian Therapeutic Goods Administration (TGA), US Food and Drug Administration (FDA), Japanese Pharmaceuticals and Medical Device Administration (PMDA) and the European Medicines Agency (EMA). Similarly, the nonclinical support industry is small in global terms, but offers fully cGLP-compliant studies conducted to standards that major regulatory authorities will accept for evaluations.

The population of Australia exceeds 22 million and represents a relatively large market for globally-based pharmaceutical companies. Australian-based biotechnology and pharmaceutical companies choose either to undertake initial phase clinical trials in Australia and complete clinical development and seek marketing approval off-shore, or

Nonclinical Safety Assessment: A Guide to International Pharmaceutical Regulations, First Edition.
Edited by William J. Brock, Kenneth L. Hastings and Kathy M. McGown.

complete clinical development and gain marketing approval in Australia before making application for market approval in areas of larger market size such as the USA or Europe. An increasing number of overseas companies are conducting early phase clinical trials in Australia due to the more time and cost efficient approval process compared to their country of origin.

The TGA operates under relevant legislation in Australia to assess the quality, safety and efficacy of pharmaceutical medicines produced locally or being introduced to Australia by overseas pharmaceutical companies.

This chapter provides an outline of the legislative framework within which the TGA operates, and the method by which therapeutic goods are registered and gain marketing authorization in Australia. In addition, the structure and organization of the Australian clinical trial schemes, together with the nonclinical data required to support the conduct of clinical trials and registration applications, will be considered.

Legislative and data requirement to support clinical trials and registration of medicines within Australia will be discussed in detail. No attempt has been made to incorporate information relating to use or registration of other therapeutic goods such as medical devices or blood and blood products, for example – products derived from the plasma components of blood.

11.2 Australian Therapeutic Goods Administration (TGA)

11.2.1 Introduction

The Australian Therapeutic Goods Administration (TGA) is a division of the Australian Department of Health and Ageing and is responsible for the regulation of therapeutic goods including medicines, biologicals and medical devices within Australia. The TGA administers and operates under, the Australian Commonwealth Therapeutic Goods Act 1989. Overseas regulatory agencies with similar roles include the US FDA, the Japanese PMDA and the EMA.

Products making a therapeutic claim through methods such as labelling or advertising need to be on the Australian Register of Therapeutic Goods (ARTG) prior to being supplied in Australia. Inclusion in the ARTG requires the satisfactory evaluation of manufacturing, nonclinical and clinical data by the TGA.

The TGA controls the supply of therapeutic goods in Australia by undertaking:

- Evaluation of quality and nonclinical data when clinical trials are being conducted through the Clinical Trial Exemption (CTX) scheme (see below);
- The pre-market evaluation and approval of products;
- The licensing of pharmaceutical manufacturers; and
- Post-market surveillance.

11.2.2 Legislative Backing

The TGA operates under the Therapeutics Good Act (the Act) and the Therapeutic Goods Regulations (the Regulations). The Act is administered by the Australian Commonwealth Government and sets out the legal requirements for the import, export, manufacture and supply of medicines in Australia and provides a substantially uniform national system of control over therapeutic goods.

The Act defines **therapeutic goods** as:

(a) Goods that are represented in any way to be, or that are, whether because of the way in which the goods are presented or for any other reason, likely to be taken to be:
  (i) for therapeutic use; or
  (ii) for use as an ingredient or component in the manufacture of therapeutic goods; or
  (iii) for use as a container or part of a container for goods of the kind referred to in subparagraph (i) or (ii); or

(b) included in a class of goods the sole or principal use of which is, or ordinarily is, therapeutic use or a use of a kind referred to in subparagraph (a)(ii) or (iii);

and **therapeutic use** as:

(a) preventing, diagnosing, curing or alleviating a disease, ailment, defect or injury in persons; or
(b) influencing, inhibiting or modifying a physiological process in persons; or
(c) testing the susceptibility of persons to a disease or ailment; or
(d) influencing, controlling or preventing conception in persons; or
(e) testing for pregnancy in persons; or
(f) the replacement or modification of parts of the anatomy in persons.

The TGA defines therapeutic goods as:

- preventing, diagnosing, curing or alleviating a disease, ailment, defect or injury;
- influencing inhibiting or modifying a physiological process;
- testing the susceptibility of persons to a disease or ailment;
- influencing, controlling or preventing conception;
- testing for pregnancy.

11.2.2.1 Australian Register of Therapeutic Goods (ARTG)

Use and/or sale of therapeutic goods in Australia require that they appear in the ARTG, and the manufacturer of such goods be licensed by the TGA. Within the regulatory framework, medicines are classified into several categories (Figure 11.1):

- Registered medicines which are either prescription (high risk) or non-prescription (low risk);
- Listed medicines that include most over-the-counter medicines; and
- Complementary medicines.

In January 2011 there were approximately 62 000 products in the ARTG. The Act (as defined above) details the requirements for listing, registering or including medicines and biological products in the ARTG as well as many other aspects of the law including advertising, labelling, and product appearance. The ARTG is defined as a register for the purpose of compiling information in relation to, and providing for evaluation of, therapeutic goods for use in humans. The TGA plays a vital role in the entry of products in the ARTG through the evaluation of manufacturing, nonclinical and/or clinical data prior to ARTG entry.

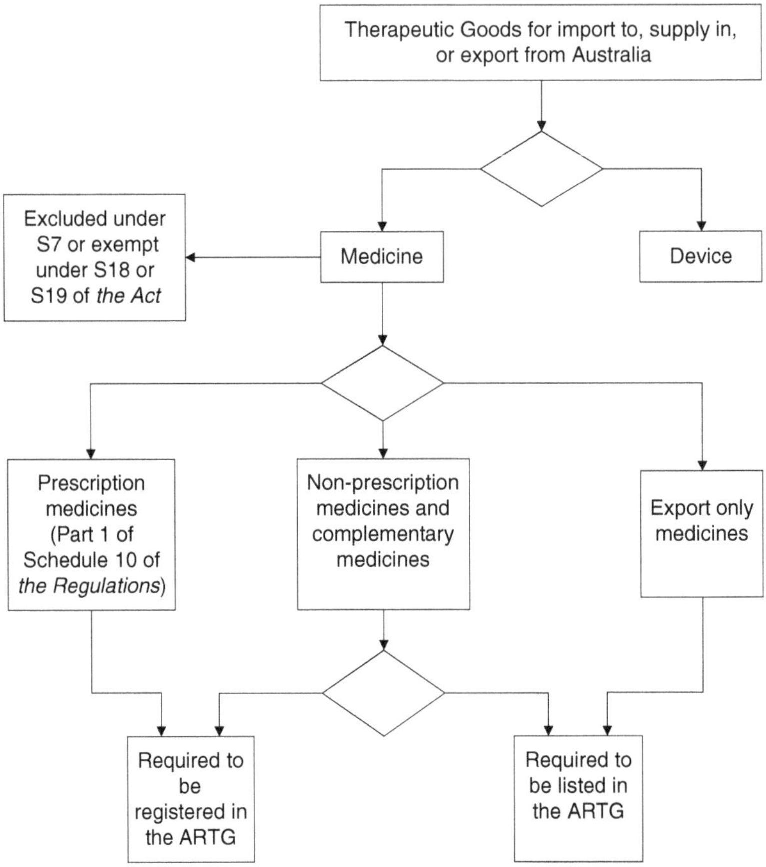

Figure 11.1 *Goods required to be included in the ARTG (Australian regulatory guidelines for prescription medicines (ARGPM), June 2004).*

Sponsors must progress through the regulatory system to have their therapeutic good appear in the ARTG before it can be used or supplied within Australia. However, there are a number of ways to gain access to therapeutic goods not appearing in the ARTG as outlined in Figure 11.2. These include:

- the special access scheme;
- the personal import scheme;
- authorized prescriber; and
- for use in clinical trials

11.2.3 Information to be Supplied to the TGA to Support Inclusion of Therapeutic Goods in the ARTG

Under the Act and appropriate Regulations, the TGA, completes evaluation of quality (chemistry, manufacturing and control), nonclinical and clinical data to support marketing applications and inclusion of therapeutic goods in the ARTG.

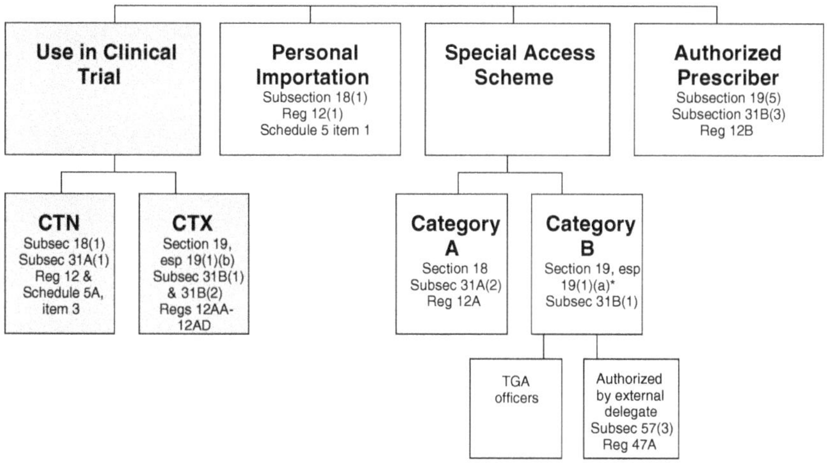

* Section 19 (1)(a) allows supply for Category A and Category B patients but, in practice, category A cases are dealt with under s18 and Reg12A.

Reg = Therapeutic Goods Regulations 1990

Figure 11.2 *Outlines the methods through which access can be gained to unapproved medicines in Australia. Includes the Sections of the Act and Regulations pertinent to their operation (Access to unapproved therapeutic goods. Clinical trials in Australia, October 2004).*

There are two categories of medicines within the TGA:

Prescription medicines and other specified medicines are regulated and evaluated by the Drug Safety and Evaluation Branch (DSEB) of the TGA (Part 1 of Schedule 10 of the Regulations). The Australian Regulatory Guidelines for Prescription Medicines (ARGPM), June 2004, describes the information to be supplied with an application to include a new medicine in the ARTG. This document applies to medicines that are evaluated by the DSEB of the TGA, in accordance with Section 25 of the Therapeutic Goods Act 1989.

Non-prescription medicines (over-the-counter medicines and complementary medicines) regulated and evaluated by the Non-prescription Medicines Branch or the Office of Complementary Medicines of the TGA.

The majority of the discussion that follows is pertinent to the evaluation of prescription medicines by the DSEB of the TGA for inclusion in the ARTG.

Therapeutics goods that require evaluation by the DSEB include:

- therapeutic goods containing a substance mentioned in Schedule 4, 8 or 9 of the Poisons Standard, or which meet the criteria for mention in any of those Schedules;
- a medical gas;
- a vaccine;
- an allergen, except an allergen for skin patch testing on unbroken skin;
- a biotechnology medicine;
- an immunoglobulin;

- a radiocontrast agent, except barium sulfate for radiological use;
- a radiopharmaceutical;
- a dialysis solution, except a haemodialysis solution;
- a special dosage form, such as a transdermal system and osmotic pump;
- an injectable medicine dosage form;
- a blood product, unless coated on a therapeutic device;
- goods referred to the DSEB for evaluation;
- an excipient in therapeutic goods mentioned in this part; and
- a therapeutic device that depends upon the release of a substance for some or all of its action.

11.2.4 Evaluation Categories

The TGA has developed assessment categories for the evaluation of applications for inclusion of new medicines in the ARTG. The categories are as follows:

Category 1 applications – An application for a new medicine or a change to a medicine constitutes a Category 1 application if it does not meet the specific requirements for Category 2 or 3. Applications for new dosage forms, new strengths and new generic products are usually Category 1 applications. Extensions of indications and amendments to the Product Information (PI) are also normally Category 1 applications.

Category 2 applications – Category 2 application provisions can only be utilized when an application has been previously approved in two *acceptable countries*, such as the USA and England. These applications have a shorter statutory time frame for evaluation.

Two independent evaluation reports from *acceptable countries*, where the product is already approved, are required to be provided at the time of application.

Category 3 applications – Category 3 applications involve changes to the quality data of medicines already included on the ARTG which might not need to be supported by clinical, nonclinical or bioequivalence data.

All submission dossiers for Category 1, 2 and 3 applications to the TGA must appear in the Common Technical Document (CTD) format as follows:

Module 1: Administrative Information and Prescribing Information for Australia
Module 2: Summaries
Module 3: Quality
Module 4: Nonclinical study reports
Module 5: Clinical study reports

The CTD is based on the International Conference on Harmonization (ICH) M4(R3) guidance document and is organized into five modules. Module 1 (Administrative Information and Prescribing Information), not strictly considered part of the CTD, is region specific and for Australia is detailed in "Administrative Information and Prescribing Information for Australia, Notice to Applicants, CTD-Module 1, January 2011". Modules 2, 3, 4 and 5 (Summaries, Quality, Nonclinical, and Clinical modules respectively) are intended to be common for all regions. Organization of the CDT is detailed in

"Organisation of the Common Technical Document for the Registration of Pharmaceuticals for Human Use, M4, ICH, January, 2004" and quality, nonclinical, and clinical data to be included in Modules 2–5 is outlined in the ICH M4 guidance documents (http://www.ich.org/products/ctd.html).

The TGA encourages a pre-submission meeting that is attended by the sponsor, supporting consultants and representatives from all relevant divisions of the Administration to discuss aspects of the proposed submission. It is recommended to present all quality, nonclinical and clinical data and seek comment from the TGA on the suitability of the data for submission and identify any obvious deficiencies. Such a practice will minimize the risk of submission rejection at the time of pre-submission assessment. The outcomes from such meetings are non-binding.

In 2010, the TGA introduced a streamlined submission process for prescription medicine applications that require the evaluation of nonclinical, clinical and/or bioequivalence information (category 1 and category 2 submissions) (see Transitional Prescription Medicine Streamlined Submission Process, January 2011). Known as the Business Process Reform (BPR) scheme it is designed to improve the flow of submissions through the TGA, and is hoped to minimize delays in the submission and assessment process. The BPR scheme not only aims to streamline efficiency of the evaluation process but also to increase access to product information and consumer medicine information, and to make available Australian Public Assessment Record (AusPAR) documents that provide information about the evaluation of a prescription medicine and the considerations that led the TGA to approve or not approve a prescription medicine submission.

The BPR scheme has introduced a pre-submission screening process to initially evaluate the submission dossier and identify any sections that have not been supplied. The legislated TGA evaluation period of 255 working days from the point of submission acceptance to when the delegate issues a decision is effectively unchanged under the new scheme. The submission format (CTD) and data requirements for submissions have not altered under the BPR scheme. A summary of the TGA streamline submission process is shown in Table 11.1.

Under the new BPR scheme, the TGA requires a pre-submission planning form (PSF) (http://www.tga.gov.au/industry/pm-forms-presubmission-planning.htm) to be submitted through the TGA eBS online site (https://www.ebs.tga.gov.au/). The PSF outlines the type of submission, data to be submitted and the proposed date for dossier submission. All category 1 and category 2 prescription medicine submission dossiers must be lodged in paper (hard copy) and electronic format.

The TGA will accept electronic copies of the submission dossier in either non-eCTD electronic submission (NeeS) format or eCTD format. The TGA prefers electronic submission dossiers to be lodged in NeeS format as it does not yet have the ability to fully manipulate eCTD format submission dossiers.

Recently, the TGA released the Australian Regulatory Guidelines for Biologicals (ARGB) (http://www.tga.gov.au/industry/biologicals-argb.htm). The guideline is empowered by the Biologicals Regulatory Framework that came into effect on 31 May 2011 with an amendment to the Australian Therapeutic Goods Act 1989. The ARGB provides information on the legal arrangements in Australia for the supply and use of human cell and

Table 11.1 *Summary of the TGA streamline submission process (BPR scheme) introduced in 2010 (http://www.tga.gov.au/industry/pm-ssp.htm).*

Phases and milestones	The streamlined submission process consists of eight phases with eight milestones, allowing effective planning and tracking by the TGA and sponsors.
Presubmission	During the presubmission phase, sponsors complete and lodge a presubmission planning form (PPF). The PPF provides information on the scope and scale of a submission, including details of the quality, nonclinical, and clinical evidence. The information provided in the PPF allows the TGA to effectively assign resources for the evaluation process.
Submission quality	Sponsors must lodge well-planned, high-quality, complete submission dossiers. Sponsors must ensure submissions meet the TGA requirements for format and content. Where sponsors submit incomplete, delayed, or poor-quality submissions, the submission will be considered not effective and therefore not accepted for evaluation.
Submission consideration	The previous 40 working-day period for the screening of submissions on receipt has been replaced by a shorter period for ascertaining whether the submission will be considered effective and therefore accepted for evaluation; or not effective and not accepted for evaluation. For straightforward submissions, this process will generally be completed in a 15 calendar-day period. Complex submissions could take longer.
Consolidated s. 31 request for information	At the completion of the 1st round assessment phase, the TGA will prepare a consolidated s.31 request for information. This request will be sent at the predesignated date specified in the planning letter so sponsors can conduct any necessary preparation activities.
No additional or supplementary data after submission lodgement	The documentation lodged in the submission dossier will be taken as the complete application.

tissue-based therapeutic goods (collectively defined as "biologicals") and how biologicals will gain entry into the ARTG. The guideline:

- explains which products are included in the Biologicals Regulatory Framework, and why;
- describes transition arrangements that apply for up to three years to allow all biologicals to meet the new arrangements;
- explains the Australian regulatory requirements for supplying biologicals; and
- sets out what is required for making an application to the TGA for biologicals.

11.2.5 Evaluation Fees and Timeframes

Evaluation fees for a new chemical entity is approximately AUD160 000. The full range of fees charged by the TGA is shown on the TGA website: http://www.tga.gov.au/about/fees-110701.htm. If a category 1 application is accepted, the legislated timeframe for evaluation is 255 working days. If a category 2 application is accepted the application must be evaluated in 175 working days from the date of acceptance. The BPR scheme recently introduced by the TGA aims to improve evaluation efficacy and possibly reduce evaluation timeframes.

Following evaluation of a prescription medicine data dossier, the TGA prepares a report that is submitted to, and reviewed by the Advisory Committee on Prescription Medicines (ACPM). The ACPM advise on:

- inclusion of a prescription medicine on the ARTG (the Register);
- changes to an entry of a prescription medicine on the Register; and
- removal or retention of a prescription medicine on the Register.

The ACPM makes a recommendation to the delegate of the DSEB who subsequently makes a recommendation to accept or reject the application for inclusion of the entry of prescription medicine in the ARTG.

11.3 Clinical Trials in Australia

11.3.1 Introduction

Clinical trials in Australia are cGCP-compliant as described in the ICH guidance document ICH E6(R1) and are undertaken to answer questions about efficacy and safety of medicines following nonclinical evaluation. It is one of the few ways to access unapproved therapeutic goods in Australia (Figure 11.2). Clinical trials need to be carefully designed to ensure safe use of the medicine by trial participants, in addition to maximizing the amount of safety and efficacy data generated from each patient. The ongoing discussion focuses on the conduct of clinical trials using investigational medicines, not medical devices within Australia.

11.3.2 Clinical Trial Schemes in Australia

Australia has two clinical trial schemes in operation which are described in some detail in "Access to Unapproved Therapeutic Goods Clinical Trials in Australia". The first of the schemes, the Clinical Trial Exemption (CTX) scheme, is largely administered through the TGA that evaluates the quality, nonclinical and clinical data relevant to the trial and makes a recommendation relating to the initiation of the trial. The second scheme, the Clinical Trial Notification (CTN) scheme, is largely operated independent of the TGA and is administered by the trial site Human Research Ethics Committee (HREC). The HREC role and responsibilities are similar to those of the US Institutional Review Board (IRB). The TGA is advised of the clinical trial once HREC approval is given. If the TGA has safety concerns relating to the clinical trial test item or trial design, they can request to review relevant quality, nonclinical and clinical summary data (contained in the investigator brochure (IB) and clinical trial protocol) and can direct questions to the sponsor relating to these data. Both the CTX and CTN schemes have their legal basis in the Therapeutic Good Act 1989 and appropriate Regulations; however, their operation is under different sections of the Act to that of the TGA.

A document has been released by the Australian government that outlines the operation of clinical trials within Australia (*The Australian Clinical Trial Handbook, March 2006*). This is a simple, practical guide to the conduct of clinical trials to international standards of Good Clinical Practice (GCP) in the Australian context and contains the following statement that outlines, in many respects, the high standard to which clinical trials in Australia are conducted:

> Through the efforts of the International Conference on Harmonisation (ICH), standards of conduct for clinical trials have been determined that are now essentially uniform for all the major regulatory agencies world-wide, including Australia's TGA. These comprise the so-called principles of "Good Clinical Practice" or GCP. Although the methods for implementing and enforcing these principles vary across regulatory agencies, the end result, it is hoped, are trials that collect high quality, credible data that contribute to the answering of specific scientific questions, while most importantly protecting the rights, safety and well-being of clinical trial participants. All these principles have their origin in the World Medical Association's Declaration of Helsinki.

Within both clinical trial schemes, the HREC plays a pivotal role. The document titled "Human Research Ethics Committees and the Therapeutic Goods Legislation (June 2001)" outlines the role and responsibilities of the HREC under the Therapeutic Goods legislation. It describes the role of the HREC in the supply of unapproved therapeutic goods for use in the CTX and CTN clinical trial schemes. A HREC operates under the guidelines contained in the "National Statement on Ethical Conduct in Human Research (March 2007)" that operates in accordance with the National Health and Medical Research Council Act, 1992. In Australia, the National Health and Medical Research Council (NHMRC) plays a vital role by providing guidance and advice to HRECs.

In summary, the HREC:

- reviews the scientific and ethical aspects of clinical trial proposals; and
- undertakes the chief role of ongoing monitoring of such research. This is crucial in delivering a number of the requirements of GCP-standard research, and highlights one way in which Australia differs from other regulatory agencies in the provision of GCP standards, with many other jurisdictions using the regulator for initial trial documentation review.

11.3.3 Clinical Trial Process

The sponsor initially selects either the CTN or CTX scheme through which to conduct their clinical trial. The CTN scheme is largely independent of the TGA and incurs relatively low lodgement fees. In general, a clinical trial to be conducted through the CTN scheme can expect to be initiated within 30–60 days of HREC application.

The decision to accept an application to conduct a clinical trial through the CTN scheme rests with the HREC. The Committee considers whether it has sufficient scientific and technical skills to satisfactorily evaluate the application. If the HREC considers it does not have sufficient skills to adequately evaluate an application under the CTN scheme, it will refer the application to the CTX scheme.

Of the clinical trials conducted in Australia, 90–95% are through the CTN scheme. In general terms, trials are conducted through the CTX scheme when the therapeutic good is considered high risk and/or it is felt that an HREC and associated advisory committees lack sufficient expertise to fully assess the safety and clinical aspects of the investigational drug product. It should be noted that under the new Biologicals Regulatory Framework, all clinical trials using high-risk biologicals would need to be evaluated through the CTX scheme.

11.3.4 CTN Scheme

Application to conduct clinical trials through the CTN scheme is made directly to the trial site HREC. HRECs generally meet to consider clinical trial applications 12 times a year, with some committees meeting more frequently.

The HREC must be supplied with an IB, a clinical trial protocol and required clinical trial patient consent forms and insurance statements. The format and content of the IB needs are described in Section 11.7 of the regulatory guidance documents CPMP/ICH/135/95 and ICH E6(R1).

Data contained in the IB is in summary form and should include the names of the study sites and the standard (non-GLP or GLP) to which the nonclinical data was generated. The following are section headings of the IB that provide an indication of the type of data required:

- Summary
- Introduction
- Physical, Chemical, and Pharmaceutical Properties of the Investigational Drug Substance and Drug Product
- Nonclinical Studies Overview
- Nonclinical Pharmacology
- Nonclinical Pharmacokinetics and Absorption, Distribution, Metabolism and Excretion (ADME)
- Nonclinical Toxicology
- Effects in Humans (if applicable)
- Pharmacokinetics and ADME in Humans (if applicable)
- Clinical Safety and Efficacy (if applicable)
- Marketing Experience (if applicable)
- Summary of Data and Guidance for the Investigator

The primary responsibility of the HREC and associated advisory committees is to ensure the safe administration of the investigational medicine during the clinical trial. The investigational drug substance and drug product should be fully characterized in terms of the physicochemical properties and stability studies sufficient to support the duration of the investigational drug product storage for the clinical trial, should be completed. The HREC or the associated scientific advisory committee expect that the information provided is in accordance with European Union (EU) or ICH (ICH M3(R2)) guidelines.

Data contained in these guidance documents are required for review, or a scientific argument presented for their absence.

Following evaluation of the IB and clinical trial protocol, the HREC provides advice to the clinical trial site as to the suitability of the application to support the conduct of the proposed trial. Once clinical trial approval is given by the HREC, the sponsor, principal investigator, Chairman of the supporting HREC, and a representative of the clinical trial site complete and sign the "Notification of Intent to Supply Unapproved Therapeutic Goods under the Clinical Trial Notification Scheme form" (CTN form) that outlines the investigational drug, the clinical trial design and proposed site. This form is submitted to the TGA together with the appropriate application fee (AUD280). Following processing and acknowledgement of the CTN form by the TGA, the clinical trial can commence. The TGA, following review of the appropriately signed CTN form, can request a copy of the IB and clinical trial protocol from the applicant for review if they have safety concerns associated with use of the investigational product. If deemed necessary, the TGA can place a clinical trial on hold that will remain in place until such time as the sponsor supplies sufficient data to the TGA to alleviate their concerns.

The TGA is not required to review data contained in an IB submitted to the HREC, and generally relies on expertise within the HREC, advisory scientific committees or independent expert reviewers to evaluate the suitability of the submitted data to support the clinical trial. As all phases of clinical trials can be conducted through the CTN scheme, the TGA cannot evaluate nonclinical and clinical data generated to support a product's registration until the point of marketing application.

The TGA maintains a record of clinical trials that have been initiated under the CTN scheme and need to be advised on completion of the clinical trial and of any deviations to the trial information originally supplied.

11.3.5 CTX Scheme

Application to conduct a clinical trial through the CTX scheme is made directly to the TGA. An application form (http://www.tga.gov.au/pdf/forms/clinical-trials-forms-ctx-part1.pdf) and supporting data as outlined in "Access to Unapproved Therapeutic Goods, Clinical Trials in Australia, October 2004", is made directly to the TGA by the sponsor.

The TGA is primarily concerned with safety assessment of the investigational product. Data submitted (four copies) to support the application should be contained in the following parts:

Part 1: Administrative information and information complementary to the summaries of scientific information.
Part 2: Summary of chemical, pharmaceutical and biological information.
Part 3: Summary of pharmaco-toxicological data.
Part 4: Summary of clinical use.
Part 5: Documentation on all fatal or life–threatening adverse events that have been associated.
Part 6: Information for Human Research Ethics Committees that included summary of overseas registration and use status, summary data sheets of the chemical,

pharmaceutical and biological information, pharmaco-toxicological data, clinical use and proposed usage guidelines.

It should be noted that clinical protocols are not submitted to the TGA as part of the CTX application. The clinical trial protocol is assessed by the HREC of the clinical trial institution following TGA review of the quality and nonclinical data as outlined above.

The TGA applies a 50-working-day period for evaluation of chemical, pharmaceutical and biological, and pharmaco-toxicological data supporting a CTX application. As at 1 July 2010, the TGA fee to complete a full evaluation to support a clinical trial conducted through the CTX scheme was AUD17 300.

If the TGA does not object to clinical trial initiation following review of the submitted data, the supporting TGA documentation that includes a summary of the application and the proposed clinical trial protocol, is submitted to the trial site HREC for consideration. A clinical trial can commence following approval by the HREC and the institution through which the clinical trial will be evaluated. The TGA must be advised within 28 days of the start of a clinical trial under the CTX scheme using the appropriate form obtained from the TGA (http://www.tga.gov.au/pdf/forms/clinical-trials-forms-ctx-part2.pdf).

11.3.6 Conducting Clinical Trials in Australia

Marketing applications to the TGA do not need to contain clinical trial data generated through the Australian CTX or CTN schemes, although there are a number of issues to be considered prior to undertaking clinical trials outside Australia:

- Clinical trial standards in Australia are high and practices are similar to those in Western Europe and North America, but with less bureaucracy and lower costs. Clinical trials conducted through the CTX or CTN schemes must be fully compliant with current GCP and analytical procedures compliant with current GLP, making the data generated of high standard and accepted by all major regulatory agencies.
- The language, healthcare system and clinical practices are similar to the majority of other developed regions in the world (USA, Europe).
- The time to commence a clinical trial through the CTN scheme in Australia is relatively short. The IB and clinical trial review cycle by an HREC is normally 4–8 weeks. Following completion of a successful HREC review and receipt of notification from the TGA, initiation of the trial can take as little as 7–10 days.
- Australia has a large European population base and many skilled clinicians, therefore minimizing the delay in patient recruitment for Phase II, III, and IV clinical trials.
- For Phase I clinical trials conducted in Australia, the investigational drug product does not need to be fully developed, and Good Manufacturing Practice (GMP) grade product is not required. However, if the drug product is not fully GMP-compliant, it should be manufactured at a quality site that follows the principles of GMP.
- Phase I clinical trial data generated through the CTX or CTN schemes can be used to conduct further trials through a US IND, or in Europe.

11.4 Nonclinical Data to Support the Conduct of Clinical Trials in Australia and Marketing Application to the TGA

11.4.1 Introduction

Much of the nonclinical data required to support clinical trials (contained in the IB or CTX data document) and marketing applications (contained in the CTD), are mandated in general terms in the Act and the Regulations. The TGA has adopted (and occasionally annotates) many of the EU regulatory guidance documents relating to nonclinical data requirements. US FDA guidance documents can be used with justification, when no equivalent EU guideline has been adopted by the TGA. In certain cases, scientific argument can be substituted for specific data to address a particular nonclinical requirement in the IB or CTD. Each argument will be assessed on a case-by-case basis for its ability to address the particular requirement. It is recommended that advice relating to Australian nonclinical data requirements be obtained from preclinical consultants and regulatory contract research organizations (CROs) at an early stage of drug development. In addition, it is recommended to meet with the TGA to discuss proposed clinical development programs prior to initiating supporting nonclinical programs.

11.4.2 Chemistry, Manufacturing and Controls

Detailed discussion relating to the Quality or Chemistry, Manufacturing and Controls (CMC) aspect of the investigational product is beyond the scope of this chapter. In general terms, information listed in the Physical, Chemical, and Pharmaceutical Properties and Formulation portion of the section devoted to the IB (Section 11.7) in ICH E6(R1) can be used as a guide to the extent of Quality/CMC data required for the IB. Similarly, the ICH M4Q(R1) guidance document outlines the Quality/CMC data to be included in the CTD submitted to the TGA for product marketing authorization and entry in the ARTG.

There is no legislated requirement in Australia for the investigational drug product used in phase I clinical trials to be manufactured to current GMP (cGMP) standard. Although cGMP product is not required, it is strongly recommended that the product be manufactured at a reputable site and in the "spirit of cGMP". The investigational drug product used in early phase clinical trials should not significantly differ from that to be marketed. Beyond Phase I clinical trials, the investigational product needs to be manufactured to cGMP standard. For marketing application and entry in the ARTG, the therapeutic good must be manufactured in a cGMP-compliant facility that is licensed by the TGA and contains an active pharmaceutical ingredient (API) and excipients that are manufactured under cGMP or to Pharmacopeia standards.

The API, and the formulation of the investigation drug product, needs to be well characterized in terms of their physicochemical properties and impurity profiles. The purity of the API in the investigational drug product used in early phase clinical trials should not exceed 93–95% and it should increase to 98–99% or greater purity for use in Phase III clinical trials and for market applications. The impurity profile (see ICH Q3A(R2) and ICH Q3B(R2) guidelines) of the API should improve as the clinical program advances, and the manufacturer of the API must be able to demonstrate that they are capable of controlling the level of impurities during the manufacturing process. For listing in the ARTG, active substances should be described in a pharmacopoeial monograph (USP, European Pharmacopeia (Ph.Eur) or equivalent). If the active ingredient is new or not described in a pharmacopoeia monograph, the sponsor should ensure that the manufacturing process is well controlled and the active substance is well described in terms of physicochemical composition and impurity profile.

Initial stability studies of the API in the investigational product, in addition to information on the formation of degradation products in the formulation over time, need to be completed prior to initiation of clinical trials. These studies should cover, at a minimum, the duration of the proposed clinical trial. Prior to registration application to the TGA, more extensive stability data as detailed in the guidance documents CPMP/QWP/122/02, rev 1 and CPMP/ICH/421/02 (ICH Q1F), are required.

11.4.3 Nonclinical Pharmacology and Pharmacokinetics

Primary and secondary *in vitro* and *in vivo* pharmacodynamic studies are required, conducted to determine how, at a cellular and biological level, the investigative molecule functions. Such studies include those to elucidate the mode of action and biological interaction at a molecular level, in addition to *in vivo* efficacy models examining the primary therapeutic activity of the investigational drug product. Such information is of value when assessing the ability of the investigational drug to induce "off-target" effects with the possible induction of unwanted toxicities. Studies, in summary form, are required for the IB (see ICH E6(R1) and for incorporation into the TGA CTD marketing application submission dossier.

Safety pharmacology data should be generated and evaluated prior to human exposure. The three areas of primary concern are the central nervous system (CNS), respiratory system and the cardiovascular (CV) system. *In vitro* (hERG assay) and *in vivo* studies (including the Irwin study) to evaluate these systems are described in the EU guidance documents, CPMP/ICH/539/00 and CHMP/ICH/423/02.

Certain safety pharmacology endpoints can be incorporated into repeat-dose nonclinical toxicology studies or clinical trial designs, whereas other end-points might be better assessed in nonclinical stand-alone studies. The use of telemetry in nonclinical stand-alone safety pharmacology studies enables a thorough assessment of respiratory and CV function following drug administration. The need or otherwise, for stand-alone safety pharmacology studies vary with the investigational drug product and its proposed clinical use and should be discussed with the TGA (or a regulatory toxicology consultant) prior to such studies being embarked upon.

In vitro metabolic and plasma binding data are recommended prior to the first human exposure and should be included in IB (in summary form) or TGA data submissions. In addition, an understanding of the ADME of the active drug substance in rodents and nonrodents is of value prior to use of the investigational drug product in clinical trials. Such pharmacokinetic (PK) studies, and the generation of PK exposure parameters are generally part of the discovery phase of a drug development program. Additional drug exposure and distribution data are gained from the toxicokinetic (TK) portion of repeat-dose toxicology studies. Comparison of animal/human drug systemic exposure data, in terms of maximum concentration (C_{max}) in plasma and area under the plasma level-time curve (AUC), is important in assessing the applicability of animal model pharmacology/toxicology data to humans.

11.4.4 Nonclinical Toxicology

Safety considerations are vital when moving an investigational drug from the preclinical to the clinical phase. Initial safety of the investigational product is addressed using well-designed and conducted nonclinical toxicology studies, the majority of which are driven by the need to support the use of the drug. The nonclinical program and design of the studies are largely driven initially by the design of the proposed clinical trial program, and ultimately by the disease being targeted, the population that the drug will be used in and the route of administration. Within the Australian system, the HREC and TGA expect that the sponsor consider the ICH and EU guidance documents relating to nonclinical toxicology data requirements. Australia is a signatory to the ICH and therefore adheres to many of the guidelines developed by this organization. The TGA has adopted the majority of the EU nonclinical guidance documents and has annotated a number of the documents with requirements pertinent to Australia. In addition, the TGA has noted that:

> Where EU guidelines adopted in Australia include references to EU legislation (including EC Directives and Regulations), the requirements contained in the referenced EU legislation are not applicable to the evaluation of prescription medicines by the TGA. The Australian legislative requirements applying to prescription medicines are contained in the Therapeutic Goods Act 1989 and the *Therapeutic Goods Regulations 1990*, as well as in various legislative instruments such as Therapeutic Goods Orders, Notices and Determinations. (http://www.tga.gov.au/industry/pm-euguidelines-adopted-nonclinical.htm).

Where relevant EU guidance documents are not available, the TGA and HREC will consider guidance documents from other recognized regulatory agencies such as the US FDA. Although each area is outlined in the relevant nonclinical guidance documents, sound scientific argument can be presented for consideration in place of actual toxicology study data. The arguments will be considered by the TGA or HREC on a case-by-case basis.

Nonclinical toxicology or safety data are required prior to the initiation of clinical trials. Toxicology studies generate biological safety data in a controlled environment, as opposed to the less controlled environment of the clinical trial. Toxicology nonclinical studies are completed to identify target organs and systems that could be affected in humans, to identify a safe starting dose for early phase clinical trials and identify systems that need to be closely monitored during clinical trials. Nonclinical toxicology studies conducted should be so designed to be predictive of the activity of the investigational drug activity in humans. It is important from a predictive perspective to assess the degree of systemic drug exposure achieved in the nonclinical studies and compare the values to those achieved in humans when the investigational drug is administered at a similar dose and route. Maximum predictive value of the nonclinical study will be gained when systemic exposure in the nonclinical and clinical studies is similar.

In addition to the degree of systemic exposure, the species used in nonclinical toxicology studies should be considered as appropriate in terms of the biological activity of the investigational drug. Similar activity in terms of receptor interaction or induction of biological activity should be demonstrated to validate the choice of species selected for the nonclinical toxicology studies.

Toxicology studies during early drug development phases tend to focus on the activity of the active ingredient and are not required to comply with Good Laboratory Practice (GLP) principles. However, later pivotal nonclinical toxicology studies that will be adopted to support the initiation of clinical trials or for marketing application should use the formulated drug product that will be used clinically, and be conducted using GLP principles. If significant changes occur in the formulation during the clinical trial program, and scientific argument cannot be generated relating to the toxicological equivalence of the two formulations, additional toxicology testing could be required in order to "bridge" the two data sets. In addition to formulation, attention should be paid to the impurity profiles of investigational drugs used in nonclinical studies as discussed above (Section 11.4.2).

Good Laboratory Practice is a quality system concerned with the organizational process and the conditions under which nonclinical health and environmental safety studies are planned, performed, monitored, recorded, archived and reported. Compliance to GLP as described in the Organization for Economic Cooperation and Development (OCED) Principles of Good Laboratory Practice is the preferred guideline in Australia. The National Association of Testing Authorities (NATA) administers the OECD Principles of Good Laboratory Practice in Australia. The OECD permits a number of non-member countries (under the mutual acceptance of data (MAD) agreement) to use the data generated in OECD member counties adhering to the OECD Principles of Good Laboratory Practice. The TGA and HREC accept GLP-compliant data generated under the GLP guidelines outlined in the US FDA 21 CFR, part 58.

Analytical methods for testing the concentration of an active ingredient in the investigational drug product and in the plasma of the species to be used in the toxicology studies are to be completed prior to initiation of toxicology studies. The analytical methods are required for dose formulation analysis used in pivotal toxicology studies and for analysis of API levels in toxicokinetic (TK) plasma samples. The data generated from the TK study component will be used to demonstrate drug exposure, important for pivotal toxicology studies, and for generating TK/pharmacokinetic (PK) parameters following drug administration. It is preferable that these analytical studies (development and validation) be GLP-compliant when samples being analyzed are part of a GLP-compliant toxicology study.

Prior to initiation of nonclinical toxicology studies, sufficient quantities of the investigational drug substance or product (as discussed above) should be available to complete the study. There is no requirement for the drug substance or drug product used in the toxicology studies to be produced under GMP. However, the test article used in the regulatory toxicology studies should be similar to, in terms of composition and manufacturing method, the product intended for use in the clinical trials. The impurity profile (in terms of number and concentration of impurities) of the clinical trial product should be reduced compared to the material used in the nonclinical toxicology studies.

11.4.5 Nonclinical Toxicology Studies

A general overview of the toxicology studies required to support clinical trials (evaluated by HREC or TGA) and marketing application (evaluated by TGA) in Australia is contained in the guidance documents CPMP/ICH/286/95 (ICH M3(R2)) and are similar to the requirements in other regions of the developed world, for example, USA, Canada, Japan and Europe. The categories of toxicological testing are described below.

Nonclinical studies, both in terms of design and duration, need to support proposed clinical trials. It is therefore recommended that the intended clinical trial designs be considered prior to designing the nonclinical toxicology testing program.

Scientific argument can be presented where a sponsor considers that the nonclinical safety/toxicology data requirements outlined in CPMP/ICH/286/95 (ICH M3(R2)) to support a "proof of concept" or early phase clinical trial are not required. In the case of a clinical trial being conducted through the CTN scheme, the institutional HREC and advising toxicologist will consider such scientific arguments on a case-by-case basis.

The discussion that follows is relevant to the nonclinical toxicology evaluation of small molecules. A number of special considerations for biological agents are discussed in the regulatory ICH guidance documents ICH S6 and ICH S6(R1) and the reader is directed to these documents and relevant consultants prior to embarking on a nonclinical program to support clinical trials or for a marketing application using a biological agent.

11.4.5.1 Genotoxicology

Genotoxicity studies are conducted to assess the tumorigenic potential of the investigational compound. Detailed description of the genotoxicity studies required for initiation of clinical trials and for product registration can be found in Chapter 16 of this book and the reader is referred to this chapter.

As these studies will be used for regulatory submission purposes, it is recommended that they be GLP-compliant. The genotoxicity studies required to support clinical trials and marketing authority application of prescription medicines are outlined in the ICH guidance document ICH M3(R2) and further described in ICH S2A and S2B. In brief, the standard battery of genotoxicity studies as recommended by the ICH (ICH S2B) is:

- A test for gene mutation in bacteria (Ames test);
- An *in vitro* test with cytogenetic evaluation of chromosomal damage in mammalian cells or an *in vitro* L5178Y tk± mouse lymphoma forward mutation assay;
- An *in vivo* test for chromosomal damage using rodent hematopoietic cells (e.g., mouse or rat bone marrow or blood).

In November 2011, the ICH finalized under Step 4 the document ICH S2(R1). The guidance document largely replaces ICH S2A and S2B and proposes a minor variation in the genotoxicity testing strategy, in addition to recommendations on data evaluation and result interpretation.

Option 1

- A test for gene mutation in bacteria (Ames test);
- A cytogenetic test for chromosomal damage (the *in vitro* metaphase chromosome aberration test or *in vitro* micronucleus test), or an *in vitro* L5178Y tk± mouse lymphoma forward mutation assay;
- An *in vivo* test for genotoxicity, generally a test for chromosomal damage using rodent hematopoietic cells, either for micronuclei or for chromosomal aberrations in metaphase cells.

Option 2

- A test for gene mutation in bacteria;
- An *in vivo* assessment of genotoxicity with two tissues, usually an assay for micronuclei using rodent hematopoietic cells and a second *in vivo* assay. Typically this would be a DNA strand breakage assay in liver, unless otherwise justified.

Genotoxicity studies assessing mutagenicity are recommended prior to the initiation of single-dose clinical trials. Assessment of chromosome damage in mammalian cells should be completed prior to multi-dose clinical trials. A complete battery of genotoxicity assessment needs to be completed prior to commencing Phase II clinical trials.

11.4.5.2 Acute and Repeat-Dose Toxicology Studies

Separate acute, single-dose toxicology studies are no longer required if such data are generated during dose range finding (DRF) or maximum tolerated dose (MTD) studies that are completed prior to the longer-term repeat-dose studies. In general, there is no requirement for GLP compliance for DRF or MTD studies.

The route of administration for acute and repeat-dosing studies should be the same as that to be used clinically. The test item should be comparable, or similar in terms of composition to that intended for clinical use, and the number and percentage of impurities should be the same or greater than those to be used in the clinical setting.

Repeat-dose studies are generally considered pivotal for regulatory agency consideration. They should be GLP-compliant, and completed in rodent (usually rat) and nonrodent species unless a valid scientific reason can be presented for use of a single species. Selection of the most appropriate nonrodent species should be based on consideration of factors such as systemic exposure and receptor binding or *in vivo* test drug activity as discussed above.

The duration and frequency of administration in the repeat-dose studies will vary with the proposed duration of treatment in the clinical trials, the PK profile of the test item and the therapeutic indication. Below are the ICH recommendations for the duration of repeat-dose toxicology studies based on the length of the proposed clinical trial (ICH M3 (R2)). These recommendations have been adopted by the TGA, and are considered suitable by most HRECs.

Maximum duration of clinical trial	Minimum duration of repeat-dose toxicology studies to support clinical trials	
	Rodent	Nonrodent
Up to 2 week	2 week	2 week
Between 2 week and 6 months	Same as clinical trial	Same as clinical trial
>6 months	6 months	6–9 months

The duration of nonclinical studies required to support market applications through the TGA are marginally longer, as shown in the table below (ICH M3(R2).

Duration of indicated treatment	Rodent	Nonrodent
Up to 2 week	1 month	1 month
>2 week to 1 month	3 months	3 months
>1 month to 3 months	6 months	6 months
>3 months	6 months	9 months

Dose selection for the studies is generally based on results of DRF or MTD studies completed in rodents and nonrodents respectively. Recommended maximum dosing levels for toxicology studies is 2000 mg/kg for rodents, and 1000 mg/kg for nonrodents. As a general design, three dose levels should be used, with the top dose inducing signs of toxicity and the bottom dose not inducing signs of toxicity. Ideally, the no observed adverse effect level (NOAEL) generated in the toxicology studies should have an exposure multiple (in terms of human equivalent dose, scaled on body surface area, or systemic exposure in terms of AUC) of at least 10-fold.

All repeat-dose studies should include appropriate recovery, nontreatment groups, and assessment of test item exposure by the incorporation of TK evaluation in the study design.

11.4.5.3 Reproduction Studies

Relevant development and reproductive toxicology (DART) studies (as outlined in ICH S5(R2) are to be completed prior to marketing application. On the assumption that male reproduction organs have been examined as part of a repeat-dose study, male fertility studies are not specifically required prior to large-scale Phase III clinical trials.

All female reproduction studies need to be completed prior to inclusion of women of child-bearing potential, or breast feeding or pregnant women into clinical trials.

11.4.5.4 Carcinogenicity Studies

Carcinogenicity studies are completed prior to marketing application and are designed to assess the tumorigenic potential of pharmaceutical products in animals and are used on the assumption that the findings are predictive for humans. The ICH discusses study design and consideration for such studies, and the reader is referred to the guidance documents ICH S1A, S1B and S1C.

11.4.5.5 Nonclinical Evaluation to Support Exploratory Clinical Trials

A guideline released by the FDA in 2006 (Guidance for Industry, Investigators, and Reviewers Exploratory IND Studies) outlines an approach whereby sponsors can conduct limited clinical trials using small amounts of a product to identify, early in the development process, those products that lack promise as therapeutic agents. As exploratory clinical trials use limited amounts of product and pose minimal potential risk, the preclinical data required to support such studies are often less than the traditional clinical trials as recommended in ICH M3(R2). The TGA has adopted the EU guidance document CPMP/SWP/2599/02/Rev1 (with amendment) and the guidance outlined in ICH M3(R2) in relation to this topic. The TGA and HREC may therefore consider reduced nonclinical testing (such as extended single-dose study in an appropriate species) to support exploratory clinical trials which adopt a number of dosing regimes that are not aimed at identifying dose limiting toxicities. The application should be accompanied by a thorough review of literature in the public domain that discusses the biological activity and safety of the test article and related compounds and will be considered on a case-by-case basis.

Application to undertake an "exploratory clinical trial" through the CTX or CTN scheme would be considered on a case-by-case basis, and it is recommended that the potential sponsor seek advice from the TGA or relevant consultants prior to embarking on a program to support such a clinical trial.

References

Access to unapproved therapeutic goods. Clinical trials in Australia, October 2004. Australian Government. Department of Health and Ageing, Therapeutic Goods Administration.

Administrative Information and Prescribing Information for Australia. Notice to Applicants, CTD-Module 1, January 2011. Australian Government. Department of Health and Ageing, Therapeutic Goods Administration.

Australian Regulatory Guidelines for Prescription Medicines (ARGPM) (June 2004) Australian Government. Department of Health and Ageing, Therapeutic Goods Administration.

CPMP/ICH/135/95. Notes for Guidance on Good Clinical Practice. Annotated with TGA comments, July 2000. Australian Government. Department of Health and Ageing, Therapeutic Goods Administration.

CHMP/ICH/423/02. Note for Guidance on the Nonclinical Evaluation of the Potential for Delayed Ventricular Repolarization (QT Interval Prolongation) by Human Pharmaceuticals (ICH 7B), May 2005.

CPMP/ICH/286/95. Note for Guidance on Non-Clinical Safety Studies for the Conduct of Human Clinical Trials and Marketing Authorization for Pharmaceuticals (ICH M4(R2)). June 2009.

CPMP/ICH/421/02. Note for Guidance on Stability Data Package for Registration in Climatic Zones III and IV (ICH Q1F), 20 February 2003 (with TGA annotation).

CPMP/ICH/539/00. Note for guidance on Safety Pharmacology studies for Human Pharmaceuticals (ICH 7A), November 2000.

CPMP/QWP/122/02, rev 1. Guideline on Stability Testing: Stability Testing of Existing Active Substances and Related Finished Products, 17 December 2003.

CPMP/SWP/2599/02/Rev1. Position paper on non-clinical safety studies to support clinical dosing with a single microdose, June 2004. Committee for Medical Products for Human Use (CHMP).

Guidance for Industry, Investigators, and Reviewers Exploratory IND Studies, January 2006, CDER.

Human Research Ethics Committees and the Therapeutic Goods Legislation (June 2001). Australian Government. Department of Health and Ageing. Therapeutic Goods Administration.

ICH E6(R1). Guideline for Good Clinical Practice. Notes for Guidance on Good Clinical Practice, June 1996. International Conference on Harmonisation of Technical Requirements for Registration of Pharmaceuticals for Human Use.

ICH M4Q(R1). The Common Technical Document for the Registration of Pharmaceuticals for Human Use: Quality – Module 3: Quality, September 2002. International Conference on Harmonisation of Technical Requirements for Registration of Pharmaceuticals for Human Use.

ICH Q3A(R2). Impurities in New Drug Substances, October 2006. International Conference on Harmonisation of Technical Requirements for Registration of Pharmaceuticals for Human Use.

ICH Q3B(R2). Impurities in New Drug Products, June 2006. International Conference on Harmonisation of Technical Requirements for Registration of Pharmaceuticals for Human Use.

ICH S2A. Guidance on Specific Aspects of Regulatory Genotoxicity Tests for Pharmaceuticals, July 1995. International Conference on Harmonisation of Technical Requirements for Registration of Pharmaceuticals for Human Use.

ICH S2B. Genotoxicity: A Standard Battery for Genotoxicity Testing of Pharmaceuticals. July 1997. International Conference on Harmonisation of Technical Requirements for Registration of Pharmaceuticals for Human Use.

ICH S5(R2). Detection of Toxicity to Reproduction for Medicinal Products and Toxicity to Male Fertility. Parent Guideline dated 24 June 1993 (Addendum dated 9 November 2000 incorporated in November 2005). International Conference on Harmonisation of Technical Requirements for Registration of Pharmaceuticals for Human Use.

ICH S6. Preclinical Safety Evaluation of Biotechnology-Derived Pharmaceuticals, 1997. International Conference on Harmonisation of Technical Requirements for Registration of Pharmaceuticals for Human Use.

ICH S6(R1). Guidance on Genotoxicity Testing and Data Interpretation for Pharmaceuticals Intended for Human Use, March 2008. International Conference on Harmonisation of Technical Requirements for Registration of Pharmaceuticals for Human Use.

ICH S6(R1). Addendum to ICH S6: Preclinical Safety Evaluation of Biotechnology-Derived Pharmaceuticals (Draft). October 2009. International Conference on Harmonisation of Technical Requirements for Registration of Pharmaceuticals for Human Use.

National Statement on Ethical Conduct in Human Research (March 2007). Developed by the National Health and Medical Research Council, the Australian Research Council and the Australian Vice Chancellor Committee.

OCED Principles of Good Laboratory Practice, as reviewed in 1997 (ENV/MC/CHEM(98)17, OECD Principles of Good Laboratory Practice (as revised in 1997)).

Organisation Of The Common Technical Document For The Registration Of Pharmaceuticals For Human Use M4, ICH, January 2004. (http://www.ich.org/fileadmin/Public_Web_Site/ICH_Products/CTD/M4_R3_Organisation/M4_R3__organisation.pdf).

The Australian Clinical Trial Handbook. A simple, practical guide to the conduct of clinical trials to International standards of Good Clinical Practice (GCP) in the Australian context. March 2006. Australian Government. Department of Health and Ageing. Therapeutic Goods Administration.

Therapeutics Good Act 1989 (http://www.comlaw.gov.au/Series/C2004A03952).

Therapeutic Goods Regulations 1990. (http://www.comlaw.gov.au/Details/F2011C00308).

Transitional Prescription Medicine Streamlined Submission Process, Version 1.5. Australian Government. Department of Health and Ageing. Therapeutic Goods Administration. January 2011.

21 CFR, Part 58, Good Laboratory Practice for Nonclinical Laboratory studies. (http://www.accessdata.fda.gov/scripts/cdrh/cfdocs/cfcfr/cfrsearch.cfm?cfrpart=58).

Part II

Toxicology Studies Supporting Clinical Development

12

Repeated-Dose Toxicity Studies in Nonclinical Drug Development

Shana Azri-Meehan[1] *and Louise Latriano*[2]
[1]*Forest Research Institute, Jersey City, USA*
[2]*ToxPharm Consulting LLC, Scotch Plains, USA*

12.1 Introduction

Repeated-dose toxicology studies are integral to the nonclinical testing programme for safety assessment of drug candidates. The results of animal studies are used to evaluate its toxicological profile to support clinical trial initiation, progression, and eventual marketing. Chronic repeated-dose studies are designed to characterize potential toxicological effects with respect to target organ toxicity, dose-dependency, relationship to exposure, and potential reversibility. In addition, these studies can be used to identify potential adverse events that should be monitored in clinical studies. Although the nonclinical protocols for repeated-dose toxicity studies are relatively standard overall, there are several aspects that need to be considered during study design to provide information that is scientifically appropriate and relevant to the type of pharmaceutical under development. These include – but are not limited to – selection of animal models, route of administration, study duration, nature of the test article, and systemic exposure. All pivotal, IND (Investigational New Drug)-enabling studies to be used to support a clinical trial need to be conducted in compliance with Good Laboratory Practice (GLP) regulations.

Nonclinical Safety Assessment: A Guide to International Pharmaceutical Regulations, First Edition.
Edited by William J. Brock, Kenneth L. Hastings and Kathy M. McGown.

12.2 General Considerations

12.2.1 Duration and Timing of Repeated-Dose Toxicology Studies

Prior to initiation of repeated-dose studies, a dose-escalation study in a rodent and nonrodent species is typically conducted to determine the spectrum of toxicity. This approach has replaced the typical acute toxicity study design to determine a LD_{50} (OECD, 2001). Dose escalation studies provide a window into how well a new chemical or molecular entity (NCE/NME) is tolerated and entails administration of a single dose, an observation period, followed by administration of a higher dose. Typically, the maximum tolerated dose (MTD) is determined in these studies that will allow selection of the doses for repeated-dose studies (Carey and Spurling, 1994).

In order for a NCE to be administered to humans, the completion of longer-term repeated-dose toxicology studies are required (Lumley and Walker, 2008). The duration of a nonclinical study to support human clinical trials of a given scope and direction in specific regions and countries has been specified in several international regulations and discussed in several chapters of this book. Within a conventional drug development programme (i.e., molecules not derived from biotechnology), the key recommendations are discussed in the International Conference on Harmonization (ICH) Guidance M3R2 (2009). These are considered to be the standard for determining the duration and timing of the repeated dose toxicology studies needed to support clinical trials of increasing dose, duration, and/or size of the exposed patient population to support a submission/registration. Table 12.1 shows the duration of dosing need to support clinical trials as they progress from Phase 1 through Phase 3.

In general, a repeated-dose study equal to or greater than the duration of a clinical trial is generally required in two species (rodent and nonrodent) prior to initiation of the clinical trial. For instance, therapeutics that will be administered for more than 28 days in a Phase II clinical study will require a 90-day or 6-month toxicology study. In the European Union (EU), data from a 6-month study in nonrodents should be available prior to clinical trials longer than 3 months. If the clinical trial exceeds this duration, then a 9-month nonrodent study should be completed. Final audited study reports must be available to the relevant regulatory authorities in order for a clinical trial to be approved.

For the US and Japan, there are some exceptions where a 6-month toxicology study is considered adequate to support longer-term/chronic clinical studies. Such exceptions include agents that induce immunogenicity or intolerance prevents prolonged exposure.

Table 12.1 *Duration of Repeated Dose Toxicity Studies to Support the Conduct of Clinical Trials.*

Duration of Clinical Trials	Minimal Duration of Repeated Dose Toxicity Studies	
	Rodents	Non-Rodents
Up to 2 week	2 week	2 week
Between 2 week and 6 months	Same as clinical trial	Same as clinical trial
>6 months	6 months	9 months

Source: ICH M3R2, 2009.

Additional examples include drugs to treat intermittent conditions that entail short-term exposure over prolonged periods of time (e.g., treatment of migraine, erectile dysfunction), drugs used in cancer therapy, and/or drugs to treat conditions where life expectancy is short.

In addition to supporting clinical trials, chronic studies (90-day for US and 6 months in the EU) are required prior to the conduct of carcinogenicity studies (ICH S1A, 1995). Dose selection for carcinogenicity studies are based on data from longer-term repeated-dose studies. In the US, the carcinogenicity protocols are reviewed by the Food and Drug Administration (FDA) under the auspices of a special protocol assessment (SPA; see Chapter 15; FDA, 2002).

12.2.2 Anticancer Therapeutics

For therapeutics used to treat serious and life-threatening malignancies, the timing and duration of the nonclinical evaluation differ from other drugs. As with all drugs, the primary objective in Phase 1 clinical trials in patients is to assess safety of the drug. For drugs used to treat patients with advanced cancer, preclinical dosing could involve administration of the clinical maximum tolerated dose (MTD) or demonstration of dose-limiting toxicity. This end-point need not be death provided that the doses administered induce severe, life-threatening toxicity. For many small molecule anticancer agents, the starting dose for the first-in-humans study is often set at 1/10 of the severely toxic dose in 10% (STD_{10}) based on body surface area (mg/m^2) based on rodent studies or at the highest non-severely toxic dose (HNSTD) from nonrodent studies (see Chapter 3). If irreversible toxicity is induced in the nonrodent species and it is a more appropriate animal model, then the starting dose would be 1/6 of the highest dose tested in the dose-range finding study (DeGeorge *et al.*, 1997). In toxicity studies with oncologics, the NOAEL or no observed effect level (NOEL) is not considered essential (ICH S9, 2010). A new or separate toxicology study is not needed to support higher clinical doses or continued treatment beyond the duration of the clinical trial. In support of continued development for patients with advanced cancer, results from repeated dose studies of three months' duration following the intended clinical schedule should be provided before initiating Phase 3 studies (ICH S9, 2010).

The dosing regimen and/or treatment schedule for oncologic products is often different than conventional products as well. Dosing can range from a single dose every 3–4 weeks to daily or weekly dosing for a specified time period. How the designs from a preclinical study are used to support clinical dosing regiments for oncologics is provided in Table 12.2.

This regimen can then be tailored to the patient population and repeated for a specified duration based on the clinical indication (ICH S9, 2010; Chhabra *et al.*, 1990). However, for advanced cancer where there might be limited options for a patient, the nonclinical study duration of more than four weeks is not usual. This clearly depends on the intended indication. For most pharmaceuticals to treat advanced cancer, nonclinical studies of three months' duration are considered sufficient support registration and marketing.

In a conventional drug development programme, repeated dose toxicology studies are conducted to support Phase 3 clinical trials and fulfil regulatory requirements for subsequent registration and approval. If, during development, there are significant changes in the clinical dosing regimen or new/additional manufacturing processes of the drug

Table 12.2 Examples of Oncology Treatment Schedules and Duration of Toxicology Studies to Support Initial Clinical Trials.

Clinical Schedule	Examples of Nonclinical Treatment Schedule
Once every 3-4 week	Single Dose
Daily for 5 days every 3 week	Daily for 5 days
Daily for 5–7 days, alternating week	Daily for 5–7 days, alternating weeks (2-dose cycles)
Once a week for 3 week, 1 week off	Once a week for 3 week
Two or three times a week	Two or three times a week for 4 week
Daily	Daily for 4 week
Weekly	Once a week for 4–5 doses

Reproduced from http://www.ema.europa.eu/docs/en_GB/document_library/Scientific_guideline/2010/01/WC500043471.pdf Copyright (2009) European Medicines Agency.
Source: ICH S9, 2010.

substance/drug product formulation, an additional repeated-dose study might be necessary. Changes of this magnitude could alter the chemical nature of the pharmaceutical and/or impact exposure which, in turn, could alter its safety profile. Regulatory agencies consider such changes to be major, and therefore require generation of new data to confirm the drug safety.

12.2.3 Assessment of Systemic Exposure

The relevance to exposure is an essential consideration in preclinical studies, is clinically relevant and an integral part of the drug development process. Toxicokinetics (TK) is defined as the generation of pharmacokinetic data (PK), either as an integral component of the nonclinical study (concomitant TK) or in specially designed supportive studies to assess systemic exposure (bridging study) (ICH S3A, 1994). Furthermore, this guidance states that TK information could allow better interspecies comparisons than simple dose/-body weight (or surface area) comparisons. Therefore, when human PK data become available, the TK data from preclinical toxicology studies allow an understanding of the level of exposure where toxicity occurs in animal studies and how this can be related to the clinic. A ratio is used to calculate human versus animal exposure (to drug and metabolites) allowing for the calculation of a margin of safety (MOS) or margin of exposure (MOE) based on area under the plasma concentration curve (AUC). Comparison of dose is not always relevant. The quantification of systemic exposure also provides an assessment of the body burden and assists in the interpretation of similarities and differences in toxicity across species, dose groups, and sexes.

TK assessment of a NCE in a repeat-dose study is used to determine whether the kinetics are linear and if drug accumulation occurs over time. Both the parent compound and main metabolites are evaluated. The key TK parameters are similar to those determined in a single PK study and include (ICH S3A, 1994):

Cmax: Maximum (peak) plasma/serum concentration
Tmax: Time to achieve maximum plasma/serum concentration
AUC0-t: Area under the plasma concentration vs. time curve from time zero to specified time (t)

Specific examples of AUC values of interest in toxicology studies include:

AUC0–24: Area under the curve for 24-hour dosing period. For many substances, the AUC_{0-24} after the last dose in a repeated-dose study represents the total daily exposure to drug under steady-state conditions. This value is often reported in both nonclinical and clinical studies and used for calculation of MOS.

AUC0-∞: Area under the plasma concentration curve vs. time curve from time 0 to infinity (i.e., time of last quantifiable sample), accounting for total exposure from the dose. This value is usually calculated after a single dose, or after the last dose of a multi-dose study.

Additional TK parameters can be determined using these data that include volume of distribution, clearance, and half-life. To calculate these end-points, it is critical to collect enough blood samples following dosing to fully characterize the concentration versus time profile.

Results from single-dose kinetic studies could also provide guidance regarding formulation selection and in the prediction of rate and duration of exposure during the dosing interval (ICH S3A, 1994). These data might also assist in the selection of appropriate dose levels and provide justification that the study TK sampling scheme is adequate to estimate exposure following repeat dosing. TK assessments in repeated-dose studies are based on multiple and chronological blood collections following dosing and are typically evaluated on Day 1 and the final day of dosing prior to necropsy.

12.2.4 Qualification of Drug Substance and Product

Repeated-dose studies are also pivotal for the evaluation and qualification of impurities or degradants that couldy be present in the drug substance and/or drug product. It is advisable to first identify all potential impurities, including those generated by the synthetic process and degradants. Once identified, the structures should be subject to *in silico* structure-activity analysis (SAR) to determine if there are structural alerts on the molecule with the potential to induce genotoxicity and/or carcinogenicity. There are several commercially-available software programs such as DEREK® and Multicase®.

These impurities/degradants will then need to be qualified in order for the drug to be considered safe. Qualification is the process of acquiring and evaluating data that establishes the biological safety of an individual impurity/degradant. In addition to altering the synthetic process to reduce levels of these entities, repeated-dose and genotoxicity studies could also be conducted to establish that the impurities, degradants or even excipients do not have the potential to induce toxicity degradants (ICH Q3A, 2006; ICH Q3B, 2006; EMA, 2003; FDA, 2005; FDA, 2008). These guidelines call for limits of specified and unspecified impurities/degradants in the drug product batches administered to humans and required toxicology studies to support their safe use. Safe use can be defined as being in below or at the Threshold of Toxicological Concern (TTC) as described in EMA (2006) and Munro *et al.* (2008).

12.2.5 Other Types of Applications/Submissions

12.2.5.1 Changes in Previously-Approved Products

Previously-approved drug products may require a new approval due to changes in indication, dosage form, strength, route of administration, regulatory status (e.g., switch to over-the-counter (OTC) status). To implement these changes in the US and acquire approval, an application could initially rely on the FDA's decision regarding the safety and effectiveness of the previously-approved product. This could then be coupled with the new information that will be used to support the "new" product. The additional information could result from new study results or published data from the scientific literature. If safety information to support the change or modification from the listed drug(s) is not available in the public domain, data from appropriate bridging studies can provide an adequate basis for assessing any new impact on safety. This can include – but is not limited to – a 4-week repeated-dose study in rodents (FDA, 1999). The study should compare the product in the new application to the previously-approved product to determine whether the toxicity profile has changed (such as target organ toxicity).

The drug substance used in repeated-dose studies should be representative, both qualitatively and quantitatively, of the material to be used in the clinic, starting from the first-in-human study that requires GMP grade material. It is important to have an adequate level of characterization of the drug early in the development process. Since studies are conducted in compliance with GLP, typical parameters such as identity, homogeneity, and stability, including quantification of the drug degradation profile and process-related impurities need to be evaluated and documented.

12.2.5.2 Exploratory IND and Microdosing

Efforts to reduce the number and breadth of toxicology studies needed to permit a clinical evaluation of low pharmaceutical doses have resulted in a guidance document from FDA (1996) and a position paper from EMA (2004) on the concept of microdosing. The FDA defines a *microdose* as less than 1/100th of the dose of a compound calculated (based on animal data) to yield a pharmacologic effect of the test substance, with a maximum dose of <100 micrograms. In both the UK and US, an "extended" single-dose toxicology study is required to support administration of a single microdose to humans. In the US, administration of repeated microdoses in clinical trials lasting up to seven days can be supported by a 2-week repeated-dose toxicology study in a sensitive species accompanied by TK evaluations. The goal of this study would be to select an optimal dosing range for the clinical trial. The rat is the usual species chosen for this purpose. Additional studies in nonrodents, most often dogs, can also be used to determine whether the rodent is an appropriately sensitive species. This "confirmatory" study can include only one sex if no gender differences were noted in the rodent study, and/or if only a single sex will be studied in the clinical trial. It can use fewer animals and include a dose that approximates the rat NOAEL. The end-points should be identical to those assessed in the rodent study. If the data from the confirmatory study suggest that the rodent is not the more sensitive species, then a 2-week repeated-dose toxicity study should be performed in the nonrodent species to select doses for human trials.

12.2.5.3 Drugs Used in Combination and Combination Drug Products

A combination product is defined as a product comprised of any combination of a drug and a device, a biological product and a device, a drug and a biological product, or a drug, device, and a biological product (FDA, 2006). Development of these products is clearly more complex based on what the drug is being combined with, for example, another drug, biological, device, contrast image agent A key factor is whether one of the individual components is an already-approved product. If this is not the case and one of the compounds is an early stage NCE, then a limited toxicology study should first be conducted using end-points such as mortality, body weight, and clinical observations in addition to a pharmacology study to demonstrate its increased potency (ICH S9, 2010). In these studies, the dose of the approved product should remain constant (and at a sufficient multiple of the clinical dose) and the dose of NCE may vary. In addition, it would be worthwhile to have one dose group contain the approved drug alone at the same fixed dose to confirm the drug toxicity profile in the test system. Oncology drugs are frequently used and evaluated in combination. It is noteworthy that additional toxicology studies are not warranted if the toxicity profile of the individual pharmaceuticals is well characterized.

12.3 Study Design Considerations

12.3.1 Selection of Animal Model

There are several critical factors that need to be considered when selecting the appropriate animal model for repeat-dose toxicology studies (Olson *et al.*, 2000). Critical parameters that should be addressed are outlined in Table 12.3. Regulatory requirements need also to be addressed.

Regulatory guidance documents (FDA, ICH) typically require the use of a rodent and one nonrodent species for longer-term studies. The rodent species used is typically the rat and, less commonly, the mouse. The nonrodent species can be dogs (beagles), minipigs, or nonhuman primates, depending upon which species is the most appropriate in terms of how the drug is handled metabolically relative to humans. Dogs are often the more common nonrodent species from a cost perspective. For all of these species, the availability of historical control data is an important consideration when evaluating the relationship of the drug relative to toxicity.

With regard to the strain for use in rodent studies, there are several that are typically used in GLP studies. For rats, the typical strains are Sprague-Dawley, CD, Fisher 344 (F344), or Wistar rats. The strains of mice that are used are CD-1, BALB/c, B6C3F1, or Swiss-Webster. Generally, very little differences in toxicity are observed across strains within a species.

Dog studies typically use beagles. Other breeds have also been used for specialized applications such as the greyhound for their well-defined muscle and nerve systems, and

Table 12.3 *Considerations in Selecting Animal Models for Toxicology Studies.*

Target organ toxicity is comparable to that observed in humans
Biosimilarity in regard to PK/ADME profile
The pharmacological target is the same as that in humans
There is a dose-response relationship[a]
Responsive to the primary pharmacodynamic effect of the substance, if possible[b]
Availability of morphological, biochemical and physiological historical control data[b]

ADME: absorption, distribution, metabolism, and excretion.

[a]Tibbits *et al.*, 2010.

[b]EMA, 2010.

large chest cavity, the Dalmatian for its gastrointestinal system being similar to humans, and the German Shepherd for its bone and joint configuration (Haggerty *et al.*, 2008).

Minipigs are the preferred nonrodent model for evaluating the repeated-dose toxicity of pharmaceuticals administered topically. The body weight/surface area ratio, surface texture, and skin architecture of the minipig are similar to humans (Makin *et al.*, 2012). This species is also finding use in phototoxicity, safety pharmacology and reproductive toxicity studies.

When the dog is not an appropriate choice, due either to different metabolic profile or other physiological reasons, nonhuman primates, such as the Cynomolgus monkey, are the species of choice. Baboons could also be used as well as marmosets, or squirrel monkeys (Walker *et al.*, 2008). The most common route of administration in these species is oral (gavage or nasogastric administration).

In studies conducted to determine the safety of an NCE in drug discovery, selection of the nonrodent species hinges on several critical factors. A key consideration is how comparable is the metabolism in the chosen species to that expected in humans based on *in vitro* metabolism studies (hepatocytes). Are the pathways similar or is there a species-specific pathway that results in formation of a different metabolite or a higher level of a potentially toxic metabolite? This will clearly impact the toxicity profile of the molecule and the interpretation of the findings. Once the programme progresses, resulting in better characterization, it is acceptable to change species for chronic studies to ensure that the ADME profile is similar to humans representing the most appropriate animal model.

12.3.2 Size of Treatment Groups

12.3.2.1 Toxicology

The number of animals per dose group is usually dependent on the animal model used but should include both genders to assess any potential sex differences. For rodents, there should be enough animals to account for potential mortality. The typical number of animals used to evaluate toxicity in rodent studies is 10–15/animals/sex/dose group for the main study (dosing period). This does not include TK and recovery group animals (discussed below). With nonrodent studies, the number of animals is much lower. The recommended number of animals per dose group in chronic studies recommended in ICH M3 (2009) is 3/sex/dose, but 4–5 animals/sex/dose is recommended by OECD (2008), and is preferred by the FDA.

12.3.2.2 Toxicokinetic Evaluation

Appropriate monitoring of the plasma or serum levels of the parent compound and metabolites is critical within any pivotal repeat-dose toxicology study to assess exposure (Cayen, 1995). As noted previously, determining the PK parameters, for example, C_{max} or AUC, is integral to the study design and will need to be incorporated into all repeated-dose study protocols. The time points for collecting blood in concomitant TK studies should not interfere with the normal conduct of the study or cause undue physiological stress to the animals. Rodent studies, due to their size and blood volume limitation, typically employ satellite groups of animals used for TK evaluation. It is strongly recommended that a TK satellite group be used in the study since repeated blood sampling of rodents can result in undesirable impact on haematological end-points, for example, haematocrit (Young *et al.*, 2011). The evaluation of toxicokinetics in chronic toxicology studies is typically conducted on Day 1 following dosing and again at the end of the treatment period. The number of individual time points that can be collected sequentially from rodents is dependent on several factors including assay blood volume requirements for analysis, method of collection, and approval by the laboratory's animal welfare committee. In many cases, rodents can be bled 2–3 times over a >24 hour dosing interval, and 2–3 times over the course of ≥90 day study, if needed, provided appropriate recovery time is allowed between collections. A TK profile with 4–8 time points typically requires 6–10 animals/sex/dose to produce a sample value in triplicate for each time point. TK monitoring and/or profiling is usually done for all treatment groups, including controls. Although it is often considered unnecessary to assay samples from control animals, these could be collected and assayed to determine if contamination occurred or for method validation. For long-term studies, collection of samples from control animals is required by the EU.

The recommended number of matrix samples to be collected for AUC determination is 4–8 time points during a dosing interval. Justification of the sampling schedule is recommended to ensure adequate characterization of exposure (ICH S3A, 1994). This is especially important for estimating C_{max} as it a major determinant of the AUC value. For drugs that are rapidly distributed, the early time points following dosing are particularly critical in order to capture a fleeting C_{max}. Later time points commonly collected include a TK sample between 8–12 hour post dose, and 24 hour postdose sample, which must be taken before the administration of the next dose. The last sample taken could vary based on the half-life of the drug.

12.3.2.3 Recovery

The study duration cited in Table 12.1 only covers the dosing period. It is advisable to include a recovery period in a chronic repeat-dose study. Recovery entails the use of a second subset of animals that have undergone treatment for the designated dosing period and are then maintained without drug treatment for a predetermined time. This allows evaluation of whether there is reversibility of treatment-induced toxicity or to determine if there is delayed toxicity over this period. There is no specific guidance for the number of recovery animals in a study, but the general practice is to use 5–10 animals/sex/dose for rodents and 2–3 animals/sex for nonrodents.

In the recovery phase, all of the standard parameters measured in the main study (dosing phase) should be assessed with toxicokinetics being optional, considering the recovery period would likely result in complete drug elimination. The duration of the recovery period is dependent upon the treatment phase and is typically equal to or shorter in duration to the main study. Factors that impact the duration of the recovery phase are the pharmacokinetics of the test agent, the nature of the findings including clinical signs, and an understanding of the biology and potential for recovery of the target tissue. Older study protocols evaluated only the control and high dose groups in the recovery phase, but all dose groups should be evaluated in order to have a complete recovery profile, especially if there is evidence of a dose response. To control cost of the study, however, usually the control and high-dose animals are evaluated with evaluation of the intermediate doses dependent on findings at the high dose.

The total of number of animals in a rodent repeated-dose study that includes evaluation of both TK and recovery is approximately 25–35 animals/sex/dose, In nonrodents, 3–5 animals/sex/dose is commonly used. The control group in rodent studies could have a smaller number of animals if TK time points are evaluated.

12.3.3 Dose and Administration

The dose regimen and the route of administration should be chosen based on its intended use in humans allowing sufficient exposure to the drug and its metabolites. Other routes of administration can be used if justified by pharmacological, TK/PK considerations, and/or toxicity of the test substance (EMA, 2010).

For drugs administered orally in the clinic, the mode of drug administration in rodents is typically via gavage or food/water. For the latter, however, calibration in regard to daily ingestion is necessary in order to calculate the daily dose. According to FDA, for oral administration, the volume of an aqueous solution in rodents should not exceed 1 mL/100 g body weight and 0.4/100 g body weight for an oil-based vehicle. For the latter case, a low-fat diet could be considered. The volume should be adjusted every 1–3 days based on body weight (FDA, 2007). Gavage is also used for dogs. Tablets or gelatine capsules containing an excipient is also an acceptable mode of administration in this species. Nasogastric gavage is the most commonly-used route in monkeys as capsule administration is not recommended for longer-term studies (Gad *et al.*, 2008).

When administering a drug via the IV route, there are several critical considerations that should be addressed. In the clinic, will the test material be administered by bolus or via infusion? This could have a direct impact on the safety profile of the drug if toxicity is dependent on C_{max}, which would be evident if toxicity is evident immediately following dosing. It is advisable to review the PK profile of the drug when designing repeat-dose studies. To prevent C_{max} dependent toxicity, the drug could be administered via a slow bolus or slow infusion. This will likely allay the immediate toxicity and will provide data as to how the drug will be administered clinically.

Repeat IV dosing of rodents for more than four weeks becomes challenging, particularly for bolus administration, due to local inflammation and potential necrosis at the tail injection site.

Use of cannulated animals could resolve this issue to avoid local irritation at the injection site. However, this alternative is more costly and the presence of an in-dwelling catheter over extended periods of time could lead to additional toxicity such as inflammation of the infusion site leading to mild-to-moderate spleen or local lymph node enlargement and increased organ weights. This could include thrombosis and chronic-active inflammation and secondary findings associated with catheterization. These findings are well-documented due to cannulation and might not be treatment-related.

For drugs targeting the respiratory system, the route of administration is either intranasal or via inhalation. The choice of animal model should allow administration using the clinically relevant drug-delivery device, provide a similar pulmonary or nasal deposition profile, and demonstrate a metabolic profile expected to be similar in humans. Another aspect that is unique using this route is that if the level of exposure, based on TK/PK studies, is lower in animals relative to humans, different routes of administration could be combined such as via oral administration. However, for drugs such as corticosteroids, where the oral route produces a low deposition and systemic exposure, the IV route could be the best mode of administration to achieve an exposure that is toxicologically relevant (DeGeorge *et al.*, 1997).

Dermal/topical preparations present several unique considerations and challenges. Dose levels can be calculated based on body weight (mg/kg) or body surface area (mg/m^3) (Makin *et al.*, 2012). In rodents, and even in minipigs, it is difficult to achieve doses that are significantly higher than the intended human dose due to limits in the amount of drug that can be applied via this route. Many topical drugs have limited solubility and cannot be formulated at higher concentrations. In these cases, high doses can be achieved by drug application several times a day or by increasing the treated dermal surface area. Absorption will only occur at the skin interface and therefore layering drug material will have little impact on the overall penetration of the drug through the skin. In addition, the application site needs to be protected by gauze or bandage to minimize the potential for unintended oral ingestion or cross-contamination, which also could increase absorption. Due to the difficulty of testing a topical product at doses that provide adequate safety margins of systemic exposure, topical drug programmes could include a systemic chronic rodent repeated-dose study, for example, 28 days or longer using the oral or parenteral (subcutaneous, intraperitoneal) routes of administration to fully characterize systemic toxicity at higher exposures.

Administration via the intrathecal, intrarticular, intraocular, and other routes is not optimal for long-term repeated dosing in animals and, therefore, alternative routes of administration might need to be considered. However, many of these alternative routes of administration are to examine therapies that are not usually administered for long periods of time, for example, antibiotics and cytotoxic oncologics.

12.3.4 Dose Selection

Longer-term repeated dose studies are designed to support the progression of extended clinical trials, resulting in prolonged exposure and/or to increase the number of patients enrolled. Dose selection for each repeat dose clinical study is dependent on the toxicity observed on the preceding, shorter, respective dose-range finding study, for example, doses for a 90-day study are contingent on data from the 28-day repeat-dose study. Dose levels are typically selected as multiples of one another in order to determine whether a dose/concentration response will be evident. Dose levels should achieve, at the low end, a dose that produces the pharmacodynamic or therapeutic effect and systemic exposure comparable to what is expected in patients at the intended clinical dose (EMA, 2010). One critical goal of toxicology repeated-dose studies is to identify a high dose which enables identification of target organ toxicity or other non-specific toxicity. If the drug is difficult to formulate, then the highest dose could be limited by the maximum volume that can be administered and/or solubility. The high dose should not induce high mortality rates, which then could complicate interpretation (FDA, 2007). In regard to carcinogenicity studies where a 3-month repeated-dose study in rodents is first conducted, it is important to demonstrate the MTD for each species as well as to try to obtain a 25-fold multiple of the highest anticipated clinical exposure (ICH S1C(R2), 1994). As previously mentioned, in cancer clinical trials, doses could exceed those tested in the preclinical toxicology studies.

In the early stage of a drug development programme, there is typically limited toxicology information available on a NCE. The available data might be limited to the evaluation of single and/or pharmacological doses in rodents. This is partly due to the limited availability of test substance in the discovery phase of drug development. Dose-range finding studies can help address any potential technical challenges in drug formulation and delivery, identify a potential lethal dose, and provide an initial assessment of any relationship between toxicity and dose. In such cases, it is advisable to conduct a non-GLP dose range-finding study to support dose selection prior to initiation of GLP repeated-dose studies, for example, those that enable the opening of an IND/eCTD. The non-GLP study typically uses a smaller number of animals/group, and/or could evaluate only one sex. Use of a single sex is recommended for gender-specific drugs only – this practice could lead to missing potential androgenic effects. The duration of these studies can range from 3–7 days of dosing. In nonrodents, a dose-escalation scheme could be used to reduce animal numbers and blood samples can be collected to determine the multi-dose TK profile. Histopathology evaluation is usually not conducted in non-GLP range-finding studies and, if so, are limited to a known or suspected target organ.

When a novel vehicle is being used in the toxicology studies, and its effects are unknown, it could be beneficial to include a secondary control group with a known vehicle as a comparator (Levine, 2009). Upon completion of the study, data from both control groups should be compared to each other as well as relative to the conducting laboratory's historical control data to ensure that there were no confounding factors. This will allow selection of the optimal vehicle.

12.3.5 Test Article (Drug Substance) and Drug Formulation

12.3.5.1 Drug Substance Quality

As stated earlier, the material used in nonclinical studies should be representative of the material to be used in the clinic and be in compliance with GLP. At this point in the development process, the test material does not need to be GMP grade, as is required for clinical studies. However, all of the supporting documentation to support its GLP status (including identification and levels of impurities) should be in place and included in the final report. Each batch used in the repeated-dose toxicity studies should be identified as well as the specifications for known impurities. The physiochemical characteristics of the batch should be presented and certified for each one, and the stability of the drug substance stated. A certificate of analysis (CoA) should be available for each batch used in the study and included in the final report.

12.3.5.2 Drug Formulations

Typical vehicles for oral administration include carboxymethylcellulose (CMC), Tween 80, propylene glycol, polysorbate, and hydroxypropyl-beta-cyclodextrin (Thackaberry *et al.*, 2010). These are usually used alone or in combination, depending on the solubility of the test material. The formulations should be characterized with validated analytical methods prior to study start, with recovery levels within the designated specification. Both long-term and short-term stability should be established under use conditions (ambient or under refrigeration). When deciding how long to collect stability data, consideration should be given to how often the formulation will be prepared at the test site (e.g., daily/weekly), and the time to complete the analysis of the dose solution. Both actual and accelerated stability should be conducted.

For poorly soluble oral drugs, achieving reasonable multiples of clinical doses can be a challenge. In some cases, the amount of the vehicle needed to deliver high toxicology doses could be greater than the dose used to establish safety. Poorly soluble test substances are also a challenge in dosing dermal drug products, as previously discussed. Oral suspensions are also limited by volume. The drug could be administered twice daily (BID) or three times daily (TID) in order to acquire the optimal doses. PK evaluations should precede the actual study to ensure adequate exposure.

Intravenous formulations should be sterile solutions. Suspensions cannot be administered via this route. Prior to the conduct of repeated-dose studies, it is wise to determine whether there is a potential for local irritation and red blood cell haemolysis at the infusion site to avoid tissue damage following repeated long-term administration. If irritation potential is evident, then the mode of administration might need to be changed as previously discussed in Section 12.2.3.

12.4 Study Observations and Assessments

12.4.1 General

There are many critical parameters that need to be assessed in a chronic study in order to fully evaluate the potential toxicity of a test material. These include – but are not limited to – clinical observations, clinical chemistry, haematology, toxicokinetics, urinalysis, ophthalmology, macroscopic, and microscopic assessments. Repeat-dose juvenile studies should include neurobehavioural parameters as well. Protocols using nonrodents typically include electrocardiograms (ECG), which cannot be performed routinely on rodents. Standard parameters are summarized in Table 12.4.

For both rodents and nonrodents, historical control data from the laboratory should be available for morphological, biochemical, and physiological parameters that are evaluated in these studies. In the case of nonrodents, pre-treatment values should also be obtained from the animals used in the study (EMA, 2010). Over the course of the study, the in-life observations should be monitored with a frequency which allows an assessment of the changes that occur over time without inducing any undue physiological stress on study animals. Control and treated animals are subject to identical assessments and examinations. Animals that die or are sacrificed during the study should be autopsied and, if feasible, subjected to microscopic examination in order to determine the cause of death/morbidity.

12.4.2 Clinical Observations

Cage-side clinical observations should be conducted at least twice daily following dosing to determine whether there are immediate signs of toxicity as well as morbidity and mortality. These should be conducted consistently, preferably at the same time each day, with an interval of at least six hours or near the T_{max} (FDA, 2007). Observations include, but are not limited to, changes in respiration, clonic, tonic movements, emesis, salivation,

Table 12.4 *Parameters Examined in Repeated Dose Chronic Toxicology Studies.*

Haematology/Coagulation	Tissue Preservation
leucocyte count	adrenal (2)
erythrocyte count	aorta
haemoglobin	brain
haematocrit	caecum
MCH	colon
MCV	duodenum
MCHC	oesophagus
platelet count	epididymis (2)
differential count	eye(2) with optic nerve*
cellular morphology (prepare slide/hold)	femur (articular surface of the distal end)
reticulocyte count	gallbladder[e]
PT[a]	gross lesions
APTT[a]	Harderian gland[d]
Clinical Chemistry	heart
alanine aminotransferase[f]	ileum
sodium[a]	jejunum
potassium[a]	kidney (2)
chloride[a]	lacrimal gland[c]
total protein	lesions
albumin	liver
calcium[a]	lung with bronchi
phosphorus[a]	lymph node (mesenteric)
total bilirubin[a]	mammary gland
urea nitrogen	ovary (2)
creatinine[a]	pancreas
glucose[a]	pituitary
total cholesterol[a]	prostate
ALT[a]	rectum
AST[a]	salivary gland (2) (mandibular)
alkaline phosphatase[a]	sciatic nerve
triglycerides[a]	seminal vesicles[b]
globulin	skeletal muscle (thigh)
A/G ratio (calculated) serum protein electrophoresis (MHLW only)[a]	skin
Urinalysis/ Urine Chemistry	spinal cord - thoracic, lumbar, cervical
appearance[a]	spleen
specific gravity[a]	sternum with bone marrow
pH[a]	stomach
protein[a]	testis (2)*
ketones[a]	thymus
bilirubin[a]	thyroid (2) with parathyroid
glucose[a]	tongue
occult blood[a]	trachea
volume[a]	urinary bladder
micro examination of sediment[a]	uterus
sodium(MHLW only)[a]	vagina
chloride(MHLW only)[a]	
potassium(MHLW only)[a]	
tissues fixed in neutral buffered formalin	

The above table lists the tissues, blood and urine parameters collected for most general toxicity studies. Tissues are generally fixed in neutral buffered formalin with the exception of the testis and eyes which are fixed in modified Davidson's solution. Some tissues are present only in some species. For example, rats do not possess a gallbladder, dogs do not have seminal vesicles, Harderian glands are only collected from rodents while lacrimal glands are only collected from dogs and primates. Blood and urine parameters are consistent between rats, dogs and primates however due to the limited blood volume available from a mouse and due the limited urine output of a mouse these parameters are abbreviated for this species. If these parameters are needed for scientific purposes related to the test compound additional animals will need to be added to the study in order to measure these parameters.

*Fixed in Modified Davidson's solution.

[a]Not collected from mice.

[b]Not collected/found in dogs.

[c]Dogs and primates only.

[d]Rodents only.

[e]Not found in rats.

[f]Mouse only.

lacrimation, lethargy, piloerection, alopecia, changes in fur, eyes including changes in pupil size, changes in gait, posture, and bizarre behaviour such as grooming, and self-mutilation. In the cases where there is clear abnormal behaviour, the animal should be examined more extensively. These parameters are also examined during the recovery phase of the study to determine reversibility or delayed toxicity.

12.4.3 Food Consumption/Body Weight

Body weight and food consumption should be recorded individually for all animals prior to the start of dosing and at least once weekly thereafter. This is a critical parameter as it is reflective of any potential general toxicity effects that could be induced by treatment. If animals exhibit excess thirst following treatment, then water consumption should be monitored as well.

12.4.4 Clinical Chemistry

Clinical chemistry parameters can reflect organ-specific toxicity that can precede and/or confirm histopathological findings. These analyses generally measure electrolyte balance, carbohydrate and lipid metabolism as well as kidney and liver function and are measured at the end of the treatment and recovery periods. The list of parameters is cited in Table 12.4. Furthermore, specific biomarkers in a target organ can be added to determine potential functional endpoints.

12.4.5 Haematology

Similar to clinical chemistry parameters, haematological parameters should be measured at study termination as well as following the recovery phase. Coagulation parameters should also be assessed. If additional blood samples are required in rodents, then collections should be carefully planned due to limited blood volume in these animals. Collections should not impact haematological parameters and should be toxicologically relevant (Young, 2011). Inclusion of additional animals in each dose group to ensure that adequate blood can be drawn could resolve this issue. Standard haematological parameters are listed in Table 12.4.

12.4.6 Urinalysis

Although urinalysis is a standard measure in chronic studies to assess urogenital function and can be used to assess general systemic health in the animal, it is not a particularly sensitive measure in toxicology studies and several factors need to be considered. Urine volume might be small in rodent species such as mice and specimens collected are not sterile. Furthermore, measurements could be prone to error. The presence of blood cells, crystals and casts is not uncommon in animal urine and could be pH-dependent making it difficult to discern if such findings are test article-related.

On the other hand, urinalysis provides information pertinent to renal function, which is particularly important when it is the primary route of excretion. Specific gravity assessment examines overall kidney function as it measures the ability to concentrate urine. High levels of protein in the urine (proteinuria) might indicate glomerular injury, poor tubular resorption, inflammation, or secreted protein downstream from the kidney in the urogenital tract (Hall, 2001). These parameters should be considered to be confirmatory of renal toxicity when there are also changes in clinical chemistry and/or histopathology. Typical parameters are listed in Table 12.4.

12.4.7 Ophthalmologic Examinations

Ophthalmologic examinations should be conducted on both rodents and nonrodents in all groups, including controls, prior to the start of dosing as well as prior to terminal sacrifice. If no changes are observed following the treatment phase, then ophthalmologic evaluations during the recovery period can be optional. Eyelids, lacrimal apparatus, and conjunctiva are examined grossly. A slit lamp or an indirect ophthalmoscope is typically used to examine the cornea, anterior chamber, iris, lens, vitreous humour, retina, and optic disc. It is not uncommon to use a short-acting mydriatic such as tropicamide for these evaluations. For ophthalmic drugs, funduscopy and tonometry canalso be conducted (FDA, 2008).

12.4.8 Electrocardiographic Examinations

To evaluate the potential for cardiotoxicity, nonrodents are subject to electrocardiographic (ECG) examination. ECGs are not often conducted on rodents. The standard parameters are the RR, PR, and QT intervals that measure the time between the specific waves, as well as the QRS duration which is reflective of the rate of depolarization of the right and left ventricles. If the heart rate is increased or decreased by any dose level, then the QT interval should be corrected (QTc). Blood pressure is not usually measured in chronic toxicology studies due to high variability. Data are collected prior to initiation of dosing (pre-dose) and again prior to necropsy. The timing of ECG assessments following treatment is dependent on the T_{max} of the drug being administered. Data should also be collected following the recovery period if changes are evident following termination of the treatment phase to measure reversibility. These measurements are particularly important if a cardiovascular signal has been observed in single-dose safety pharmacology studies (hERG assay, Purkinje fibre assay and/or telemetry) or the drug class has known cardiovascular effects.

12.4.9 Macroscopic Examination

Following necropsy, organs are systematically removed for weighing. They are then examined macroscopically for visual changes. Parameters examined include organ surface (evidence of rough appearance or pitting), as well as alterations in colour and shape (Wilson *et al.*, 2001). All changes should be noted and further microscopic evaluation should be conducted to determine whether these gross observations reflect whether these changes are treatment-related.

12.4.10 Organ Weights

Changes in organ weights could be indicative of target organ toxicity. In addition to the standard tissue list typically examined, additional organs can be added based on the mechanism of action of the test material, absorption, distribution, metabolic profile, route of elimination, toxicokinetics, and/or the physiology of the test species (Sellers *et al.*, 2007).

In a position paper publication from the Society of Toxicologic Pathology for a GLP repeated-dose study, the liver, heart, kidneys, brain, adrenal glands, and sexual organs from sexually mature animals were considered to be critical organs (Baily *et al.*, 2004). Organ weights are typically also normalized using body and brain weights (relative body weight), which is important when assessing whether terminal body weights were affected by treatment. In nonrodents, this is particularly important as a means to normalize intra-group variation. Absolute and relative organ weights are recommended for studies where the test material is administered for at least seven days. The thyroid and pituitary glands are also typically weighed (Levine, 2009).

12.4.11 Histopathology

Upon macroscopic evaluation, tissues are preserved and prepared for microscopic examination typically using a 10% formalin solution. Certain organs require specific fixatives based on the nature of the tissue such as Bouin's fluid for the testes, Davidson's fixative for the eyes and paraformaldeyde in 0.1M phosphate buffer for *in situ* perfusion (Latendresse *et al.*, 2002; Levine, 2009).

The tissues collected are typically those cited in the 1981 OECD toxicology test guidelines, which are reflected in the EMA (2010) guideline. A list of tissues is provided in Table 12.4 that includes the core list based on a proposal by the Society of Toxicological Pathologists (Bregman *et al.*, 2003). Often, additional tissues are collected depending on the route of administration, mechanism of action, and/or known or suspected toxicity of the test material. For example, the addition of nasal cavity and turbinates, larynx, and tracheobronchial lymph nodes can be included in the protocol for inhalation studies. For locally administered products, including IV, a tissue sample of the injection site should be evaluated.

Histopathological examination of all animals is critical, including controls and those that died prematurely or were sacrificed during the study. In cases where there are clear histopathological changes that are not easily interpreted, electron microscopy is typically used to better assess the findings. In addition, specific stains can be used to better understand target organ toxicity such as the Nissl or Golgi stains for drugs causing neurotoxicity (Pilati *et al.*, 2008).

12.4.12 Additional Parameters

The repeated-dose studies represent an opportunity to incorporate the evaluation of parameters of interest based on the pharmacology and/or toxicity of the test substance. For anticancer products, an evaluation of some of the safety pharmacology parameters could be included. This includes an assessment of cardiovascular safety by EKG monitoring, and central nervous system effects conducted using the Irwin Assay. For drugs that modulate the immune system, additional haematology, clinical chemistry, target organ weight, and histopathology can be conducted as suggested by ICH.

12.4.13 Medical Devices

The testing regimen for medical devices is substantially different from that of pharmaceuticals. The purpose of preclinical testing is typically to evaluate biocompatibility *in vivo* and is governed by the guidelines outlined in ISO 10993-1. Chronic studies for medical devices are recommended for devices that entail permanent exposure (>30 days). Surface medical devices that are in contact with mucosal membranes and breached or compromised surfaces (e.g., wound care) require chronic toxicity studies, as do those with indirect and direct contact with blood and h tissue, bone and dentin as are implantable devices. For implanted devices, the duration of devices comprised of bio-absorbable polymers (such as dissolving sutures) might vary based on the absorption rates of the component polymers. The tissue impacted by the implant should be examined at several intervals over the course of the study to determine the level of inflammation, bioabsorption, and recovery.

Acknowledgement

The authors would like to thank Dr Christina Carruthers for her valuable input.

References

Baily, S.A., Zidell, R.H., and Perry, R.W. (2004) Relationship between organ weight and body/brain weight in the rat: What is the best analytical endpoint. *Toxicol. Pathol.*, **32**, 448–466.

Bregman, C.L., Adler, R.R. Morton, D.G. *et al.* (2003) Recommended tissue list for histopathological examination in repeat-dose toxicity and carcinogenicity studies: A proposal of the society of toxicological pathology (STP). *Toxicol. Pathol.*, **31**, 252–253.

Carey, P.F. and Spurling, N.W. (1994) Maximum tolerated dose studies. *Drug Inf. J.*, **28**(1), 203–211.

Cayen, M.N. (1995) Considerations in the design of toxicokinetic programs. *Toxicol. Pathol.*, **23**(2), 148–157.

Chhabra, R.S., Hyff, J.E., Schwetz, B.S., and Selkirk, J. (1990) An overview of prechronic and chronic toxicity/carcinogenicity experimental study designs and criteria used by the National Toxicology Program. *Environ. Health Perspec.*, **86**, 313–321.

DeGeorge, J.J., Ahn, C.H. Andrews, P.A. *et al.* (1997) Considerations for toxicology studies of respiratory drug products. *Reg. Toxicol. Pharmacol.*, **25**(2), 189–1983.

DeGeorge, J.J., Ahn, C.H. Andrews, P.A. *et al.* (1997) Regulatory considerations for preclinical development of anticancer drugs. *Cancer Chemother Phamacol*, **41**(3), 173–185.

EMA (2003) Guideline on the Limits of Genotoxic Impurities.

EMA (2004) Position Paper on Non-Clinical Safety Studies to Support clinical Trials with a Single Microdose CPMP/SWP/2599/02/Rev 1.

EMA (2010) Guideline on Repeated Dose Toxicity. CPMP/SWP/1042/99 Rev 1.

FDA (1999) Draft Guidance for Industry: Applications Covered by Section 505(b)2.

FDA (2002) Guidance for Industry: Special Protocol Assessment.

FDA (2005) Guidance for Industry: Estimating the Maximum Safe Starting Dose in Initial Clinical Trials for Therapeutics in Adult Healthy Volunteers.

FDA (2006) Guidance for Industry: Early Development Considerations for Innovative Combination Products.

FDA Guidance for Industry and Other Stakeholders 2000, revised July 2007. Toxicological Principles for the Safety Assessment of Food Ingredients. *Redbook*.

FDA (2008) Draft Guidance for Industry: Genotoxic and Carcinogenic Impurities in Drug Substances and Products: Recommended Approaches.

FDA March (2008) Guidance for Industry and Review Staff: Nonclinical safety evaluation of reformulated drug products and products intended for administration by an alternate route.

Gad, S.C., Cassidy, C.D. Aubert, N. *et al.* (2008) Nonclinical vehicle use in studies by multiple routes in multiple species. *Intl. J. Toxicol.*, **25**, 499–521.

Haggerty, G.C., Peckham, J.C., Thomassen, R.W., and Gad, S.C. (2008) The dog, in *Animal Models in Toxicology*, 2nd edn (ed. S.C. Gad), Informa Healthcare, New York, NY, p. 563.

Hall, R.L. (2001) Principles of clinical pathology for toxicology studies, in *Principles and Methods of Toxicology*, 4th edn (ed. A.W. Hayes), Taylor and Francis, Philadelphia, Pa.

ICH Guidance M3 (R2) (2009) Nonclinical Safety Studies for the Conduct of Human Clinical Trials and Marketing Authorization for Pharmaceuticals.

ICH Guidance Q3A (2006) Note for Guidance in Impurities Testing: Impurities in new Drug Substances.

ICH Guidance Q3B (2006) Note for Guidance in Impurities Testing: Impurities in New Drug Products.

ICH Guidance S1A (1995) Guideline for the Need for Carcinogenicity Studies of Pharmaceuticals.

ICH Guidance S1C(R2) (1994) Dose Selection for Carcinogenicity Assessment of Pharmaceuticals.

ICH Guidance S3A (1994) The Assessment of Systemic Exposure in Toxicity Studies.

ICH Guidance S9 (2010) Nonclinical Evaluation for Anticancer Pharmaceuticals.

ISO 10993-1 (2009) Biological evaluation of medical devices Part 1: Evaluation and testing in the risk management process.

Latendresse, J.R., Warbritton, A.R., Jonassen, H., and Creasy, D. (2002) Fixation of testes and eyes using modified Davidson's Fluid: Comparison with Bouin's Fluid and conventional Davisson's Fluid. *Toxicol Pathol.*, **30**(4), 524–533.

Levine, B.S. (2009) Single and repeated dose toxicity, in *International Pharmaceutical Product Registration*, 2nd edn (eds A.C. Cartwright and B.R. Matthews), Informa Healthcare, New York, NY, p. 377.

Lumley, C.E. and Walker, S.R. (1985) The value of chronic animal toxicity studies of pharmaceutical compounds: A retrospective analysis. *Fund. Appl. Toxicol.*, **5**, 1007–1024.

Makin, A., Mortensen, J.T., and Brock, W.J. (2012) Dermal toxicity studies. Skin architecture, metabolism, penetration, and toxicological and pharmacological methods, in *The Minipig in Biomedical Research* (eds P.A. McAnulty, A.D. Dyan, N.C. Ganderup, and K.L. Hastings), CRC Press, New York, Chapter 12. OECD Guidance Document for the performance of chronic toxicity and carcinogenicity studies supporting TG 451, 452, and 453. 2008.

Munro, I.C. and Renwick, A.G., and Danielewska-Nikiel, B. (2008) The threshold of toxicological concern (TTC) in risk assessment. *Toxicol Lett.*, **180**(2), 151–156.

OECD Guideline for Testing of Chemicals: Acute Oral Toxicity–Acute Toxic Class Method. 2001. 423.

OECD Guidance Document for the Performance of Chronic Toxicity and Carcinogenicity Studies, Supporting TG 451, 452 and 453. (Draft) 2008.

Olson, H., Betton, G. Robinson, D. *et al.* (2000) Concordance of the toxicity of pharmaceuticals in humans and in animals. *Reg. Toxicol. Pharmacol.*, **32**, 56–67.

Pilati, N., Barker, M. Panteleimonitis, S. *et al.* (2008) A rapid method combining Golgi and Nissl staining to study neuronal morphology and cytoarchitecture. *J. Histochem. Cytochem.*, **56**(6), 539–550.

Sellers, R.S., Morton, D. Michael, B. *et al.* (2007) Society of Toxicology pathology position paper: Organ weight recommendations for toxicology studies. *Toxicol. Pathol.*, **35**(5), 751–755.

Thackaberry, E.A., Kopytek, S. Sherratt, P. *et al.* (2010) Comprehensive investigation of hydroxypropyl methylcellulose, propylene glycol, polysorbate 80, and hydroxypropyl-beta-cyclodextrin for use in general toxicology studies. *Toxicol. Sci.*, **117**(2), 485–492.

Tibbits, J., Cavagno, J.A. Haller, C.A. *et al.* (2010) Practical approaches to dose selection for first in-human clinical trials with novel biopharmaceuticals. *Reg. Toxicol. Pharmacol.*, **58**, 243–251.

Walker, M.D., Nelson, J.K. Bernal, J.C. *et al.* (2008) Primates, in *Animal Models in Toxicology*, 2nd edn (ed. S.C. Gad), Informa Healthcare, New York, NY, p. 663.

Wilson, N.H., Hardisty, J.F., and Hayes, J.R. (2001) Short-term, subchronic, and chronic toxicology studies, in *Principles and Methods of Toxicology*, 4th edn (ed. A.W. Hayes), Taylor and Francis, Philadelphia, PA, p. 917.

Young, J.K., Hall, R.L. O'Brein, P. *et al.* (2011) Best practices for clinical pathology testing in carcinogenicity studies. *Toxicol. Pathol.*, **39**(2), 429–434.

13

Evaluation of Potential Carcinogenicity

James A. Popp[1] *and Matthew S. Bogdanffy*[2]
[1]*Stratoxon, Lancaster, USA*
[2]*Boehringer Ingelheim Pharmaceuticals, Ridgefield, USA*

13.1 Introduction

13.1.1 Short History of Carcinogenicity Testing

Over 225 years ago, the seminal work of Percival Pot laid the foundation for the concept that chemicals could be the cause of human cancer (Pot, 1775). In Pot's publication in 1775, the high incidence of scrotal cancer in British chimney sweeps was attributed to the soot from chimneys. The fundamental observation that an external agent could contribute to, if not cause, cancer was not experimentally explored for 143 years until Yamagiwa and Ichikawa (1918) demonstrated the production of skin tumors on the ears of rabbits painted with coal tars. Approaches to carcinogenicity testing and evaluation in animals have been steadily refined during the past century (Figure 13.1). Follow-up work to the original coal tar studies resulted in the identification of specific chemicals in the coal tar that had carcinogenic properties. By the 1950s, additional publications identified carcinogenicity of various chemicals unrelated to coal tar. Through the 1950s and 1960s, most carcinogenicity studies could be characterized as observational studies in which animals received the potential carcinogenic agent for varying periods of time with incomplete evaluation for carcinogenicity that generally included incomplete histopathological evaluation of tissues. In addition, the evaluation of various agents followed vastly different protocols. As experimental studies, the results rarely, if ever, resulted in a comprehensive evaluation of potential animal carcinogenicity.

Nonclinical Safety Assessment: A Guide to International Pharmaceutical Regulations, First Edition.
Edited by William J. Brock, Kenneth L. Hastings and Kathy M. McGown.

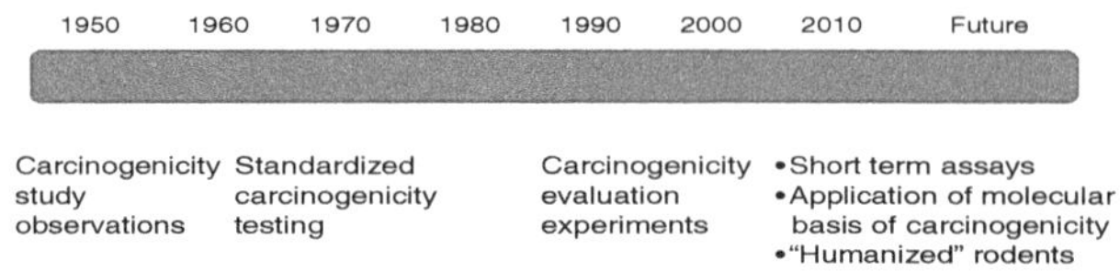

Figure 13.1 *Carcinogenicity testing: Historical perspective.*

Standardized approaches to evaluation of carcinogenicity using rats and mice started to emerge in the 1960s and early 1970s when there was an increased awareness that chemicals can cause cancer, with the major focus on environmental chemicals and a lesser but important interest in drugs. Consequently, the evaluation for potential carcinogenicity expanded from the research laboratories into a testing scenario in which studies were being designed to address a broader question of whether a given agent could cause cancer at any site within an exposed animal. Therefore, it was realized that comparison of carcinogenicity study results from one study to another required standardized approaches. A "Standard Chronic Bioassay" for the evaluation of carcinogenicity was started in the 1960s through multiple efforts but was clearly enhanced by the National Cancer Institute programme which was the predecessor to the National Toxicology Program (NTP). While there have been numerous contributors to the standardization of carcinogenicity testing, the NTP has had a significant, if not predominant, role in setting the standards for carcinogenicity testing that are used worldwide today. The NTP, mandated by the US Congress in 1978, has evaluated over 500 compounds using standardized protocols and methods for the evaluation and documentation of tumour findings. In the 1990s, the ICH Guidelines for carcinogenicity testing provided specific direction on critical aspects of carcinogenicity study design in addition to specific information on when carcinogenicity testing was required for pharmaceuticals.

The 1980s and 1990s ushered in an era with increased focus on trying to understand the human relevance of animal tumors. This effort required experimental approaches, added to basic testing paradigms of administration and standard tumour evaluation, to provide critical information on the mechanism of the tumour induction. Based on the more advanced understanding of tumour mechanisms, certain tumours in rodents are now considered by many to be irrelevant as an indication of human cancer risk. Most importantly, the basic concepts developed over the past several decades allow incorporation of specific end-points such as evaluation of TSH and thyroid hormones into the carcinogenicity study if tumours are anticipated in the thyroid. The modern carcinogenicity testing protocol should be designed to obtain as much relevant information as possible considering the time, cost and animal usage inherent in a carcinogenicity testing study.

Obviously, the current paradigm for carcinogenicity testing as discussed throughout this chapter has not reached a pinnacle of success for effectively and efficiently determining the potential carcinogenic risk of a drug to humans. Refinement continues, as has occurred over the past decade when the use of transgenic mice has been introduced for the assessment of animal carcinogenicity. The quest for better approaches continues with the evaluation of other short-term and, hopefully, more predictive assays for carcinogenicity. The ultimate goal would, of course, be to accurately identify every human carcinogen with no or very few false positives. Today, extensive attention is being paid to developing such predictive systems using molecular techniques leading to the identification of specific carcinogenicity pathways in the cell. However, such techniques are not currently validated for the determination of carcinogenicity, resulting in the continued use of the rodent bioassay until better approaches become available and are validated. However, it is imperative that rodent bioassay studies are thoughtfully designed, performed with minimal to no flaws and the tumour response be critically evaluated at the end of the study. If a tumour response is identified in the study, it is important that a reasonable understanding of the mechanism of carcinogenicity be developed to contribute to the evaluation of potential risk to humans. This chapter is intended to provide a summary of expected standard approaches in carcinogenicity studies to be used until toxicologists are able to move to more advanced approaches.

13.1.2 Objective of Carcinogenicity Testing

The objective of a carcinogenicity test is succinctly stated by the ICH Guideline S1A (ICH, 1995): "The objective of carcinogenicity studies is to identify a carcinogenic potential in animals and to assess the relevant risk in humans". It is important to note the two components of this objective. The first component, that is, ". . . to identify a tumorigenic potential in animals" is relatively clear. The study must be designed to allow adequate assessment of the carcinogenic response in animals taking into consideration such parameters as number of animals, doses, length of dosing period, animal survival and full tumour characterization through histopathology that will withstand scrutiny and appropriate statistical evaluation. The second component is indeed much more difficult and complex, that is, ". . . to assess the relevant risk to humans". If a tumour response occurs in the study, this second component generally demands that additional insight into the tumour response is required beyond the simple identification of a statistically elevated tumour incidence in treated versus control animals. Several of the most important aspects of this component are outlined in Figure 13.2. It is important that tumour incidence is related to administered dose and systemic exposure. For pharmaceuticals, a "yes/no" answer to carcinogenicity in animals has very limited value in assessing human risk, particularly since most are nongenotoxic, which is very important in determining if there is an apparent threshold for a carcinogenic response. The identification of a threshold is very important in assessing risk. However, the limited number of animals in each dose group does not permit the identification of an absolute threshold in animals that can be utilized for assessing risk. Nevertheless, the shape of the exposure-to-tumour response curve provides information to strongly suggest that, below a defined exposure, a carcinogenic response is very unlikely in animals and therefore unlikely to occur in humans. The relationship of the occurrence of the tumours in animals related to defined animal drug

- Characterize the tumour incidence related to administered dose and internal exposure
- Define the apparent threshold for a tumor response within the limits of power of study
- Provide tumour incidence in relation to human exposure, i.e. exposure, margin
- Provide data related to mode of action

Adapted from *Critical Reviews in Toxicology* **37**:729-837, 2007

Figure 13.2 *Objectives of carcinogenicity study relevant to human risk.*

exposures is important information to compare with human exposures. If the tumour response is clearly restricted to a high-dose group and this group has a substantially higher exposure than humans receiving therapeutic doses, the concern for human risk is greatly reduced. Additional information that could define the mode of carcinogenic action should be obtained from a carcinogenicity study whenever possible, but being cautious to not compromise the primary goal for determining whether the drug causes a carcinogenic response in animals.

13.1.3 Overview of Regulatory Guidelines for Testing Carcinogenicity of Pharmaceuticals

For many years, the requirement for carcinogenicity evaluation, study design and general approaches for the evaluation of carcinogenicity was based on different requirements in different parts of the world. The specific design of the studies was largely determined based on the experience and precedent of previous approaches that were used and accepted by regulatory agencies and the varying opinions of regulatory and pharmaceutical industry scientists. This informal system resulted in differences in expectations in various parts of the world, and in misunderstandings of expectations amongst toxicologists in general and between pharmaceutical and regulatory scientists specifically.

The ICH S1A guideline entitled "Guideline on the Need for Carcinogenicity Studies of Pharmaceuticals" (ICH, 1995) has clarified the criteria used to determine if a carcinogenicity study is required for drug registration. These criteria include the duration and exposure of human treatment, concern of carcinogenicity based on a number of scientific parameters related to the drug or related drugs, genotoxicity, the indication and patient population, route of exposure and extent of systemic exposure. While all of these criteria must be considered, there are several key points that frequently determine the need for a carcinogenicity study in animals, most frequently rodents. A carcinogenicity study is usually required when the drug is indicated for chronic use, defined as daily administration for six months. Also, carcinogenicity studies are generally needed when a drug will be frequently used in intermittent cycles resulting in exposure equivalent to six months' duration. Carcinogenicity studies might not be required where the life expectancy of the treated population is less than 2–3 years. Consistent with this point, ICH S9 guideline notes that carcinogenicity studies are not required for therapies for advanced cancer (ICH, 2009a, 2009b).

The ICH S1B guideline entitled "Testing for Carcinogenicity of Pharmaceuticals" provides a very important perspective on approaches for evaluation of carcinogenicity (ICH, 1997). This guideline indicates how species for evaluation of carcinogenicity should be selected. The guideline also presents a statement on the acceptability of various short- and mid-term rodent test systems which is the basis for the use of transgenic mouse assays that are frequently used today in lieu of the traditional 2-year mouse study. For additional information on the use of a transgenic mouse model for assessing the carcinogenicity of a pharmaceutical, the EMA document should be consulted (EMA website). The ICH S1B guideline also discusses the importance and significance of mechanistic studies in the interpretation of carcinogenicity study results. While mechanistic studies are most frequently initiated after the identification of a carcinogenic response, the possibility of including study parameters related to mechanism of carcinogenicity should be considered in the design of a carcinogenicity study when there is good reason to suspect a positive carcinogenic response.

The ICH S1C(R2) guideline entitled "Dose Selection for Carcinogenicity Studies of Pharmaceuticals" should be reviewed when the carcinogenicity study protocol is being developed. This revision of the original guideline focuses on the selection of the high dose which is critical for a carcinogenicity study to be considered acceptable by regulatory agencies. This guideline outlines multiple approaches for the selection of a high dose in addition to the possible use of a maximum tolerated dose (MTD) which was the primary, if not the solely, accepted approach for the evaluation of carcinogenicity of pharmaceuticals in the past. This guideline also defines multiple points for consideration of selection of the mid and low doses in carcinogenicity studies. It should be noted that this guideline addresses the selection of doses in 2-year carcinogenicity studies and does not necessarily apply to transgenic mouse studies where the use of an MTD for the high dose continues to be the only accepted approach.

FDA will review and comment on protocols for carcinogenicity studies prior to the initiation of the studies as outlined in a Guidance for Industry entitled "Carcinogenicity Study Protocol Submissions" (FDA, 2002). This guidance should be utilized to make certain that the specific criteria used by the FDA for evaluation of a study plan have been appropriately addressed and included in the submission for protocol review. This guidance also provides information on the specific submission procedures.

13.2 Preparation for the Carcinogenicity Study

13.2.1 Timing in Relation to the Regulatory Submission

When to initiate the carcinogenicity studies is frequently a drug development decision rather than a scientific decision. According to ICH M3(R2), the results of the carcinogenicity study are needed to support market authorization and, unless there is significant cause for concern of a carcinogenic risk, the results are not required to support clinical trials (ICH, 2009a, 2009b). In drug development, the project plan, which frequently includes a series of Gantt charts outlining the critical work packages necessary for regulatory approval, is the road map to final submission of the Market Authorization Application (MAA) or New Drug Application (NDA). Approval of the MAA or NDA is often the anchor point for a drug development plan because it marks the point in time at which the drug is available to patients, revenue flows and offsets research and development investments, the period of patent exclusivity is marked, and the total value of the project can be estimated. Given that the cost of the carcinogenicity study will be in the range of US$1–2 million dollars per species, the carcinogenicity study is one of the most expensive nonclinical safety investments made during drug development and therefore is often staged so that the final reports are available at the end of the project but in time for submission of the MAA or NDA. Thus the time for initiating the carcinogenicity study is often based on the anticipated regulatory submission date. Since the investment in the carcinogenicity study is significant and initiating the study too early could lead to loss of investment if the project does not continue, the typical drug development plan will stage the carcinogenicity study to run in parallel with Phase III clinical trials. This approach can put the carcinogenicity study on the critical path to MAA or NDA submission and therefore proper planning is crucial to the entire project.

There are also scientific and safety reasons that dictate when the carcinogenicity studies should be completed and these are often related to the therapeutics' mode of action or to the primary therapeutic indication. The mode of therapeutic action or results from subchronic toxicity studies could suggest the new drug has carcinogenic potential, for example, severe immunosuppressive therapies or if highly proliferative lesions were observed in subchronic studies. Especially in cases where the drug is intended to treat a non-life threatening disease, it may be necessary to submit the results of the carcinogenicity study prior to entering into large-scale clinical trials, such as Phase III trials, where patients can number in the thousands. On the other hand, in some instances, the drug being developed is intended to treat an important unmet medical need. Because the carcinogenicity study can take three years from time of study initiation to final report, regulatory authorities might, in rare instances, allow the carcinogenicity study results to be submitted after MAA or NDA approval as a post-approval commitment, in order to expedite delivery of the new drug to patients in need. This was the case during the early years of HIV drug discovery and development when, for example, nevirapine was approved under the condition that the results of the carcinogenicity study would be submitted after the NDA approval. Ultimately, the most effective strategy for determining the timing of the submission of the carcinogenicity study results is to prepare a plan and submit the plan to the regulatory authorities for their comment. This can be done as early as the pre-IND submission or at any time after the IND is opened through a Type C correspondence (FDA, 2009).

13.2.2 Evaluation of Available Toxicology Data

In a typical drug development programme, toxicology studies will be completed to support clinical trials through Phase II prior to the consideration of a carcinogenic study. Depending on the indication and clinical plan, Phase II clinical trials are generally supported by a GLP genetic toxicology package, and rat and nonrodent studies through 4-weeks' duration and sometimes through 13- or 26-weeks' duration. Although these studies are designed to support clinical trials, the rat data will also be used to support design and interpretation of the carcinogenicity study, a fact which must be considered at the earliest stages of a drug development programme. As discussed below, the carcinogenicity study plan will be submitted to the FDA Carcinogen Assessment Committee (CAC) for review and therefore the critical data bearing on dose level selection, including these earlier studies, must be evaluated and integrated into an overall proposal for doses and study design. Each critical data set is discussed below.

13.2.2.1 General Toxicology Data

General toxicology data available at the time of preparation for the rat and mouse carcinogenicity studies are often not sufficient to select doses. The doses used in the rat studies through 4 or 13 weeks sometimes are not maximized for exposure or tolerability and generally there is very little, if any, toxicology data in mouse. As a result, an additional 13-week rat study might be necessary and a 13-week mouse study is usually necessary as dose range finding studies to support selection of doses for the carcinogenicity study. These studies are often called MTD studies; their design has been described elsewhere in this text.

As discussed in more detail in later sections, the results of the 13-week study are critical to setting dose levels for the carcinogenicity study. Data on body weight gain, food consumption, clinical pathology and histopathology need to be evaluated in an integrated fashion. These data should also be evaluated in light of published data on markers predictive of carcinogenic potential. For example, in rat studies of 6-months' duration on non-genotoxic compounds, the absence of hyperplasia, hypertrophy, or eosinophilic and basophilic foci of cellular phenotypic alteration can yield a strong predictivity of a negative carcinogenicity study (Reddy *et al.*, 2010; Sistare *et al.*, 2011).

In addition to routine general toxicology end-points, other more specialized end-points could be included in the general toxicology studies. These end-points can prove to be highly valuable when planning the carcinogenicity study, but proactive planning in the toxicology programme is necessary in order to generate these data. It is important that the toxicologist responsible for the drug development safety programme considers how the results from the general toxicology studies will be used to design the carcinogenicity studies.

13.2.2.2 Indicators of Cellular Proliferation

The results of the subchronic studies should be evaluated for tissue responses suggestive of cellular proliferation. It is has long been established that conditions promoting sustained cellular proliferation will enhance the probability of tumour development (Ames and Gold, 1990). If those conditions are not relevant to the intended therapeutic modality, then positive results from the cancer bioassay that are difficult to interpret could be generated, particularly if the increased cell proliferation only occurs in rodents at plasma concentrations that are substantially higher than plasma concentrations in humans at the maximum recommended human dose (MRHD).

Enhanced cellular proliferation could be induced by chronic cytotoxicity, which has been referred to as a regenerative state of proliferation. Chemical-induced hepatic necrosis is one of the classic mechanisms by which non-genotoxic agents given chronically results in liver tumors (Butterworth *et al.*, 1992). Necrosis is accompanied by influx of inflammatory cells and pro-inflammatory cytokines, resulting in proliferation of hepatocytes in a regenerative, reparative state ultimately leading to errors in DNA replication at critical sites in the genome that transform the cell into a malignant state. Chronic cytotoxicity and necrosis have been shown to contribute to tumours in tissues such as liver, kidney, lung, spleen, bladder and lung.

The second type of cellular proliferation has been referred to as augmentative proliferation and is typically a state of hyperplasia in the absence of cytotoxicity or necrosis. Phenobarbital-induced liver tumours in rats is the classic example in which induction of cytochrome P450 and proliferation of smooth endoplasmic reticulum result in both a hypertrophic state and a hyperplastic response concomitant with enhanced rates of cellular proliferation (Williams and Iatropoulos, 2002). Aside from histopathological evidence of such a response, organ weights and toxicokinetic results suggestive of induced drug metabolism can provide a hint of carcinogenicity.

Measures of cellular proliferation have long been established and improvements in immunohistochemical techniques have rendered these studies routine. Cells that are undergoing rapid DNA replication can be marked by pulse label (i.v. injection) or continuous label (osmotic mini-pump infusion) approaches using ^{3}H-thymidine or its analogue bromodeoxyuridine (Bogdanffy and Connolly, 1993). Replicating DNA incorporates these nucleobases and their presence in nuclei can be visualized by autoradiography or immunohistochemistry. These techniques must be included in the general toxicology studies, generally as satellite groups; therefore requiring prior planning and knowledge of the affected target organ (methodologies may vary depending on the target organ of interest). Alternatively, natural markers of cellular proliferation such as the Ki-67 protein and proliferating cell nuclear antigen (PCNA), which is a cofactor of DNA polymerase δ, can also be immunohistochemically visualized and their cellular expression quantified. Antigen retrieval methods are often used to reveal latent antigen, which make these approaches extremely useful for retrospective evaluations of tissues from general toxicology studies (D'Amico *et al.*, 2009).

Cellular apoptosis is the process of programmed cell death in which intracellular signalling pathways orchestrate a controlled sequence of events that is quite different from necrosis. The pro-inflammatory process is greatly subdued but an enhanced rate of apoptosis can also signal events related to carcinogenesis. The homoeostatic balance of cells within an organ is managed via cellular proliferation (mitosis) and apoptosis. Enhanced apoptosis can therefore result in compensatory enhanced rates of cellular proliferation or selective expansion of apoptosis-resistant mutant clones. The process of apoptosis produces small DNA fragments whose nucleotide ends can be labelled as an *in situ* marker. The histochemical technique is referred to as TUNEL (terminal deoxynucleotidyl transferase (dUTP) nick end labelling) and can be applied to fixed tissue.

13.2.2.3 Hormonal Imbalance

Because hormones control the trophic state of many organs, hormonal imbalances can lead to hypertrophic and hyperplastic pathology that might appear to be primary drug effects but are in fact secondary. Organs of the reproductive tract and metabolic endocrine tissues such as thyroid and adrenal gland are responsive to imbalances in hormones. The rat is particularly sensitive to changes in thyroid hormone levels due to its naturally low levels of circulating thyroid hormone-binding globulin and therefore perturbations in the mechanisms regulating thyroxine levels, such as enhanced clearance of T3 or T4, can promote thyroid follicular cell proliferation (Burns-Naas *et al.*, 2005). Similarly, alterations in the hypothalamic pituitary-adrenal, or –testis axes could also result in proliferative tissue responses. Suppression of ovulation due to sustained high plasma levels of luteinizing hormone and oestradiol can result in hyperplasia of granulosa cells in the retained follicles and potentially neoplasia, as was described for the selective oestrogen receptor modulator raloxifene (Long *et al.*, 2001). The rat mammary gland is susceptible to hormonal imbalances that originate in the pituitary and result in sustained elevations in serum prolactin. Aripiprazole and other antipsychotic agents induce pituitary and mammary gland proliferation and tumours. Serum prolactin levels in mice are elevated as early as 13 weeks at doses associated with tumours. Although sometimes evident from short-term treatments, generally these types of responses become more evident during 4- and 13-week dosing durations and therefore collection of samples for hormonal analyses during the general toxicology studies of these durations can be of value when designing and interpreting results from the carcinogenicity study.

13.2.2.4 Immunosuppression

ICH S8 lists immunosuppression as a mechanism of carcinogenesis (ICH, 2005). Chronic exposure to immunosuppressive drugs such as azathioprine and cyclosporin A increases the risk of certain cancers in humans (Bugelski *et al.*, 2010). In rat studies, cyclosporin was shown to induce lymphocytic lymphoma and hepatocellular carcinoma. Presumably the mechanism of carcinogenic action involves suppressed immunosurveillance of spontaneous malignancies. Although difficult to specify what preclinical toxicology study parameters might be most useful for evaluation when preparing for the carcinogenicity study, clearly off-target effects of the immune system should be considered. Such responses would generally be detected in routine haematological and histopathological evaluations but also in more specialized and directed end-points such as immunophenotyping of peripheral blood white cells and lymphoreticular organs or functional assays such as the T-cell dependent antibody response (TDAR) test.

13.2.2.5 Gene Expression Profiling

More recently, gene expression profiling approaches have been used to inform the likelihood of carcinogenic outcome and these evaluations are being included more routinely in subchronic general toxicology studies (Foster *et al.*, 2007). In this approach, target organ tissue is typically collected at the end of the drug administration phase and snap frozen in liquid nitrogen. Tissue selection is based on histological findings from short-term (e.g., 2- or 4-week duration) studies. RNA extracts are prepared and gene expression profiles developed using any of a number of hybridization platforms. These profiles are compared to training data sets derived from gene expression signatures of known genotoxic and non-genotoxic carcinogens. Although still in development, these approaches show promise for the identification of key genes known to be associated with carcinogenic pathways and could prove useful to making decisions regarding the timing of the carcinogenicity study and the dose levels used. Ideally, gene expression signatures could signal the need for earlier testing for carcinogenic potential to better define the liability or could even obviate the need for testing when the gene signature suggests a strong signal of carcinogenic risk. Gene signatures for hepatic tumours have reportedly given sensitivity and predictivity of 86% and 81%, respectively (Fielden *et al.*, 2007). A well-designed toxicology programme will consider the future utility of gene expression profiling and include tissue collection in the general toxicology studies and banking the tissues for future analysis.

13.2.2.6 Toxicokinetics

As discussed above, the primary goal of the carcinogenicity study is to evaluate the carcinogenic hazard of the new drug. The carcinogenicity study is minimally a qualitative test but seldom with a definitive "yes/no" outcome. Of greater importance is a quantitative assessment of exposure-response behaviour so that the human risk of carcinogenicity can be assessed in the context of the expected therapeutic plasma exposures. Thus, toxicokinetic data are critical to the overall goals of the carcinogenicity study in that they (1) provide a means for demonstrating maximal exposure of rodents to the drug, thereby assuring a robust qualitative assessment of carcinogenic potential, and (2) provide data on the dose-exposure-response relationship so that the tumour incidence results, if any, can be evaluated in the context of therapeutic exposures.

Toxicokinetic data obtained from subchronic studies should be evaluated first to ensure that exposures have been maximized. An effective toxicology programme will establish in the early phases of development the vehicles to be used throughout the programme. Typically, this involves collaboration with colleagues in pharmaceutical sciences to develop a range of vehicles that can be evaluated in single-dose toxicokinetic studies. These studies will incorporate the drug in several formulations, including suspensions and solutions, given at several dose levels in order to determine Cmax and AUC for each. From those studies, the optimal dose in terms of exposure and vehicle tolerability will be used in the general toxicology programme. Dose-dependent exposure is then evaluated in each general toxicology study and especially in the 13-week dose range finding studies in rodents. Exposure data collected at the end of the dosing phase are most important but data collected after the first day of dosing, and ideally also during the middle of the subchronic study, can be used to evaluate time-dependent autoinduction and more effectively predict exposures expected during the carcinogenicity study. These data should be organized and evaluated to determine if exposure is dose-dependent up to the limits of tolerability, or to determine the dose at which exposure saturation occurs. Calculating dose-normalized Cmax or AUC can also reveal dose-exposure non-proportionality and inflections in the dose-exposure curve where saturation is approached. From these data, an assessment of the dose-exposure relationship can be developed in order to inform dose selection for the carcinogenicity study.

13.2.2.7 Metabolite Profile

The purpose of animal toxicology studies is not only to assess safety of the drug substance but also the safety of the metabolites derived from the drug substance. However, drug metabolizing enzymes differ across species and consequently the metabolite profile of a drug in rodents is occasionally qualitatively dissimilar and often quantitatively dissimilar from that of humans. To ensure the rat or mouse carcinogenicity study will adequately assess human metabolite safety, the major human metabolites should be identified and tabulated. ICH M3(R2) defines a major human metabolite as any metabolite that represents 10% of the drug-related material, preferably when exposures are at steady state, as generally derived from evaluation of plasma samples from human clinical trials or from a human metabolism study with ^{14}C-labelled drug (ICH, 2009a, 2009b). The systemic levels of these metabolites are then assessed in rat and/or mouse at steady state and at dose levels equal to or less than those anticipated for the carcinogenicity study. Metabolite exposures in the rat and mouse should be approximately equal to or greater than that in humans at the (FDA, 2008). Bioanalytical assessments of rat and mouse metabolites can use plasma samples collected during the 4- or 13-week studies. These evaluations have the disadvantage of relying on non-isotopic means of metabolite identification but have the advantage of providing an early assessment of metabolite coverage in the rodent species.

13.3 Elements of the Protocol/Study Plan

13.3.1 Species and Strain Selection

Theoretically, the choice of the test species should be based on biochemical and physiological similarity to humans in metabolite profile and pharmacologic response. In practical terms, however, species selection is limited to the rat and mouse or, on rare occasions,

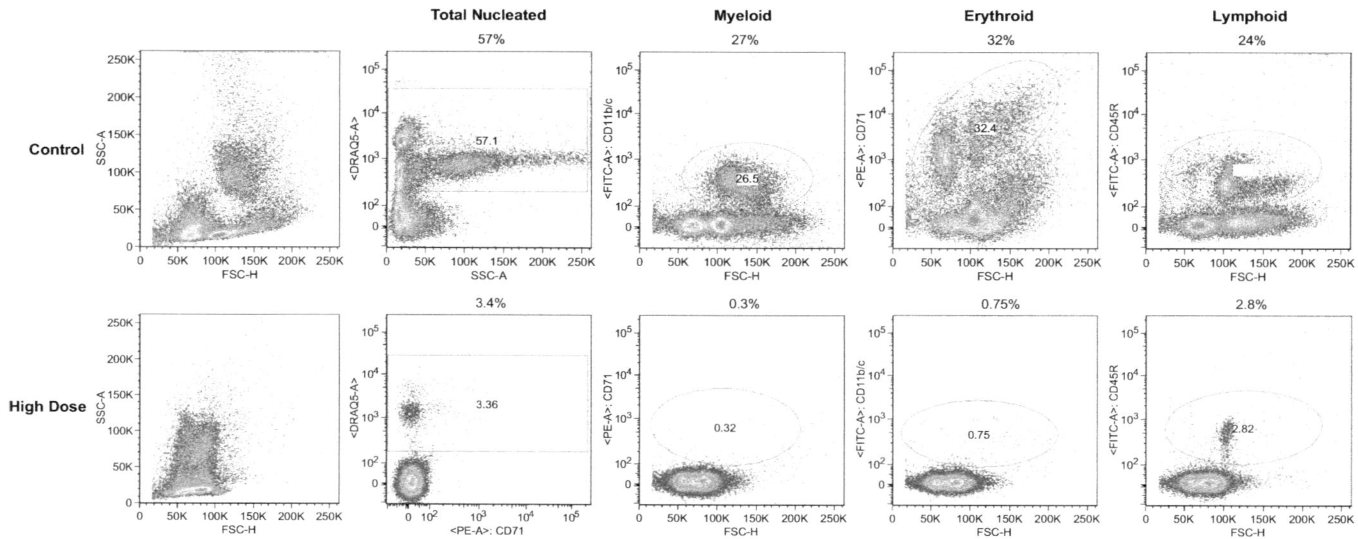

Figure 17.2 *Flow cytometric evaluation of bone marrow. Rats were dosed with the vehicle (control) or a high dose of a cell cycle inhibitor agent. At the end of the study, bone marrow was harvested from the femur and the various lineages in the bone marrow evaluated by flow cytometry. Data provided with the compliments of the Biomarkers Group, Drug Safety Research and Development, Pfizer (San Diego).*

Nonclinical Safety Assessment: A Guide to International Pharmaceutical Regulations, First Edition.
Edited by William J. Brock, Kenneth L. Hastings and Kathy M. McGown.

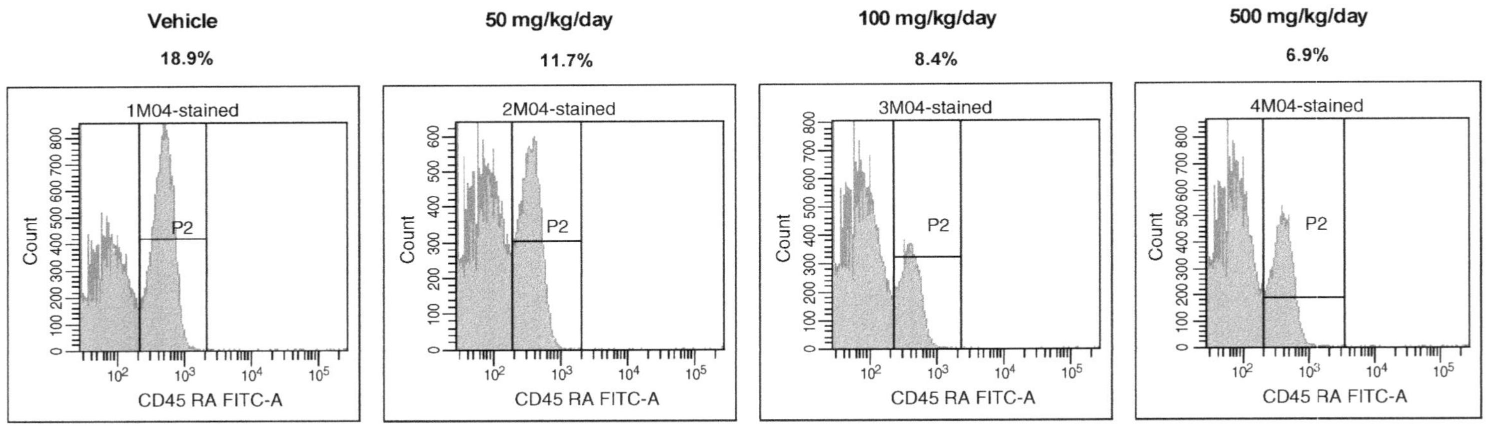

Figure 17.4 *Immunophenotyping evaluation of drug-induced alteration in circulating B cells. Rats were treated for two weeks with increasing concentrations of a drug which demonstrated altered splenic histology in the marginal zone region in a standard toxicology study. Data provided with the compliments of the Biomarkers Group, Drug Safety Research and Development, Pfizer (San Diego).*

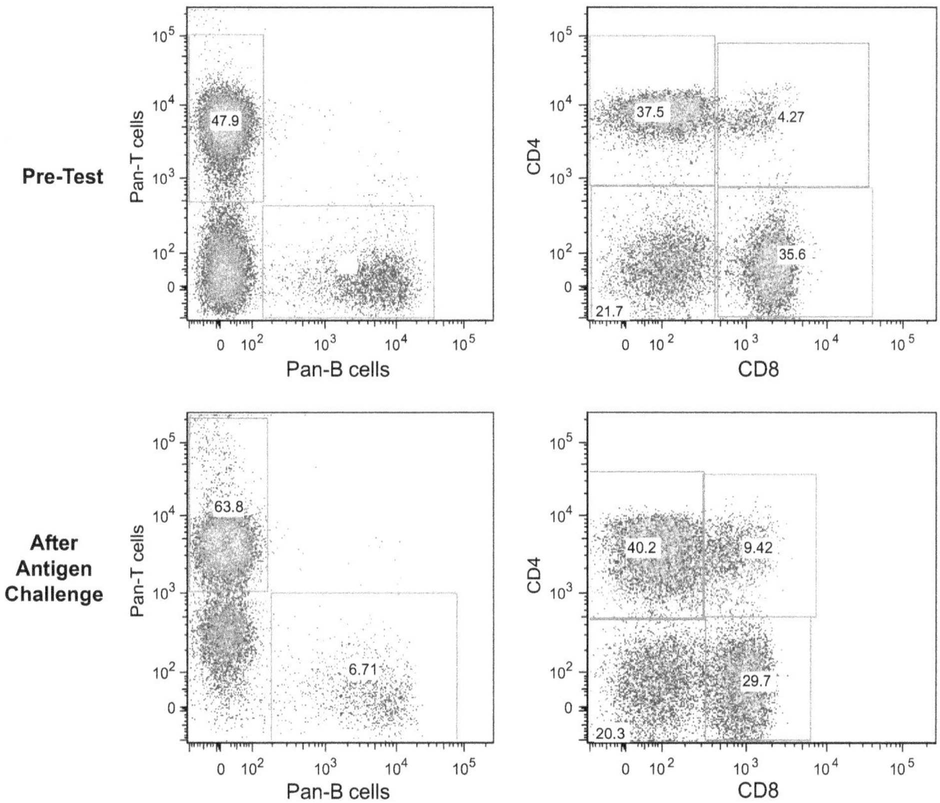

Figure 17.5 *Evaluation of hypersensitivity response in dogs. Dogs which were determined to be hypersensitive to a specific allergen were challenged with the allergen and the changes in peripheral T and B cell populations were evaluated in an effort to develop potential biomarkers for future therapeutic intervention studies. Data provided with the compliments of the Biomarkers Group, Drug Safety Research and Development, Pfizer (San Diego).*

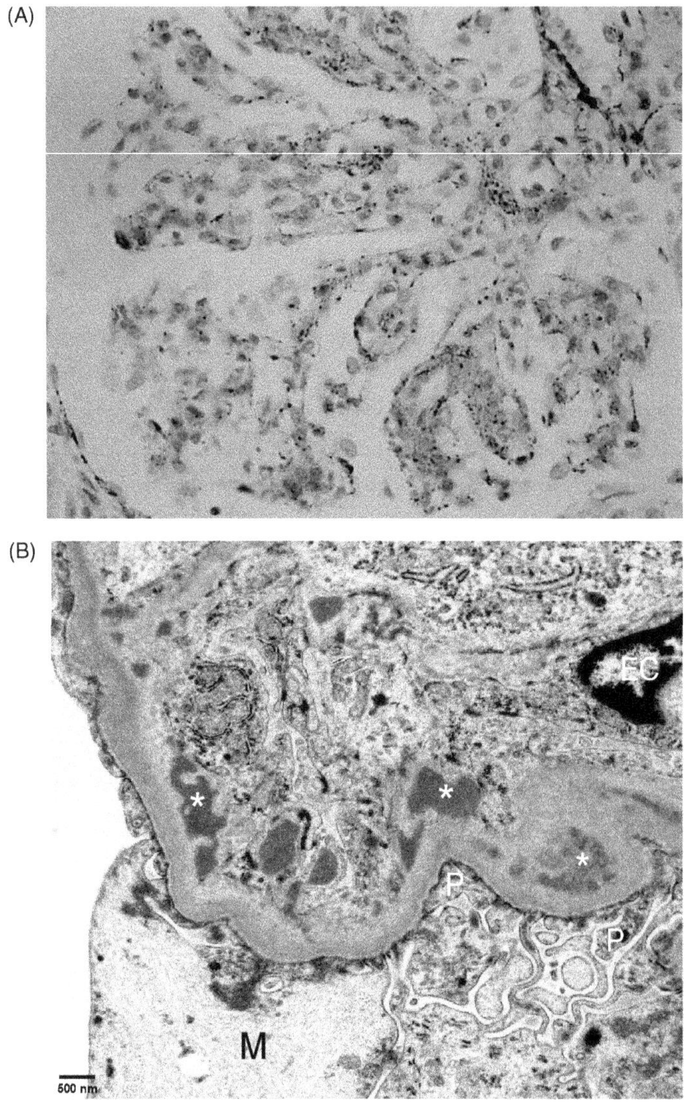

Figure 17.7 *Evaluation of Systemic Immune Complex Disease. (a) Renal glomerulus of Cynomolgus Monkey. Brown-staining granular pigment consistent with immune complex deposits is evident along the contours of the glomerular capillary network (immunohistochemical staining for SC5b-9; 600X). (b) Electron micrograph of renal glomerulus. Many electron-dense, immune-type deposits (*) of variable morphology and sizes are present in the subendothelial region of the glomerular capillary wall. An endothelial cell (EC) is evident projecting into the capillary lumen that is filled with undulating folds of endothelial cellular processes. Mesangial matrix (M) and foot processes (P) of podocytes are evident (5000X). Data with the compliments of Charles River Laboratories and the Pathology Group, Drug Safety Research and Development, Pfizer.*

the hamster. These species provide the optimum combination of life-span and husbandry requirements. The more critical choice is rodent strain. Amongst rat strains, inbred Fisher-344, and outbred strains such as Wistar (including several substrains) and Sprague Dawley, are most commonly used. In a 2005 report of the CDER/FDA database, these strains were used in 13%, 18%, and 68% of studies, respectively (Jacobs, 2005). While the Sprague Dawley is the most commonly-used amongst US pharmaceutical companies, the Wistar rat (particularly the WistarHan) is frequently used by European companies. Amongst mouse carcinogenicity studies, 87% used the CD-1 and 13% the B6C3F1 strains (Jacobs, 2005). All strains have advantages and disadvantages, but it is most important to use the same rat and mouse strains consistently throughout the toxicology programme for the new drug. Since strain-specific responses to toxicants and strain-specific metabolite patterns are encountered, the choice of strain is an important decision to be made early in the toxicology programme.

Spontaneous tumour incidence differs amongst strains and can often be a confounding factor when assessing drug-related tumour responses. The rat strain traditionally used by the NTP, the F344/N, has been plagued with high incidence of spontaneous tumours such as leukaemia and testicular interstitial cell tumours, poor fertility and other diseases, while the Sprague Dawley rat has a high spontaneous incidence of mammary tumours. The Wistar Han rat, on the other hand, has a relatively low spontaneous tumour incidence and high survival rate (Tennekes *et al.*, 2004; King-Hebert and Thayer, 2006).

It is important that the same strain of rat is used in the carcinogenicity study as was used in the dose ranging study. The supplier should be maintained across studies since differences have been noted in animals of the same strain from different suppliers.

13.3.2 Route of Administration

Route of administration in rodent carcinogenicity studies should be the same as the route for clinical administration of the pharmaceutical agent (ICH, 1995). Thus, inhalation, dermal and even intravenous products are best evaluated by the inhalation, dermal and intravenous routes, respectively. For inhalation studies, metered dose inhalers (i.e., drug product) can be used to deliver test atmospheres through nose-only exposure apparatus. The need for generation of respirable aerosols should be considered. For orally administered drugs, options for administration include oral gavage, dietary admix, and administration in drinking water. Administration in drinking water is rarely used since many drugs are poorly soluble or unstable in water; it is difficult to control the administered dose and large amounts of the drug are necessary. Oral gavage administration has the advantage of minimizing the amount of drug needed and being able to adjust and control administered doses easily by simply adjusting the dose volume based on body weight. These adjustments are particularly important in the first three months of the carcinogenicity study when rats and mice are in their rapid growth phase. Also, if the intended oral treatment regimen is less than daily administration, oral gavage application is the only viable option. The disadvantage of oral gavage administration is that it is labour intensive.

An alternative approach to oral gavage administration is dietary admix in which the drug is formulated into a powdered rodent chow that is fed directly or pressed into pellets and then fed. In all cases, test formulations should be prepared in which the drug is shown to be mixed homogeneously and is stable during the period of use of the formulation. During the first three months of the study, dietary formulations are generally prepared in batches to supply one week of administration. The concentration of drug in diet is adjusted weekly based on group average body weight and feed consumption data in order to deliver a constant dose in mg/kg/day. The rate of body weight gain in rats and mice diminishes beyond three months such that bi-weekly diet formulations can be prepared. When dietary intake is reduced due to palatability issues, it might be necessary to pair-feed control groups in order to control for effects related to decreased food consumption. However, palatability of drug in diet should be investigated as part of the dose range finding studies and, in the case of poor palatability, alternative methods of administration, such as gavage dosing, might be more appropriate. The concentration of the drug in diet should normally not exceed 5% in order to avoid nutritional imbalances. Dietary administration has the advantage of being convenient and less labour intensive but has the disadvantages of yielding only estimates of administered dose (cage spillage needs to be estimated), and requires large amounts of drug much of which is either wasted in unconsumed feed or is recovered and repurified. While dietary administration can be used in carcinogenicity studies, the oral gavage route is generally preferred since this approach best approximates human exposure. Oral gavage typically results in a noted peak level of drug consistent with a peak level of drug in humans. In contrast, dietary administration in the carcinogenicity study minimizes or ablates the peak which could be relevant to identification of a toxicity including carcinogenicity.

13.3.3 Analysis of Drug and Dosage Formulation

A complete certificate of analysis of the drug substance and the components of the vehicle formulation should be available. Physico-chemical tests should document the identity, purity and stability of these materials over the course of the in-life phase of the study. Suitability of the dose formulation preparation method and the stability of the drug in the formulation should be demonstrated (i.e., homogeneity or formulation methods that ensure homogeneity of the drug in the formulation and stability of formulation over the intended use period such as weekly formulation preparation). Dose formulations should be analyzed periodically (e.g., every three months) to ensure formulations are prepared within acceptable target ranges.

13.3.4 Age of Animals

Rats and mice should be between 4–8 weeks of age at the start of dosing in order to ensure hardiness post-weaning and to allow for two years of treatment, which approximates a lifetime of drug exposure. In the case of nose-only inhalation studies, several weeks of acclimation to restraint tubes may be necessary prior to beginning drug administration.

13.3.5 Group Size

Tumour development is typically a function of age, but obviously survival decreases with age and therefore a challenge in the carcinogenicity study is to complete the dosing period with enough animals remaining to ensure a statistically robust analysis of tumour incidence. To have an adequate carcinogenicity study, it is generally accepted that at least 15–20 animals should survive until the end of the 2-year dosing period. The number of animals per group at the beginning of the study must therefore be determined based on survival experience of the strain of rodent and the laboratory. It is well known that different strains of rats have different survival rates and that housing, handling and feeding conditions will impact the survival of control animals. When all of these factors are considered, group size in most rodent carcinogenicity studies is between 50 and 70 animals/sex/group. Animals that die of non-drug-related deaths (e.g., dosing accidents) during the first two weeks of the study are generally replaced. For this reason, additional animals could be assigned to the study to serve as replacements during this period. If not used, those animals could be added to a group of sentinels that are not dosed but are sampled for bacterial and viral infection periodically during the in-life phase of the study. Additional satellite groups could be added for other purposes, such as toxicokinetic measures or mechanistic toxicology studies.

13.3.6 Control Groups

Vehicle control groups are required but, in addition, sham-dosed control groups are also occasionally included. In the case of an inhalation study where the drug might be administered as a liquid aerosol, the liquid vehicle would serve as one control group while an air-only group could also be included in order to assess responses, such as respiratory tract irritation that is due to the vehicle. Similarly, when exotic vehicles are required for gavage administration of poorly-soluble drugs or if there is a lack of historical control data for the particular vehicle, an aqueous vehicle control might also be necessary.

Whereas a single control group is acceptable by regulatory authorities, use of dual control groups has gained wide acceptance in industry. In reviews of 13 rat and 10 mouse studies, notable inter-study variation occurred in background tumour incidences and, together with robust contemporary data gleaned from the use of two control groups, an easier interpretation of drug-treatment findings was possible (Baldrick, 2005; Baldrick and Reeve, 2007). Given the cost of the carcinogenicity study, the incremental cost of dual control groups is warranted.

13.3.7 Food Restriction

The CPMP Note for Guidance on Carcinogenic Potential states that dietary restriction should be considered if a low survival rate is anticipated (EMA, 2003). As mentioned above, lifespan of standard rat strains has been declining for decades, in part due to genetic drift and breeding practices. *Ad libitum* feeding, which is the standard approach in carcinogenicity bioassays, has been shown clearly to exacerbate poor survival amongst standard strains. In contrast, moderate dietary restriction of approximately 25–35% results in a better toxicology model by significantly improving survival, controlling adult body weight and obesity, reducing the onset, severity, and morbidity of age-related renal, endocrine, metabolic, and cardiac diseases, reduces inter-study variability, increases treatment exposure time, and increases the ability to distinguish true treatment effects from spontaneous ageing (Keenan *et al.*, 2005). Therefore, while food restriction should be considered, it is infrequently used for a variety of logistical reasons that result in increased cost. In addition, the dose range finding studies must also use feed restriction to provide appropriate data for dose selection in the carcinogenicity study.

13.3.8 Routine Measurements

Routine measurements include body weight and feed consumption, which typically are collected weekly during the first three months of the study when the animals are in rapid growth phase and monthly thereafter. Cage-side observations for morbidity/mortality are made twice daily (a.m. and p.m.) and detailed clinical observations of toxicity are collected at the time of body weight collection. Palpation for masses begins in week 13; the time of onset, location, size, appearance and notes on progression are recorded. Mapping of the location of the mass becomes important since other masses could appear in the same location, original masses will sometimes regress, and collection of the mass at necropsy is required. Since the spontaneous incidence of mammary gland masses is high in several rat strains, careful tracking of the time of onset is important. Ophthalmological exams are conducted pre-test and then once during drug phase, usually near week 52 and prior to necropsy.

13.3.9 Dose Selection

The doses chosen for the carcinogenicity study must be maximized in terms of exposure and/or tolerability without resulting in a level of mortality that would compromise overall survival and interpretation of tumour incidences. For this reason, the maximum tolerated dose (MTD) is generally defined as a dose estimated from the 13-week dose range-finding study that is predicted to produce a minimum toxic effect over the course of the carcinogenicity study. While testing for carcinogenic potential at the MTD has been the subject of debate for decades, inclusion of dose based on MTD is still the most frequently-used basis for setting the high dose in carcinogenicity studies.

13.3.9.1 High Dose

FDA guidance states that the highest dose to be included in a carcinogenicity study should be based on one of six criteria established in ICH S1C(R2) (ICH, 2008):

- Toxicity
- Dose-limiting pharmacodynamic effects
- Exposure 25 times human AUC
- Saturation of absorption
- Maximum feasible dose
- Limit dose of 1500 mg/kg/day.

Minimum signs of toxicity include a 10% decrease in absolute body weight relative to controls, target organ toxicity of a severity that would not interfere with survival and study interpretation, and significant alterations in clinical pathology parameters that indicate failure of physiological function.

Dose-limiting pharmacodynamic effects would be highly dependent on the pharmacologic mode of action of the drug and include responses that either would not enable survival over the 2-year period of dosing, such as severe diuresis, or limit the physiological function of the rodent, such as depressants of CNS function or blood pressure. The highest dose for which these pharmacodynamic responses could be tolerated, as defined by the 13-week study, would be considered dose-limiting pharmacodynamic effects.

Except in the case of a genotoxic drug, exposures that achieve 25-fold multiples over the MRHD are considered adequate to test the carcinogenic potential of a drug. The value of 25 was derived through a retrospective analysis of drugs tested for carcinogenicity at the MTD. Exposure multiples of 10–15 were identified for those carcinogens designated by IARC as "known" or "probable" human carcinogen (i.e., category 1 and 2A carcinogens), depending on whether exposure was estimated using body surface area scaling or actual systemic exposure data. Therefore, the exposure multiple of 25 was deemed acceptable. It should be noted that the exposure multiple applies to free drug (i.e., non-protein bound) and in some cases, especially a pro-drug, might also include metabolites. Clinical exposures at the MRHD must be known and since Phase III clinical trials typically assess efficacy at several doses/exposures, justification of the high dose in the carcinogenicity study based on the 25x criterion must encompass the highest anticipated clinical dose.

Saturation of absorption at the highest dose is also an acceptable justification for setting the high dose. Saturated absorption would be demonstrated through toxicokinetic analyses across multiple dose levels. However, if saturation of absorption is used as a justification for setting the high dose, it is necessary to make a concerted effort to achieve a maximum exposure through the evaluation of toxicokinetics using multiple vehicles, particularly where the animal exposure is a small multiple of human exposure at the MRHD. Until such effort has been demonstrated, the use of saturation of absorption to set the high dose would likely be unacceptable.

The maximal feasible dose in dietary studies is currently considered to be 5% as higher concentrations negatively impact nutrition, but for other routes of administration, the dose might be limited by local tolerance. As discussed above, in some rare cases the maximum feasible dose could be limited by acceptable formulations and the maximum dose volume for rodents, which is typically considered to be 10 mL/Kg.

Finally, where there is no evidence of genotoxicity, where other criteria have not been met, and where the maximum recommended human dose does not exceed 500 mg/day, a limit dose of 1500 mg/kg/day is justified. However, the limit dose can only be applied if the lower 95th percent confidence limit on systemic exposure in the rodent is at least an order of magnitude greater than human exposure measured at the human therapeutic dose.

The high dose can sometimes be increased by toleration to the drug by increasing the dose progressively over several weeks at the beginning of the dosing period. This approach can be used in cases where the drug is administered orally and is impalatable and the palatability issue decreases with time. In these cases, escalating the dose over a period of two weeks can reduce struggling of the animals and the potential for dosing accidents and thereby enable a higher MTD. This approach could also be successfully used to obtain maximum dosing and thereby exposure when animals become tolerant to pharmacologic effects that wane with continued dosing or, in cases where exposure is decreased, secondary to enzyme induction occurring over the first several weeks.

13.3.9.2 Mid and Low Doses

Multiple factors should be considered in the selection of mid and low doses, including the relationship of animal exposure to human exposure at the MRHD. Ideally, all doses in the carcinogenicity study would yield exposure multiples greater than one compared to human exposure at the MRHD but a balance must be achieved between maximizing the exposure multiple at the mid and low dose and creating dose and exposure separation from the high dose. Standard fractions of the high dose, such as ½ and ¼ of the high dose, are generally acceptable and at least offer a starting place for refining the choice of mid and low doses. However, the dose-exposure and dose-response relationships need to be taken into account, particularly when the slopes of those relationships are not steep. Thus it may be necessary to select doses that are smaller fractions of the high dose in order to ensure separation of exposure across doses and to ensure a dose-response continuum producing lower incidences of toxicity. Since these doses are selected primarily based on dose-range finding studies of 13-weeks' duration, expectations for treatment duration-related progression of toxicity beyond 13 weeks should also be taken into account. Any available ancillary data should also be considered when establishing the mid and low dose. For example, when cell proliferation data are available, it is advisable to select a mid dose that produces minimal increases and a low dose that has no effect over a 13-week treatment period. In some drug development programmes, where clinical trials have required toxicity studies greater than 13-weeks' duration (e.g., 26-week chronic studies), use of those results should also be part of the rationale for dose selection. Finally, the low dose should be selected in order to obtain a no-observed adverse effect level, or anticipated tumour-free dose.

13.3.10 Toxicokinetics

The results of the carcinogenicity study will be included in the package insert, or label, in terms of multiples of MRHD exposures. Ideally, the exposures achieved should be multiples >1x the MRHD exposure (see Section 13.3.9). Satellite groups should be included in the carcinogenicity study expressly for collection of toxicokinetic data (ICH, 1994). No other data are collected from these animals other than cage-side observations for mortality/morbundity and possibly gross examination of tissues at necropsy. Typically, an additional 12/sex/group will be added to the study so that 3/sex can be sampled twice in order to collect toxicokinetic data at six sampling intervals. When the drug is to be administered by dietary admix, it is critical to establish dietary concentration-exposure targets during the design phase and prior to start of the study, especially if prior general toxicology studies have been conducted using a different route of administration. Toxicokinetic parameters to be collected include Cmax and AUC at steady state as these parameters will be compared most readily to clinical exposure data. Alternatively, if it can be shown that exposure is constant with minimal or well-described diurnal variation, single point concentrations can be obtained at steady state but those samples must be collected consistently at the same time of day. Measures of drug exposure should be collected at multiple points during the in-life phase but generally measures near drug day one, and months 3 and 6 are adequate. These data should demonstrate steady state conditions and therefore collection of toxicokinetic data at later intervals is unnecessary. Exposure to major metabolites should also be measured to ensure their qualification for carcinogenic hazard.

13.3.11 Clinical Pathology

Routine clinical chemistry, haematology and urinalysis evaluations are not recommended for carcinogenicity studies (Young *et al.*, 2011). These end-points are included in all general toxicology studies where doses, treatment durations and data interpretation are more readily translatable to the clinical setting. Blood smears should be routinely collected from all sacrificed animals but evaluated only after assessment of tissue histopathology as an adjunct to making diagnosis of possible hematopoietic neoplasms (Young *et al.*, 2011). Collection of bone marrow smears or other special clinical pathology assessment should be considered if warranted to address issues identified in previous toxicity studies. Clinical chemistry and urinalysis parameters measured in aged rodents do not aid in the interpretation of tumour findings and their quantitative interpretation is obscured by high inter-animal variability late in life.

While not included in the protocol, it is sometimes very tempting to collect blood samples for clinical pathology from debilitated animals, particularly when such debilitation was unexpected. However, the hope that such clinical pathology evaluation will be helpful is generally not fulfilled. A severely debilitated animal has such extensive alteration of physiology that substantial changes from normal are frequently found for multiple clinical pathology parameters but such information is generally not interpretable in defining the cause of debilitation. Assessment of clinical pathology in other animals in the group that had debilitated animals is more likely to result in useful data.

13.3.12 Pathology

Since the final interpretation of a carcinogenicity study is based on the results of histological evaluation of tissues for the identification of neoplasms, it is essential that the evaluation of gross and microscopic pathology be adequately considered and detailed in the study plan and protocol.

Necropsy scheduling is a critical factor. All animals that die during the study should be necropsied and appropriate tissues collected under conditions that allow for the adequate histological evaluation of tissues. The daily check of animals in the in-life phase should identify those that are in a state of reduced or questionable health. Such animals should be observed closely to ensure that they are necropsied as soon as possible after death. This check should also identify animals that are in a moribund state and should be euthanized for humane reasons. Dead animals should be necropsied within several hours after death whenever possible and should be held at refrigerator temperature until necropsied. Moribund animals should be necropsied immediately after euthanasia. Specific information on time of collection of tissue in relation to death should be included in the study record. Animals that survive to the end of the 2-year time period should be humanely euthanized and necropsied immediately, using a schedule that includes an equal number of animals from each group on each necropsy day since the large number of animals in the study will require multiple days for completion of necropsy.

While tissue weights can be very useful in assisting the interpretation of histopathological effects in toxicity studies up to one year of dosing, tissue weights are considered inappropriate in carcinogenicity studies (Sellers *et al.*, 2007), for several reasons. At the end of two years of treatment, which approaches the lifespan of rodents, numerous neoplasms are expected even in control groups due to the spontaneous tumour occurrence in older rodents resulting in meaningless organ weight data. In treated animals where neoplasms could be the result of the treatment, data on organ weight will not be of assistance in determining the carcinogenicity of the treatment regimen. Two-year-old rodents also have a high incidence of spontaneous non-neoplastic lesions which will be dependent on the species and the strain of rodent used in the carcinogenicity study. Again, these spontaneous non-neoplastic lesions will vary from animal to animal and will therefore result in meaningless organ weight data. Debilitated animals also have changes in the weight of various organs related to debilitation that may or may not be associated with the molecule being evaluated. In rare instances, organ weights could be collected for a specific tissue based on results of shorter-term toxicology studies and where spontaneous hyperplastic or neoplastic lesions are rarely observed in the species and strain of animals used.

An extensive number of different tissues should be collected and properly fixed for histological evaluation with the specific tissues listed in the study protocol. A recommended tissue list has been published by the Society of Toxicologic Pathology (STP) (Bregman *et al.*, 2010) and should be used as a reference. Special attention should be given to the tissue lists that have been developed by the European community and by Japan as referenced in the STP publication. All grossly observed abnormalities should be histologically evaluated. The final tissue list selected for a given study must also take into consideration the route of administration and previous knowledge of histological effects caused by the agent being evaluated. For example, injection sites in vessels or subcutaneous tissue should be included in the tissue list. Nasally-applied pharmaceuticals would require a more extensive assessment of the nasal cavity than would be normally included for a study using oral administration.

Complete and accurate histological evaluation of the tissues is essential and should therefore be performed by a pathologist with previous experience in assessing tissue from carcinogenicity studies. Specific experience with carcinogenicity studies is important since the pathologist must be familiar with the myriad of spontaneous lesions that occur in aged rodents and which would not have been experienced by a pathologist that has evaluated tissues only from subchronic and chronic rodent studies. It is also preferable to have a single pathologist assess the tissues from all animals in the study to maintain consistency in diagnosis and to have a single pathologist knowledgeable of the findings in all groups and in both sexes. If multiple pathologists are involved in the histological assessment of tissues from a single study, it is imperative that the protocol and the subsequent report outline the steps taken to assure consistency between or amongst the various pathologists.

It is generally recommended that all tissues of all animals be evaluated histologically although other approaches could be acceptable. Some sponsors select to first evaluate all tissues from the control and high-dose group in addition to all gross lesions and then make a decision on which tissues to evaluate from the mid- and low-dose groups. This approach is certainly not appropriate if the high-dose group has a reduced survival that could result in an undetected neoplastic response related to treatment. Assuming there is no treatment-related reduced survival, the histological data from the control and high-dose groups would be evaluated for the identification of "target organs" with these organs being subsequently evaluated in the lower-dose groups. There are several potential issues related to the approach of evaluation of tissues from control and high-dose animals followed by the evaluation of target tissues. First, the designation of target tissues is based on judgement that might differ from the judgement of a subsequent reviewer. If a reviewer requires the evaluation of additional tissues during the regulatory review, there is a reasonable probability that marketing approval will be delayed. Second, this sequential process rarely, if ever, results in the anticipated saving in either time or money that was expected by doing less histological evaluation. The process of identification of "target organs" and the subsequent slide preparation and tissue evaluation minimizes potential savings and could actually take longer than if all tissues had been evaluated in the original pathology assessment. Third, the lack of data in all dose groups limits the statistical analysis of the data. Specifically, it is not possible to determine a statistical trend in increased incidence of neoplasms in treated animals unless all animals in the study have been evaluated histologically.

13.3.13 Satellite Groups for Mechanistic Studies

Satellite groups are frequently included in the carcinogenicity study when it is anticipated that tissue, plasma, or urine samples would be useful to further investigate mechanisms of carcinogenicity. Since the carcinogenicity study is a lifetime treatment duration, it might be the only opportunity to collect samples in studies of greater than 26 weeks' duration and obviate the need to repeat a very expensive and time-consuming long-term study. These samples can be stored frozen and utilized to investigate findings following the histopathology evaluation as may be useful. When adding satellite groups, care needs to be given to not overly complicate the study design, potentially compromising the main objectives.

13.3.14 Review of Study Plan

The development of a plan including a protocol for a carcinogenicity study is very complex and is dependent upon the inclusion and interrelationship of many different components. After the expenditure of a substantial amount of time and energy to develop the plan, there could be a desire to initiate the study and proceed as quickly as possible, particularly due to the time pressures related to drug development. However, adequate time and effort should be reserved for comprehensive review of the carcinogenicity study plan prior to study start.

Internal review of a carcinogenicity study plan should occur within the organization that is developing the new drug and should have at least two components. First, the completed draft documents outlining a carcinogenicity study plan prepared for later submission for regulatory review should be distributed to all individuals who have contributed in any way to the material included in the plan. The number of people involved will depend on the size and complexity of the organization but would obviously include the toxicologists, pathologists, drug metabolism specialists and the staff responsible for the performance of the animal component of the study. The first focus of review by the staff preparing the plan is to make certain that the pieces of information contributed to the plan are included in the appropriate context and that there is no obvious opportunity for misinterpretation. The second focus of review by the staff preparing the plan is to make certain that the documents provide a clear and complete presentation of the plan. In other words, a reviewer who was not involved in the development of the plan should readily understand the rationale and design of the study including the various parameters to be evaluated, for example toxicokinetics at specific time points in the study, and the inclusion of any special assessment such as thyroid hormone assay.

The second component of internal review of a carcinogenicity study plan should be performed by a group of scientists who have not been involved in the development of the plan. These scientists should have significant experience in the design, performance and interpretation of carcinogenicity studies in the recent past. In smaller organizations which may have a limited number of staff with experience in carcinogenicity study design and performance, this review step might need to be completed by toxicologist outside of the immediate company. This should be a scientific and feasibility review and not a perfunctory review to determine if the documents are well written. Scientific review in this context is the determination of whether the study is appropriately designed to achieve its objective. For example, the selection of inappropriate doses can render a study unacceptable by a regulatory agency or, alternatively, the selection of inappropriate doses could result in data that are not optimized to support human risk assessment. Feasibility in this context is the determination of whether the study can be performed with minimal risk of performance error that can occur due to the inclusion of special end-points that may be warranted but increase the study complexity, rendering it likely to result in performance errors.

While the inclusion of a rather extensive internal review might at first seem to be cumbersome and time consuming, experience has demonstrated that such reviews often identify opportunities for refinement and, in some cases, significant improvement in the study approach. In some cases, such reviews identify deficiencies that could have seriously compromised the study outcome if they had not been corrected. The extra time and resources to perform a detailed internal review of the carcinogenicity plan is well warranted when the consequences of a study deficiency are fully considered. At a cost of approximately US $2 million dollars per species, the economic incentive to have the study correct the first time is obvious. However, the more important cost of a failed study due to poor design or planning is the potential delay in drug approval.

Due to the negative consequences of performing a carcinogenicity study that might be unacceptable to a regulatory agency to support marketing approval, study plans should be reviewed by a regulatory agency prior to initiation of the study wherever such an agency is willing to perform such reviews. Review of carcinogenicity study plans by the FDA has been available for many years and provides an important opportunity for a check on both scientific and performance aspects of carcinogenicity studies. The FDA review process is outlined in Guidance for Industry entitled "Carcinogenicity Study Protocol Submission" (FDA, 2002).

Under the Prescription Drug User Act of 1992, the FDA should evaluate and comment on certain protocols within 45 days. Animal carcinogenicity studies are included in this special protocol assessment. Submitted protocols should be complete and appropriate for initiating the study with the exception of an actual study start date. However, the submission of protocols must be accompanied by additional detail to provide the regulatory reviewer with adequate information for review. Since the preparation and organization of this material is critical, the following section outlines the specific information to be included in most reviews although there may be some variation in required material based on the specific conditions related to the molecule under investigation. The specific type of data required will be dependent on the dose selection end-point as outlined in the FDA Guidance (FDA, 2002) and discussed previously. Thirty days prior to submitting the protocol to the FDA for review, the Agency should be notified in writing of the sponsor's intended submission.

The submission should immediately and clearly identify the proposed doses in the planned carcinogenicity study and should include the bases for the selection of the high dose from amongst the possible options outlined in the ICH S1C(R2) guideline (ICH, 2008). The regulatory reviewer should be aware of the basis for dose selection prior to reviewing the specific information used for the selection of the high dose.

Specific toxicity data are required to provide a basis for selection of doses. The type of data useful for evaluating carcinogenicity bioassay protocols is described in the FDA Guidance (FDA, 2002). Table 13.1 provides an outline for organizing these data in the

Table 13.1 *Elements of an effective carcinogenicity protocol review submission.*

Element of the CAC proposal	Comment
Summary	A brief summary of the indication, mode of action, expected exposures at the MRHD, the basis for selecting the doses, the doses chosen for the carcinogenicity study and the expected exposure multiples for each dose.
Introduction	Brief introductory paragraphs giving the indication, mode of therapeutic action, anticipated MRHD, a statement regarding the design of the carcinogenicity study, applicable regulatory requirements, and a final brief statement giving the basis or criteria that will be used to support the proposed doses.
Species/Strain Selection Rationale	This brief section should provide details of the rodent strain to be used in the carcinogenicity study. The strain should be identical to the strain used in the 13 wk dose range finding study.
Dose Selection Rationale	This section focuses on data supporting dose selection and should provide detailed information that justifies the high dose. Tables summarizing the supporting facts (e.g., body weight gain, histopathology incidence data) and the expected exposure multiples at the high dose, relative to the MRHD should be included. Exposure multiples should be adjusted for protein binding. When exposure limitations (e.g., saturable absorption or exposure 25x human AUC) support selection of the high dose, detailed graphical presentation and discussion of the dose-exposure relationship should be included. A rationale is also given for the low and intermediate doses.
Overview of Supporting Toxicology Studies	This section provides additional details on the available rodent studies and should include a tabular summary and text description of the key findings of each dose range finding study and genetic toxicology study. Studies shorter than 13 wk duration require only brief summary. Summary descriptions should closely match the individual study report summaries. The presentation should be organized by study duration in order to emphasize repeated findings, and dose- and treatment duration-related trends.
Comparative Assessment of Rodent and Human Metabolism	A description of the key metabolic pathways in human, rat and mouse, identified from *in vitro* and *in vivo* studies, and a tabular listing of each that highlights which human metabolites, if any, are not produced in the rodent strains. If available, quantitative information on each metabolite for each species should be included in order to assess whether human exposures at the MRHD will be covered by either of the rodent species. Species differences in protein binding should be discussed. A brief paragraph summarizing clinical exposure data should be included.
Study Outline	An outline of the rat and mouse carcinogenicity study protocols should be summarized in tabular format. The outline should include details such as strain, housing conditions, dose formulation volumes in order to demonstrate comparability to the conditions used in the 13 wk dose range finding studies.
Study Protocols	Draft protocols should be included in the appendix.
Relevant Reports	To facilitate the review, all reports cited in the submission should be attached as appendixes.

submission. Although toxicity information from dose range finding studies can be summarized, the submission should also include a copy of the full study report. The summary document should clearly summarize the major toxicity findings that would limit the use of higher doses in a carcinogenicity study if toxicity including the MTD is being used to set the high dose. It is very helpful if the relevant findings are presented in a text table to clearly show the dose response relationship of the finding. The text should clearly articulate why the finding is appropriate for limiting the dose in the high-dose group which can be based on several factors including a probable negative impact on survival that would limit the number of animals expected to survive to the end of study at 24 months.

The submission to the FDA should include information on the metabolic profiles in humans and the species proposed for use in the carcinogenicity study. This information is assessed to determine whether the selected species and strain of animal chosen for the carcinogenicity study adequately assesses the metabolites found in humans. Metabolite information should demonstrate that the selected rodent will test the parent and major metabolites identified in humans. If the rodent does not have all of the human metabolites, this point should be addressed in the submission. Again, a simple text table could be very helpful in presenting data on parent and metabolite in the rodent compared to humans.

Steady state toxicokinetic data, especially AUC, in the animals from the dose range finding studies should be reported and compared to the exposure data from humans that received the MRHD. It is important to present and discuss any gender-specific differences in exposure that could occur in either animals or humans.

Plasma protein binding in both the animal species selected for the carcinogenicity study and in humans should be presented. It is important that this data include information over a range of concentrations observed in the animal dose range finding studies and in humans at concentrations encountered in clinical trials. Plasma protein binding in animals and humans should also be provided for any identified major human metabolites.

A summary of the genotoxicity findings should be presented. If studies were negative, the description of each genotoxicity study should clearly demonstrate that the studies were adequately designed and performed. Positive or equivocal genotoxicity study results can impact the acceptability of the use of certain approaches for selection of the high dose in 2-year studies and can also impact the use of specific transgenic mouse models for the second carcinogenicity study.

An understanding of the submission and review process is very important. First, the sponsor should notify the FDA in writing 30 days prior to protocol submission. The primary responsibility for review of carcinogenicity study protocols remains in the reviewing division within CDER. Therefore, all correspondence and interaction with the FDA should be addressed to the appropriate individual in the reviewing division. The reviewing division generally, if not always, interacts with CDER's Carcinogenicity Assessment Committee (CAC) or CDER's Executive Carcinogenicity Assessment Committee (ECAC). The CAC and ECAC provide a very important function by assuring a level of consistency in the Agency's review of animal carcinogenicity study plans. The CAC or ECAC will provide written comments that will be forwarded to the sponsor by the reviewing division. Any response or clarification requested by the sponsor must be submitted to the reviewing division.

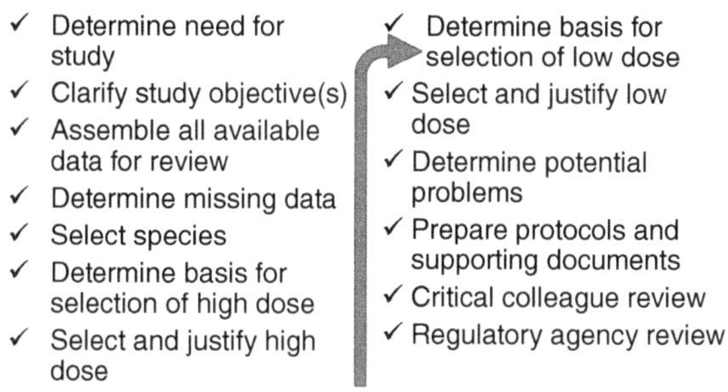

Figure 13.3 *Design of carcinogenicity study: Sequential checklist.*

13.3.15 Summary of Development of a Study Plan

Planning a 2-year study is a very complex process requiring the consideration of multiple scientific and logistical points as outlined above. Due to this complexity, it is important that the design of a carcinogenicity study is started at a time point that allows adequate time for completion of all of these steps. Figure 13.3 provides a sequential list of items for consideration and completion to assist in planning.

13.4 Study Performance

13.4.1 Study Oversight During the In-Life Phase

While the study planning and initiation phases of the carcinogenicity study are intense, the in-life phase of a well-designed, planned and executed study should be more routine. Most importantly, the lines of communication between the Study Director and Study Sponsor's Study Monitor during this time should be open and include weekly, if not daily, updates. A study communication plan should be established between the Study Monitor and the Study Director. The first month of the study demands significant attention to ensure the plans come to fruition. During the first several weeks, close attention is paid to in-life parameters (e.g., clinical signs, feed consumption and body weight data) to ensure that the study is performing as expected and findings are tracking with those of previous studies. Acclimation of the animals to routine dosing can cause the occasional dosing accident death and, if this happens within the first several weeks of study, those animals should be replaced. Toxicokinetic data obtained from sampling during the first week should be generated as soon as possible to ensure that drug systemic exposures are as expected.

During the later phase of the in-life segment, in-life data should be monitored routinely. Prior to study start, it should be decided between the Study Monitor, Study Director and Study Pathologist whether the histopathology results of intercurrent deaths should be evaluated immediately or after the final necropsy. Test article-related data such as periodic dose formulation analyses should be reviewed. Toxicokinetic data should be evaluated to ensure systemic exposures are at or near the targeted levels. On rare occasions, it might be necessary to adjust dose levels but, if necessary, this should be done within the first month of the study and should be done with caution since such an important change in study design has the potential to confound final interpretations and risk assessments. Finally, palpable mass and mortality data should be monitored routinely and at weekly intervals during the last six months of the study, which is when mortality rates rise exponentially. In general, a 50% survival rate to weeks 80–90 is considered adequate (FDA, 2001). Therefore, projections of survival should be made with the aim of determining if and when the number of survivors will drop to 20–30. When mortality in a group approaches 20–30 survivors, it is advised to approach regulatory authorities with a recommendation about how to proceed. The proposal could be to proceed with an early final necropsy for that group or the entire study, or to stop dosing the treatment group(s) and allow the animals to remain on study. A proposal for early termination of a single-dose group or the entire study will depend on various factors, especially the survival rate amongst controls. Whatever the approach taken, it must be emphasized that early termination should be done with concurrence of the FDA since it is difficult to devise a rule that covers every situation.

13.4.2 Pathological Evaluation

13.4.2.1 Gross Pathology

The necropsy of animals should be performed by trained and experienced prosectors under the immediate direction and oversight of an experienced toxicologic pathologist. The pathologist should be in the necropsy room during the performance of necropsy. Any unusual observations that exceed the experience of the prosectors should be referred to the pathologist to make the final recorded observation. Adequate time must be allocated for animal dissections and recording of observations considering the numerous observations that will be present due to frequent occurrence of spontaneous lesions in addition to any compound-related lesions that might occur. Since the necropsy must extend over multiple days due to the large numbers of animals, a subset of animals from each group should be terminated on each necropsy day to avoid any unanticipated variations that could occur from day to day. Also to prevent bias across treatment groups, animals necropsied on a single day should be taken randomly from the different groups in the study. This approach prevents bias that could occur as a result of one group being necropsied and observed in the morning when staff attention is high in comparison to animals necropsied at a later time of day when staff may not be as attentive.

Tissues must be immediately fixed in appropriate fixative, which is generally 10% formalin, although special fixatives are routinely used for some tissues such as eyes and testis. Tissues should not be allowed to dry even on the surface to prevent artifacts that will hinder histological diagnosis.

In the event that organ weights were included in the protocol for selected tissues, it is important that these tissues are collected carefully and uniformly. Specifically, the extraneous adipose tissue and fascia must be trimmed from the tissue since inclusion can result in unacceptable and misleading variation in organ weights, particularly when small tissues are being collected, for example, endocrine organs. The interpretation of the results of organ weights must be done in conjunction with a review of histopathology, particularly where unusually high or low weights are recorded in individual animals.

13.4.2.2 Histopathology

Histopathology is the ultimate basis for determining the carcinogenicity of a molecule. The experienced pathologist identifies proliferative lesions in histological sections that meet established and acceptable criteria for neoplasia considering the species and strain of animal that is being examined. The primary diagnostic issue is to distinguish neoplastic lesions from hyperplastic lesions. Hyperplastic lesions are defined as a proliferation of normal cells that retain normal growth control characteristics. In contrast, neoplasms are proliferative lesions in which the cell proliferation is no longer restrained by normal growth control mechanisms. While the definitions are fairly simple, the determination of biological potential from a histological pattern noted on the microscopic slide is much more difficult. However, experience of pathologists has established criteria for distinguishing hyperplastic from neoplastic lesions. Neoplastic lesions can be either benign or malignant. Benign tumours will continue to proliferate locally and might result in compression but not invasion of local tissue. In contrast, malignant tumours will invade local tissues and could also metastasize to distant sites either through seeding on a surface or through dissemination to distant sites following invasion of either blood or lymphatic vessels. Diagnostic criteria for rodent neoplasms are generally well established through the publication of standardized diagnostic criteria and terminology. To adequately review carcinogenicity data, whether the reviewer is from a regulatory agency or a pharmaceutical company, it is important that standardized diagnostic terminology be used to allow comparison of the results to the results from other carcinogenicity studies. (Society of Toxicologic Pathology website, 2010.)

Older rodents, as with older individuals in any other species including human, have a background of spontaneous neoplasms that will complicate the interpretation of a carcinogenic response. It is important for the pathologist to determine if the tumours noted in the treated groups are similar to tumours noted in control groups or whether the neoplasms associated with treatment have a morphology that differs from the morphology of spontaneous neoplasms found in the control animals. However, it is rare for treatment to be related to the appearance of a unique neoplastic type. Most frequently, the neoplasms associated with treatment are histologically similar to tumours that are commonly found as background tumours and which occur at an incidence of greater than 1%. The appearance of tumours in treated animals that are rarely found as background spontaneous lesions in controls (incidence less than 1%) at the end of a 2-year study require special consideration in study interpretation. The histological type and incidence of spontaneous tumours in control animals will be dependent on the species and strain of rodent used in the study. For example, female Sprague Dawley rats will have much higher spontaneous background incidence of mammary tumors than female Fischer-344 rats. In contrast, male Fischer-344 rats will have a very high incidence of interstitial cell tumours of the testicle compared to a very low background incidence in the male Sprague Dawley rat. The source of the rat diet can also significantly impact the background incidence of neoplasms in rodents. Therefore, the pathologist, toxicologist and statistician should be familiar with the incidence of the background or spontaneous neoplasms.

While the diagnostic terminology and criteria for rodent neoplasms have been standardized over the last 20 years, histopathological diagnosis continues to be and will always be subjective, for the simple reason that neoplasms within a single diagnostic category are not identical. To assure the best possible and consistent diagnosis of neoplasm, it is important that the pathologist be experienced in diagnosis of neoplasms of the species and strain under study as stressed above. Despite the best of experience and the diligence of the individual pathologist, it is highly recommended that the pathology of all carcinogenicity studies undergo a Pathology Peer Review performed by a second qualified and experienced pathologist. The Pathology Peer Review concepts and process have been defined for more than 15 years (Black, 1991; Ward *et al.*, 1995) and currently include the following level of review of a carcinogenicity study. All neoplastic lesions and hyperplastic lesions that might result in a diagnostic quandary in distinguishing hyperplasia from neoplasia should be examined. All tissues of a subset of animals (generally 10%) from all groups should be examined to assure that lesions were not missed in the original pathology assessment. The peer review pathologist should have all information available from the study including the diagnoses from the primary pathologist. The peer review pathologist is responsible for validating that the neoplastic lesions have been diagnosed correctly with appropriate distinction between neoplasms and hyperplastic lesions and to assure that neoplastic lesions have been identified in the study. Since all diagnostic pathology is subjective, it is common that the primary and peer review pathologists will have different diagnoses on a small subset of tissues. The primary pathologist and peer review pathologist review the lesions and reach a consensus that is included in the final report. The final report should include a Pathology Peer Review statement identifying the tissues examined and the process followed, including a description of how diagnostic differences were addressed.

On very rare occasions, the primary pathologist and the peer review pathologist cannot agree on the diagnosis. However, this generally occurs when there is difficulty in distinguishing lesions that are on the borderline between neoplasia and hyperplasia or, very rarely, when the lesion is uncommon and outside the experience of one or both pathologists. To resolve these issues, a Pathology Working Group (PWG) should be formed to provide perspective to the primary and peer review pathologist. The PWG is organized and chaired by an experienced pathologist who has not been previously involved in the assessment of slides from the study and generally includes three to five pathologists selected for expertise in the tissue or neoplastic type in question. The review focuses on the tissue diagnosis where disagreement has occurred or where a neoplasm of unusual histological type has been identified. The slides are reviewed in sets and then discussed by the group of reviewing pathologists. A consensus diagnosis is sought from this process to be conveyed to the primary and peer review pathologist. A PWG report is prepared as well as a statement of the process. The PWG statement and the peer review pathologist's reports are filed with the study raw data and are generally not included in the final pathology report which does include the statement of the peer review pathologist and the PWG.

The well-established pathology process, including pathology peer review and a pathology working group, if necessary, ensures that the best possible data have been generated from what is a subjective science. This data provides the basis for the determination of whether a given molecule causes cancer in animals which in turn provides the basis for assessing potential human carcinogenic risk.

13.5 Alternative Models to Evaluate Potential Carcinogenicity in Lieu of a 2-Year Mouse Study

For many decades, the evaluation of potential carcinogenicity of drugs in development relied primarily on the performance of 2-year studies in two species, most frequently rats and mice although other species such as hamster were occasionally used for specific scientific reasons. The reliability, predictivity and cost of such studies have been continually questioned and challenged. The mouse study usually generated more detractors than the rat study for a variety of reasons but certainly including the frequent increase in liver tumours that were present at a high background incidence in most mouse strains used. The continuing development of better mechanistic understandings of the origin of tumours fuelled this debate while the development of potential alternative models was considered to provide a possible alternative to the 2-year studies. In the early 1990s, several transgenic mice were being evaluated in experimental laboratories as tools to define cancer development. These models soon started to generate interest as possible animal models for the assessment of chemical- and drug-induced carcinogenicity. Since only limited data were available from several mouse models in which a very limited number of compounds had been evaluated in the early 1990s, regulatory agencies were justifiably reticent about allowing substitution of these newer models for the currently-accepted 2-year carcinogenicity studies. To address this issue, an industry/government joint effort to assess the performance of alternative models for assessing carcinogenicity was designed and performed under the auspices of the Health and Environmental Sciences Institute (HESI). It should be noted that the HESI effort primarily evaluated five potential alternative models including:

- initiation-promotion models in rats;
- newborn mouse model;
- a $P53^{+/-}$ knockout mouse;
- a TG.AC transgenic mouse; and
- a Hras2 transgenic mouse.

For details of this effort, including a description of the models, the reader is referred to the special issue of the journal *Toxicological Pathology* in which the design and results of the studies performed (*Toxicological Pathology*, 2001) are described. The reader must be aware that several aspects of study design have been modified (see below for current study design parameters for selected models). However, the results of the HESI effort were considered in addition to the developing published literature in the preparation of the ICH S1B Guideline promulgated in 1997 which stated that the 2-year mouse study could be replaced by a "short or medium term *in vivo* rodent test system".

Since the publication of the ICH S1B Guideline, the use of alternative models for assessment of carcinogenicity in mice has focused on a few models that primarily rely on the Hras2 model although the $P53^{+/-}$ and TG.AC models are selectively used under special circumstances. It is interesting to note that approximately 20% of the mouse cancer bioassays use transgenic mice based on protocols submitted to the FDA for review and this percentage has not changed over the past eight years (Jacobson-Kram, 2010).

The newborn mouse model is rarely used in lieu of a 2-year carcinogenicity study primarily due to the limitations of sensitivity and to the fact that it is most appropriate for genotoxic compounds which are very rarely evaluated for carcinogenicity in drug development. The initiation promotion system has great value for elucidating the mechanism of carcinogenicity, specifically to determine if the molecule has unusually potent tumour promotion activity. However, this model is rarely used for the basic assessment of carcinogenicity in lieu of a 2-year study.

The following statements provide guidance for the current use of the various alternative models for assessing potential carcinogenicity. For detail about the molecular constructs and characterization of the models the reader is referred to *Toxicological Pathology*, 2001; Rhomberg *et al.*, 2007).

The Hras 2 model is currently the most frequently-used transgenic model for the evaluation of carcinogenicity in both the United States and Europe. It is acceptable for use when the molecule under investigation has no suggestion of genotoxicity or when there is a questionable genotoxicity finding.

The $P53^{+/-}$ model is accepted by regulators in the United States when there is a question of potential genotoxicity which might occur when a genotoxicity study result is equivocal. This model can also be used for clearly genotoxic compounds although such molecules are rarely assessed for carcinogenicity. In contrast to the United States, the $P53^{+/-}$ mouse and the Hras 2 model are considered equally acceptable irrespective of the genotoxic status of the molecule.

The TG.AC mouse model was originally developed to assess a carcinogenic response in the skin by first identifying proliferative lesions by visual inspection followed by histological confirmation of the neoplastic characteristics of the lesion. While this model has been considered as a potential model for assessing carcinogenicity that could occur at any site in the body, use of the model today is appropriately restricted to the evaluation of skin products particularly where the product has been demonstrated to have poor skin penetration.

While the alternative models for assessing carcinogenicity were accepted through the ICH programme as early as 1997, alternative models were used to a very limited degree for the next several years and primarily limited to a few of the larger pharmaceutical companies. There were several reasons for this slow implementation, including the lack of familiarity of the models and uncertainty on the part of many pharmaceutical companies as to what results might be generated. Ever since the first experimental introduction of these models, there was a concern that transgenic models would be "over sensitive" or that they would result in the identification of numerous "false positives". The data from the HESI programme reduced this concern somewhat, based on a simple review of the data. However, the very analytical assessment of results from the HESI programme as well as the increasing published literature data base (Pritchard *et al.*, 2003) have satisfactorily addressed concern regarding the sensitivity of mouse transgenic models. This publication noted that individual transgenic models made a "correct" determination of carcinogenicity at least as frequently as standard 2-year bioassays when "correct" was based on a comparison of animal study data with accepted human carcinogens. Additional experience from the studies performed with pharmaceuticals and discussed in aggregate at public meeting has greatly reduced the concern for "false positives" with transgenic models.

The study design for the most widely-used models, Hras 2 and $P53^{+/-}$ models, have become relatively standardized and in some instances changed from early study design through agreement of scientists and through iterations between pharmaceutical sponsors and regulatory agencies. Several important points are addressed here, although it is highly recommended that study design is reviewed and/or discussed with the regulatory agency prior to study initiation. This is particularly important since approaches may change as additional experience is obtained through more extensive use of transgenic model systems. In the Hras2 and $P53^{+/-}$ models, the animals are dosed for six months followed by termination of the animals at the end of dosing. A positive control group should be included in each study unless the regulatory reviewers indicate that a positive control is not required. In general, a positive control will likely be required unless the laboratory has performed multiple studies with the model and had a consistent neoplastic response to the positive control material. As with any other carcinogenicity study, adequate data must be available to set the doses for the carcinogenicity study. It should be noted that the only generally recognized basis for setting the high dose is the MTD. The dose ranging study can utilize the wild type mouse since there has not been a significant difference noted in the toxicity response including the MTD between the transgenic and wild type animal. At the end of the 6-month dosing period, a complete necropsy should be performed with collection of a complete tissue list similar to the performance of a 2-year study. All tissues of all animals in the study should be histologically examined for the control group and the groups treated with the molecule under investigation. It is appropriate to histologically examine only the tissues where tumours are expected in the positive control group to simply assess the performance of the study. The lack of neoplasms in the tissues where tumours are expected in the positive control group raises a serious question regarding the adequacy of the study.

13.6 Special Consideration for Carcinogenicity Evaluation of Biotherapeutics

Biotherapeutic drugs, such as monoclonal antibodies, replacement proteins, nanobodies and peptides, present a unique set of considerations when assessing their carcinogenic potential. As with small molecules, the need for a carcinogenicity assessment is first driven by the indication, treatment duration and target population. However, unlike many small molecules, protein- and peptide-based drugs are generally considered non-reactive, are not metabolized to reactive intermediates, have modes of action that are highly target-specific with few off-target responses and, importantly, are often immunogenic in traditional rodent carcinogenic bioassay species. While biotherapeutics may be non-genotoxic, the biological pathways they modulate could be involved with cellular growth and replication, which could promote epigenetic mechanisms for tumour growth, or the biotherapeutic might be immune suppressive. Understanding the potential of a biotherapeutic to modulate pathways of cellular proliferation or immune suppression through careful literature search, including data from knock-out animals and computer-based systems analysis, is the first step in the carcinogenicity assessment of a biotherapeutic. In some cases, a literature-based assessment is all that is necessary to determine the carcinogenic hazard (ICH, 2009a, 2009b, 2011). A review of carcinogenicity assessments of biotherapeutic proteins is given in Vahle *et al.* (2010).

Experimental evaluation for carcinogenic potential may rely on nontraditional *in vitro* and *in vivo* methods. ICH S6(R1) states that products having the ability to support or induce proliferation of transformed cells and clonal expansion possibly leading to neoplasia should be evaluated with respect to receptor expression in various malignant and normal cells. A variety of insulin-like products, haematology factors and interferon products have been assessed using *in vitro* approaches that employ transformed cell lines (Vahle *et al.*, 2010). Similarly, several growth factors have been evaluated in *in vivo* immune-suppressed xenograft models but the reliability of data derived from these models is often questionable. Bioassays using homologous products that are not immunogenic in rodents but are not the clinical candidate are generally considered of limited value for assessing carcinogenic potential. Similarly, although evaluations of carcinogenic potential using transgenic animals expressing the human target are possible and have been conducted, these studies can be complicated by limited background tumour information.

Data from general toxicology studies should be evaluated for indicators of neoplastic progression. Evidence of proliferative lesions observed during long-term repeat dosing (e.g., 6-month chronic) studies could be suggestive of a carcinogenic hazard upon chronic exposure. These observations are often subsequently pursued experimentally using end-point-direct studies to further evaluate the carcinogenic hazard.

When the results of the literature and class-based biology assessment, together with the results of chronic toxicity studies, suggest a carcinogenic hazard, the information might be sufficient to characterize the carcinogenic risk in the label or additional studies could be conducted to mitigate the concern (ICH, 2009a, 2009b). When the carcinogenic hazard cannot be adequately evaluated without a rodent bioassay and when the product is biologically active and non-immunogenic, a study in a single species should be considered. When the weight of evidence does not suggest a concern for carcinogenicity, a rodent bioassay is not recommended.

13.7 Regulatory Implications of a Study Identifying an Animal Carcinogenic Response

In the performance of carcinogenicity studies in drug development, it is relatively common to identify a "positive" response, that is, an increase in neoplasms in treated as compared to control animals. Since it is very uncommon for genotoxic molecules to be pursued in drug development, most of the positive carcinogenic responses are apparently the result of non-genotoxic mechanisms. There are numerous non-genotoxic mechanisms for rodent tumour induction with variable relevance as an indicator of human risk. A human risk assessment must be performed, taking into account the results of the carcinogenicity study, the information obtained from mechanistic studies in rodents and information from the experimental literature. While there are several cases where it is generally accepted that the tumour response observed in rodents will qualitatively not occur in humans (e.g., renal tubular cell tumours in male rats associated with accumulation of alpha 2-globulin in the renal tubular epithelium), such cases are uncommon. In most instances, the consideration of human risk is largely based on an evaluation of the doses and, more importantly, the internal exposures in rodents compared to humans receiving a maximum recommended therapeutic dose. A safety margin between plasma concentrations in animals at doses where neoplasms were not observed compared to human plasma concentrations at the MRHD provides a level of reassurance of minimal risk in humans receiving therapy since non-genotoxic neoplastic responses are generally believed to have a threshold.

However, the final determination of acceptability of a drug considered for marketing approval that has a demonstrated neoplastic response in rodents is ultimately dependent on a risk-benefit analysis and not simply a risk analysis as is common practice for non-therapeutic agents such as chemicals and agri-chemicals that are regulated under different legal statutes. If a drug has a demonstrated human benefit for an unmet medical need (i.e., other effective medications are not available), the acceptable relative risk may be higher than if a drug is simply providing an additional therapeutic agent that has similar efficacy as a marketed drug that does not have a demonstrated rodent carcinogenic liability. The final decision of the risk-benefit analysis is made based on professional judgement, first by FDA staff followed by input from an FDA Advisory Committee in the United States.

13.8 Interpreting the Relevance of Positive Results for Human Safety

Surveys of marketed drugs suggest that 38–47% have positive or equivocal results in carcinogenicity tests (Snyder and Green, 2001; Brambilla and Martelli, 2009) yet a relatively small number of pharmaceuticals are known human carcinogens (MacDonald, 2004). Therefore, it is essential to make the best possible assessment of human risk based on the animal carcinogenicity study utilizing all available data.

In the absence of evidence to the contrary, it is assumed that tumour responses observed in rodent studies are relevant for humans.

ICH S1B recognizes the importance of mechanistic studies to the interpretation of carcinogenicity bioassay results and for providing perspective of relevance to human risk assessment (ICH, 1997). Since most drugs evaluated in carcinogenicity studies have been demonstrated to be non-genotoxic by traditional genetic toxicology tests, it is generally assumed that the mechanism of tumourigenesis in rodents is via non-genotoxic or epigenetic mechanisms. The guidance discusses specifically the potential need for supplementary studies at the cellular and biochemical levels and, in the absence of clear evidence for an epigenetic mechanism, additional genetic toxicology studies that focus on the organ(s) showing a tumourigenic response.

Cellular-based studies useful for elaborating a non-genotoxic mechanism are manifold and would be quite specific for the target tissue. Since there are many factors that could impact the ability to extrapolate results from isolated cell systems, these approaches are useful for assessing mechanism and less useful for quantitative risk extrapolation. *In vivo* studies of cellular changes related to carcinogenesis on the other hand are useful in both contexts. For example, dose- and time-course studies of cellular proliferation and apoptosis using the methods discussed above can reveal subtle changes in cellular homoeostasis that may not be evident by routine histopathological evaluation. Bursts of cellular proliferation that occur early in the course of a 2-year treatment could expand clones of cells having stable spontaneous mutations in oncogenes and tumour suppressor genes and alter expression of proteins involved in signal transduction pathways. These mutant clones might then progress, perhaps through additional mutation, to yield a fully malignant phenotype. Similarly, alterations in apoptotic pathways can, over long-term treatments, result in non-genotoxic pathways to tumourigenesis.

Foci of cellular alteration, especially in liver, have been considered in the interpretation of rodent carcinogenicity studies and have been extensively evaluated in experimental studies. Foci of cellular alteration tend to be less than the size of a normal hepatocellular lobule and occur spontaneously in control animals with an increase in number of foci per liver with increasing age (Popp *et al.*, 1985). These foci can be identified by standard hematoxylin and eosin stain but are more easily noted by changes in the levels of expression of cellular markers such as gamma glutamyl transpeptidase and ATPase. Thus, clusters of highly proliferating non-neoplastic hepatocytes (Marsman and Popp, 2004) will precede tumour formation and the progression or lack of progression of the foci to tumours is different with various non genotoxic liver tumour promoting agents (Cattley and Popp, 1989). Although eosinophilic hepatocellular foci are less likely to convert to malignant hepatocellular carcinoma compared to basophilic foci, the increased number of foci in treated compared to control animals of either type of foci cannot be automatically considered a predictor of rodent carcinogenicity (Wood *et al.*, 1991). In addition, in the presence of a strongly negative weight of evidence for genotoxic activity, liver tumours related to such foci are not necessarily an indication of human carcinogenic risk. Phenobarbital is the classic example of a drug that induces liver enlargement, enzyme induction, eosinophilic foci and neoplasm in the liver of rodents, yet extensive epidemiology studies show no evidence of liver tumour risk in humans.

Biochemical measurements mentioned in ICH S1B include many of the hormonal evaluations discussed above. The more common rodent tumour types, such as pituitary adenoma, Leydig cell carcinoma, mammary gland fibroadenoma and adenocarcinoma, and thyroid adenoma and carcinoma, often can be explained by hormonal dysregulation that is related to the pharmacologic mechanism of action or induction of drug clearance pathways that are also involved in the regulation of hormonal status. The sensitivity of rodents to these tumours is well known and generally recognized as having questionable or unknown relevance to humans.

When unusual tumour types are observed it can be very difficult to develop a drug-specific mode of action, especially one that can be concluded as being relevant or irrelevant for human risk. In these cases, hypotheses must be generated from the available data on the drug, its mechanism of pharmacologic action, and available literature. Four approaches useful to hypothesis generation are:

- Literature mining tools that broadly scan publications, patents and publicly-available regulatory submission documents and reports and visualize relationships between pharmacologic mechanisms and biochemical pathways related to carcinogenesis;
- Systems biology (*in silico*) approaches that develop computer-based models of potential carcinogenic pathways related to the drug's pharmacologic mechanisms and organize information into testable hypotheses;
- Gene expression profiling techniques where gene signatures and annotations can be developed from toxicogenomic evaluations of tissues. As discussed above, transcriptomes are often generated from short-term dosing ($\leq$4 weeks) under conditions where

tissue histopathology would not obfuscate underlying and subtle mRNA expression patterns. From these data, hypotheses for carcinogenic mechanism of action can be developed and further tested (Pennie *et al.*, 2004).
- Electron microscopic evaluation of target tissues during the early phases of drug treatment is an often overlooked but information-rich source of hypotheses. For example, alteration of mitochondrial structure could provide critical information to focus on a drug-induced biochemical perturbation of the mitochondria.

Special studies designed to provide interpretation of and mechanistic insights into results of carcinogenicity studies should follow the conditions of the original carcinogenicity bioassay. A weight of evidence for the mode of action should be developed and its relevance for humans assessed. A generic framework for this evaluation has been proposed and involves three questions (Meek *et al.*, 2003):

1. Is the weight of evidence sufficient to establish the mode of action in animals? What is the postulated mode of action, what are the key events, what is the animal evidence?
2. Are the key events in the animal mode of action plausible in humans?
3. Taking into account kinetic and dynamic factors, is the animal mode of action plausible?

The framework for human relevance has been applied to multiple compounds, including peroxisome proliferators. The value of the framework is the step-by-step analytical process for considering animal and human data. In particular, the second question prompts an in-depth evaluation of mode of action. For pharmaceutical compounds the mode of pharmacologic action is generally well understood. The nonclinical pharmacology data should be considered especially with regard to the potential for the mode of action to affect cell cycling and intracellular signalling pathways or to perturb hormonal pathways that could result in enhanced cellular proliferation. The result of the analysis is a documented qualitative evaluation of relevance of the tumours for humans. The evaluation could be useful when presenting the results of the carcinogenicity bioassay to regulatory authorities.

13.9 Communicating the Results in the Product Label

The product label, or package insert, is the primary means for communicating the risks and benefits of a therapeutic to the physician who, together with the patient, can make an informed decision. Statements regarding animal carcinogenicity studies are relatively brief and generally found in the label section entitled "Precautions" or "Nonclinical Toxicology". Information will generally include, but be limited to, tumour response of males and females if different, tumour type, animal dose and exposure associated with the dose expressed as multiples of the human exposure at the MRHD. Tumour incidence data is not included. The reader is encouraged to look at package inserts, many of which are available via the internet including the FDA and EMA websites (Drugs@FDA, European Public Assessment Reports). Genetic toxicology data are summarized briefly in this section. This brief paragraph thus summarizes the salient animal carcinogenicity information that is important to the clinician.

References

Ames, B.N. and Gold, L.S. (1990) Too many rodent carcinogens: mitogenesis increases mutagenesis. *Science*, **249**, 970–971.

Baldrick, P. (2005) Carcinogenicity evaluation: comparison of tumor data from dual control groups in the Sprague-Dawley rat. *Toxicol Pathol.*, **33**, 283–291.

Baldrick, P. and Reeve, L. (2007) Carcinogenicity evaluation: comparison of tumor data from dual control groups in the CD-1 mouse. *Toxicol. Pathol.*, **35**, 562–569.

Black, H.E. (1991) Peer review in toxicologic pathology: some recommendations. *Toxicol Pathol.*, **19**, 290–292.

Bogdanffy, M.S. and Connolly, K.M. (1993) Evaluation of proliferating cell nuclear antigen (PCNA) as an endogenous marker of cell proliferation in rat liver: a Dual-stain comparison with 5-bromo-2′-deoxyuridine. *J. Histochem. Cytochem.*, **41**, 1–6.

Brambilla, G. and Martelli, A. (2009) Update on genotoxicity and carcinogenicity testing of 472 marketed pharmaceuticals. *Mutation Res.*, **681**, 109–229.

Bregman, C.L., Adler, R.R., Morton, D.G. *et al.* (2003) Recommended tissue list for histopathological examination in repeat-dose and carcinogenicity studies: a proposal of the Society of Toxicologic Pathology (STP). *Toxicol Pathol.*, **31**, 252–253.

Bugelski, P.J., Volk, A., Walker, M.R. *et al.* (2010) Critical review of preclinical approaches to evaluate the potential of immunosuppressive drugs to influence human neoplasia. *Int. J. Toxicol.*, **29**(5), 435–466.

Burns-Naas, L.A., Zorbas, M., Jessen, B. *et al.* (2005) Increase in thyroid follicular cell tumors in nelfinavir-treated rats observed in a 2-year carcinogenicity study is consistent with a rat-specific mechanism of thyroid neoplasia. *Hum. Exp. Toxicol.*, **24**, 643–654.

Butterworth, B.E., Popp, J.A., Conolly, R.B., and Goldsworthy, T.L. (1992) Chemically-induced cell proliferation in carcinogenesis, in *Mechanisms of Carcinogenesis in Risk Identification*, vol. **116** (eds H. Vainio, P.N. Magee, D.B. McGregor, and A.J. McMichael), IARC Scientific Publications, pp. 279–305.

Cattley, R.C. and Popp, J.A. (1989) Difference between the promoting activities of the peroxisome proliferator WY-14,643 and Phenobarbital in rat liver. *Cancer Res.*, **49**, 3246–3251.

D'Amico, F., Skarmoutsou, E., and Stivala, F. (2009) State of the art in antigen retrieval for immunohistochemistry. *J. Immunochem. Methods*, **341**, 1–18.

FMA (2003) Note for Guidance on Carcinogenic Potential. European Agency for Evaluation of Medicinal Products, Committee for Proprietary Medicinal Products (CPMP). January 2003.

FDA (2001) Guidance for Industry. Statistical aspects of the design, analysis, and interpretation of chronic rodent carcinogenicity studies of pharmaceuticals. Draft. May 2001.

FDA (2002) Guidance for Industry; Carcinogenicity Study Protocol Submissions. U.S. Food and Drug Administration, May 2002.

FDA (2008) Guidance for Industry. Safety testing of drug metabolites. U.S. Food and Drug Administration. February 2008.

FDA (2009) Guidance for Industry. Formal meetings between the FDA and sponsors or applicants. U.S. Food and Drug Administration. May 2009.

Fielden, M.R., Brennan, R., and Gollub, J. (2007) A gene expression biomarker provides early prediction and mechanistic assessment of hepatic tumor induction by nongenotoxic chemicals. *Toxicol. Sci.*, **99**, 90–100.

Foster, W.R., Chen, S.-J., He, A. *et al.* (2007) A retrospective analysis of toxicogenomics in the safety assessment of drug candidates. *Toxicol. Pathol.*, **35**, 621–635.

ICH Website http://www.ich.org/products/guidelines.html Accessed 2/6/2011.

ICH (1994) Note for guidance on toxicokinetics: the assessment of systemic exposure in toxicity studies. S3A. International Conference on Harmonization of Technical Requirements for Registration of Pharmaceuticals for Human Use. October 2004.

ICH (1995) Guideline on the need for carcinogenicity studies of pharmaceuticals S1A. International Conference on Harmonization of Technical Requirements for Registration of Pharmaceuticals for Human Use. November 1995.

ICH (1997) Testing for carcinogenicity of pharmaceuticals. S1B International Conference on Harmonization of Technical Requirements for Registration of Pharmaceuticals for Human Use. July 1997.

ICH (2005) Immunotoxicity studies for human pharmaceuticals. S8. International Conference on Harmonization of Technical Requirements for Registration of Pharmaceuticals for Human Use. September 2005.

ICH (2008) Dose selection for carcinogenicity studies of pharmaceuticals S1C(R2). International Conference on Harmonization of Technical Requirements for Registration of Pharmaceuticals for Human Use. March 2008.

ICH (2009a) Note for guidance on non-clinical safety studies for the conduct of human clinical trials and marketing authorization for pharmaceuticals. M3(R2). International Conference on Harmonization of Technical Requirements for Registration of Pharmaceuticals for Human Use. June 2009.

ICH (2009b) Nonclinical evaluation for anticancer pharmaceuticals. S9. International Conference on Harmonization of Technical Requirements for Registration of Pharmaceuticals for Human Use. October 2009.

ICH (2011) Preclinical safety evaluation of biotechnology-derived pharmaceuticals S6(R1). International Conference on Harmonization of Technical Requirements for Registration of Pharmaceuticals for Human Use. June 2011.

Jacobs, A. (2005) Prediction of 2-year carcinogenicity study results for pharmaceutical products: How are we doing? *Toxicol. Sci.*, **88**, 18–23.

Jacobson-Kram, D. (2010) Cancer risk assessment approaches at the FDA/CEDR: is the era of the 2-year bioassay drawing to a close? *Toxicol. Pathol.*, **38**, 169–170.

Keenan, K.P., Hoe, C.-M., Mixson, L. *et al.* (2005) Diabesity: a polygenic model of dietary-induced obesity from ad libitum overfeeding of Sprague Dawley rats and its modulation by moderate and marked dietary restriction. *Toxicol Pathol.*, **33**, 650–674.

King-Hebert, A. and Thayer, K. (2006) NTP Workshop: Animal models for the NTP rodent cancer bioassay: Stocks and strains – should we switch? *Toxicol. Pathol.*, **34**, 802–805.

Long, G.G., Cohen, I.R., Gries, C.L. *et al.* (2001) Proliferative lesions of ovarian granulose cells and reversible hormonal changes induced in rats by a selective estrogen receptor modulator. *Toxicol. Pathol.*, **29**, 403–410.

MacDonald, J.S. (2004) Human carcinogenic risk evaluation , part IV: Assessment of human risk of cancer from chemical exposure using global weight of evidence approach. *Toxicol. Sci.*, **82**, 3–8.

Marsman, D.S. and Popp, J.A. (1994) Biological potential of basophilic hepatocellular foci and hepatocellular adenoma induced by peroxisome proliferator, WY-14, 643. *Carcinogenesis.*, **15**, 111–117.

Meek, M.E., Bucher, J.R., Cohen, S.M. *et al.* (2003) A framework for human relevance analysis of information on carcinogenic modes of action. *Crit. Rev. Toxicol.*, **33**(6), 591–653.

Pennie, W., Pettit, S., and Lord, P.G. (2004) Toxicogenomics in risk assessment: An overview of an HESI collaborative research program. *Environ. Health Persp.*, **112**(4), 417–419.

Popp, J.A., Scortichini, B.H., and Garvey, L.K. (1985) Quantitative evaluation of hepatic foci of cellular alteration occurring spontaneously in Fischer-344 rats. *Fundam. Appli. Toxicol.*, **5**, 314–319.

Pot, P. (1775) Cancer scroti, in *Chirurgical Observations Relative to the Cataract, the Polypus of the Nose, the Cancer of the Scrotum, the Different Kinds of Ruptures and the Modification of Toes and Feet*, Hawes, Clarke, Collin, London, pp. 63–68.

Pritchard, J.B., French, J.E., Davis, B.J., and Haseman, J.K. (2003) The role of transgenic mouse models in carcinogen identification. *Environ. Health Persp.*, **111**, 444–454.

Reddy, V.M., Sistare, F.D., Christensen, J.S. *et al.* (2010) An evaluation of chronic 6- and 12-month rat toxicology studies as predictors of 2-year tumor outcome. *Vet. Pathol.*, **47**, 614–629.

Rhomberg, R.L., Baetche, K., Blancato, J. *et al.* (2007) Issues in the design and interpretation of chronic toxicity and carcinogenicity studies: approaches to dose selection. *Crit. Rev. Toxicol.*, **37**, 729–837.

Sellers, R.S., Morton, D., Michael, B. *et al.* (2007) Society of toxicologic pathology position paper: organ weight recommendations for toxicology studies. *Toxicol. Pathol.*, **35**(5), 751–755.

Sistare, F.D., Morton, D., Alden, C. *et al.* (2011) An analysis of pharmaceutical experience with decades of rat carcinogenicity testing: support for a proposal to modify current regulatory guidelines. *Toxicol. Pathol.*, **39**, 716–744.

Snyder, R.D. and Green, J.W. (2001) A review of the genotoxicity of marketed pharmaceuticals. *Mutation Res.*, **488**, 151–169.

Society of Toxicologic Pathology website http://www.toxpath.org/ssndc.asp Accessed 2/6/2010.

Tennekes, H., Kaufmann, W., Dammann, M., and Van Ravenzwaay, B. (2004) The stability of historical control data for common neoplasms in laboratory rats and the implications for carcinogenic risk assessment. *Reg. Tox. Pharmacol.*, **40**, 293–304.

Toxicol. Pathol. (2001) **29** (suppl 1), 1–351.

Vahle, J.L., Finch, G.L., Heidel, S.M. *et al.* (2010) Carcinogenicity assessment of biotechnology-derived pharmaceuticals: a review of approved molecules and best practices recommendations. *Toxicol. Pathol.*, **38**, 522–553.

Ward, J.M., Hardisty, J.F., Hailey, J.R., and Street, C.S. (1995) Peer review in toxicologic pathology. *Toxicol. Pathol.*, **23**, 226–233.

Williams, G.M. and Iatropoulos, M.J. (2002) Alteration of liver cell function and proliferation: differentiation between adaptation and toxicity. *Toxicol. Pathol.*, **30**, 41–53.

Wood, F.E., Tierney, W.J., Knezevich, A.L. *et al.* (1991) Chronic toxicity and carcinogenicity studies of olestra in Fischer 344 rats. *Food Chem. Toxicol.*, **29**, 223–230.

Yamagiwa, K. and Ichikawa, K. (1918) Experimental study of the pathogenesis of carcinoma. *J. Cancer Res.*, **3**, 1–21.

Young, J.K., Hall, R.L., O'Brien, P. *et al.* (2011) Best practices for clinical pathology testing in carcinogenicity studies. *Toxicol. Pathol.*, **39**, 429–434.

14

Genetic Toxicology

Mark W. Powley
CDER, Office of New Drugs, FDA, Silver Spring, USA

14.1 Background

As a subdiscipline within toxicology, genetic toxicology focuses on the ability of agents to induce genetic damage. Unrepaired or misrepaired genetic damage could be replicated and passed on to daughter cells, a process resulting in a genetic mutation (i.e., change in the DNA sequence). Genetic mutations, such as those that result in oncogene activation or tumour suppressor gene deactivation, contribute to the multistep process of carcinogenesis.

Genetic effects are associated with a number of adverse health outcomes such as birth defects and ageing. However, the primary application of genetic toxicology in drug development is hazard identification for the purpose of predicting potential for human carcinogenicity. Because of the duration involved in carcinogenesis (i.e., carcinogenic effects will not be evident for many years) it is impractical to monitor this end-point in clinical trials. The data obtained from rodent carcinogenicity studies serve as a surrogate for human carcinogenicity resulting from exposure to drugs in accordance with the International Conference for Harmonization (ICH) S1A (ICH, 1995). However, per ICH M3(R2) (ICH, 2009) data from these studies is not required until the submission of a marketing application. Because rodent carcinogenicity studies are resource intensive, investigators routinely delay initiation until later stages of development. Therefore, genetic toxicology data serve as the basis for assessing the potential carcinogenic risk of drugs until rodent carcinogenicity data are available.

Genetic toxicology studies are often used to screen candidate drugs with the goal of excluding genotoxic compounds from entering development. Genotoxic potential

Nonclinical Safety Assessment: A Guide to International Pharmaceutical Regulations, First Edition.
Edited by William J. Brock, Kenneth L. Hastings and Kathy M. McGown.

is also considered during the qualification of major drug metabolites, impurities, and excipients.

14.2 Regulations Guiding Drug Development

Globally-adopted regulations for genotoxicity testing of small molecule drugs were previously described in ICH S2A (ICH, 1996a) and ICH S2B (ICH, 1996b). These guidelines provided details including the recommended battery of genetic toxicology assays, conduct of assays (e.g., test conditions, appropriate test systems, etc.) and evaluation of results. The information provided in ICH S2A and S2B was recently updated and combined into a single guideline referred to as ICH S2(R1) (ICH, 2011). The evaluation and integration of genetic toxicology data has also been described in an FDA guidance document (FDA, 2006). The information below is intended to summarize key aspects of regulatory genetic toxicology testing conducted during drug development.

14.2.1 Genetic Toxicology Assays

Genetic damage impacts DNA at both the gene and the chromosome level. Gene mutations are the result of events such as nucleotide substitutions, additions, and deletions leading to change in the nucleotide sequence. A change in the nucleotide sequence could result in expression of a non-functional or poorly functional protein. Besides impacting the structural integrity of chromosomes, chromosomal damage can affect the number of whole (i.e., polyploidy) or partial (i.e., aneuploidy) chromosome sets. Potential outcomes of chromosome damage include loss or gain of genetic information as well as unintended changes in gene expression.

Genetic toxicology assays conducted to support drug development are intended to evaluate drug candidates for their ability to induce gene mutations, structural chromosomal damage (i.e., clastogenicity), and numerical chromosomal damage (e.g., aneugenicity). Because genotoxicity could be attributable to a metabolite and/or the parent compound, *in vitro* assays are conducted with and without metabolic activation. Subcellular liver fractions from rats treated with agents designed to maximize, or induce, enzymatic activity are routinely used. Alternative sources of metabolic activation might be justified, based on the human relevance of the metabolite profile. *In vivo* assays have the advantage of accounting for pharmacokinetic and ADME (absorption, distribution, metabolism and excretion) properties of a drug.

The various end-points measured by commonly-used *in vitro* and *in vivo* genotoxicity assays are summarized below (Tables 14.1 and 14.2). With the exception of DNA adduct evaluations and the *in vivo* single cell gel electrophoresis/comet assay, formally standardized protocols (i.e., OECD guidelines) are available for the other assays. The use of the standard protocols assures experiments are conducted by globally-accepted methodology, a critical consideration for regulatory use.

The ability of several commonly-used genetic toxicology assays to predict rodent carcinogens has been described in published literature. Kirkland *et al.* (2005) calculated that the bacterial reverse mutation assay had a sensitivity of 59% and a specificity of 74%. These authors also showed that *in vitro* mammalian cells assays had sensitivity ranging

Table 14.1 *Commonly used* in vitro *assays.*

Assay	Damage detected	Standard methods
Bacterial Reverse Mutation Assay	• gene mutations	OECD 471 (OECD, 1997a)
Chromosomal Aberration Assay	• chromosomal damage • structural • numerical	OECD 473 (OECD, 1997b)
Mouse Lymphoma Assay	• gene mutations • chromosomal damage • structural • numerical • sizing of mutant colonies can be used to differentiate between gene mutations (large colonies) and clastogenicity (small colonies)	OECD 476 (OECD, 1997c)
Micronucleus Assay	• chromosomal damage • structural • numerical • special procedures can be applied to differentiate between clastogenic and aneugenic mechanisms	OECD 487 (2010a)
DNA Adducts	• covalent binding to DNA	N/A

N/A – not applicable.

from 66–79% with a specificity of 31–45%. The *in vivo* rodent micronucleus has a sensitivity of 40% and specificity of 75% (Benigni *et al.*, 2010). Although genetic toxicology assays appear to be imperfect predictors of rodent carcinogenicity, it is important to note that both genotoxic and non-genotoxic rodent carcinogens are included in the

Table 14.2 *Commonly used* in vivo *assays.*

Assay	Damage detected	Standard methods
Single Cell Gel Electrophoresis (Comet Assay)	• DNA strand breaks	N/A
Chromosomal Aberration Assay	• chromosomal damage • structural • numerical	OECD 475 (OECD, 1997d)
DNA Adducts	• covalent binding to DNA	N/A
Liver Unscheduled DNA Synthesis (UDS)	• repair of DNA damage	OECD 486 (OECD,1997e)
Micronucleus Assay	• chromosomal damage • structural • numerical • special procedures can be applied to differentiate between clastogenic and aneugenic mechanisms	OECD 474 (OECD,1977f)
Transgenic Mouse Gene Mutation Assay	• gene mutations	OECD 488 (OECD, 2011)

N/A – not applicable.

comparison. The predictive performance of the assays would likely increase if only compared against genotoxic carcinogens.

As with all toxicology studies, an important consideration in genetic toxicology testing is the selection of an appropriate dose range. When selecting a top dose, it is necessary to balance the need to fully characterize the genotoxic potential with assuring the relevance of the assessment. Data generated at doses yielding excessive toxicity *in vitro* or *in vivo* are of questionable utility. Likewise, data obtained from low *in vitro* concentrations or from *in vivo* studies where the target tissue may not have been adequately exposed are also not useful. To avoid these situations, ICH S2(R1) provides criteria for high-dose selection for *in vitro* and *in vivo* assays. In the *in vitro* assays, the default top dose for bacterial reverse mutation assay is 5000 μg/plate and 1 mM or 0.5 mg/mL for assays conducted in mammalian cells. The top dose can also be limited by cytotoxicity, a critical consideration for mammalian cells assays, or solubility of the test article.

The selection of an appropriate limit dose for *in vivo* assays depends on the duration of dosing and whether genetic toxicology end-points are combined with a general toxicology study. For instance, an acute micronucleus study should include a top dose of 2000 mg/kg compared to 1000 mg/kg which is an appropriate top dose when evaluating micronuclei following $\geq$14 days of dosing. Other important considerations when choosing a top dose for an *in vivo* genetic toxicology study are issues such as maximum tolerated dose (MTD), maximum feasible dose (MFD), saturation of systemic exposure, and target tissue toxicity. When combining a genetic toxicology end-point with a general toxicity study, top dose selection to support clinical development as described in ICH M3(R2) should be followed.

14.2.2 ICH Genetic Toxicology Battery

While quantitative risk assessment is possible in some cases, the primary application of genetic toxicology assays in drug development is hazard identification. In order to maximize the potential to identify genotoxicity arising from a wide variety of mechanisms, ICH recommends conducting a battery of genetic toxicology tests. Two options are included in order to provide flexibility in testing (Table 14.3). The Option 1 battery includes *in vitro* assays designed to detect gene mutations (i.e., the bacterial reverse mutation assay) and chromosomal damage as well as an *in vivo* genotoxicity evaluation. The *in vitro* assessment of chromosomal damage can be accomplished through one of three different mammalian cell-based assays. The assays mentioned are the chromosomal aberration assay, micronucleus assay, or mouse lymphoma assay. The *in vitro* micronucleus assay can provide mechanistic information to differentiate clastogens and

Table 14.3 *ICH battery of genotoxicity studies.*

Option 1	Option 2
bacterial reverse mutation assay	bacterial reverse mutation assay
in vitro mammalian cell assay to detect chromosomal damage	*in vivo* genotoxicity in rodent hematopoietic cells
in vivo genotoxicity in rodent hematopoietic cells, either micronuclei or chromosomal aberrations	second *in vivo* assay/endpoint in a second tissue

aneugens. The mouse lymphoma assay has the advantage of being able to detect gene mutations versus chromosomal effects based on collection of colony sizing data. Option 1 also includes an *in vivo* assay to detect chromosomal damage, most often including an evaluation of micronuclei in rodent hematopoietic cells although an evaluation of chromosomal aberrations is also acceptable. The ICH guideline suggests that this option is more desirable in cases where the bacterial reverse mutation assay is not appropriate (e.g., testing of antibacterials) or when systemic exposure in rodents is much lower than that measured or expected in the clinic.

Option 2 also includes an assessment of gene mutations using the *in vitro* bacterial reverse mutation assay but instead of an evaluation of chromosomal damage *in vitro* it allows two *in vivo* assays or two end-points in a single assay. The expectation is that the *in vivo* assays will measure different end-points in different tissues. The most likely combination will be micronuclei in rodent hematopoietic cells and the single cell gel electrophoresis assay (i.e., Comet assay) in liver. With an understanding of metabolism and target organ toxicity, other end-points and other tissues could also be scientifically justified. The ICH guideline recommends this option when reactive metabolites are formed in the liver and might not reach the bone marrow.

14.2.3 Positive Results and Follow-up

It is critical to evaluate genetic toxicology in the context of the intended clinical use of the drug. Both the clinical development phase, when patients and/or healthy volunteers could be administered the drug, and marketing should be considered. Negative results in the ICH genotoxicity battery allow drugs to enter into and proceed in clinical trials. Information obtained at later stages of development could result in additional testing. For instance, if systemic exposure is found to be substantially higher in humans versus the chosen rodent species, the utility of an *in vivo* genetic toxicology assay could be questioned. Also, qualitative differences in metabolite profiles could warrant concern, especially when a potentially reactive metabolite is formed uniquely or disproportionately in humans. When metabolite concerns are encountered, a genetic toxicology assessment in another species or with directly administered synthesized metabolite might be warranted.

Although positive results obtained from one or more genetic toxicology assays can be problematic, the scenario does not necessarily lead to the termination of the development of the drug. This was confirmed in a recent review that found 7% of marketed drugs were positive in the Ames assay, 19.1–26.1% were positive in an *in vitro* mammalian cell assay, and 11.1% were positive for *in vivo* clastogenicity (Snyder, 2009). Strategies for mitigating a positive genotoxicity finding are described in general terms by ICH and FDA and include evaluation of biological relevance, establishing a mechanism, and experimental follow-up.

The first step in placing a positive genetic toxicology assay result in perspective is to evaluate the biological relevance. Establishing relevance primarily involves determining whether the conditions leading to the positive are likely to occur in humans. For instance, a positive in the bacterial reverse mutation assay due to the action of bacterial specific enzymes (e.g., nitroreductases) is not informative with regard to potential clinical outcome. Likewise, extreme experimental conditions, such as excessive cytotoxicity or nucleotide pool imbalance, can result in a positive *in vitro* result in a mammalian cell assay with questionable human relevance. Micronuclei can form *in vivo* as a result of changes in body temperature, altered erythropoiesis, or stimulatory effects on cell division (Tweats *et al.*, 2007). Different drug batches are likely to have different impurity profiles. Therefore, genotoxic impurities present in the drug batch used for genetic toxicology testing lack relevance for a drug batch with a different impurity profile. *In vitro* positives generated in the presence of induced rat S9 and *in vivo* positives in rodents could potentially be due to metabolites unlikely to be formed in humans.

After determining that a positive finding is clinically relevant, it is helpful to also investigate the mechanism before deciding on experimental follow-up. Confirming that a drug induces a gene mutation event, structural chromosomal damage or numerical chromosomal damage will help guide selection of additional genetic toxicology assays. A likely mechanism of action will be evident when dealing with a positive bacterial gene mutation assay or mouse lymphoma assay primarily causing either small or large colonies. While definitive information cannot always be obtained from a single assay, a potential mechanism can be inferred based on the overall genotoxicity profile. As an example, a compound that is negative in the bacterial reverse mutation assay, negative in an *in vitro* chromosomal aberration assay, but causes *in vivo* micronuclei suggests the possibility of an aneugenic mechanism.

Once perspective is gained by assessing the biological relevance and potential mechanism related to the positive finding, it might be necessary to conduct additional genetic toxicology assays. The critical consideration is to conduct assays that will provide information to help further describe the positive finding. The best experimental follow-up to a positive micronucleus assay thought to be due to an aneugenic mechanism is a second micronucleus assay to look at the presence of kinetochores. The presence of these proteins associated with the mitotic spindle apparatus confirms that micronuclei contain whole chromosomes generated through an aneugenic mechanism while absence indicates a chromosomal fragment arising from a clastogenic mechanism. Another relatively common follow-up is to conduct an *in vivo* Comet assay to evaluate DNA damage after identifying chromosomal effects in an *in vitro* mammalian cell assay. A similar strategy is now described in ICH S2(R1) as Option 2. Although compounds that give a positive bacterial reverse mutation assay are difficult to develop, several assays could be used to potentially mitigate this outcome. These include gene mutation assays in mammalian cells, an evaluation of DNA adduct formation, the transgenic mouse gene mutation assay, and the Comet assay.

A practical assumption in drug development is that direct effects (e.g., gene mutations and chromosomal breaks) are the result of mechanisms lacking a threshold. In contrast, there are well-established threshold-based mechanisms for non-direct acting genotoxic compounds. These include some of the mechanisms previously described such as nucleotide pool imbalance, inhibition of topoisomerase, impairment of the mitotic spindle apparatus, extreme *in vitro* experimental conditions, and *in vivo* temperature changes. Because of the risks involved in developing genotoxic drugs, it is rare for sponsors to perform the evaluation necessary to properly establish a threshold. However, *in vivo* tests can be performed to identify no observed effect levels (NOELs) for genotoxic end-points. When adequate margins of safety are established, the genotoxic risk is minimized and development may proceed.

14.2.4 Timing

Although not required, the prevailing practice in drug development is to submit results of the genotoxicity battery in support of the initial Phase 1 clinical trial. According to ICH M3(R2) the *in vitro* assays are required to support a typical Phase 1 trial while the *in vivo* assay could be submitted prior to Phase 2. Exploratory trials could require a reverse bacterial mutation assay and *in vitro* mammalian cell assay, a bacterial reverse mutation assay alone, or in some require no genetic toxicology data. With the acceptance of ICH S2(R1), Option 1 follows the timing recommended in ICH M3(R2). A general assumption is that all assays conducted per Option 2 will be submitted to support Phase 1. The timing of follow-up assays will vary but it is worth noting that in some instances, a positive genotoxicity finding could result in a clinical hold until the risk is mitigated.

14.3 Genotoxic Impurities

Another application of genetic toxicology data in drug development is impurity qualification. Impurities include everything except the active pharmaceutical ingredient and excipients. Because impurities offer no benefit to clinical trial subjects or patients, a conservative approach is taken for risk assessment with these compounds.

ICH Q3A(R2) (ICH, 2006a) and ICH Q3B(R2) (ICH, 2006b) are applicable for impurities described at the marketing application stage. When impurities are present in drug substances or products at levels greater than the ICH Q3A and B qualification thresholds, empirical testing is generally recommended. An appropriate testing strategy would include an *in vitro* assessment for potential to cause point mutations and chromosomal aberrations. Impurities tested and shown to lack genotoxic potential are considered qualified based on the empirical data. Impurities possessing genotoxic potential should be controlled to appropriate safe levels.

While ICH Q3A(R2) and Q3B(R2) are useful in addressing testing of high-level impurities at the marketing stage, these guidelines do not provide specific criteria for establishing safe exposures to genotoxic impurities. In 2006, the Committee for Medicinal Products for Human Use of the European Medicines Agency's addressed this issue (EMA, 2006) and provided subsequent clarification in a question-and-answer document (EMA, 2010). The FDA has also published a draft guidance on the topic of genotoxic and carcinogenic impurities (FDA, 2008). Important considerations also covered in these regulatory documents are *in silico* predictions and empirical testing of impurities. Although differences exist, the various sources of regulatory recommendations are generally in close agreement. Several key components of the regulatory recommendations are outlined below.

14.3.1 *In Silico* Predictions

Structural alerts are features of a molecule (e.g., functional groups) that are associated with potential for genotoxicity. Per regulatory recommendations (EMA, 2010; FDA, 2008), an evaluation for structural alerts can serve as the basis of qualification for impurities that fall below the ICH Q3A and Q3B qualification thresholds. The assessment of structural alerts is routinely based on *in silico* predictions for the bacterial reverse mutation assay. Predictions are made by expert systems that detect structural features known to be associated with genotoxicity and statistically-based models that derive alerts from trainings sets populated with structures and associated empirical data. Collectively these assessments are termed (Quantitative) Structural Activity Relationships or (Q)SAR. An evaluation of structural alerts could also include a visual inspection for published alerts or known reactive groups based on the viewer's experience. In addition to an expert review of the (Q)SAR prediction, supporting information such as data for either public or proprietary structural analogs should be taken into account.

An important consideration is the degree to which the chemistry of the impurity is represented in training set molecules (i.e., domain of applicability). Impurities that fall outside a model's domain of applicability are not covered and cannot be qualified by *in silico* methods. Overall, impurities that lack structural alerts based on an adequate *in silico* evaluation are considered qualified. However, when a structural alert is identified, the impurity should be empirically tested to definitively establish mutagenic potential or assumed to be mutagenic and controlled to the appropriate level.

14.3.2 Empirical Testing

As previously mentioned, impurities above the ICH Q3A/B qualification threshold require *in vitro* testing for point mutations (e.g., bacterial reverse mutation assay) as well as chromosomal aberrations. A bacterial reverse mutation assay will suffice for establishing mutagenic potential of impurities with structural alerts that are below the ICH qualification threshold. When evaluating impurities, an additional consideration is the genotoxicity profile of the parent drug. There is little justification for empirical testing of an impurity if the parent molecule is mutagenic.

ICH Q3A/B indicates that impurity present in drug substance product are considered to be tested and qualified. In contrast, the EMA and FDA (EMA, 2006; FDA, 2008) recommend that isolated impurities be tested. An appropriate default testing strategy is that the evaluation will be conducted with an isolated impurity in an OECD-compliant assay, including an appropriate limit dose level. This is supported by published data including Kenyon *et al.* (2007) who found that while ~85% of the molecules in a database of mutagens were detected at levels ≤ 250 μg/plate, 15% required higher levels. These authors also showed that some mutagens were classified as non-mutagenic when tested in the presence of other chemicals. In spite of the default testing strategy described, it is recognized that impurities might not be synthesized in quantities that allow testing in isolation or in a fully compliant assay. When scientifically justified, suboptimal testing conditions (e.g., truncated dose range, limited number of bacterial strains, etc.) could be applied.

14.3.3 Safe Levels of Genotoxic Impurities

Safe levels of genotoxic impurities are based on the threshold of toxicological concern (TTC), an approach developed by the US FDA CFSAN to regulate exposure to potential carcinogens through the diet (Cheeseman *et al.*, 1999). Using this approach, a TTC of 1.5 μg/day will result in a minimal carcinogenic risk (i.e., 1×10^{-5}) due to exposure to genotoxic impurities in drugs. This TTC derived from a large publicly-available dataset of carcinogenic potencies expressed as the TD_{50} (http://potency.berkely.edu). TD_{50} is the dose producing a 50% tumour incidence in rodent carcinogenicity studies. The value used is the most sensitive species, sex, and tumour site. Lower exposures are warranted for impurities that structurally resemble particularly potent carcinogens. Deviation from the default TTC is also warranted when carcinogenicity data are available allowing for a chemical specific risk assessment.

The 1.5 μg/day is considered an acceptable level to support a marketing application. However, both the EMA Q&A document and FDA draft guidance provide recommendations for appropriate levels during clinical development. Muller *et al.* (2006) have also proposed appropriate levels for the development phase. While specific limits differ, all recommendations are based on the staged TTC concept. This concept takes into account less-than-lifetime exposures and assigns limits based on the duration of clinical use.

Other factors impacting regulatory view of safe limits include practical considerations of controlling the impurity, the drug's intended indication, availability of other drugs, patient population.

14.4 Regulatory Decision Making

An important aspect of regulatory decision making is consideration of supporting information and benefits of the drug. Concern with genotoxicity is minimized for drugs indicated for serious or life-threatening indications. In contrast, genotoxicity is a major liability for a drug with a less serious indication. Duration of use will also weigh into a regulatory decision as genotoxic potential of a drug designed for short-term use will be less critically viewed compared to a chronically administered drug. Other factors include the patient population, availability of alternative drugs, standard of care, and so on. Similar considerations are weighed when evaluating impurities.

In summary, genetic toxicology testing serves as a surrogate for carcinogenicity data until results of rodent carcinogenicity assays are available. In this regard, evaluation of genotoxic potential is critical to minimizing risk to clinical trial subjects and patients who will receive a marketed drug. There are multiple sources of regulatory recommendations available to guide genetic toxicology testing in drug development but, ultimately, regulatory decisions will be made based on the totality of information and good science.

Disclaimer

The views expressed are those of the author. No official support or endorsements by the US Food and Drug Administration are provided.

References

Benigni, R., Bossa, C., and Worth, A. (2010) Structural analysis and predictive value of the rodent *in vivo* micronucleus assay results. *Mutagenesis*, **25**, 335–341.

Cheeseman, M.A., Machuga, E.J., and Bailey, A.B. (1999) A tiered approach to threshold of regulation. *Food Chemicol. Toxicol.*, **37**, 387–412.

EMA (2006) Guideline on the limits of genotoxic impurities.

EMA (2010) Questions and answers on the guideline on the limits of genotoxic impurities.

FDA (2006) Recommended approaches to integration of genetic toxicology study results.

FDA (2008) Guidance for industry genotoxic and carcinogenic impurities in drug substances and products: recommended approaches.

ICH (1995) Guideline on the need for carcinogenicity studies of pharmaceuticals. ICH S1A.

ICH (1996a) Specific aspects of regulatory genotoxicity tests for pharmaceuticals. ICH S2A.

ICH (1996b) A standard battery for genotoxicity testing for pharmaceuticals. ICH S2B.

ICH (2006) Impurities in new drug substances. ICH Q3A(R2).

ICH (2009) Guidance on nonclinical safety studies for the conduct of human clinical trials and marketing authorization for pharmaceuticals. ICH M3(R2).

ICH (2011) Guidance on genotoxicity testing and data interpretation for pharmaceuticals intended for human use. ICH S2(R1).

Kenyon, M.O., Cheung, J.R., Dobo, K.L., and Ku, W.W., (2007) An evaluation of the sensitivity of the Ames assay to discern low-level mutagenic impurities. *Reg. Toxicol. Pharmacol.*, **48**, 75–86.

Kirkland, D., Aardema, M., Henderson, L., and Muller, L., (2005) Evaluation of the ability of a battery of three *in vitro* genotoxicity tests to discriminate rodent carcinogens and non-carcinogens I. Sensitivity, specificity, and relative predictivity. *Mutat. Res.*, **584**, 1–256.

Muller, L., Mauthe, R.J., Riley, C.M., Andino, M.M., Antonis, D.D., Beels, C., DeGeorge, J., De Knaep, A.G., Ellison, D., Fagerland, J.A., Frank, R., Fritschel, B., Galloway, S., Harpur, E., Humfrey, C.D., Jacks, A.S., Jagota, N., Mackinnon, J., Mohan, G., Ness, D.K., O'Donovan, M. R., Smith, M.D., Vudathala, G., and Yotti, L., (2006) A rationale for determining, testing, and controlling specific impurities in pharmaceuticals that possess potential for genotoxicity. *Regul. Toxicol. Pharmacol.* **44**, 198–211.

OECD (1997a) Bacterial reverse mutation assay. OECD Guideline for the Testing of Chemicals, 471.

OECD (1997b) *In vitro* mammalian chromosome aberration test. OECD Guideline for the Testing of Chemicals, 473.

OECD (1997c) *In vitro* mammalian cell gene mutation test. OECD Guideline for the Testing of Chemicals, 476.

OECD (1997) Mammalian bone marrow chromosome aberration test. OECD Guideline for the Testing of Chemicals, 475.

OECD (1997) Unscheduled DNA synthesis (UDS) test with mammalian liver cells *in vivo*. OECD Guideline for the Testing of Chemicals, 486.

OECD (1997) Mammalian erythrocyte micronucleus test. OECD Guideline for the Testing of Chemicals, 474.

OECD (2010) *In vitro* mammalian cell micronucleus test. OECD Guideline for the Testing of Chemicals, 487.

OECD (2010b) *In vitro* mammalian cell micronucleus test. OECD Guideline for the Testing of Chemicals, 487.

OECD (2011) Transgenic rodent somatic and germ cell gene mutation assays. OECD Guideline for the Testing of Chemicals, 488.

Snyder, R., (2009) An update on the genotoxicity and carcinogenicity of marketed pharmaceuticals with reference to *in silico* predictivity. *Environ. Mol. Mutagen.*, **50**, 435–450.

Tweats, D.J., Blakey, D., Heflich, R.H., Jacobs, A., Jacobson, S.D., Morita, T., Nohmi, T., O'Donovan, M.R., Sasaki, Y.F., Sofuni, T., and Tice, R., (2007) Report of the IWGT working group on strategies and interpretation of regulatory *in vivo* tests I. Increases in micronucleated bone marrow cells in rodents that do not indicate genotoxic hazards. *Mutat. Res.*, **627**, 78–91.

15

Developmental and Reproductive Toxicology

Robert M. Parker[1] *and Raymond G. York*[2]
[1]*Huntingdon Life Sciences, East Millstone, USA*
[2]*RG York & Associates LLC, Manlius, USA*

15.1 Introduction

The objective of this chapter is to provide the methodologies used during the performance of developmental and reproductive safety toxicity testing for evaluation of pharmaceuticals, compliant with the latest international guidelines. Traditionally, multiple agencies and countries promulgated their own developmental and reproductive testing guidelines resulting in time-consuming and overlapping testing and data sets, high use of animal resources, and high testing costs for worldwide registration. In 1994, three pharmaceutical industry associations and three government agencies of Europe, USA and Japan came together to harmonize preclinical testing guidelines and eliminate these burdens of global registration. According to the ICH S5(R2) document, Guideline for Industry, Detection of Toxicity to Reproduction for Medicinal Products (US FDA, 1994), a reproductive and developmental toxicity testing regimen should be selected that would "allow exposure of mature adults and all stages of development from conception to sexual maturity. To allow detection of immediate and latent effects of exposure, observations should be continued through one complete life cycle, that is, from conception in one generation through conception in the following generation". The document further suggests that an integrated test sequence can be subdivided into the following stages:

Nonclinical Safety Assessment: A Guide to International Pharmaceutical Regulations, First Edition.
Edited by William J. Brock, Kenneth L. Hastings and Kathy M. McGown.

- **Stage A:** Premating to conception (adult male and female reproductive functions, development and maturation of gametes, mating behaviour, fertilization);
- **Stage B:** Conception to implantation (adult female reproductive functions, pre-implantation development, implantation);
- **Stage C:** Implantation to closure of the hard palate (adult female reproductive functions, embryonic development, major organ formation);
- **Stage D:** Closure of the hard palate to the end of pregnancy (adult female reproductive functions, foetal development and growth, organ development and growth)
- **Stage E:** Birth to weaning (adult female reproductive functions, neonate adaptation to extrauterine life, preweaning development and growth);
- **Stage F:** Weaning to sexual maturity (postweaning development and growth, adaptation to independent life, attainment of full sexual function).

Nevertheless, in most cases those six stages are assessed by means of just three studies:

1. ICH 4.1.1 The Fertility and General Reproductive Performance Study ("Segment I"; Stages A to B).
2. ICH 4.1.2 The Prenatal and Postnatal Study ("Segment III"; Stages C to F).
3. ICH 4.1.3 The Developmental Toxicity or Embryotoxicity Study ("Segment II"; Stages C to D).

In addition, in recent years increased emphasis has been placed on direct toxicity studies in juvenile animals (Hurtt *et al.*, 2004; US FDA, 2006a) and developmental immunotoxicity (Dietert and Hopsapple, 2007). All of these study types are discussed in some detail in other chapters in this book.

Although the United States, the European Community and Japan have worked together to harmonize their test guidelines via the International Conferences on Harmonization (ICH), there still remain differences on the timing of these studies in relation to the clinical trials. These differences will also be highlighted in this chapter. Recently, a series of review articles concerning the three principle ICH Developmental and Reproductive Toxicology study designs were published and these have also been incorporated into the discussion below (Lerman *et al.*, 2009; Wise *et al.*, 2009; Bailey *et al.*, 2009). The Non-human Primate Developmental and Reproductive Toxicity and Juvenile Toxicity study designs will not be discussed but are reviewed in other chapters in this book. Also, the topic has been thoroughly reviewed in recent publications (Chellman *et al.*, 2009; Cappon *et al.*, 2009; Martin and Weinbauer, 2010).

15.2 Standard Reproduction and Developmental Toxicity Study Designs

15.2.1 ICH 4.1.1 The Fertility and General Reproductive Performance Study ("Segment I"; Stages A to B)

15.2.1.1 Aim

The aim of this study is to test for toxic effects/disturbances resulting from treatment before mating (males/females) through mating and implantation (Stages A and B of the reproductive process). For females, this should detect effects on the oestrous cycle, tubal transport, mating, implantation, and development of preimplantation stages of the

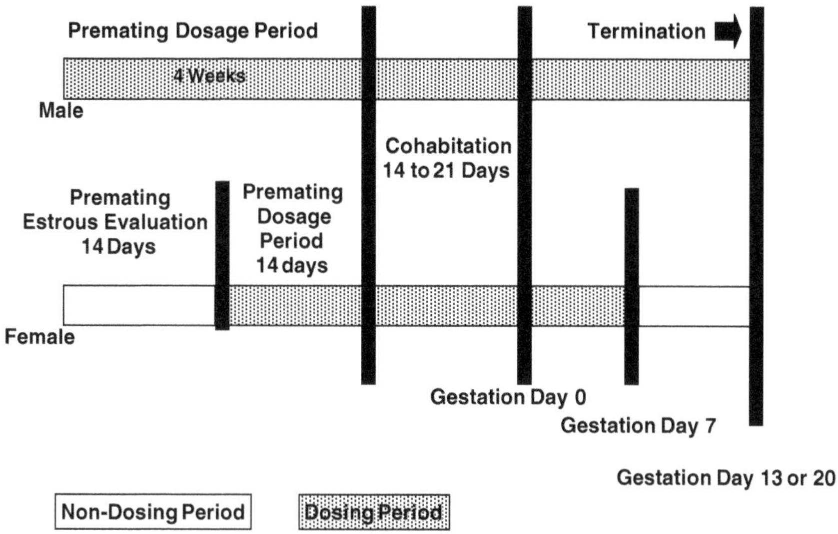

Figure 15.1 *ICH 4.1.1 The Fertility and General Reproductive Performance Study ("Segment I"; Stages A to B).*

embryo. For males, it will permit detection of functional effects (e.g., on libido, epididymal sperm maturation) that might not be detected by histological examinations of the male reproductive organs. For a schematic of the study design for a Fertility and General Reproductive Performance Study ("Segment I"; Stages A to B), see Figure 15.1.

15.2.1.2 Species and Number of Animals

At least one species, preferably rats with evaluation of between 16 to 20 litters per group for rodents, provides sufficient numbers to allow meaningful interpretation of the data. Advantages and disadvantages of species (strains) should be considered in relation to the substance to be tested, the selected study design and in the subsequent interpretation of the results. Rats, and to lesser extent mice, are good, general-purpose models. Mice have a fast metabolic rate, stress sensitivity, malformation clusters, limited size for toxicokinetic blood sampling, and small foetuses. The rabbit has been somewhat underused as a "nonrodent" species for reproduction studies other than embryotoxicity testing. The rabbit has attributes that would make it a useful model for fertility studies, especially male fertility. For both rabbits and dogs (which are often used as a second species for repeat-dose toxicity studies) semen samples can easily be obtained (electro ejaculation) for longitudinal semen analysis. For most other species, disadvantages outweigh the advantages.

15.2.1.3 Administration Period

Provided no effects have been found in repeated-dose toxicity studies of at least one month duration, a premating treatment interval of two weeks for females and 2–4 weeks for males can be used. Selection of the length of the premating administration period should be stated and justified in the protocol. However, if repeated-dose toxicity studies (general toxicity studies) show effects to the male reproductive system, then treatment of the male for up to 10 weeks prior to cohabitation might be necessary. This duration is based on the duration of spermatogenesis in the rodent (Hood and Parker, 2008). Treatment should continue throughout mating to termination of males and at least through implantation for females (Gestation Day [GD] 6). The Fertility Study has three designs: male treated only, female treated only, or both genders treated.

15.2.1.4 Mating

A 1 : 1 mating ratio is advisable and procedures should allow identification of both parents of a litter. Most laboratories use a mating period of 2–3 weeks; however, the minimum mating period is five consecutive nights. Routinely, if mating is not confirmed within two weeks, the unsuccessful male is replaced with another male from the same group that has had a successful mating and the new pair will continue cohabitation for one additional week or until mating is confirmed.

15.2.1.5 Terminal Sacrifice

Females can be sacrificed at any point after mid-pregnancy. When treatment of the females ceases at implantation (GD 6), termination of females between GD 13 to 17 is adequate to differentiate between implantation and resorption sites. Males can be sacrificed at any time after mating but it is advisable to ensure successful induction of pregnancy before taking such an irrevocable step. In the event of an equivocal result, males could be mated with untreated females to ascertain their fertility or infertility.

15.2.1.5.1 Observations

During study:

Oestrous cycle monitoring: 2 weeks pretreatment, 2 weeks during treatment prior to cohabitation and during cohabitation until confirmed mating.

At terminal examination:

Necropsy: macroscopic examination of all adults,

Males (if treated): Testes (weighed separately), epididymides (weighed separately), seminal vesicles with coagulating gland (weighed together), prostate, abnormal tissues, and any target organs are weighed and retained for possible histopathological evaluation;

Sperm motility, epididymal sperm and testicular spermatids counts, and sperm morphology is optional but should be performed if the repeated-dose toxicity studies showed effects to the male reproductive system.

Females (if treated): Ovaries (weighed separately), uterus with oviducts, and cervix and vagina, abnormal tissues, and any target organs are weighed and retained for possible histopathological evaluation;

Corpora lutea and implantation sites counts (pre- and post-implantation losses), and live and dead conceptuses (early and late resorptions) are recorded.

15.2.2 ICH 4.1.2. The Prenatal and Postnatal Study ("Segment III"; Stages C to F)

15.2.2.1 Aim

The aim of this study is to detect adverse effects on the pregnant/lactating female and on development of the conceptus and the offspring following exposure of the female from

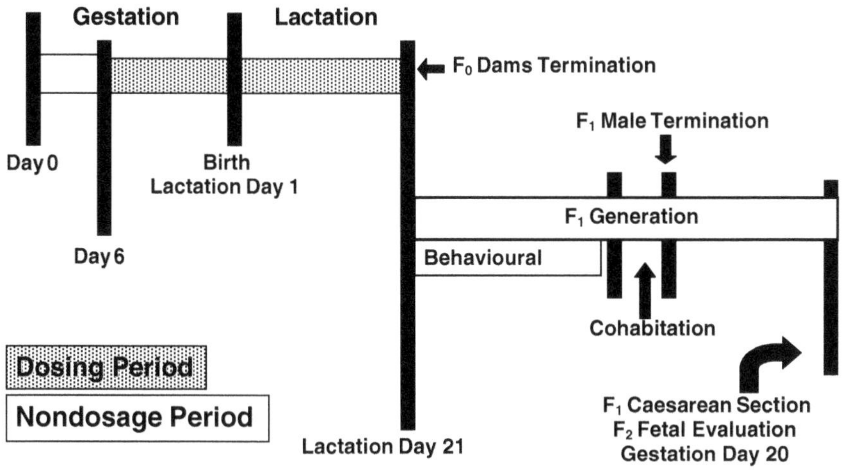

Figure 15.2 *ICH 4.1.2. The Prenatal and Postnatal Study ("Segment III"; Stages C to F).*

implantation through weaning. Since manifestations of effect induced during this period could be delayed, observations should be continued through sexual maturity (i.e., Stages C to F). For a schematic of the study design for a Prenatal and Postnatal Study ("Segment III"; Stages C to F), see Figure 15.2.

15.2.2.2 Species and Number of Animals

At least one species, preferably rats, with evaluation of between 16 to 20 litters per group for rodents, provides sufficient numbers to allow for meaningful interpretation of the data.

15.2.2.3 Administration Period

Females are exposed to the test substance from implantation to the end of lactation (Lactation Day [LD 20]).

15.2.2.4 Experimental Procedure

The females are allowed to deliver and rear their offspring to weaning, at which time one male and one female offspring per litter are selected for rearing to adulthood and mating to assess reproductive competence.

15.2.2.4.1 Observations

During study (for maternal and offspring):

F_0 litter and F_1 pre-weaning observations:

Duration of gestation, abnormal parturition, maternal behaviour

Live litter size: Daily from Postnatal Day (PND) 0/1 to PND 21

Pup abnormalities, sex ratio – PND 0/1, 4 and 21

Reflex development (at least two measures: for example, surface righting (from PND 2), mid-air righting (from PND 14), auditory startle reflex (from PND 10), and/or visual function (pupillary reflex) on PND 20; body weight is recorded at achievement.

F_1 post-weaning observations (1 male + 1 female from each litter) [Examples]:
Open field evaluation (for posture, gait, and abnormal behaviour) on PND 22/23
Motor activity (1-hour, in-cage, automated device) on PND 28 ± 1
Sexual maturation (vaginal opening monitored from PND 30 and balano-preputial separation from PND 40; body weight is recorded at achievement).
Learning ability and memory from approximately 8 weeks of age will be evaluated.
Daily monitoring of oestrous cycle for 2 weeks prior to pairing for mating in a reproductive function test (mating trial at approximately 10 weeks of age, cohabitation up to 20 days with termination and pregnancy evaluation on Day 14 of presumed gestation).
At terminal examination (for maternal animals and where applicable for offspring)
Necropsy (macroscopic examination) of all adults.
Preservation and possibly histological evaluation of organs with macroscopic findings.
Implantations (pre-and post-implantation losses for F_1 and F_2).
Live, dead or stillborn F_1 offspring and body weights at birth.
Pre- and postweaning survival and growth/body weight.

15.2.3 ICH 4.1.3 The Developmental Toxicity or Embryotoxicity Study ("Segment II"; Stages C to D)

15.2.3.1 Preliminary (Dose Range-Finding) Developmental Toxicity or Embryotoxicity Studies

15.2.3.1.1 Aim

The preliminary study is designed to assess any gross maternal and/or embryo-foetal toxicity of the test article in the rats and rabbits, following daily administration during the period of major organogenesis, from implantation to the approximate day of closure of the hard palate, GDs 6 to 17 in the rat, GDs 6 to 15 in the mouse, and GDs 6 to 18 or GDs 7 to 19 in the rabbit. Caesarean sections will be performed on GD 20/21 in the rat, GD 18 in the mouse and GD 29 in the rabbit. This study is used to determine the appropriate dose levels for the main embryotoxicity study. For a schematic of the study design for developmental toxicity or embryotoxicity studies ("Segment II"; Stages C to D) using rats and rabbits (Figure 15.3).

15.2.3.2 Species and Number of Animals

Usually, two species are used with one rodent, preferably rats and one nonrodent, preferably rabbits. Justification should be provided when using one species. For evaluation, 5–8 litters per group for rodents and rabbits should provide sufficient numbers to allow for meaningful interpretation of the data. Mice have also been used, usually because the test article requirement is less, and are acceptable if pharmacologically relevant. On occasion, the transgenic mouse (knock-ins and knock-outs), guinea pig, hamster, dog and nonhuman primate may be used because they demonstrate efficacy and cross-reactivity (Martin and Weinbauer, 2010).

15.2.3.2.1 Administration Period

The treatment period extends from implantation to the closure of the hard palate (i.e., end of Stage C).

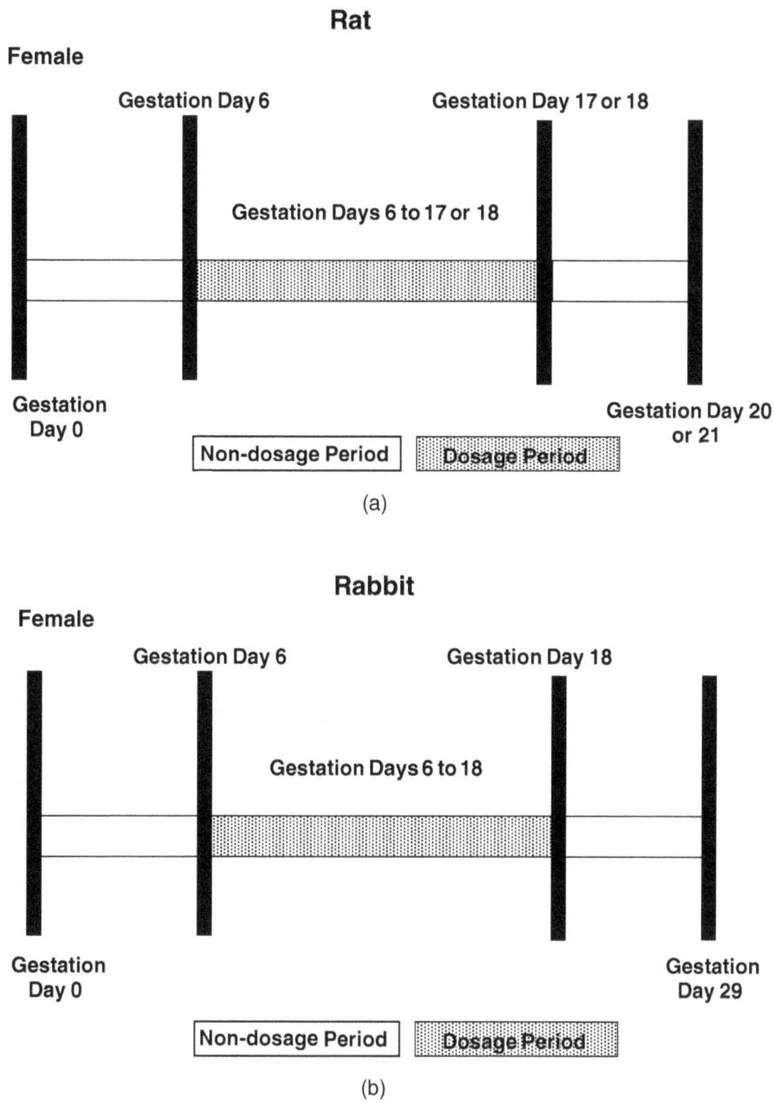

Figure 15.3 *(a) ICH 4.1.3. The Rat Developmental Toxicity or Embryotoxicity Study ("Segment II"; Stages C to D). (b) ICH 4.1.3. The Rabbit Developmental Toxicity or Embryotoxicity Study ("Segment II"; Stages C to D).*

15.2.3.2.2 Experimental Procedure

Females should be killed and examined about one day prior to parturition. All foetuses should be individually identified and be examined for viability and external abnormalities.

15.2.3.2.3 Observations

During study:

Toxicokinetic evaluation: Sampling on first and last days of dosing is recommended.

Terminal examination:

Macroscopic examination (dams): gravid uterus weight, pregnancies evaluated (corpora lutea, pre- and post-implantation losses), abnormal tissues preserved, as appropriate.

Fetuses are externally examined and live fetuses sexed and weighed.

Placentas are examined and weighed.

15.2.3.3 Main Developmental Toxicity or Embryotoxicity Studies

15.2.3.3.1 Aim

The aim of the main embryotoxicity study is to detect adverse effects on the pregnant female and development of the embryo and foetus consequent to exposure of the female from implantation to closure of the hard palate (i.e., Stages C to D).

15.2.3.3.2 Species and Number of Animals

Usually, two species are included with one rodent, preferably rats, and one nonrodent, preferably rabbits. Justification should be provided when using one species. Evaluation of between 16 and 20 litters per group for rodents and rabbits should provide sufficient numbers to allow for meaningful interpretation of the data.

15.2.3.3.3 Administration Period

The treatment period extends from implantation to the closure of the hard palate (i.e., end of Stage C)

15.2.3.3.4 Experimental Procedure

Females should be killed and examined about one day prior to parturition. All foetuses should be individually identified and examined for viability and abnormalities.

When using techniques requiring allocation to separate examination for soft tissue or skeletal changes, it is preferable that 50% of foetuses from each litter be allocated for skeletal examination. A minimum of 50% rat foetuses should be examined for visceral alterations, regardless of the technique used. When using fresh micro-dissection techniques for soft tissue alterations – which is the strongly preferred method for rabbits – 100% of rabbit foetuses should be examined for soft tissue and skeletal abnormalities.

15.2.3.3.5 Observations

During study:

Toxicokinetic evaluation: Sampling on first and last days of dosing is recommended.

Terminal examination:

Macroscopic examination (dams): gravid uterus weight, pregnancies evaluated (corpora lutea, pre- and post-implantation losses), abnormal tissues preserved, as appropriate. Foetuses are externally examined and live foetuses sexed and weighed.

Placentas are examined and weighed.

Rat and mouse foetuses are examined internally, sexed and processed: half for visceral abnormalities and half for skeletal abnormalities and state of skeletal ossification.

Rabbit foetuses are examined internally sexed and processed for visceral and skeletal abnormalities and state of skeletal ossification.

15.3 Timing of Preclinical Developmental and Reproductive Toxicity Studies

15.3.1 Based on Sex and Reproductive Potential

As discussed in ICH Guidance M3(R2) (ICH, 2009a), the timing of the conduct of the reproduction toxicity studies is based on two factors: (1) the population in which the clinical trials are going to be performed; and (2) the ICH countries to which the regulatory dossier will be submitted.

15.3.1.1 Men

Men can be included in Phase I and II clinical trials prior to the conduct of the male fertility study since an evaluation of the male reproductive organs is performed in the repeated-dose toxicity studies. An assessment of male and female fertility by thorough standard histopathological examination on the testis and ovary in a repeated-dose toxicity study (generally rodent) of at least 2-weeks' duration is considered to be as sensitive as fertility studies in detecting toxic effects on male and female reproductive organs (Sakai *et al.*, 2000; Sanbuissho *et al.*, 2009). A male fertility study should be completed prior to the initiation of large-scale or long duration clinical trials (e.g., Phase III trials) (NC3Rs, 2007; Robinson *et al.*, 2008).

15.3.1.2 Women Not of Childbearing Potential

Women who do not have childbearing potential (i.e., permanently sterilized, post-menopausal) can be included in clinical trials without reproduction toxicity studies if the relevant repeated-dose toxicity studies (which include an evaluation of the female reproductive organs as described above) have been conducted. Post-menopausal is defined as 12 months with no menses without an alternative medical cause.

15.3.1.3 Women of Childbearing Potential (WOCBP)

A high level of concern exists for the unintentional exposure of an embryo or foetus of WOCBP before information concerning the potential risk/benefit ratio is available. Therefore it is imperative that the risk to the embryo or foetus when including WOCBP in clinical trials be minimized. Minimizing risk can be achieved in several ways. Preclinical reproduction toxicity studies can be conducted to understand the inherent risk of a drug and appropriate precautions can be taken during exposure. Likewise, the risk can be limited by taking precautions to prevent pregnancy during clinical trials. Either way, precautions should include pregnancy testing, use of a highly effective method of birth control (i.e., barrier contraceptive), and only allowing study entry of WOCBP after a confirmed menstrual period. Highly effective methods of birth control are defined as those, alone or in combination, that result in a low failure rate (i.e., less than 1% per year) when used consistently and correctly (ICH, 2009b). For subjects using a hormonal contraceptive method, information regarding the product under evaluation and its potential effect on the contraceptive should be addressed. Testing for pregnancy during the clinical trial and subject/patient education should be sufficient to ensure compliance with the measures designed to prevent pregnancy during the period of drug exposure (which could exceed the length of study).

Informed consent should be based on any known pertinent information related to reproduction toxicity, such as a general assessment of potential toxicity of pharmaceuticals with related structures or pharmacological effects. If no relevant reproductive information is available, the potential for risks should be communicated.

The recommendations on timing of reproduction toxicity studies to support the inclusion of WOCBP in clinical trials are similar in all ICH regions (US, EU and Japan). WOCBP can be included in clinical trials without nonclinical developmental toxicity studies (e.g., embryotoxicity studies) in certain circumstances.

WOCBP can be enrolled in clinical trials of short duration (such as two weeks) with intensive control of pregnancy risk. WOCBP can also be enrolled in longer duration clinical trials when the objectives of the clinical trial cannot be effectively met without their inclusion, when the disease occurs predominantly in women, and when pregnancy risk can be adequately controlled.

WOCBP without the nonclinical developmental toxicity studies can also be considered for inclusion in early clinical studies based on the knowledge of the type of pharmaceutical agent (e.g., an antibody), its mechanism of action of the agent, its Absorption, Distribution, Metabolism and Excretion (ADME) characteristics (such as half-life, AUC, C_{max}), and difficulty of conducting developmental toxicity studies in an appropriate animal model.

Generally, where appropriate, preliminary reproduction toxicity data are available from two species but the definitive reproduction toxicity testing has not been completed, and where adequate birth control methods are used, WOCBP can be included in clinical trials for a relatively short duration (up to three months) and a relatively small size (consisting of 150 subjects). An appropriate preliminary embryo-foetal study is defined as a study with adequate dose levels with a minimum of six dams per group that are treated over the period of organogenesis; assessment of foetal survival, body weight, and external and visceral examinations; and the ability of adequately designed preliminary studies to detect most developmental toxicity findings that could raise concern for enrollment of WOCBP in clinical trials. The preliminary nonclinical studies should be conducted under GLP conditions or under high-quality scientific standards with data collection records readily available.

The inclusion of WOCBP in these studies is based on the very low rate of pregnancy in controlled clinical trials of this size and duration. The number of WOCBP and the duration of the study can be influenced by characteristics of the population that alter pregnancy rates (e.g., age, disease). The pregnancy rate of women who are attempting to become pregnant is approximately 17% per menstrual cycle. Pregnancy rates estimated from Phase III studies conducted in WOCBP, where the subjects were encouraged to avoid pregnancy and measures were instituted to prevent pregnancy, were observed to be <0.1% per menstrual cycle. Based on the Phase III experience, Phase II trials enrolling 150 WOCBP for three months are estimated to result in significantly less than 0.5 pregnancies per pharmaceutical under development.

The timing of the conduct of the reproductive toxicity studies varies by region:

- In the US, assessment of embryo–foetal development can be deferred until prior to Phase III for WOCBP using highly effective contraceptive methods.

- In the EU and Japan, definitive nonclinical developmental toxicity studies should be completed prior to exposure to WOCBP.
- In all ICH regions, nonclinical studies that specifically address female fertility should be completed to support inclusion of WOCBP in Phase III trials.
- In all ICH regions, the pre- and postnatal development study should be submitted for marketing approval or earlier if there is cause of concern.

For WOCBP not using highly effective birth control or whose pregnancy status is unknown, all female reproduction toxicity studies and the standard battery of genotoxicity tests (ICH, 2011a) should be completed prior to the inclusion in any clinical trial.

15.3.1.4 Pregnant Women

All of the reproduction toxicity studies and the standard battery of genotoxicity tests should be conducted prior to the inclusion of pregnant women in clinical trials. In addition, safety data from previous human exposure should be evaluated.

15.3.1.5 Paediatric Populations

Reproduction toxicity studies relevant to the age and gender of the paediatric patient populations under study can also be important to provide information on direct toxic or developmental risks (e.g., fertility and prenatal and postnatal developmental studies). Embryotoxicity studies are not critical to support clinical studies for males or prepubescent females (ICH, 2009a). Results from repeated-dose toxicity studies of appropriate duration in adult animals, the core safety pharmacology package (ICH, 2000), and the standard battery of genotoxicity tests should be available prior to the initiation of trials in paediatric populations.

15.4 Based on Disease Indication

15.4.1 Anticancer Pharmaceuticals

There have been no internationally accepted objectives or recommendations on the design and conduct of nonclinical studies to support the development of anticancer pharmaceuticals in patients with advanced disease and limited therapeutic options. The purpose of the S9 guidance (ICH, 2009c) is to provide information to assist in the design of an appropriate programme of nonclinical studies for the development of anticancer pharmaceuticals (see Farrell *et al.*, 2006, for review).

Since malignant tumours are life-threatening, the death rate from these diseases is high, and existing therapies have limited effectiveness, it is desired to provide new effective anticancer drugs to patients more expeditiously. Nonclinical evaluations are intended to: (1) identify the pharmacologic properties of a pharmaceutical; (2) establish a safe initial dose level for the first human exposure; and (3) understand the toxicological profile of a pharmaceutical, for example, identification of the target organ, estimation of the safety margin, and reversibility. In the development of anticancer drugs, most often the clinical studies involve cancer patients whose disease condition is often progressive and fatal. In addition, the clinical dose levels often are close to or at the adverse effect dose levels. For these reasons, the type and timing and flexibility called for in designing nonclinical developmental toxicity studies of anticancer pharmaceuticals can have a different pattern from those for other pharmaceuticals.

An embryo–foetal toxicology assessment is warranted to communicate potential risk for the developing embryo or foetus to patients who are or might become pregnant. Embryotoxicity studies of anticancer pharmaceuticals should be available when the marketing application is submitted, but these studies are not considered essential to support clinical trials intended for the treatment of patients with late stage or advanced cancer. These studies are also not considered essential for pharmaceuticals that target rapidly-dividing cells in general toxicity studies or belong to a class which has been well characterized in causing developmental toxicity. Embryotoxicity studies are typically conducted in two species. In cases where an embryotoxicity study is positive for embryo–foetal lethality or is teratogenic, a confirmatory study in a second species is usually not warranted. For biopharmaceuticals, an embryo–foetal toxicity study might not always be feasible. Generally, no fertility study is warranted to support the treatment of patients with late stage or advanced cancer. Information available from general toxicology studies on reproductive organs should be incorporated into the assessment of reproductive toxicology. A prenatal and postnatal toxicology study is generally not warranted to support the treatment of patients with late stage or advanced cancer (ICH, 2009c).

15.4.1.1 Nonclinical Studies to Support Trials in Paediatric Populations

Studies in juvenile animals (Chapter 18) are not usually conducted in order to support inclusion of paediatric populations for the treatment of cancer. The recommendations for nonclinical testing outlined elsewhere in this book also apply to this population. Conduct of studies in juvenile animals should be considered when human safety data and previous animal studies are considered insufficient for a safety evaluation in the intended paediatric age group.

15.4.1.2 Evaluation of Drug Metabolites in Anticancer Drugs

In some cases, metabolites have been identified in humans that have not been qualified in nonclinical studies. For these metabolites, a separate general toxicology evaluation might not be warranted for patients with late stage or advanced cancer, as the human safety of the metabolite would have been assessed in Phase I clinical trials. If the parent compound is considered positive in an evaluation for embryo–foetal toxicity or genotoxicity then separate studies for the disproportionate metabolite might not be warranted. Unless there is a specific cause for concern, nonclinical testing of the metabolite is not usually warranted.

15.4.1.3 Evaluation of Impurities in Anticancer Drugs

It is recognized that impurities are not expected to have any therapeutic benefit, that impurity standards have been based on a negligible risk (e.g., an increase in lifetime risk of cancer of one in 10^5 or 10^6 for genotoxic impurities), and that such standards might not be appropriate for anticancer pharmaceuticals intended to treat advanced stage patients. The limits on impurities in other ICH guidances might be exceeded as justified on a case by case basis.

15.4.2 Topical Microbicides Intended for Prevention of Viral Sexually Transmitted Diseases Including Human Immunodeficiency Virus (HIV)

Vaginal products intended to prevent transmission of the HIV represent a category of topical agents with important public health applications. Included in this category are a highly diverse group of drugs and biologics that vary not only in terms of chemical composition, but also with respect to their ability to support other indications (e.g., contraception, broad spectrum STD prophylaxis). Vaginal products seeking an HIV prevention claim can travel a unique and often multifaceted, regulatory path to approval. The primary reason for this multidisciplinary approach is that vaginal HIV prophylaxis is generally not a "stand-alone" indication. Many potentially useful topical microbicides are active against a variety of different pathogens and, hence, might seek a more global STD prevention indication. Furthermore, vaginal prophylaxis products can take a number of different forms (i.e., simple chemical barrier, chemical and physical barrier, immunologic + chemical barrier, etc.). Finally, from a regulatory standpoint, potential reproductive effects are an important consideration when evaluating a topical agent intended for vaginal use during sexual intercourse. Each of these factors can influence the type of data required for marketing approval and will dictate which groups at the FDA will participate in the product review process (US FDA, 2012).

To support the safety of proposed clinical trials with vaginal products, preclinical safety studies in mammals must be designed to adequately model the intended clinical use of the drug (US FDA, 2005a). Bearing in mind the site of administration, a special emphasis should be placed on conducting preclinical reproductive toxicology studies as early as possible in the clinical development of the drug. ICH guideline developmental and reproductive toxicology studies should be conducted using the intended route of exposure (i.e., vaginal administration). These studies should employ the final formulation, if possible, intended for clinical use in doses that are comparable, based on appropriate methods of interspecies extrapolation, to intended clinical doses. These studies should also include experimental groups which will receive doses significantly higher than proposed clinical doses.

15.4.3 Drugs Intended to Prevent the Transmission of Sexually Transmitted Diseases (STD) and/or for the Development of Drugs Intended to Act as Vaginal Contraceptives

There are several nonclinical pharmacology/toxicology issues that are inherent with the development of topical drugs which are intended to prevent sexually transmitted diseases (STD) or with the development of drugs proposed to act as vaginal contraceptives (US FDA, 2005a). The cited FDA guidance was not meant to replace existing guidance concerning the nonclinical pharmacology/toxicology safety data required to support the submission of Investigational New Drug (IND) applications. Rather, it offers insight into some aspects of these classes of drugs that make them unique from systemically administered drugs, namely, the topical sites of their administration and action and the prophylactic nature of the indications.

15.4.3.1 Toxicology Studies

To support the safety of the individual phases of clinical development, studies in at least two animal species (one being a nonrodent) should be used to assess acute, subchronic and chronic toxicity at the proposed site of exposure. Potential sites of exposure to topical microbicides for the prevention of STDs include vaginal, cervical, penile, oral and rectal mucosal areas. For the purpose of this document, contraceptives are considered to expose vaginal and penile tissue. All toxicology studies should use at least three dose levels of the drug and an appropriate control, with the high dose showing frank toxicity (it is understood that there may be limits to the ability to achieve a toxic dose), and the low dose showing little or no toxicity. With the exception of the varying concentrations of the active product, the drug to be applied should be in its final formulation and the study duration should be equal to, or longer than, the proposed duration of treatment in the clinical trial. However, if in an early clinical trial the duration of treatment is less than two weeks, nonclinical safety study duration of two weeks should generally be used. All nonclinical studies carried out to assess safety of a drug should be performed according to Good Laboratory Practices (GLP; 21 CFR 58). Sponsors should consult with the FDA reviewing division concerning approaches and protocols regarding these issues.

Because the topical microbicides are intended for intermittent use during periods in which the individual will be at risk of contracting a STD and contraceptives are intended for intermittent use over long periods of reproductive competence, they are, for regulatory purposes, considered to be chronically administered drugs.

15.4.3.2 Reproductive Toxicology

Reproductive toxicology studies should be carried out to explore the possible effects of the drug on fertility and reproductive performance. Additional studies should be performed to examine whether the drug is teratogenic or has an effect on perinatal/postnatal development. Studies designed to assess the teratogenic potential should be carried out in two species, usually rats and rabbits. It is expected that reproductive toxicology studies will be completed prior to Phase II/III trials.

15.4.4 Human Insulin Analogues

In 2002, the Committee for Proprietary Medicinal Products of the EMA adopted the "Points to Consider on the Need for Assessment of Reproductive Toxicity of Human Insulin Analogues" (EMA, 2002). New insulin analogues are being developed with the aim of improving the duration of activity and/or the ease of administration. Some of these insulin analogues are fast acting while others have a prolonged activity giving patients overnight coverage. Women of childbearing potential (WOCBP) with diabetes mellitus need special and careful control of their glucose levels if they become pregnant. Human insulin administration is the treatment of choice in pregnant diabetic women, even in Type 2 diabetes. Depending on the phase of pregnancy, the effects of loss of control of glucose levels are different. Lack of glucose control around conception has been associated with a high risk of spontaneous abortion and foetal cardiovascular and respiratory changes, while glucose imbalance later in pregnancy increases the risk of dwarfism or small body.

In view of the differences in pharmacokinetics in different species and use of supratherapeutic doses in preclinical safety studies, it is difficult to model the impact of insulin analogues in healthy euglycemic animals (rats and rabbits) as employed in current reproductive toxicity safety studies. While insulin administration at therapeutic doses in pregnant diabetic women might decrease birth defects, the opposite has been shown in studies using normal healthy animals where insulin administrations at high doses have caused hypoglycemia and teratogenic effects. It is generally accepted that the teratogenic response is related to the hypoglycemia induced by insulin and not the hormone as such. Therefore, selection of dose levels in these reproductive and developmental toxicity studies is extremely important. The maximum dose should be chosen on the basis of the pharmacodynamic end-point. The high dose should be at the high end of the effect span, affecting the glucose concentration without causing a non-physiological prolonged hypoglycemia. According to the "Points to Consider" document, several unpublished studies using insulin analogues and human insulin positive controls have shown that the incidence of abnormalities in animals was essentially unaffected at doses at the high end of the effect span without causing undue mortality due to hypoglycemia. Based on these data, study designs based on ICH guideline S5(R2) can be used.

Since diabetic rat models are available, it would be possible to test insulin analogues for reproductive toxicity using these models. Since the insulin analogue would normalize the glucose levels in these models, this would mimic the human insulin-controlled diabetic pregnancy. The usefulness of these models is uncertain due to the lack of experience with these models and the subsequent lack of historical control data.

15.5 Based on Pharmaceutical Characteristic

15.5.1 Biotechnology-derived Products

Biopharmaceuticals (biotherapeutics) are medical drugs, usually large molecular, weight recombinant proteins and peptides, produced by biotechnology. They can be derived from cell cultures or produced using recombinant DNA technology including transgenic production by plants or animals (e.g., cytokines, growth factors, enzymes, hormones, plasminogens, fusion proteins, receptors and monoclonal antibodies). In general, the ICH S5(R2) regulatory developmental and reproductive toxicity testing guidelines for biopharmaceuticals are similar to those for small-molecule pharmaceuticals; however, because biopharmaceuticals are designed to be specific for a human target, they show limited or no pharmacological activity in traditional animal models (see review article Martin *et al.*, 2009). ICH S6(R1) defines a pharmacologically-relevant species as "one in which the test material is pharmacologically active due to expression of the receptor or an epitope (in the case of monoclonal antibodies)". Alternative approaches to evaluate developmental and reproductive toxicity potential of biotechnology-derived pharmaceuticals are outlined in ICH S6(R1) (ICH, 2011b) and include evaluation of biological activity, animal model selection, number and gender of animals, selection of administered dose and immunogenicity (see review article, Bussiere *et al.*, 2009).

The traditional animal species used to evaluate developmental and reproductive toxicity potential of small molecules has been the rat and rabbit (ICH S5(R2)) and these also have been used to evaluate some large molecules (e.g., enzymes and hormones) if they are pharmacologically relevant. In some cases, one relevant species could suffice (e.g., if only one species can be identified and the biological activity is well understood and characterized). In other cases, the guinea pig or hamster were used as the animal model. The rat and rabbit can still be used, even if the binding affinity or pharmacological activity is less than humans or nonhuman primates, as long as the exposure levels in the rat and rabbits can be increased to compensate for the reduced potency during the critical time periods. The advantages of using the rat and rabbit are the availability of historical control data, short gestation times, larger litters, ease of breeding and overall study costs. The disadvantage is the immunogenicity of antidrug antibodies.

Immunogenicity of testing biopharmaceuticals using traditional animal species in developmental and reproductive toxicity evaluations has been overcome by dosing at a higher level or, more frequently, to overcome the antidrug antibodies, as long as there is adequate drug exposure during the critical time periods. If only a portion of the traditional animals develop antidrug antibodies, increasing the group size could yield an adequate number of non-affected animals for evaluation. If the biopharmaceutical is highly immunogenic, evaluation could be accomplished by dosing subgroups of the animals during different critical windows of development (the shorter periods of exposure could produce less neutralizing antibodies) and then combining the results (Faustman *et al.*, 2006). The advantage is the traditional animal species is still being used, however, there is a concomitant increase in the number of animals used, study costs and study length.

Biopharmaceuticals that show species-specific cross-reactivity restricted to only humans and nonhuman primates may require the developmental and reproductive toxicity testing being conducted in nonhuman primates (mostly macaques although marmosets have been used) (Zuhike *et al.*, 2009). The potential effects of biopharmaceuticals on fertility using nonhuman primates are of limited value. Fertility *per se* is not assessed. However, reproductive status (menstrual cycles, hormone levels, semen parameters, and testicular size and standard histopathological evaluation of reproductive organs) can be assessed in repeat-dose toxicity studies of at least 3-months' duration using sexually mature non-mated NHPs. For products pharmacologically active only in NHPs, one well-designed developmental toxicity study (stage C to E ICH S5a) which includes dosing from day 20 of gestation to birth can be considered. No caesarean section group is warranted in this study, but assessment of pregnancy outcome at natural delivery should be performed. This study should also evaluate offspring viability and survival, external malformations, skeletal effects (e.g., by X-ray) and, ultimately, visceral morphology at necropsy. Ultrasound could be useful to track maintenance of pregnancy but not for monitoring embryo–foetal development or detecting malformations. CT-scans and other imaging techniques can be used for embryo–foetal development or detecting malformations. Other end-points in the offspring can also be evaluated if relevant for the pharmacological activity (e.g., immune function or neurobehavioural assessment). The duration of the postnatal phase will be dependent on which additional end-points are considered relevant for the pharmacological activity. The numbers of confirmed pregnant cynomolgus monkeys per group should be sufficient to detect threefold increase in pregnancy/parturition-associated losses with 80% power with 95% confidence interval (Jarvis *et al.*, 2009). The sponsor should justify the study design if other NHP species are used. Because the developmental toxicity study in NHP is a hazard identification study, it might be possible to conduct these studies using a control group and only one dose group, provided there is a scientific justification for the dose level selected.

If there is a cause for concern, the use of a surrogate molecule or genetically-modified animal might be appropriate to reduce the nonhuman primate usage (see below). The advantages of using nonhuman primates are that the biology, physiology, pharmacology, endocrinology and placentation are similar to humans and well characterized, and clinical samples sizes are larger and can be collected more frequently. The disadvantages are lower reproduction rates and statistical power, longer and more costly studies, limited number of breeding nonhuman primates, historical control data and facilities, larger test article requirements, and animal welfare concerns.

In cases where the biopharmaceutical cross-reacts with only chimpanzees or humans, the use of surrogate molecules could be considered to evaluate developmental and reproductive toxicity (Clark *et al.*, 2004). Surrogate molecules are usually a mouse protein, although it could be developed for any species that has similar pharmacology to the human biopharmaceutical. The development of a surrogate molecule allows all developmental and reproductive toxicity testing to be conducted in the traditional animal species. The disadvantage is the cost, resources and time of full development of a second molecule that will never be marketed and the regulatory hurdle of using a molecule that will not be used in the clinic. If an adverse finding is observed in the rodent embryo–foetal developmental study using a surrogate molecule, then it is likely the regulatory authority will require that an assessment is conducted again using the human therapeutic in nonhuman primates to confirm the observation. Ensuring regulatory acceptance for this approach is strongly encouraged.

The use of genetically-modified mice (knock-outs, knock-ins and transgenic) has been used to evaluate developmental and reproductive toxicity when the cross-reactivity is limited to only nonhuman primates and humans (Bolon *et al.*, 2008). Knock-out (KO) mice have selective genetic deletions (specific receptor or pathway) that fail to express the related target protein(s). Knock-in (KI) or "humanized" mice have a human gene inserted into the mouse genome that expresses one or a few human proteins of interest. Transgenic mice (Tg) have been engineered to overexpress target protein(s). Many KO, KI and Tg mice appear morphologically normal; however, functionally they may be abnormal (Inoue, 1998). The advantage to this approach is that the genetically-modified mouse can be used to collect developmental and reproductive toxicity data. However, the modified mice are often generated on nontypical strains (e.g., C57Bl/6 and S129). To date, there are no approved biopharmaceuticals that have relied solely on genetically-modified animals, mainly because this data represents the worst-case scenario that might not be applicable to the clinical situation. The genetically-modified animal might also develop compensatory pathways, feedback mechanisms or messengers that could limit interpretation (Bolon and Galbreath, 2002; Tanabe *et al.*, 2005). Ensuring regulatory acceptance for this approach is strongly encouraged.

Finding a relevant species for a biopharmaceutical whose target is expressed or upregulated only in certain disease states presents some unique challenges (e.g., viral or bacterial antigens that are not expressed in healthy animals; unique cancer antigens, mutated host proteins). These animal models are not only useful in evaluating the pharmacology of the biopharmaceutical, but provide some insight for safety testing, including appropriate safety margins. Haemophilic dogs have been used to evaluate factor VIII and VIIa products (Lewis, 2008). The selection of an animal disease model for toxicity testing should be accompanied by sound scientific justification (Cavagnaro, 2008; Inoue, 1997).

For monoclonal antibodies for which embryo–foetal exposure during organogenesis is low in humans, the embryo–foetal development toxicity study can be conducted during Phase III (ICH M3 (R2)). The completed reports should be available to support submission of a marketing application. For other biological products where embryo–foetal exposure is demonstrated to be low during organogenesis, the same timing for testing can be applicable.

Where there is embryo–foetal exposure during organogenesis and the product is pharmacologically active only in NHPs and a sponsor elects to use the extended Pre- & Postnatal Development (ePPND) study design, an interim report for data to day 7 post-partum for all animals is called for to support Phase III. End-points to be included in an interim report of ePPND study in nonhuman primates:

- Dam data such as survival, clinical observations, body weight, gestational exposure data, and any specific pharmacodynamic (PD) end-points;
- Pregnancy data such as number of pregnant animals started on study, pregnancy status at end of organogenesis (GD50) and at GD100 as a minimum, abortions and timing of abortions;
- Pregnancy outcome data such as number of live births/still births, infant birth weight, infant survival and bodyweight at day 7 post-partum, qualitative external morphological assessment (i.e., confirming appearance is within normal limits), infant exposure data, any specific PD end-points in the infant if appropriate.

If the rodent or rabbit is a relevant species and embryo–foetal exposure is demonstrated, use the ICH M3 (R2) guidance for timing of reproductive toxicity studies. ICH M3 (R2) should also be followed for the timing of data on fertility for products where rodents are relevant species.

Abbreviated, deferred or omitted developmental and reproductive toxicity testing might be required for: a biopharmaceutical if it is a life-saving therapy (advanced cancer, resistant HIV infection, congenital enzyme deficiency diseases); if it is used in combination with another molecule that has developmental and reproductive liabilities; if sufficient product class information is available for labelling; or if additional animal testing would not change the product label.

15.5.2 Biosimilars

Biosimilars or follow-on biologics are terms used to describe officially-approved new versions of innovator biopharmaceutical drugs, following patent expiry. Biosimilar is an official term used by the European medical authorities; the US terminology is follow-on protein products (FOPPs). A reproductive and developmental toxicity testing regimen would typically follow the ICH S5(R2) document, "Guideline for Industry, Detection of Toxicity to Reproduction for Medicinal Products".

To date, a limited number of biosimilars have been approved in the world, with the European Union, which has approved seven, having the most active market (EMA, 2005). The Patient Protection and Affordable Care Act (PPAC Act), signed into law 23 March 2010, amends the Public Health Service Act (PHS Act) to create an abbreviated approval pathway for biological products that are demonstrated to be "highly similar" (biosimilar) to or "interchangeable" with an FDA-approved biological product. These new statutory provisions can also be referred to as the Biologics Price Competition and Innovation Act of 2009 (BPCI Act).

Unlike the more common small-molecule drugs, biologics generally exhibit high molecular complexity, and can be quite sensitive to manufacturing process changes (Table 15.1).

The follow-on manufacturer does not have access to the originator's molecular clone and original cell bank, nor to the exact fermentation and purification process. Finally, nearly undetectable differences in impurities and/or breakdown products are known to have serious health implications. The industry already has an example: Amgen's Epogen and Johnson & Johnson's Eprex. Amgen had licensed the active chemical in Epogen, erythropoietin, to J&J, which manufactured and marketed the drug in Europe. Although Epogen and Eprex is the same molecule, some variation in the way Eprex was manufactured (Deechongkit *et al.*, 2006) or packaged caused patients who took the drug to develop antibodies against it (Locatelli *et al.*, 2004). No-one could tell ahead of time that this could be the case, because J&J did not have to run clinical studies.

15.5.2.1 Bio-Betters or Bio-Superiors

Bio-betters or bio-superiors are existing biologics but differ enough to qualify for regulatory approval as new biological entities under existing regulations. They are second-generation, improved versions of approved biologics – that is, longer half-lives, more convenient administration schedules, more targeted approach, and a more user-friendly or innovative delivery system or formulation.

15.5.3 Vaccines

For the purpose of this document, vaccines are a heterogeneous class of preventive, in some cases therapeutic, medicinal products, the administration of which is intended to elicit an immune response(s) that can prevent and/or lessen the severity of one or more infectious diseases (US FDA, 2006b). A vaccine can be a live attenuated preparation of bacteria, viruses, or parasites, inactivated (killed) whole organisms, living irradiated cells, crude fractions or purified immunogens, including those derived from recombinant deoxyribonucleic acid (DNA) in a host cell, conjugates formed by covalent linkage of components, synthetic antigens, polynucleotides (such as plasmid DNA vaccines), living vectored cells expressing specific heterologous immunogens, or cells pulsed with immunogen. It can also be a combination of vaccines listed above. Antigens can be presented plain or delivered in combination with other antigens, adjuvants, additives and other excipients. Therapeutic vaccines for non-infectious diseases and monoclonal antibodies used as immunogens are not considered in this guidance (Wise *et al.*, 2009).

Developmental toxicity studies are usually not necessary for vaccines indicated for immunization during childhood. However, for vaccines indicated for adolescents and adults and for vaccines that are indicated or may have the potential to be indicated for immunization of pregnant women, it is recommended that developmental toxicity studies be performed.

There are currently differences in the timing of these developmental toxicity studies (see below), to support inclusion of either pregnant individuals or females of childbearing potential in clinical trials.

Table 15.1 *Comparing Small Molecule to Biosimilar Drugs.*

	Small molecule	Biosimilar
Product characteristics	• Small molecules • ~ <1000 Daltons • Often very stable • Administered without a device	• Large, complex molecules • Often > 10 000 Daltons • Stability requires special handling • Device is often a key differentiator
Physiology characteristics	• Diffuses across placenta	• Not expected to gain access to conceptus except by specific active transport
Manufacturing	• Produced by chemical synthesis • Generally oral solids • Relatively lower costs	• Produced in living organisms; highly sensitive to manufacturing changes • Often injected or infused • Often comparatively high costs
R&D	• Very limited clinical trials (often only Phase I PK/PD studies)	• Significant R&D (i.e., cell lines) • Extensive clinical trials, including Phase I and Phase III studies
Regulations	• Abbreviated registration procedures in Europe and US • Usually enjoy "inter-changeability" status	• Regulatory pathway now defined by EMA • Abbreviated pathway in US (BPCI Act)

Maternal immunization: For products indicated specifically for immunization of pregnant women, it is recommended that the data from nonclinical developmental toxicity studies be available prior to the initiation of any clinical trial enrolling pregnant women.

Females of childbearing potential: For vaccines indicated for females of childbearing potential, subjects can be included in clinical trials without nonclinical developmental toxicity studies, provided that appropriate precautions are taken by subjects enrolled in these trials to avoid vaccination during pregnancy, such as pregnancy testing and use of birth control. For these products, it is recommended that data from developmental toxicity studies be included with the initial BLA submission, regardless of whether such studies have been submitted earlier to the IND.

Males: Currently, males can be included in Phase I, II, and III clinical trials in the absence of nonclinical male fertility studies, although such studies may be recommended for certain products in the future.

15.5.3.1 Application of ICH Guidance Document S5(R2)

For preventive and therapeutic vaccines for infectious diseases, the primary concern is potential untoward effects of the test article on development and growth of the embryo and foetus. The ICH S5(R2) guidance document entitled "Detection of Toxicity to Reproduction for Medicinal Products" addresses the design of animal studies primarily for detection of toxicity on reproduction, dividing the reproductive cycle into different segments, defined as Stages A to F. The ICH S5(R2) guidance suggests that different studies can be conducted to address the various segments of the reproduction cycle. Thus, the primary focus is on developmental toxicity studies to detect adverse effects on the pregnant/lactating female and development of the embryo/foetus and the offspring following exposure of the female to the vaccine from implantation through the end of pregnancy, with follow-up of the offspring through weaning. These stages are defined as Stages C, D, and E in the ICH S5(R2) document. Depending on the product and on a case-by-case basis, additional studies may be required to address additional segments of the reproductive cycle.

The ICH S5(R2) guidance is recommended as a general point of reference to assist in the general design of developmental toxicity studies and evaluation of end-points. However, it should be emphasized that there are distinguishable factors relevant to vaccines. The most important feature distinguishing vaccines from other pharmaceutical products is the intended vaccine-induced immune response. Also, vaccines are usually administered in limited, episodic dosages with months or even years between doses. Vaccines include a broad range of product categories such as live attenuated, inactivated, recombinant, polynucleotide, polysaccharide, protein antigens, vectored vaccines, and conjugate vaccines. These could be adjuvanted or consist of a combination of different vaccine antigens. Thus, given the complexity of these issues, the nonclinical testing strategies outlined in the ICH S5(R2) document might not be directly applicable to vaccines, and study designs outlined in the document may need to be tailored to the vaccine product under consideration. Outlined below are specific considerations that should be taken into account when designing developmental toxicity studies for vaccines. It is also recommended that, prior to the conduct of the study, there is an early dialogue with CBER to reach agreement on a specific protocol including study endpoints.

15.5.3.2 Specific Considerations

15.5.3.2.1 Animal Model

It is recommended that the initial clinical trial submission, for example, IND, provides a justification for the choice of the animal model to be used in the developmental toxicity study. This should include a demonstration that the species is able to develop an immune response to the vaccine antigen, even though there may be quantitative and qualitative differences in immune responses between species. The laboratory species most often used for developmental toxicity studies, on the basis of availability of background data and historical experience, are rats, rabbits and mice. Most human vaccines are immunogenic in rodents or rabbits. In some cases, only nonhuman primates might show an adequate immune response. However, because of the technical and logistic difficulties involved in using nonhuman primates for developmental toxicity studies, it is recommended that these nonhuman primates should only be used if no alternative models are available.

In addition to demonstrating an immune response in the pregnant female, it is recommended that the exposure of the foetus to maternal antibodies be verified. Since there are differences between primates, nonrodents, and rodent animal species in terms of timing of maternal antibody transfer to the offspring, it is recommended that the prenatal and postnatal exposure of the offspring to maternal antibody be evaluated as a criterion for selecting the most appropriate experimental model. In addition, the species selected should be amenable to foetal and postnatal examinations.

In cases where lack of an appropriate animal model hinders the assessment of an immune response, developmental toxicity studies could still provide important information regarding potential embryo/foetal toxic effects of the vaccine components/formulation and safety of the product in the pregnant animal.

In most cases, it is sufficient to conduct developmental toxicity studies using only one species. Thus, there is no requirement for the routine use of two species, that is, one rodent and one nonrodent, described in ICH S5(R2).

The number of animals per group should be sufficient to allow meaningful interpretation of the data. For example, for a developmental toxicity study using rats or rabbits, guidelines recommend that an adequate number of animals is assigned to each group to allow an evaluation of at least 40 animals per group. These animals can be further allocated to the Caesarean and littering subgroups using 20 animals each.

15.5.3.2.2 Pharmacodynamics

It is recommended that information is obtained about the onset and duration of the antibody response in pilot studies because these data are helpful in selecting the proper species, study design, and dosing schedules. Initial information can be derived from non-pregnant animals. However, it might also be necessary to perform these pilot studies in a small group of pregnant animals to evaluate antibody formation in relation to test article exposure and placental antibody transfer to the foetus if there is evidence that antibody formation could differ in pregnant versus non-pregnant animals.

It is recognized that antibody induction presents only one aspect of the overall immune response induced by the vaccine and that other immunological parameters, such as cytokines and induction of cytotoxic T cells, could be as important. However, given the relative lack of validated assays to assess the induction of these other parameters, antibody assessments are currently used as a marker for vaccine-induced effects in these studies. This does not exclude the evaluation of additional immunologic parameters on a case-by-case basis. For example, if data are available which indicate that a vaccine antigen induces a particular cytokine response, respective cytokine measurements could be included, especially if the cytokine is one that might affect pregnancy.

15.5.3.2.3 Experimental Procedure

In order to detect adverse effects on the pregnant/lactating female animal and development and growth of the embryo/foetus and the offspring, the female should be exposed to the vaccine during the interval from implantation through closure of the hard palate and also at later stages of pregnancy. The offspring should be followed to weaning and observed for normal growth and development. One subgroup of pregnant females should be submitted to Caesarean examination at the end of pregnancy for routine uterine and foetal examinations, and the other subgroup should be allowed to litter and rear their offspring to weaning in order to monitor the post-natal development of the offspring up to weaning.

15.5.3.2.4 Dosage

Studies have shown that a single-dose level that is capable of inducing an immune response in the animal model can be used. Where possible, animals should be administered the maximum human dose (e.g., 1 human dose = 1 rabbit dose) regardless of body weight. If it is not feasible to administer the maximum human dose (e.g., limitation in total volume that can be administered; dosing-induced local toxicity affecting pregnancy), the administration of a dose that exceeds the human dose on a mg/kg basis while still capable of inducing an immune response in the animal is recommended.

15.5.3.2.5 Frequency and Route of Administration

The vaccination regimen should optimize maternal antibody titers throughout the embryonic, foetal, and early postnatal periods. Timing and number of doses will depend on the onset and duration of the immune response of the particular product. Because of concerns that a daily dosing regimen could lead to overexposure to the vaccine antigen that could potentially result in immune tolerance, episodic dosing of pregnant animals rather than daily dosing should be considered. In addition, episodic dosing appears to be more relevant, as it better mimics the clinically-proposed immunization schedule for most preventive and therapeutic vaccines for infectious disease indications. Considering the short gestational period of the animal species most frequently used, it might be necessary to administer priming doses to the animals several days or weeks prior to mating in order to elicit a peak antibody production during the critical phases of pregnancy, that is, the period of organogenesis.

When dosing prior to implantation, stress reactions might be observed in the animal that could affect the pregnancy status. Therefore, with treatment of animals prior to mating/insemination, it might be necessary to add more animals to the study to ensure that sufficient animals become pregnant for evaluation.

Administration of one or several additional doses during organogenesis (i.e., implantation to closure of the hard palate) to evaluate potential direct embryotoxic effects of the components of the vaccine formulation and to maintain a high level of antibody throughout the remainder of gestation is recommended. In certain cases, subgroups of animals that are dosed at certain time points may be included to evaluate if the vaccine acts as a selective toxicant, bearing in mind that it may be difficult to adjust vaccine administration with gestational timelines. The route of administration should mimic the clinical intended route of administration.

15.5.3.2.6 Control Groups

Control animals should be dosed with placebo at the same time and frequency as test group animals. Since the potential toxicity of each of the components presented in the vaccine formulation will need to be evaluated, consider adding additional groups if components other than the vaccine antigen contained in the vaccine formulation (e.g., excipients, preservatives) cause effects or affect the activity of the test substance. In addition, if the vaccine is formulated with adjuvant, the inclusion of an adjuvant-only control arm, particularly if the adjuvant is novel, is recommended.

15.5.3.2.7 End-points

In general, the study end-points should include those recommended for studies for effects on prenatal and postnatal development including maternal functions as stated in the ICH S5(R2) guideline. When deciding on the end-points to be evaluated, take into consideration the nature of the vaccine and particular concerns associated with that product. The following parameters listed are intended to provide a basic panel of end-points to be evaluated that are not meant to be all-inclusive.

15.5.3.2.7.1 Premating/Preinsemination Period

Clinical observations including data on general appearance, body weights and food consumption should be obtained weekly and on days of test article administration.

15.5.3.2.7.2 Gestational Period

Maternal animals should be observed during the study for signs of morbidity and mortality, and clinical observations recorded regarding general appearance and behaviour. The evaluations should include body weight and body weight change, potential signs of local toxicity, food consumption, duration of pregnancy, abortions, premature deliveries, and parturition (for maternal animals not subjected to Caesarian sectioning).

15.5.3.2.7.3 Caesarean Sectioning Group

15.5.3.2.7.3.1 Maternal Observations At terminal examination of groups subjected to Caesarean sectioning, a necropsy (macroscopic examination) should be conducted and maternal tissue with macroscopic findings should be preserved for histological evaluations as deemed necessary by the gross findings. For example, histological evaluations may be indicated if there are effects on the organ-to-body weight ratios. The number and distribution of corpora lutea, implantation sites, viable and non-viable foetuses, and early and late resorptions should be recorded and a gross evaluation of the placenta should be performed.

15.5.3.2.7.3.2 Foetal Examinations Individual body weights of live foetuses should be recorded and each viable foetus should be examined for gross external, visceral, and skeletal alterations. Late resorptions and dead foetuses should also be examined for gross external alterations to the extent possible. All foetuses should be examined internally to determine sex.

15.5.3.2.7.4 Natural Delivery Group

15.5.3.2.7.4.1 Maternal Observations The duration of gestation, and parameters such as the fertility index, gestation index, and live birth index, should be calculated. Animals that deliver a litter should be sacrificed at the end of the weaning period (LD 21). A gross necropsy of the thoracic, abdominal and pelvic viscera should be performed, and the number and distribution of implantation sites as well as any observed abnormalities should be recorded. Animals that die or are sacrificed because of moribund condition, abortion or premature delivery should be examined for the cause of death and pregnancy status recorded. Aborted foetuses and/or delivered pups should be examined to the extent possible.

15.5.3.2.7.4.2 F_1 Generation A postnatal follow-up from birth to weaning should be conducted to assess normal growth, body weight gain, and nursing activity as indicators for normal development. The study design should include tests to screen for normal neuro-development, for example, auditory and visual function tests. Individual pup counts and body weights (by sex and total) should be recorded and Viability and Lactation Indices should be calculated. At terminal sacrifice, a necropsy should be performed, recording any abnormalities and retaining gross lesions for possible histological examinations. If pups that are found dead at the first status check at birth, a lung floatation test could be performed to determine the absence of breathing indicated by sinking of the excised lung (stillborn) or the presence of breathing indicated by floating of the excised lung (died shortly after birth). These pups should be examined for malformations and/or gross lesions and a possible cause of death.

15.5.3.3 Immunological Endpoints

In addition to evaluating potential developmental adverse effects and adverse effects on the pregnant animal, vaccine-induced antibody response to verify exposure of the embryo/foetus to maternal antibodies should be assessed. Serum specimens should be collected from maternal animals prior to and at additional time points following dosing to assess the development of antibodies. Sampling is usually conducted prior to test article administration and at the day of Caesarean sectioning (where applicable), and at the end of the weaning period.

In addition, cord blood samples should be obtained to assess placental transfer of maternal antibodies from animals in the Caesarean subgroup. Antibody levels from a representative number of pups/litters at the end of the weaning period to verify exposure of the neonates to maternal antibody induced should also be assessed. Antibody evaluations in developmental toxicity studies serve the purpose of verifying an effect of the vaccine in the test species as opposed to evaluating potential immunotoxic effects. Additional immune parameters can be evaluated on a case-by-case basis. For example, if evidence exists that the vaccine antigen or other vaccine components can trigger the release of a particular cytokine potentially affecting pregnancy, respective assessments should be made.

15.5.3.4 Additional Assessments

In cases where nonclinical developmental toxicity studies reveal vaccine-induced adverse effects on the pregnant/lactating animal, embryo/foetal development, or development of the offspring, further animal studies should be conducted to evaluate the cause of the effect. Such studies can include broader immunological evaluations, for example, histochemical analysis for antibody depositions, as well as neurological assessments.

15.5.4 Botanical Drug Products

Reproductive toxicology studies, such as those on fertility/reproductive performance, teratology, and prenatal/perinatal development in animals, provide information on the potential of a botanical drug for producing toxicity during the different stages of reproductive and developmental processes. In the absence of documented data on reproductive toxicity in humans or animals, these tests should be conducted prior to expanded clinical trials.

15.5.5 Contraceptive Steroids

The Division of Metabolism and Endocrine Drug Products of the FDA has written guidelines for preclinical testing of contraceptive steroids which pertain to both male and female contraceptives. The type and duration of the preclinical studies for Phase I clinical trials are single-dose studies in rats and mice using a dose that produces overt toxicity and which is administered by the same route as intended for humans. The repeat dose studies should be in rats and monkeys (up to 200 times the human dose for rats and 50 times the human dose for monkeys) for durations of at least one month. The FDA will consider other species for toxicology testing. Contraceptives with oestrogen/progestogen combinations should use the ratio to be marketed or, if they have more than one ratio, the lowest ratio in toxicologic testing. FDA remains flexible to testing strategies for which there is a sound scientific rationale.

Reproduction and return to fertility studies are pivotal for evaluation of oral contraceptives. Since these contraceptive are to be used in women, a Segment I reproduction study is not required. The following is required for evaluating reproductive toxicity of the compound:

- Reproduction testing Segments II and III should be performed with new contraceptive steroids (Segment III testing is particularly important for long-acting injectable contraceptives).
- Rats are the preferred model for reproduction testing in Segment II and III studies.

It is necessary to demonstrate that cessation of contraceptive steroid use will result in return to fertility in animals. Although some flexibility is available for the exact design of the protocol, this study should be an essential component of the submission package. An extra 10 female rats in the control and high-dose groups of a multi-dose toxicity study should be included to determine the time required after cessation of dosing for the resumption of normal oestrous cycles. After the return of normal oestrous cycling, the female rats should be mated with males of proven fertility and the number of pregnancies and other measures of fertility assessed.

Oral contraceptive steroidal agents used in hormone replacement therapy are usually used at lower dosage levels than those used for contraception. Studies used for oral contraceptive registration can be used for hormone replacement therapy submissions provided that the ratios of the compounds are the same as, and the doses are less than, those used for contraception in humans. Nonclinical testing requirements of steroids for male contraception are similar to those for women. New esters of testosterone will need a thorough pharmacokinetic examination in animals and man to determine what additional toxicology testing is warranted.

15.5.6 Synthetic Sex Steroids Used in Food-Producing Animals

Animal testing is necessary for establishing the safety of a synthetic sex steroid used in food-producing animals. In addition to the studies recommended for evaluating the safety of residues (US FDA, 2009), it is recommended that a 180-day study in a suitable sub-human primate be included with a 90-day observation period before the 90-day dosing period, with a dose that gives no observed hormonal response. There is no need for developmental or reproductive testing in the food-producing animals; however, it is recommended that the study assess the effect of the compound on ovulation, the duration of the menstrual cycle, and changes in the concentration in the blood of the gonadotropins (luteinizing hormone [LH] and follicle stimulating hormone [FSH]) and of the endogenous sex steroids (oestradiol, oestrone and progesterone). Because of the complexity of this type of study, it is recommended that the FDA is contacted in advance of the study execution in order to reach agreement on the details of the study protocol (US FDA, 2006c).

15.6 Other Reasons to Conduct Preclinical Reproductive and Developmental Toxicity Studies

15.6.1 Drug Combinations

The Guidance for Industry Nonclinical Safety Evaluation of Drug Combinations (Draft) (US FDA, 2006d) provides recommendations on nonclinical approaches to support the clinical study and approval of combinations (fixed-dose combination products, co-packaged products, and adjunctive therapies). A *fixed-dose combination* product is one in which two or more separate drug components (active pharmaceutical ingredients) are combined in a single dosage form. A *co-packaged* product consists of two or more separate drug products in their final dosage forms, packaged together with appropriate labelling to support the combination use. An *adjunctive therapy* refers to the situation in which a patient is maintained on a second drug product that is used together with (i.e., in adjunct to) the primary treatment, although the relative doses are not fixed and the drugs need not be given at the same time. Adjunctive therapy products may or may not be labelled for concomitant use.

Drug combinations could involve: (1) previously-marketed drugs (MDs); (2) one or more new molecular entities (NMEs) and one or more previously marketed drugs; or (3) more than one NME. The nonclinical studies considered important for each type of combination can differ, depending upon the information available on each drug substance.

The nonclinical studies that FDA recommends sponsors use to characterize the combination will depend on the toxicologic and pharmacokinetic profiles of the individual drugs, the treatment indication(s), and the intended population. In this document, each of the three general types of combinations (i.e., MD-MD, MD-NME, and NME-NME) will be discussed separately.

Generally, there is sufficient clinical and nonclinical data existing for each drug product separately in a combination of two (or more) previously-marketed drugs (MD-MD). However, the indications for which each drug is marketed should be compared to that for which the combination is being proposed. If there is a possibility of a toxicologic interaction (i.e., that the target organs for toxicity are similar for each drug), then this situation could result in a lowering of the previously-determined no-effect doses for one or both drug products and/or more severe toxicities in the affected organs. The FDA will consider all known toxicology on the product (e.g., general toxicity, reproductive toxicity, carcinogenicity, and safety pharmacology studies – cardiovascular, central nervous system or CNS, respiratory). To the extent that there are gaps in the data, the FDA might recommend that additional nonclinical studies be conducted. The particular nonclinical studies recommended by the FDA will depend on a number of factors, including the nature of the toxicity. It could be important to repeat some studies, such as equivocal reproductive toxicity studies.

For assessment of general toxicity, a bridging study might be appropriate, provided the duration is sufficient to elicit the toxicity of concern. For example, a general toxicity bridging study of 3-months' duration could be considered for a chronic indication. The FDA recommends that combination studies include an assessment of several dose levels of the combination and a high dose of each drug alone. Sponsors are urged to select the doses of each drug used in combination to allow for additive or synergistic effects without unacceptable toxicity in the high-dose groups. Usually, assessment of the drug combination is conducted in only one species if one of the following conditions exists: (1) toxicity in a particular species has high concordance with human toxicity or the toxicities are similar amongst species; or (2) one species is a more relevant model for human risk based on other factors such as PK/ADME (absorption, distribution, metabolism, and excretion). There may be cases, however, in which the Agency recommends conducting studies in two species despite one or both of these conditions being met. For example, depending on the results in the first species, a new cause for concern might warrant studies in a second species.

Generally, the FDA recommends that sponsors conduct nonclinical toxicity studies before clinical studies are initiated if: (1) the drug products have similar target organ toxicity or pharmacodynamic activity; (2) either drug product causes serious or non-monitorable toxicity in animals or humans at exposures near the clinical exposure; or (3) any other reason exists for serious clinical concern. The Agency generally suggests that nonclinical studies be conducted on the NME for a combination of an NME and a previously-marketed drug substance (MD-NCE). The FDA believes that the standard battery of nonclinical studies generally will be appropriate for the NME, as described in the ICH guidance "M3 Nonclinical Safety Studies for the Conduct of Human Clinical Trials for Pharmaceuticals".

Combination developmental toxicity studies need not be conducted if one of the drug products is already known to have significant risk for developmental toxicity, because that risk will already be included in the product labelling for the combination.

For nonclinical studies for a combination of drugs when one or more is previously marketed and one is a new molecular entity, embryotoxicity studies of the combination should be conducted unless the marketed drug substance is already known to have significant risk for developmental toxicity. If there is known significant risk, embryo–foetal developmental studies on the NME would not be needed, because the labelling would not be changed in this regard for the combination.

For combination of two or more drugs when both are new molecular entities (NDE-NDE), if developmental toxicity has been assessed only on each NME separately, then the FDA recommends that developmental toxicity studies be conducted on the combination as well. Embryotoxicity studies of the combination may not be needed if one of the NMEs is known from the nonclinical studies to have significant risk for developmental toxicity.

15.6.2 Drug Metabolites

The ICH Guidance on Safety Testing for Metabolites (US FDA, 2008) encourages the identification of differences in drug metabolism between animals used in nonclinical safety assessments and humans as early as possible during the drug development process.

Identification and evaluation of the potential reproductive toxicity of the drug metabolite is considered important to ensure clinical safety, and the decision to conduct direct safety testing of a metabolite should be based on a comprehensive evaluation of the data on the parent drug and any information available for the metabolite. Drug metabolites are reviewed in another chapter in this book.

15.7 Excipients

The US FDA's guidance "Nonclinical Studies for Development of Pharmaceutical Excipients" (US FDA, 2005b), describes the reproductive toxicity testing required for excipients. According to this guidance, the reproductive toxicology of the excipient should be evaluated as discussed in the ICH S5(R2) guidance, including: (1) assessment of potential to affect fertility or early embryonic development to implantation; (2) teratology in both a rodent species and a mammalian nonrodent species; and 3) effects on prenatal and postnatal development, including maternal function. Excipients are reviewed in another chapter in this book.

15.8 Conclusion

Significant advances have already been achieved in the harmonization of the design and timing of nonclinical developmental and reproductive safety studies of pharmaceuticals for the conduct of human clinical trials, and have been detailed in this chapter. Because the "Guidelines for Toxicity to Reproduction of Medicinal Products" are so flexible, a well-designed ICH standard package of 4.1.1, 4.1.2, and 4.1.3 studies can be used for the majority of pharmaceutical, biopharmaceutical, biosimilars, and food additive INDs. However, differences remain in a few areas. Testing strategies for specific populations (paediatric, men, women not of childbearing potential, women of childbearing potential), disease state (diabetic, HIV, cancer), drug classes (combinations, contraceptives, vaccines, excipients, impurities, human metabolites, those used in food-producing animals), alternative species (nonhuman primates, knock-out, knock-in, transgenic mice), special problems (immunogenicity, surrogate molecules, prevention of viral STDs), special molecules (large-molecular-weight proteins or peptides, monoclonal antibodies), and timing of preclinical developmental and reproductive studies, have been identified and discussed. Guidelines, guidances, points to consider, advisories, workshops, and review articles have been cited where appropriate. Regulators and industry must continue to consider these differences and work towards further improving the global drug development process.

References

Bailey, G.P., Wise, L.D., Buschmann, J., Hurtt, M., and Fisher, J.E. (2009) Pre- and postnatal developmental toxicity study design for pharmaceuticals. *Birth Defects Res. B*, **86**(6), 437–445.

Bolon, B. and Galbreath, E. (2002) Use of genetically engineered mice in drug discovery and development: wielding Occam's razor to prune the product portfolio. *Int. J. Toxicol.*, **21**, 55–64.

Bolon, B., Galbreath, E., Sargent, L., and Weiss, J. (2008) Genetic engineering and molecular technology, in *The Laboratory Rat* (ed. G. Krinke), Academic Press, London, UK, pp. 60–63.

Bussiere, J.L., Martin, P., Horner, M. *et al.* (2009) Alternative strategies for toxicity testing of species-specific biopharmaceuticals. *Int. J. Tox.*, **28**(3), 230–253.

Cappon, G.D., Bailey, G.P., Buschmann, J. *et al.* (2009) Juvenile animal toxicity study designs to support pediatric drug development. *Birth Defects Res. B*, **86**(6), 463–469.

Cavagnaro, J. (2008) Implementation of ICH S6 and the case-by-case approach, in *Preclinical Safety Evaluation of Biopharmaceuticals: A Science-based Approach to Facilitating Clinical Trials* (ed. J. Cavagnaro), John Wiley & Sons, Hoboken, New Jersey, pp. 45–65.

Chellman, G.J., Bussiere, J.I., Makori, N., Martin, P.L., and Ooshima, Y. (2009) Developmental and reproductive toxicity studies in nonhuman primates. *Birth Defects Res. B*, **86**(6), 446–462.

Clark, J., Leach, W., Pippig, S. *et al.* (2004) Evaluation of a surrogate antibody for preclinical safety testing of an anti-CD11a monoclonal antibody. *Regul. Toxicol. Pharmacol.*, **40**, 219–226.

Deechongkit, S., Aoki, K.H., Park, S.S., and Kerwin, B.A. (2006) Biophysical comparability of the same protein from different manufacturers: a case study using Epoetin alfa from Epogen® and Eprex®. *J. Pharm. Sci.*, **95**, 1931–1943.

Dietert, R.R. and Hopsapple, M.P. (2007) Methodologies for developmental immunotoxicity (DIT) testing. *Methods.*, **41**(1), 123–131.

EMA, (2002) Committee for Proprietary Medicinal Products. "Points to Consider on the Need for-Assessment of Reproductive Toxicity of Human Insulin Analogues", European Medicines Agency (EMA), Evaluation of Medicines for Human Use. London, March 2002, CPMP/SMP/2600/01 Final.

EMA (2005) Guideline on Similar Biological Medicinal Products, Committee for Medicinal Products for Human Use (CHMP), European Medicines Agency (EMA), CHMP/437/04, 30 October 2005, 1–7.

Farrell, A., Papadouli, I., Hori, A. *et al.* (2006) The advisory process for anticancer drug regulation: a global perspective. *Ann. Oncol.*, **17**, 889–996.

Faustman, E., Gohike, J., Ponce, R., Lewandowski, T., Seeley, M., Whittaker, S., and Griffith, W. (2006) Experimental approaches to evaluate mechanisms of developmental toxicity, in *Developmental and Reproductive Toxicology: A Practical Approach* (ed. R.D. Hood), 2nd edn, CRC Press, Boca Raton FL, pp. 15–60.

Hood, R.D. and Parker, R.M. (2008) Reproductive and developmental toxicology, in *Preclinical Development Handbook, Toxicology* (ed. S. Gad), John Wiley & Sons, Inc, Hoboken, New Jersey, p. 373.

Hurtt, M.E., Daston, G., Davis-Bruno, K. *et al.* (2004) Workshop summary: Juvenile animal studies: testing strategies and design. *Birth Defects Res. (Part B)*, **71**, 281–288.

ICH (2000) International Conference on Harmonization of Technical Requirements for Registration of Pharmaceuticals for Human Use. ICH Harmonized Tripartite Guideline "S7A: Safety Pharmacology Studies for Human Pharmaceuticals"; November 2000.

ICH (2009a) International Conference on Harmonization of Technical Requirements for Registration of Pharmaceuticals for Human Use. ICH Harmonized Tripartite Guideline "M3(R2): Nonclinical Safety Studies for the Conduct of Human Clinical Trials and Marketing Authorization for Pharmaceuticals"; June 2009.

ICH (2009b) International Conference on Harmonization of Technical Requirements for Registration of Pharmaceuticals for Human Use. ICH Harmonized Tripartite Guideline "M3(R2): Nonclinical Safety Studies for the Conduct of Human Clinical Trials and Marketing Authorization for Pharmaceuticals", Note 3, p. 23; June 2009.

ICH (2009c) International Conference on Harmonization of Technical Requirements for Registration of Pharmaceuticals for Human Use. ICH Harmonized Tripartite Guideline "S9: Nonclinical Evaluation for Anticancer Pharmaceuticals"; October 2009.

ICH (2011a) International Conference on Harmonization of Technical Requirements for Registration of Pharmaceuticals for Human Use. ICH Harmonized Tripartite Guideline "S2(R1): Guidance on Genotoxicity Testing and Data Interpretation for Pharmaceuticals Intended for Human Use"; November 2011.

ICH (2011b) International Conference on Harmonization of Technical Requirements for Registration of Pharmaceuticals for Human Use. ICH Harmonized Tripartite Guideline: "Addendum to ICH S6: Preclinical Safety Evaluation of Biotechnology-Derived Pharmaceuticals S6(R1)"; June 2011.

Inoue, T. (1997) Biotechnologically-derived pharmaceuticals in Japan: present and future prospects, in *Safety Evaluation of Biotechnologically-derived Pharmaceuticals: Facilitating a Scientific Approach* (eds S. Griffiths and C Lumley), Kluwer Academic Press, London, pp. 51–63.

Inoue, T. (1998) Concept of a 'relevant animal model,' in *Proceedings of the Fourth International Conference on Harmonization Brussels, 1997* (eds P. D'Arcy and D. Harron), The Queen's University, Belfast, p. 209.

Jarvis, P., Srivastav, S., Vogelwedde, E., Stewart, J., Mitchard, M., and Weinbauer, G.F. (2009) The cynomolgus monkey as a model for developmental toxicity studies: variability of pregnancy losses, statistical power estimates and group size considerations (manuscript in preparation; abstract presented at European Teratology Society Meeting, 2009).

Lerman, S.A., Hew, K.W., Stewart, J., Stump, D.G., and Wise, L.D. (2009) The nonclinical fertility study design for pharmaceuticals. *Birth Defects Res. B*, **86**(6), 429–436. December 2009.

Lewis, R. (2008) Preclinical safety evaluation of blood products, in *Preclinical Safety Evaluation of Biopharmaceuticals: A Science-based Approach to Facilitating Clinical Trials* (ed. J. Cavagnaro), John Wiley & Sons, Hoboken, New Jersey, pp. 669–682.

Locatelli, F., Aljama, P., Barany, P., Canaud, B., and Carrera, F. (2004) Erythropoiesis-stimulating agents and antibody-mediated pure red-cell aplasia: here are we now and where do we go from here? *Nephrol. Dial Transpl.*, **19**, 288–293.

Martin, P.L. and Weinbauer, G.F. (2010) Developmental toxicity testing of biopharmaceuticals in nonhuman primates: previous experience and future directions. *Inter. J. Tox.*, **29**, 552–568.

Martin, P., Breslin, W., Rocca, M., Wright, D., and Cavagnaro, J. (2009) Considerations in assessing the developmental and reproductive toxicity potential of biopharmaceuticals. *Birth Defects Res. (Part B)*, **86**, 176–203.

NC3Rs (2007) National Centre for the Replacement, Refinement and Reduction of Animals in Research. "Challenging Requirements for Acute Toxicity Studies: Workshop Report", May 2007.

Robinson, S., Delongeas, J.L., Donald, E. *et al.* (2008) A European pharmaceutical company initiative challenging the regulatory requirement for acute toxicity studies in pharmaceutical drug development. *Regul. Toxicol. Pharmacol.*, **50**, 345–352.

Sakai, T., Takahashi, M., Mitsumori, K. *et al.* (2000) Collaborative work to evaluate toxicity on male reproductive organs by 2-week repeated-dose toxicity studies in rats: overview of the studies. *J. Toxicol. Sci.*, **25**, 1–21.

Sanbuissho, A., Yoshida, M., Hisada, S. *et al.* (2009) Collaborative work on evaluation of ovarian toxicity by repeated-dose and fertility studies in female rats. *J. Toxicol. Sci.*, **34**, 1–22.

Tanabe, M., Matsumoto, T., and Shibuya, K. (2005) Compensatory response of IL-1 gene knockout mice after pulmonary infection with klebsiella pneumonia. *J. Med. Microbiol.*, **54**, 7–13.

US FDA (1994) Food and Drug Administration. International conference on harmonization; guideline on detection of toxicity to reproduction for medicinal products [S5(R2)]. *Fed. Reg., Part IX*, **59**(183), 48746–48752.

US FDA (2005a) U.S. Food and Drug Administration, Center for Drug Evaluation and Research. Guidance for Industry: "Development of Topical Drugs Intended to Prevent the Transmission of Sexually Transmitted Diseases (STD) and/or for the Development of Drugs Intended to act as Vaginal Contraceptives"; July 2005.

US FDA (2005b) U.S. Food and Drug Administration, Center for Drug Evaluation and Research. Guidance for Industry "Nonclinical Studies for Development of Pharmaceutical Excipients"; May 2005.

US FDA (2006a) U.S. Food and Drug Administration, Center for Drug Evaluation and Research. Guidance for Industry: "Nonclinical Safety Evaluation of Pediatric Drug Products"; February 2006.

US FDA (2006b) United States Food and Drug Administration, Center for Biologics Evaluation and Research. Guidance for Industry: "Considerations for Developmental Toxicity Studies for Preventive and Therapeutic Vaccines for Infectious Disease Indications"; February 2006.

US FDA (2006c) U.S. Food and Drug Administration, Center for Veterinary Medicines. Guidance for Industry: "General Principles for Evaluating the Safety of Compounds Used in Food-Producing Animals"; #3, July 2006.

US FDA (2006d) U.S. Food and Drug Administration, Center for Drug Evaluation and Research. Guidance for Industry: "Nonclinical Safety Evaluation of Drug or Biologic Combinations"; March 2006.

US FDA (2008) U.S. Food and Drug Administration, Center for Drug Evaluation and Research. Guidance for Industry: "Safety Testing of Drug Metabolites"; February 2008.

US FDA (2009) U.S. Food and Drug Administration, Center for Veterinary Medicines. Guidance for Industry: "Studies to Evaluate the Safety of Residues of Veterinary Drugs in Human Food: General Approach to Testing VICH GL33", #149; March 2009.

US FDA (2012) U.S. Food and Drug Administration, Center for Drug Evaluation and Research. Guidance for Industry: "Vaginal Microbicides: Development for the Prevention of HIV Infection"; November 2012.

Wise, L.D., Buschmann, J., Feuston, M.H. *et al.* (2009) Embryo-fetal developmental toxicity study design for pharmaceuticals. *Birth Defects Res. B*, **86**(6), 418–428.

Zuhike, U., Korte, S., Niggerman, B., Fuchs, A., and Muller, W. (2002) The common marmoset (*callithrix jacchus*) as a model in biotechnology, in *Primate Models in Pharmaceutical Development* (eds R. Korte, F. Vogel, and G. Weinbauer), Waxmann Verlag GmbH, Munster, Germany, pp. 119–126.

16

Juvenile Animal Toxicity Studies: Regulatory Expectations, Decision Strategies and Role in Paediatric Drug Development

Melissa S. Tassinari[1,*], *Luc M. De Schaepdrijver*[2], *and Mark E. Hurtt*[3]
[1]*CDER, Office of New Drugs, FDA, Silver Spring, USA*
[2]*Johnson & Johnson, Belgium*
[3]*Pfizer, Groton, USA*

16.1 Introduction

In the context of regulatory testing, the juvenile animal toxicity study offers an opportunity to address specific questions of potential toxicity in the growing animal that are not evaluated in other conventional regulatory testing paradigms. The juvenile animal toxicity study can assess a safety signal noted in acute and chronic adult animal toxicity studies or test end-points not usually assessed in the adult toxicity studies, such as the potential for a medicinal product to impair growth or developmental milestones prior to the start of paediatric clinical trials. Decisions to conduct a juvenile animal study are based on data available at the time when a paediatric clinical programme is being planned. These data come from the prior toxicity studies in adult animals as well as data from adult clinical trials, literature and previous knowledge of the drug or chemical class. Included in this

[*] The views expressed in this chapter are those of the author and do not reflect the views or policies of the FDA. M.S. Tassinari current affiliation: Pediatric & Maternal Health Staff, Office of New Drugs, CDER, FDA, Silver Spring, MD.

Nonclinical Safety Assessment: A Guide to International Pharmaceutical Regulations, First Edition.
Edited by William J. Brock, Kenneth L. Hastings and Kathy M. McGown.

battery of tests are those to assess potential reproductive and developmental toxicities. The developmental toxicity studies typically include embryo–foetal and pre- and post-natal studies in which the offspring are exposed indirectly either *in utero* or postnatally through the milk. The extrapolation of these data to potential effects in juvenile animals, therefore, is limited as there is no direct exposure to the young animal.

When these data are reviewed, potential "gaps" in understanding can be identified relevant to the assessment of safety and tolerability in the preclinical population. In many cases, the data provide sufficient evidence to proceed with a paediatric clinical trial. In cases where questions remain as to the potential for a different response in a child versus an adult, a juvenile animal toxicity study can be designed and conducted. Studies in juvenile animals are most effective when particular questions are defined as a result of the existing data review and the study is designed to address a particular concern.

This chapter reviews the current regulatory expectations for the application of juvenile animal studies for the development of new medicinal products (drugs and biologics) and discuss key considerations to determine when such a study is needed and to understand what the elements of study designs are to assure meaningful data. Selected case studies have been included to illustrate the core components of a juvenile animal toxicity study design. This chapter will focus on the needs for paediatric drug development but it should be noted that, with regards to environmental chemical exposure, the Environmental Protection Agency (EPA) and the Organization for Economic Co-operation and Development (OECD) also recognize the need to perform hazard assessments in juvenile animals based on chemical-specific concerns. While there are no harmonized test guidelines for juvenile animal studies at present from either the EPA or OECD, studies in juvenile animals are undertaken when specific end-points require evaluation (Makris, 2011).

16.2 Regulatory Environment

In the current regulatory environment there are several key laws and regulations governing paediatric drug development. While an increasing number of countries and global regions have now issued regulatory expectations for paediatric drug development, the major impact continues to come from the laws and regulation set forth by the legislatures of the United States and European Union. In the US, these laws are the Best Pharmaceuticals for Children Act (BPCA) and the Pediatric Research Equity Act (PREA). Across the European Union, the regulation is "Regulation (EC) No 1901/2006 on medicinal products for paediatric use (the 'Paediatric Regulation')". Similar in scope, these regulations define expectations for evaluation of medicinal product to be used in children. Both have an obligatory component and, recognizing the added efforts required to develop medicines for children, both also provide incentives in the form of extensions to product exclusivity for companies that complete agreed-upon studies.

16.2.1 US Pediatric Laws: PREA and BPCA

PREA was first introduced into law in 2003 in response to a court challenge in which the FDA was enjoined from enforcing its Pediatric Rule issued in 1998 (Federal Register, 1998). PREA was made retroactive to April 1999 and gave the FDA statutory authority to

Table 16.1 *Age classification for pediatric patients*[a].

Preterm newborn infants	Varies
Term newborn infants	0 to 27 days
Infants and toddlers	28 days to 23 months
Children	2 to 11 yr
Adolescents	12 to 16–18 yr (region dependent)

[a]Taken from ICH E11; Note for Guidance on Clinical Investigation of Medicinal Products in the Paediatric Population (ICH E11, 2000). Ages are defined in completed days, months or years.

require paediatric assessments for all new and supplemental applications submitted for biologics and drug applications with a new active ingredient, indication, dosage form, dosing regimen or route of administration. A paediatric assessment is required at the time of submission of either a New Drug Application (NDA) or a Biologics License Application (BLA) and is expected "to assess the safety and effectiveness of the drug or the biological product for the claimed indications in all relevant pediatric subpopulations; and to support dosing and administration for each pediatric subpopulation for which the drug or the biological product is safe and effective" (PREA, 2007). In circumstances where the medicinal product is not anticipated to be used in children or it has been determined that use in children would not be safe, PREA provides for the granting of a waiver, for all or some paediatric age groups (a "full" or "partial" waiver). Table 16.1 lists the commonly-applied age classifications for paediatric patients noted in the International Conference for Harmonization (ICH) Topic E11, Clinical Investigation of Medicinal Products in the Paediatric Populations (ICH E11, 2000). In many instances, it is appropriate to wait until the new medicinal product has been sufficiently studied in adults before conducting paediatric studies. PREA therefore provides for a deferral for the conduct of paediatric studies, after the approval of the studies in adults.

BPCA was first enacted in 2002 as the renewal of original paediatric exclusivity provisions of the US Food and Drug Modernization Act (FDAMA, 1997) and provides an incentive for the conduct of paediatric studies of six months' exclusivity attached to the patent for the active moiety for the new drug product (BPCA, 2002). In order to achieve this incentive, the industry sponsor must complete a previously-agreed paediatric programme called a Written Request (WR) that is issued by the FDA. The Written Request is an optional agreement that can extend beyond the required paediatric assessments under PREA. The Written Request can either be proposed by the sponsor, via a proposed paediatric study request (PPSR) or can be issued directly by the FDA. Plans for paediatric clinical development are discussed with the FDA during the course of product development. In most cases, planning begins in clinical Phase II after early signals of efficacy are known from the adult studies (Table 16.2). This incentive was not available under BPCA for biologics. However, in March 2010, specific provisions under the Biologics Price Competition and Innovation Act were included in the Patient Protection and Affordable Care Act that allows biologics to be eligible for paediatric exclusivity through a Written Request (PPACA,).

PREA and BPCA were renewed in 2007 as Title IV and Title V, respectively, of the Food and Drug Administration Amendments Act (FDAAA). In these renewals, Congress expanded mandates for the FDA with regards to pediatrics (FDAAA, 2007). Amongst

Table 16.2 *Comparison of US and EU paediatric laws and regulation.*

	US BPCA	US PREA	EU
Requirement	Optional Written Request	Mandatory Pediatric Assessment	Mandatory[a] PIP
Waiver	na	yes	yes
Deferral	na	yes	yes
Timing (Plans)	End of Phase 2 → post approval	End of Phase 2 → NDA/BLA approval	Completion of adult PK
Reward	6 mo exclusivity	na	6 mo SPC extension
Drugs	yes	yes	yes
Biologics	yes[c]	yes	yes
Orphan drug	yes	no	yes
Decision Authority	FDA Division[b]	FDA Division[b]	EMA – Paediatric Committee (PDCO)

[a]Optional for the paediatric use marketing application (PUMA).

[b]The Division receiving the application makes final decision after consulting with internal FDA PeRC.

[c]As of March 2010, the Biologics Price Competition and Innovation Act, provision of the Patient Protection and Affordable Care Act.

na = not applicable.

other elements, the FDA can now require nonclinical studies as part of a Written Request when it is deemed necessary to more fully assess potential safety concerns in the paediatric population under study. BPCA 2007 can also require development and subsequent marketing of age-appropriate formulations. All paediatric data, clinical or nonclinical, whether positive or negative in their outcome, submitted either through PREA or a Written Request, are to be included in the product label. In 2012, there was permanent reauthorization of BPCA and PREA in the Food and Drug Administration Safety and Innovation Act (FDASIA). An important change in the new legislation under PREA requires drug developers to submit pediatric study plans earlier during drug development, at the time of the end of Phase 2. Like the EU regulation described below, this change in the law enables better integration of pediatric studies into the overall development of the medicinal product.

16.2.2 EU Regulation

In 2007, the Paediatric Regulation came into force across the European Union. This regulation contains obligatory elements for paediatric studies which, if completed, will reward the manufacturer with an additional six-month extension of the Supplementary Protection Certificate (SPC), similar to the six-month paediatric exclusivity granted under the US laws (Official Journal,). As with the US legislation, this regulation applies to all new medicinal products (biologics and drugs), new indications, new formulations or routes of administration. The work to be done, a paediatric evaluation, is filed with the Paediatric Committee (PDCO) within the European Medicines Agency (EMA) as a Paediatric Investigation Plan (PIP). An agreed PIP must be in place for the filing of a Market Authorization Application (MAA) (Table 16.2). The PDCO is responsible for the assessment of the content of the PIP (the paediatric plan, full or partial waiver, or deferrals) and adopt binding opinions on these in accordance with the provisions of the regulation. The PDCO does not, however, provide opinions on MAAs of medicinal products that were developed exclusively for paediatric use. This remains entirely within the remit of the EMAs Committee for Medicinal Products for Human Use (CHMP). The regulation also stipulates that an initial PIP must be submitted at the completion of the assessment of adult pharmacokinetics. This is early in the overall development, typically just after the end of Phase I of clinical development. While an early PIP contains little in the way of safety data for the product and is based more on a hypothetical but biologically plausible set of potential safety concerns, the initiation of interaction with the PDCO on the eventual indications and design of the paediatric plan enables these studies to be better integrated into the overall development of the medicinal product. The PIP is an evolving document which is expected to undergo several amendments as more information on the adult safety and efficacy of the drug becomes known. As with the US laws, nonclinical studies can be included in a PIP.

16.2.3 Guidances for Conduct of Juvenile Animal Studies

Under both US laws and EU regulation, a juvenile animal study can be required in the agreed paediatric plans. These studies might be needed to characterize potential toxicities that should be monitored in clinical trials or to elucidate safety signals leading to adequate labelling once the product is approved. Recognizing the importance of the juvenile animal study, both the EMA and the FDA have issued specific guidance for the conduct of these studies (FDA, 2006; EMA, 2008). The ICH guidance on nonclinical safety studies for the conduct of human clinical trials and marketing authorization for pharmaceuticals (ICH M3), also notes the role of the juvenile toxicity study (ICH M3 (R2), 2009). These guidances advocate the same principle of review and assessment of existing toxicity data as part of determining what gaps in toxicity data are present and what data should be acquired by the conduct of a study in juvenile animals. As noted in the ICH M3, " . . . The conduct of any juvenile animal toxicity studies should be considered only when previous animal data and human safety data, including effects from other drugs of the pharmacological class, are judged to be insufficient to support paediatric studies . . ." (ICH M3 (R2), 2009).

Given this guiding principle, when should juvenile animal studies be conducted? The answer to this question will be explored further in subsequent sections of this chapter, but in reference to the regulatory guidance, these studies should be planned when: (1) there are findings in nonclinical studies which indicate target organ or general toxicities relevant for developing systems; (2) there are potential effects on growth and development in the paediatric age group for whom the product is intended; (3) there are impacts on the pharmacology of the product that have a potential to impact developing organ systems; (4) there are age groups that need to be identified in which the drug should not be used or where special warnings are warranted; and (5) there are specific concerns such as long-term safety that cannot be addressed in clinical trials or there are safety margins that must be defined for the use of the product in paediatric patients.

Evaluation of the existing data is the first step to determine whether juvenile toxicity studies are needed as acknowledged in the guidances. From the US guidance,

> Standard toxicity studies with adult animals cannot assess all of the relevant endpoints, especially growth present in the immature animal. In other circumstances, however, juvenile animal studies would neither be informative nor necessary. For example, juvenile animal studies might not be necessary when: (1) data from similar therapies in a class have identified a particular hazard and additional data are unlikely to change this perspective; (2) there are adequate clinical data and adverse events of concern have not been observed during clinical use; (3) target organ toxicity would not be expected to differ in sensitivity between adult and pediatric patients because the target organ of toxicity is functionally mature in the intended pediatric population and younger children with functionally immature tissue are not expected to receive the drug.
>
> (FDA, 2006)

When and if a study is deemed necessary, its design is then based on the question or concern that is to be addressed. Regulatory guidance for timing of juvenile studies is consistent with the expectation that these studies are performed ahead of the paediatric clinical studies they are meant to inform. Decisions and planning for any juvenile animal study, therefore, need to be integrated early into the larger paediatric plan. Studies that are meant to support the assessment of safety for potential long-term developmental effects generally can be done later in the drug development programme and will impact the labelling of the approved product.

The central message in the guidances from both regulatory authorities is to evaluate existing data, both nonclinical and clinical, to determine whether an additional study in juvenile animals is needed. The guidances both indicate that a study in one species is sufficient. The rodent is normally the preferred species of choice due to its common use in the general toxicity programme. This allows for an integrated and comparative assessment of the juvenile rodent data to the adult rodent data and provides use of extensive historical data that is available for most rodent strains. However, the choice of the one appropriate species should be made on its relevance to the product and the species used in the adult toxicity studies. One example of a nonrodent species selection for paediatric evaluations is the dog for the study of fluoroquinolones (Stahlmann, 1990).

16.3 Relevance and Place in Drug Development

A paradigm change is taking place in drug development (Rose, 2008). In the past, it was believed that children needed to be protected from research and clinical trials. Today, as supported by the current legislation, there has been a shift that children need protection through, not from, research and clinical trials (Rose, 2009). This change in focus has firmly established that children have the right to benefit from research, and excluding them from the process amounts to withholding potential benefits. Additionally, continuously exposing them to medicines not properly tested in their age group is an ethical challenge (Rose, 2009). The US and EU legislation has had a positive impact in increasing the number of clinical trials in the paediatric population. In support of clinical trials in the paediatric population, an increase in the conduct of nonclinical studies has occurred to bridge the potential juvenile gap in standard nonclinical pharmacology and toxicology programmes.

Drug development is a multifaceted, complex process. Clinical safety is one major component of this process and is factored into the clinical trial design. Data from all the nonclinical studies also provide critical information for study design and, taken together, this information provides a view of the potential safety profile that may be seen in the clinical trials. This safety profile and its role in clinical trial design are really no different in the paediatric population as for the adult population.

The use of the juvenile animal data in the drug development process falls into two different but related areas. First is the potential use in supporting the design of clinical trials. Juvenile animal studies provide information that might limit adverse events in the clinic as well as inform the appropriate clinical monitoring in the trials. A publication highlighted that in a small number of cases (4/39), novel toxicity was observed compared to the routine toxicological package (Bailey and Marien, 2009). In addition, there is always the potential that biomarkers of adverse effects in the juvenile animal studies are identified that could be used in clinical studies. An example is the addition of end-points in a paediatric clinical trial to measure reproductive hormones based on data from the nonclinical toxicology package including the juvenile animal study indicating an effect on female fertility (Hurtt, personal communication). There is also the possibility, albeit infrequent, of potential effects identified from the animal study that might suggest they could not be monitored in the clinic and/or considered an unacceptable consequence of treatment. In this case, the nonclinical data would suggest that it may not be possible to conduct the clinical trial based on an unfavourable risk-benefit analysis.

The second use for data from juvenile animal toxicity studies is in product approval and labelling. The FDA Guidance for Industry on the Nonclinical Safety Evaluation of Paediatric Drug Products states that "nonclinical toxicology studies in juvenile animal models could demonstrate adverse effects that should be considered in seeking post-marketing commitments by the sponsor, in labelling a product for paediatric use, or in determining the approvability of a drug for paediatric use." (FDA, 2006) The studies could identify potential adverse effects that might impact its use in a particular paediatric population. In addition, juvenile animal studies are often conducted to evaluate potential effects on end-points that cannot be evaluated in the clinic (e.g., reproductive function, consequences on learning and memory) with the results from these assessments highlighted in the product label to help define the product's risk-benefit profile. It is also possible that the nonclinical data could result in a product label that warns against use in paediatric patients altogether.

The regulatory guidance concerning the timing for performing juvenile animal studies relative to performing clinical trials in paediatric patients allows some flexibility. In most cases, the juvenile animal studies should be conducted prior to the conduct of any large paediatric clinical trial. However, for short-term pharmacokinetic studies, for example, 1–3 doses, juvenile animal toxicity studies are generally not considered necessary (ICH M3 (R2), 2009). Flexibility enters when designing short duration, multiple-dose efficacy and safety trials. For these situations, the need for conducting a juvenile animal study is dependent on the therapeutic indication, age of the paediatric patients, and safety data from adult animal and human exposure. The lack of sufficient clinical data in the adult population will always warrant the conduct of nonclinical juvenile studies conducted prior to initiation of any paediatric clinical trials. The timing of the studies for serious or life-threatening paediatric conditions will need to be addressed with the regulatory authorities on a case-by case basis. ICH M3 (R2) guidance states that "the age of the trial participants in relation to the duration of the clinical study (i.e., the fraction of the developmental period of concern during which the clinical study participants are exposed) is among the most important considerations" (ICH M3 (R2), 2009).

16.4 Strategies for Decision Making: When are Studies Needed and Appropriate?

Much as with the situation for adult animal toxicity testing, juvenile animals offer the potential benefit of identifying possible safety concerns, ADME differences or identifying biomarkers for clinical evaluation. As noted in the previous section, the key objective of juvenile animal studies is to determine potential toxicities unique to immature animals relative to adult animals, what stage of postnatal development might be more sensitive or whether there are any resultant consequences when the animal matures (FDA, 2006; EMA, 2008; ICH M3 (R2), 2009). In addition, these studies may assess a specific concern, reversibility, aggravation of expected findings or safety margins sufficient to support dosing in human paediatric populations. They could also identify age groups in which the drug should not be used or where special warnings are needed.

There are a number of key considerations that impact the need and design of a juvenile animal toxicity study. A list of key factors is presented in Table 16.3. All these factors determine whether a study is justified and, if needed, which optimal design parameters should be used, including relevant species, age of animals at the onset of testing, study duration and study endpoints (FDA, 2006; EMA, 2008; ICH M3 (R2), 2009). It is obvious that the knowledge obtained on an investigational drug from adult clinical and nonclinical studies shape assessments in juvenile animals. Early and continuous interaction amongst the disciplines engaged in compound development including clinical, pharmacokinetics, toxicology, pharmaceutical development and regulatory affairs is key in this perspective. Also, it is highly recommended to initiate early interactions with regulatory health authorities in order to

Table 16.3 *Key considerations impacting the conduct and design of juvenile animal studies.*

Conduct Considerations
How young are the pediatric patients? (e.g., neonates, or > 6 yr old)
What is the duration of treatment? (e.g., acute vs. chronic)
Are there known target organs in an adult clinical programme?
Are there known target organs in adult animal toxicity assessments?
Are there any identified reproductive toxicities from prior studies? (e.g., from pre- and postnatal toxicity study)
Design Considerations
Pharmacokinetic and metabolism data in adult animals and humans
Species selection to address identified concerns
Route of administration appropriate to human route and technical/feasibility considerations related to age of animal to be used
Unique formulation requirements with novel excipients

come to an agreement on the study package supporting the intended paediatric population including the study design for the juvenile animal programme.

The age of the trial subjects in relation to the duration of the clinical study is amongst the most important considerations. Serious adverse effects that are irreversible are of the utmost concern, for example, those affecting organ systems with a long developmental time window such as central nervous system (CNS), skeletal, reproductive and immune systems. Clearly, for a target organ with less repair capacity, the long-term outcome of early insult during development could be devastating and a conservative approach when making a risk-benefit analysis is warranted.

In an International Life Science Institute/Health and Environmental Sciences Institute (ILSI/HESI) workshop in 2003 which brought together academia, industry and regulatory agencies from US, EU, Canada and Japan there was clear agreement on the following strategic points (Hurtt *et al.*, 2004):

1. Whether or not juvenile animal studies should be conducted needs to be considered on a case-by-case basis.
2. Testing in a single species is generally sufficient. The rat was preferred; however, consideration of other species should be made when the rat is clearly not appropriate.
3. Studies should include a toxicokinetic or pharmacokinetic assessment
4. Study designs including end-points and study duration need to be based on the individual case.

There is much debate as to how juvenile animal studies should be focused. Should they be conducted based upon a justified rationale grounded upon weight-of-evidence from accumulated data? Alternatively, should they be viewed as general screening studies designed to evaluate all possible outcomes and to avoid missing any unique toxicity? In the first case, they serve as valuable adjunct studies to address specific concerns or fill a data gap whereas, in the second case, they rarely yield meaningful data for the assessment of paediatric safety (Baldrick, 2004; Brent, 2004; Beck *et al.*, 2006; De Schaepdrijver *et al.*, 2008, 2009). A scientific strategic approach, taking into account all clinical and nonclinical data and future development plans, is key. Only when juvenile toxicity studies are embedded in a "First into Children" (FIC) strategy will they be regarded as truly value-adding studies for the clinic. Similarly, when they address existing safety questions they add value for the assessment of paediatric safety or add value to the label.

16.4.1 Study Approach and Design

Juvenile animal studies are designed to examine aspects of function or development of a particular target organ(s). The organ systems examined routinely are the CNS, skeletal, reproductive, pulmonary, cardiovascular, renal and immune systems. Study protocols should take into account the pharmacological activity of the drug, the expected target organ or system toxicity, and specific concerns from adult animal toxicity studies and adult human clinical experience. Additional considerations are species, age at start of treatment, study duration, route of administration, dose selection, study end-points, sample size, and feasibility amongst others. Technical considerations related to the route of exposure and obtaining biological samples for toxicokinetics and clinical pathology evaluations are important.

With respect to the general screen or "standard design", the juvenile studies represent a combination of a repeat-dose study design and parameters routinely found in the pre- and postnatal (PPN) study conducted as part of the developmental and reproductive toxicology (DART) regulatory testing. The routine toxicology parameters are comprised of *in vivo* monitoring of the animals, including daily examination for signs of reaction to treatment, body weight and food consumption assessment, ophthalmology, heart rate and ECG (nonrodents), laboratory investigations (haematology, biochemistry and urinalysis), gross and histopathological examinations of selected tissues and organ weights. The developmental parameters assessed in the PPN studies are also evaluated, and include physical and sexual developmental milestones, reflex ontogeny, general growth and development, effects on behaviour, learning and memory, and reproductive performance. With respect to the more specific, designed studies, screens to assess the development of particular organ systems could be added. Cappon *et al.* (2009) discuss several examples of potential study designs with a focus of a particular study design being on either CNS and reproduction or liver and reproduction as targets of concern. As would be expected with a case-by-case approach, there are many permutations of the study specifics for these studies, for example, number of animals, end-points, dosing duration and recovery duration, and so on. For more information on these specific assessments, the reader is referred to other sources (De Schaepdrijver *et al.*, 2009; Beck *et al.*, 2006).

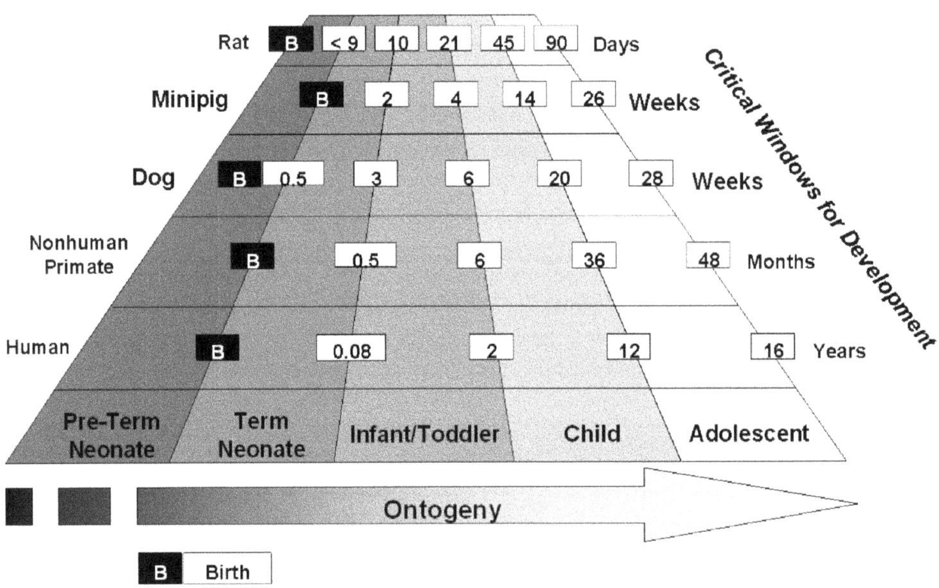

Figure 16.1 *Comparative age categories across species based on CNS and Reproductive Development. Estimates are based on combined general developmental events occurring in both sexes, and represent only the overall schedule for CNS and reproductive development in these species. Note that the end age of the comparative category to human Infant/Toddler corresponds roughly to the usual age at weaning for laboratory species (with permission, Buelke-Sam, 2003).*

A good knowledge of comparative postnatal development in animal models and humans is essential when selecting the appropriate species and study end-points. A general guide for comparative age categories between different animal species and humans with regard to central nervous system and reproductive organ development is presented in Figure 16.1 (Buelke-Sam, 2003). In addition, a series of mini-reviews has been published on the heart (Hew and Keller, 2003), lung (Zoetis and Hurtt, 2003a), kidney (Zoetis and Hurtt, 2003b), CNS (Wood, *et al.*, 2003; Watson *et al.*, 2006), immune system (Holsapple *et al.*, 2003), male (Marty *et al.*, 2003) and female (Beckman and Feuston, 2003), reproductive systems, gastrointestinal system (Walthall *et al.*, 2004) and bone and postnatal growth (Zoetis *et al.*, 2003c). These papers review the current knowledge of functional and/or physiological postnatal development, identifying stage marks for organ system development and key physiological developmental landmarks.

It is advisable to explore the absorption, distribution, metabolism and excretion (ADME) characteristics of the investigational compound in various age groups in a preliminary pharmacokinetic study or dose range finding toxicity study. Differences in toxicity between adult and neonatal/juvenile animals are often due to differences in ADME of the test compound. It is important for the efficacy/safety evaluation that the ADME characteristics in juvenile animals are comparable to the human situation at a similar stage of development. The different time frames for the ontogeny of drug metabolism enzymes and transport proteins between animals and man are an additional consideration and potential hindrance in the extrapolation of toxicological observations from juvenile animals to children (De Zwart *et al.*, 2008).

16.5 Case Studies: Application of Data Review and Decision Making

As discussed previously, unlike the standard core of reproductive toxicity studies that is required for nearly all compound registrations and which have tightly prescribed study design requirements, the need for and design of toxicity studies in juvenile animals are considered on a case-by-case basis. The importance of a case-by-case approach to study design is emphasized in both EMA and FDA regulatory guidance and also recommended by a broad group of scientists with a common interest in juvenile animal studies (EMA, 2008; FDA, 2006; Hurtt *et al.*, 2004). Several examples of juvenile animal study designs are available in the public literature (Rigdon *et al.*, 1989; Hurtt *et al.*, 2004; Beckman *et al.*, 2008; Cappon *et al.*, 2009; Anderson *et al.*, 2009) and some examples are presented below. The examples summarize experience in dealing with safety assessment of new therapeutic candidates or modalities (e.g., inhaled products) for the juvenile patient population. In some cases, the available data in adult animals were considered adequate for juvenile safety and in others special juvenile animal safety studies were appropriate.

16.5.1 Adequacy of Existing Data to Support Clinical Development in Paediatric Populations

An "inhalation formulation" of insulin was in clinical development for adults and children over the age of 6 years. Inhaled insulin was not to be recommended to children under 6 years of age due to underdeveloped coordination skills necessary to operate the inhaler apparatus. A comprehensive toxicology programme was completed to support clinical testing and registration of inhaled insulin. No target organs were identified in preclinical toxicity studies but, due to the inhalation route of exposure, effects on pulmonary function were considered to be of potential concern. Previously, no data on nonclinical safety testing of insulin existed in juvenile animals but subcutaneously injected insulin was in use in children down to 4 years of age. Based on the lack of any significant findings in adult animal toxicology studies, no other target organs of concern in adult human trials, full maturation of human lungs by 2–6 years of age, and physical limitation of children less than 6 years to use the inhaled device, the risk to young human subjects was considered minimal. Therefore, no specific juvenile animal studies were deemed necessary and none were conducted.

Another example was for a small molecule "nicotine partial agonist" that was in development for smoking cessation in adults. A comprehensive nonclinical safety programme designed to support the chronic use in adults was completed. The features of this programme included subchronic and chronic safety pharmacology, toxicology studies in rodents and nonrodents, genetic toxicity testing, carcinogenicity studies in two rodent species, and reproductive toxicity studies that addressed male and female reproductive functions beginning with mating and early pregnancy through multiple generation assessments of reproductive performance. Because the target clinical population, smokers intending to quit smoking, would not be expected to include a significant population for patients less than 18 years of age, no clinical or nonclinical safety or efficacy studies in non-adult populations were planned. At the time of US approval in adults, a post-marketing study was requested in tobacco-addicted adolescents, ages 12 through 16, to determine a safe and effective dose. Based on the age of the paediatric population, adverse events in adult clinical trials, and the toxicology profile in nonclinical studies, it was agreed that a juvenile animal toxicology study was not considered to be necessary to support the paediatric clinical plan.

16.5.2 Nonclinical Juvenile Safety Testing to Support Clinical Development

A small molecule with a "mechanistically novel approach" was in clinical development for the treatment of attention deficit hyperactivity disorder (ADHD). The paediatric programme was to follow a Phase 2b study in adults and comprised of an initial study in adolescents (ages 13–17) with ADHD followed by a study in children (ages 6–12). Because this was a novel pharmacological target for the treatment of ADHD, it was determined that a juvenile animal study could provide added information on potential safety concerns before beginning trials in children. The major target organ system identified in adult animals (dogs, rats) was the nervous system. Because of the similarity of target organs between the two animal species and the availability of validated models of neurobehavioural assessments in rats, a juvenile rat toxicology study, dosed from postnatal days 7 to 70, was considered appropriate for testing. A full neurobehavioural battery was included in the study to be performed at various development stages (acoustic startle response, motor activity, and a learning/memory test). The Regulatory Agency concurred with the nonclinical strategy and additionally recommended histopathology assessments in all tissues collected in the rat study and to potentially conduct a second juvenile toxicity study in dogs, if necessary, following review of the juvenile rat toxicity study or after review of long-term dog toxicity studies. The Regulatory Agency's response to the proposed design also indicated that "it should be specified that the juvenile animal study needs to be done only to support the younger age range (6–12 years old)". Following review of the rat study, a second study in the dog was not deemed necessary.

16.5.3 Nonclinical Juvenile Safety Testing in Two Species

On rare occasions, nonclinical juvenile testing in two species might be needed based on significant differences in the target distribution and the toxicity profiles between the animal species. As of January 2010, only two of 379 approved Paediatric Investigation Plans by the EMA had studies in multiple species (EMA, 2010).

An anti-inflammatory drug for potential clinical use in a wide age range (infant to adults) was being developed. The therapeutic target was widely distributed in various organ systems, including kidney, bone, and nervous system. The adult toxicology studies showed some common target organs of toxicity and some unique to dogs (infections and renal toxicity). Because of the potential role of the therapeutic target in growth and development and significant differences in toxicology profiles between rats and dogs, nonclinical juvenile studies were conducted in two species. Dosing in the juvenile rat study occurred between postnatal days 7 and 70 and assessments focused on effects on growth, neurobehavioural and sexual development. In order to assess safety at the neonatal and infant developmental stages, the dogs were dosed on postnatal days 5–9 (neonatal stage) and again on days 25–29 (infant stage) with particular attention on renal development.

16.6 Summary

Expectations for medicinal products have changed when it comes to children. There is recognition that the past paradigm based on an assumption that information for dosing in children could be scaled from adult safety and effectiveness data has given way to an appreciation that information on safe dosing for children must be derived from carefully designed and executed studies in children. Further, what is applicable information for the safe use of a drug in an adolescent is often not adequate for the needs of a toddler or newborn. Clinical studies must be conducted in all relevant age groups. The regulations for paediatric drugs in the US and EU have been a large impetus to achieving quality study of medicines for children as noted by the increasing integration of paediatric drug development programmes into the larger adult development programmes.

The nonclinical toxicology that supports clinical trials must adequately address safety assessments needed to enrol the population, of any age, for whom the drug is intended. Well-designed juvenile animal studies provide the ability to identify potential safety or pharmacokinetic issues, contribute to paediatric clinical trial design, and contribute to product approval and use in the paediatric population with appropriate prescribing information in the product label. Whether to conduct a juvenile animal study, or not conduct a study, is based on a careful analysis of existing data from other toxicology studies and adult clinical trials. Such decisions can be based on a "gap" in knowledge, in response to an identified safety concern or to address potential long-term effects that cannot practically be assessed in a clinical trial. To be most effective, therefore, it is a uniquely designed study. Experience with the design and conduct of juvenile animal studies, as well as an understanding of the relevance of the data to clinical settings, is growing and must continue. The product of this work is information leading to the safe and effective use of medicines in children.

References

Anderson, T., Khan, N.K., Tassinari, M.S., and Hurtt, M.E. (2009) Comparative juvenile safety testing of new therapeutic candidates: relevance of laboratory animal data to children. *J. Toxicol. Sci.*, **34**(Special Issue (II)), SP209–SP215.

Bailey, G.P. and Marien, D. (2009) What have we learned from pre-clinical juvenile toxicity studies? *Reprod. Toxicol.*, **28**(2), 226–229.

Baldrick, P. (2004) Developing drugs for paediatric use: a role for juvenile animal studies? *Regul. Toxicol. Pharmacol.*, **39**, 381–389.

Beck, M.J., Padgett, E.L., Bowman, C.J. *et al.* (2006) Nonclinical juvenile toxicity testing, in *Developmental and Reproductive Toxicology. A Practical Approach* (ed. R.D. Hood), CRC Press, Taylor & Francis Group, Boca Raton FL.

Beckman, D.A., Schneider, M., Youreneff, M., and Tse, F.L. (2008) Juvenile toxicity assessment of d,l-methylphenidate in rats. *Birth Defects Res. (Part B)*, **83**, 48–67.

BPCA (2002) Best Pharmaceuticals for Children Act of 2002, Pub. L. 107–109, 115 STAT 1408.

Brent, R.L. (2004) Utilization of juvenile animal studies to determine the human effects and risks of environmental toxicants during postnatal developmental stages. *Birth Defects Res. (Part B)*, **71**, 303–320.

Buelke-Sam, J. (2003) Comparative schedules of development in rats and humans: implications for developmental neurotoxicity testing. Presented at the 42nd Annual Meeting of the Society of Toxicology, March 9–13, 2003, Salt Lake City, Utah.

Cappon, G., Bailey, G., Buschmann, J. *et al.* (2009) Juvenile animal toxicity study designs to support pediatric drug development. *Birth Defects Res. (Part B)*, **86**, 463–469.

De Schaepdrijver, L.M., Bailey, G.P. *et al.* (2009) Preclinical juvenile toxicity assessments and study designs, in *Pediatric Drug Development. Concepts and Applications* (eds A.E. Mulberg, S.S. Silber, and J.N. van den Anker), John Wiley & Sons, Inc., Hoboken, NJ.

De Schaepdrijver, L.M., Rouan, M.C., Raoof, A. *et al.* (2008) Real life toxicity case studies: the good, the bad and the ugly. *Reprod. Toxicol.*, **26**, 54–55.

De Zwart, L., Scholten, M., Monbaliu, J.G. *et al.* (2008) The ontogeny of drug metabolizing enzymes and transporters in the rat. *Reprod. Toxicol.*, **26**, 220–230.

European Medicines Evaluation Agency (EMA), Committee for Human Medicinal Products (CHMP) (2008) Guideline on the Need for Non-clinical Testing in Juvenile Animals on Human Pharmaceuticals for Pediatric Indications, August 2008, http://www.ema.europa.eu/pdfs/human/swp/16921505en08.pdf.

European Medicines Agency (EMA) PIP data (2010) www.ema.europa.eu/htms/human/paediatrics/decisions.htm updated November 27, 2009, accessed January 16, 2010.

FDA (2006) Center for Drug Evaluation and Research, Guidance for Industry, Nonclinical Safety Evaluation of Pediatric Drug Products, U.S. Department of Health and Human Services, Rockville, MD, February 2006, http://www.fda.gov/downloads/Drugs/GuidanceCompliance RegulatoryInformation/Guidances/ucm079247.pdf.

FDAMA (1997) US Food and Drug Administration Modernization Act of 1997, Pub.S.1789, Best Pharmaceuticals for Children Act.

FDAAA (2007) US Food and Drug Administration Amendments Act (FDAAA) of 2007, Pub. L. No. 75–711, 52 Stat. 1040 (1938) as amended.

Federal Register (1998) Regulations requiring manufacturers to assess the safety and effectiveness of new drugs and biological products in pediatric patients; final rule. *Fed. Reg.*, **63**(231), 66632–66672.

Hew, K.W. and Keller, K.A. (2003) Postnatal anatomical and functional development of the heart: a species comparison. *Birth Defects Res. (Part B)*, **68**, 309–320.

Holsapple, M.P., West, L.J., and Landreth, K.S. (2003) Species comparison of anatomical and functional immune system development. *Birth Defects Res. (Part B)*, **68**, 321–334.

Hurtt, M.E., Daston, G., Davis-Bruno, K. *et al.* (2004) Juvenile animal studies: testing strategy and design. *Birth Defects Res. (Part B)*, **71**, 281–288.

ICH (2000) ICH Topic E11, Step 5, Note for Guidance on Clinical Investigation of Medicinal Products in the Paediatric Population. 2000 Federal Register, Vol. 65, No. 71, April 12, pages 19777–81.

ICH Harmonized Tripartite Guideline (2009) Guidance on the Non-Clinical Safety Studies for the Conduct of Human Clinical Trials and Marketing Authorization for Pharmaceuticals M3 (R2), June, 2009 http://www.ema.europa.eu/pdfs/human/ich/028695en.pdf.

Makris, S.L. (2011) Application of principles of non-clinical pediatric drug testing to the hazard evaluation of environmental contaminants, in *Pediatric Non-Clinical Drug Testing: Principles, Requirements and Practice* (eds A.M. Hoberman and E.M. Lewis), Wiley Press.

Marty, F M.S., Chapin, R.E., Parks, L.G. *et al.* (2003) Development and maturation of the male reproductive system. *Birth Defects Res. (Part B)*, **68**, 125–136.

Beckman, D.A. and Feuston, M. (2003) Landmarks in the development of the female reproductive system. *Birth Defects Res. (Part B)*, **68**, 137–143.

Official Journal. Regulation (EC; 2006) No 1901/2006 of the European Parliament and of the Council of 12 December 2006 on medicinal products for paediatric use and amending Regulation (EEC) No 1768/92, directive 2001/20/EC, directive 2001/83/EC and Regulation (EC) No 726/2004. Official Journal L 378, 27.12.2006.

Patient Protection and Affordable Care Act (PPACA; 2010). Pub. L. 111–148–Mar. 23, 2010 124 STAT. 119.

PREA FD&C (2007) Sec. 505B(2)(A)(i,ii) (21U.S.C. 355c) Research into Pediatric Uses for Drugs and Biological Products.

Rigdon, G.C., Boyes, W.K., and Dyer, R.S. (1989) Effects of perinatal monosodium glutamate administration on visual evoked potentials of juvenile and adult rats. *Neurotoxicol. Teratol.*, **11**, 121–128.

Rose, K. (2008) Ethical, regulatory and scientific challenges in paediatric drug development. *Pharm. Med.*, **22**(4), 221–234.

Rose, K. (2009) Challenges in pediatric drug development: a pharmaceutical industry perspective. *Pediatric Drugs*, **11**(1), 57–59.

Stahlmann, R. (1990) Safety profile of the quinolones. *J. Antimicrob. Chemother.*, **26**(Suppl (D)), 31–44.

Walthall, K., Cappon, G.D., Hurtt, M.E., and Zoetis, T. (2004) Postnatal development of the gastrointestinal system: a species comparison. *Birth Defects Res. (Part B)*, **74**, 132–156.

Watson, R.E., DeSesso, J.M., Hurtt, M.E. *et al.* (2006) Postnatal growth and morphological development of the brain: a species comparison. *Birth Defects Res. (Part B)*, **77**, 471–484.

Wood, S.L., Beyer, BK., and Cappon, G.D. (2003) Species comparison of postnatal CNS development: functional measures. *Birth Defects Res. (Part B)*, **68**, 391–407.

Zoetis, T. and Hurtt, M.E. (2003a) Species comparison of lung development. *Birth Defects Res. (Part B)*, **68**, 121–124.

Zoetis, T. and Hurtt, M.E. (2003b) Species comparison of anatomical and functional renal development. *Birth Defects Res. (Part B)*, **68**, 111–120.

Zoetis, T., Tassinari, M.S., Bagi, C. *et al.* (2003) Species comparison of postnatal bone growth and development. *Birth Defects Res. (Part B)*, **68**, 86–110.

17

Immunotoxicology

Leigh Ann Burns-Naas[1] *and Marc J. Pallardy*[2]
[1]*Gilead Sciences Inc., Foster City, USA*
[2]*School of Pharmacy and INSERM, University of Paris-Sud, Chatenay, Malabry, France*

17.1 Introduction

The immune system is a highly regulated and interdependent network able to distinguish self from non-self and thus protect the host from infectious microorganisms and neoplasms. This organ system is found throughout the body in different tissues (e.g., lymph nodes, thymus, spleen, bone marrow, blood) containing various cell types (e.g., lymphocytes, monocytes, dendritic cells, natural killer cells) and sub-types (e.g., CD4+ T-lymphocytes, CD8+ T-lymphocytes, regulatory T lymphocytes, B lymphocytes). The immune system is in a continuous state of self-renewal through proliferation, differentiation, activation, and maturation, in some cases to a long-lived memory state. As a result, the immune system can be particularly vulnerable to toxic insult. Because of its plieotropic nature (e.g., overlapping functions, "immune reserve"), the immune system is also remarkably resilient.

This chapter covers the current global regulatory status and expectations regarding the nonclinical safety assessment for drugs for immunotoxic potential. The chapter also covers non-regulatory considerations and, where appropriate, makes recommendations for follow-on testing. During the interpretation of data, two key factors should be considered. First, there can be marked differences in the immune system of different species which could result in limitations, specifically with regard to relevancy of data. Second, the immune system in humans and animals contains a great deal of redundancy or capacity to trigger compensatory mechanisms when one immune effector mechanism is inhibited. Therefore, results from nonclinical immune studies where a single end-point is affected

Nonclinical Safety Assessment: A Guide to International Pharmaceutical Regulations, First Edition.
Edited by William J. Brock, Kenneth L. Hastings and Kathy M. McGown.

may not necessarily reflect a biologically meaningful effect. These factors mean that all data, whether direct or indirect evaluations of immune function, need to be evaluated in the context of the similarities and differences of the immune systems of the nonclinical species and humans. A broad evaluation of immune effects (e.g., the totality of the data) could prove more predictive in determining the potential of a drug to induce perturbation in the immune system in humans.

17.2 Regulatory Expectations for the Immunotoxicology Evaluation of Pharmaceuticals

Regulatory requirements for the testing of pharmaceutical new molecular entities (NMEs) for potential to adversely impact the immune system are relatively new, though drug-related immunotoxic effects have been known for many years. Most commonly, this has been considered in the context of drug allergy or anaphylaxis. However, other drug-related adverse events could also be the result of primary or secondary effects on the immune system. One of the most common adverse effects observed in classic chemotherapy for cancer is neutropenia (in addition to thrombocytopenia or lymphopenia) from bone marrow suppression as a result of cytotoxic agents which target rapidly dividing cells. In an effort to develop more effective (and presumably less toxic) therapeutics and to treat newer or less well-served diseases and syndromes a vast number of highly-selective, molecularly-targeted therapeutics have entered clinical development. Many of these NMEs might have the immune system as a potential target for desired (pharmacodynamic) or undesired (adverse) effects but, unlike cytotoxic agents, their true risk to human health is not reliably predicted based solely on the target. Exaggerated pharmacology and off-target toxicity can be less obvious, and it is possible for both to occur within the same organism simultaneously. To distinguish these features, immunotoxicity testing has become an important consideration in drug development.

17.2.1 Adverse (Unintended) Immunomodulation – ICH S8, the Weight of Evidence Review, and Determination of "Cause for Concern"

Between 2000 and 2006, scientific and regulatory authorities were developing proposals for the appropriate evaluation of NMEs for their immunotoxic potential. Regional differences in requirements led to the development of a harmonized approach through the International Conference on Harmonization (ICH). ICH S8 came into force in 2006 and provided an approach to assess the need for specialized immunotoxicity testing and the timing of these studies relative to clinical development (ICH, 2006). The objective of this guidance was "to provide (1) recommendations on nonclinical testing approaches to identify compounds which have the potential to be immunotoxic, and (2) guidance on a weight-of-evidence decision making approach for immunotoxicity testing". For the purposes of the guidance, "immunotoxicity" was defined as unintended immunosuppression or enhancement, although the latter term was not precisely defined. However, since drugs can disrupt immune function with unpredictable results, it has been suggested that the term "adverse immunomodulation" may be the more appropriate descriptor (House and Hastings, 2004). ICH S8 notes that all NMEs should be evaluated for their potential to produce immunotoxicity. The key features of this guidance document are the primary reliance on data generated in standard toxicology studies (STS) and the weight of evidence review which includes the STS and other factors. Drug-induced hypersensitivity and autoimmunity were specifically excluded from ICH S8. The unexpected stimulation of the immune system (e.g., cytokine release) is also be outside of the scope of this guideline, but is considered later in this chapter.

17.2.1.1 Factors to Consider – Standard Toxicology Studies (Table 17.1)

The initial screen for immunotoxic potential involves a detailed examination of toxicity studies in rodents and nonrodents including: (1) haematology, (2) clinical chemistry, (3) immune organ weights, (4) histologic changes in lymphoid tissue, (5) presence of increased incidence of infection, and (6) the occurrence of tumours in the absence of other probable causes.

17.2.1.2 Clinical Signs

Daily observations of study animals can give clues to potential immunotoxic events. Visual observations such as blood or pus in urine on cage pans, abnormal discharge (mucoid, purulent, or haemorrhagic) from any of the orifices (nasal, ocular, vaginal, etc.),

Table 17.1 *Evaluation of Immunotoxicity (from ICH S8).*

Parameter/end-point	Potential assessment components
Standard Toxicology Studies	
Haematology[a]	Complete blood count, absolute differential white cell count
Clinical chemistry	Globulins[b], A:G ratio
Organ weights	Spleen, thymus, peripheral lymph node, draining lymph node
Histopathology[c]	Spleen, thymus, peripheral lymph node, draining lymph node, bone marrow, Peyer's patch/mesenteric lymph node (oral only), BALT (inhalation only), NALT (intranasal only)
Immune Evaluation	
Cellular characterization	Immunophenotyping, immunohistochemistry
Functional	
Innate immunity	Reticuloendothelial system assay (RES), macrophage and neutrophil function (phagocytosis, oxidative burst, chemotaxis, cytotoxicity)
Humoral immunity	T-dependent antibody response (primary and/or secondary)
Cell mediated immunity	Natural killer (NK) cell activity, delayed-type hypersensitivity (DTH), cytotoxic T cell response (CTL)
Host resistance[d]	Bacteria, fungal, viral, parasitic; may be *in vivo* or in vitro

BALT: bronchus-associated lymphoid tissue.
NALT: nasal-associated lymphoid tissue.
[a]Alterations in circulating haematologic parameters could suggest the need to specifically evaluate bone marrow cytology.
[b]Alterations in globulin levels could suggest a need to further investigate serum immunoglobulins.
[c]Semi-quantitative description of changes in the lymphoid tissue is strongly recommended for reporting treatment-related alterations in immune tissues (Haley *et al.*, 2005).
[d]An understanding of affected cell types is key to success as selection of a model whose immune component(s) is/are not impacted by the drug will provide a false answer.

dose-related diarrhoea, dermatitis or rash, respiratory alterations or distress, fever, anorexia, lethargy, or increased incidence of tumours can all be manifestations of immune alterations. None of these signs is sufficient to indicate an immune-related effect. They can, however, contribute to the overall weight of evidence evaluation.

17.2.1.3 Clinical Pathology (Table 17.2)

A thorough discussion on the intricacies of clinical pathology (both haematology and chemistry) and its interpretation is provided in Evans (2008) and Weiser (2006) and will be summarized here. Clinical pathology data are a crucial factor in the overall weight-of-

Table 17.2 *Evaluation of clinical pathology.*

Observation	Possible considerations
	Clinical Chemistry
Hyperglobulinemia	Inflammation Infection Certain lymphoid tumors
Hypoalbuminemia	Immune-mediated glomerulonephritis (when together with hypercholesterolaemia)
Hypercholesterolaemia	Immune-mediated glomerulonephritis (when together with hypoalbuminemia)
	Haematology
Pancytopenia	Direct toxicity to bone marrow architecture or stem cells Anti-mitotic effect Effects on differentiation and/or maturation Immune-mediated (antibody or cell-mediated) destruction of stem cells
MONOCYTES	
Morphology	Activated appearance (vacuolated, "fluffy") Infection/Sepsis (intracellular microorganisms)
Monocytosis	Stress (dogs) Necrosis (immune-mediated or non-immune) Inflammation (immune-related or non-immune) Immune-mediated haemolytic anaemia or thrombocytopenia Altered production or trafficking
LYMPHOCYTES	
Lymphopenia	Stress Direct toxicity (peripheral or bone marrow) Anti-proliferative effect or signal Immunosuppression Infection/Acute inflammation
Lymphocytosis	Excitability/Fear (fight or flight syndrome) Immunostimulation Lymphoid neoplasia Chronic inflammation
NEUTROPHILS	
Morphology	Bone marrow (asynchronous maturation) Infection/Sepsis (intracellular microorganisms) Trafficking/Prolonged presence in circulation (hypersegmentation) Inflammation (toxic change - vacuolation, basophilic stippling, Dohle bodies)

Table 17.2 *(Continued)*

Observation	Possible considerations
Neutropenia	Direct bone marrow suppression (including cytokine alterations
	Tissue demand exceeds production capacity (inflammation, infection)
	Increased margination/trafficking to tissues
	Immune-mediated destruction
	Inhibition of release from bone marrow
Neutrophilia	Adrenaline-induced (excitation; fear)
	Corticosteroid-induced (stress)
	Inflammation (immune-related or non-immune)
	Immune-mediated haemolytic anaemia or thrombocytopenia
	Effects on trafficking (defect in adhesion molecules/tissue migration)
EOSINOPHILS	
Eosinophilia	Hypersensitivity
	Fungal infection, parasitemia
	Tumors (e.g., mast cell, basophilic or eosinophilic)
Eosinopenia	Stress
	General bone marrow suppression
	Suppression/alteration of differentiation′
	Excitation/Fear
	Acute infection/Inflammation
BASOPHILS	
Basophilia	Persistent lipemia
	Parasitemia
	Allergy
ERYTHROCYTES	
Anaemia	Altered lipid content, oxidative damage (non-immune effects)
	Bone marrow suppression (non-regenerative)
	Monocyte activation
	Immune-mediated destruction
	Intra- or extravascular haemolysis (immune or non-immune)
	Infection/Inflammation (chronic disease)
PLATELETS	
Thrombocytopenia	Immune-mediated (often regenerative)
	Bone marrow suppression (non-regenerative)
	Disseminated intravascular coagulation (DIC)

Descriptions are taken from Evans (2008) and Stockholm and Scott (2008). Consideration are not intended to be inclusive of all possibilities.

evidence evaluation of NMEs but no one parameter should be interpreted in the absence of the totality of the data. Notably, findings considered "normal" in treated groups are not always indicative of the lack of immune effects and, similarly, alterations in haematological or serum chemistry parameters do not necessarily mean the immune system has been targeted by the NME. For example, stress as a secondary effect of treatment can cause alterations in circulating white cells as can excitation during experimental procedures such as sample collection. It is also important to remember that this evaluation is a snapshot of what is happening in this compartment within the animal at the time the sample is taken (effects on bone marrow, lymphoid tissue, vasculature may not be reflected at all).

This snapshot can be influenced by many things such as stress, excitation, relationship of the sample to feeding time and other animals (e.g., bleeding order), collection site, use of anaesthesia, circadian rhythms, and so on. Consistency in study conduct will help minimize the variability (e.g., bleeding at the same time during the day, in the same order, from the same site, and the same time relative to feeding). Additionally, when interpreting haematological data and extrapolating between species, remember that there are species-specific differences in bone marrow capacity, extramedullary hematopoiesis, longevity of circulating cells, and even in the distribution of cell types. In dogs, the predominant circulating cells are neutrophils while in rodents its lymphocytes and NHPs fall somewhere between these. Within the lymphocyte compartment, rats tend to have higher numbers of circulating B cells when compared to monkeys or humans.

The most relevant serum chemistry parameter used to evaluate potential immunotoxicity is total serum globulins. These proteins include lipoproteins and acute phase reactants (mainly from the liver), and immunoglobulins (from the immune system.) Although changes in serum globulin levels are insensitive and nonspecific, large increases or decreases could suggest immune-related effects. Large increases in globulins, especially when accompanied by leukocytosis and/or signs of inflammation, could be suggestive of an infection or autoimmunity.

Blood abnormalities can be associated with direct bone marrow toxicity or haemolysis caused by other drug-related actions such as anti-RBC autoantibody or autologous antibody generation (e.g., immune-mediated haemolytic anaemia). Notably, a direct drug-related intravascular haemolysis is frequently accompanied by increases in WBC counts, an increase in spleen weight, hemosiderosis (iron accumulation) in various tissues, and reticulocytosis. The timing of the onset of any blood dyscrasia should be carefully evaluated. Peripheral loss of one or more cell types might be the result of a direct effect on bone marrow cells and usually follows a time course that reflects the half-life of the specific cell type(s). Typically in humans, with damage to an early stem cell, neutropenia precedes thrombocytopenia, and frank anaemia appears much later, reflecting the peripheral longevity of red blood cells. Conversely, if the loss of a cell type is inconsistent with an effect on the bone marrow, a direct effect on mature circulating cells could be occurring.

The observation of anaemia or thrombocytopenia alone doesn't necessarily suggest an effect on the immune system, though generalized bone marrow suppression could cause both of these. A non-regenerative anaemia (reduced red cells and reduced or absent reticulocytes) may suggest an immune-related effect on bone marrow or a direct immune-mediated destruction of this cell type. Regenerative anemias (increased reticulocytes) suggest haemorrhage or haemolysis (intravascular or extravascular), the latter of which has the immune system as one possible mediator of the effect. Spherocytosis in the red cell compartment is suggestive of an immune-mediated haemolytic effect. The presence of either infection or inflammation can result in anaemia or chronic disease and/or thrombocytopenia from disseminated intravascular coagulation (DIC).

Monocytes are typically considered the "garbage collectors" in the body because of their role in phagocytosis and removal of cellular debris and pathogens. These cells are also antigen-presenting cells and can drive immune responses through both the innate and acquired arms of immunity. In tissues, monocytes usually differentiate into resident macrophages (e.g., alveolar and Kupffer cells). Monocytopenia is hardly ever detectable due to the very low numbers of circulating cells. However, monocytosis can be observed and

Table 17.3 *Typical leukograms in animals and humans.*

Leukogram	Description
Physiologic (adrenaline) leukocytosis[a]	Increases in all leukocytes, but most pronounced in lymphocytes Neutrophilia (resulting from de-margination) No "left shift"[b]
Stress (corticosteroid) leukogram	Neutrophilia (possibly hypersegmented) Lymphopenia +/− Monocytosis (dogs) or eosinopenia
Inflammatory leukogram	Neutropenia or neutrophilia with "left shift" +/− Toxic change, lymphopenia, monocytosis
Hematopoietic neoplasia	Cytopenias in sub-leukaemic (clinically) leukaemia Increases in affected cell type (mature or immature cells) with cytopenias in remaining lines

Descriptions are taken from Evans (2008).
[a]Generally has no direct relationship to the immune system.
[b]"Left shift" refers to a visual shift toward immature morphology typically characterized by increased banding or earlier neutrophil stages.

could suggest inflammation or infection, tissue necrosis, immune-mediated haemolytic anaemia or thrombocytopenia, and possibly activation due to cytokines or chemokines.

Circulating eosinophil and basophil numbers are very small (relative to other cells) and changes are rarely informative. The most common cause of eosinopenia is stress, but this is not a reliable indicator. A stress leukogram (Table 17.3) with absence of eosinopenia is adequately reliable. Eosinopenia can also be the result of general bone marrow suppression, suppression of differentiation, excitation/fear, and some acute infections. Eosinophilia can be associated with hypersensitivity reactions, fungal and parasitic infections, tumours (e.g., mast cell tumours, basophilic or eosinophilic leukemias) and inflammation at epithelial surfaces rich in mast cells (particularly if associated with hypersensitivity). Basophilia could be associated with persistent lipemia, parasites, and allergy.

Neutrophils are bone marrow-derived and released into the circulation where a percentage of them (species-specific) marginate and migrate into tissues. A general decision tree to evaluate neutrophilia is provided in Figure 17.1a. Neutropenia can occur as a result of bone marrow toxicity, specific effects on the ability of these cells to differentiate or be released into the circulation, or enhanced expression or activity of adhesion molecules. Immune-mediated destruction or severe infection can also be causes. In general, immune-related effects should be considered when there is neutropenia, particularly when no other cause is evident, and an evaluation of bone marrow (cytology and histology) should be performed.

Neutrophilia can be observed for a variety of reasons and should not be presumed to be an immunotoxic effect. Stress-related (corticosteroid-mediated), excitation-related (adrenaline-mediated) effects, and haemolysis/haemorrhage can result in neutrophilia. During stress, increased numbers of neutrophils are produced by the bone marrow and decreased numbers of peripheral neutrophils marginate into vessels and/or migrate into tissues. Finally, when there is peripheral destruction of erythrocytes or haemorrhage the bone marrow is stimulated to produce more cells. Neutrophilia is associated with immune-mediated haemolysis. A general decision tree to evaluate neutrophilia is provided in Figure 17.1b.

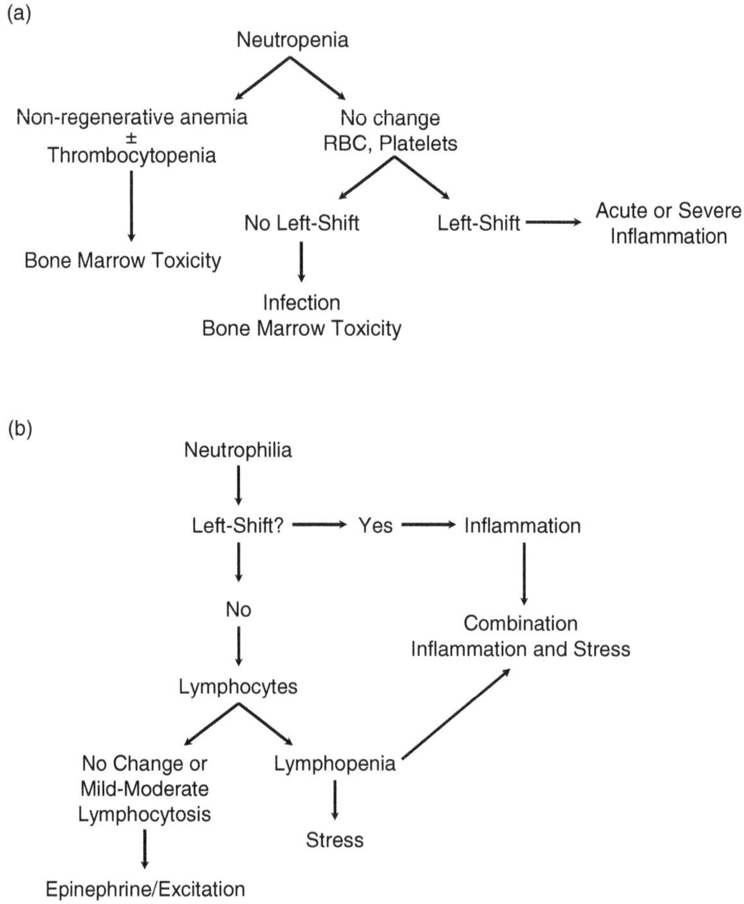

Figure 17.1 *General flow diagram consideration when alterations in neutrophils are observed. These flow diagrams are intended to stimulate the thought process. They do not represent all possibilities, just some of the more common. (a) When neutropenia is observed in clinical pathology data from standard toxicology studies, other haematology data are considered. No loss of the erythron or platelets and no left shift is suggestive of infection or bone marrow toxicity (direct or indirect). The presence of a left shift suggests a significant inflammatory response somewhere in the body. Neutropenia in the presence of a non-regenerative anaemia or thrombocytopenia suggests bone marrow toxicity. (b) When neutrophilia is observed, the data are evaluated for the presence of a left shift, which is diagnostic of an inflammatory response. If no left shift is present, the lymphocyte data are considered. Lymphopenia suggests a stress response (hence the stress leukogram being neutrophilia generally with no left shift but with lymphopenia). In the presence of a left shift, a combination of stress and inflammation is considered. If no left shift is noted and there is no change in lymphocyte numbers or they are increased, the data suggest an adrenaline/excitation response. Derived from (Weiser, 2006).*

Inflammation is a common cause of neutrophilia and can usually be distinguished from other causes by an increased number of immature cells (banded cells). This "left shift" is sometimes accompanied by the presence of neutrophil vacuolation or granulation (referred to as "toxic change") or basophilic inclusions. "Orderly left shift" means the concentration of each cell stage decreases with the degree of immaturity of the cell stage. An orderly left shift indicates an inflammatory process. Neutropenia that occurs in the presence of a left shift generally indicates a more aggressive inflammatory lesion. Inflammation can be associated with infection or immune-mediated haemolytic anaemia, thrombocytopenia, or tissue destruction. It can also be a secondary effect of direct (non-immune) toxicity. Additional neutrophil morphologic changes include the presence of microorganisms in the cells, hypersegmentation (which suggests prolonged presence in the circulation and possible inability to migrate to tissues) and asynchronous maturation (associated with bone marrow toxicity).

Like neutrophilia, a common cause of lymphocytosis is an adrenaline-induced physiologic response resulting from excitation or fear. Lymphocytosis can also be associated with a proliferative signal (increased production or altered trafficking), acute or chronic infection, antigenic stimulation such as a recent immunization/vaccination, or leukaemia. Lymphocytosis is generally not associated with chronic inflammatory disease: lymphocyte proliferation that occurs in this case is more typically confined to the lymphoid organs. Lymphopenia can result from generalized bone marrow toxicity, suppression of release from lymphoid compartments, a direct cytotoxic effect on lymphocytes, stress, trafficking from the circulation to a site of infection, or anti-proliferative agents. Neither lymphopenia nor lymphocytosis exclusively indicate an immunotoxic effect and the absence of any effect on the lymphoid compartment does not rule out an immunologic effect of the test material.

17.2.1.4 Organ Weights

All standard toxicology studies should include an assessment of immune-related organs including the thymus, spleen, and lymph nodes (draining and distant). Though these are relatively insensitive indicators of immunotoxicity, particularly in nonrodent species, significant changes can suggest an effect on the immune system. Both increases and decreases in weights are important, particularly if they are accompanied by altered histology. An increase in lymph node weight could be suggestive of immunosuppression and increased susceptibility to infection or as an indicator of autoimmune or hypersensitivity response (especially in draining lymph nodes). Decreases in the weight of immune organs could be suggestive of immunosuppression, particularly when there is an accompanying change in histology. Technical variability and species differences can impact the evaluation of lymphoid organ weights. For smaller organs, trimming differences can contribute to statistically significant differences in weight that have no reflection on immune status. Also, as the spleen in the dog functions more as a storage and filtering organ for blood, incomplete exsanguination can result in elevated spleen weight that is an artefact. Thus, organ weight changes should always be considered in the context of the histologic effects.

17.2.1.5 Histopathology

One of the more sensitive indicators of immunotoxicity is immune system histology. The concept of "enhanced histopathology", which refers to the subjective and semi-quantitative evaluation of lymphoid organs and their respective tissue compartments to identify specific changes, is important (Haley *et al.*, 2005; Kuper *et al.*, 2000; Maronpot,

Table 17.4 *Primary histomorphologic divisions of lymphoid organs.*

Bone marrow	Lymph nodes	Spleen	Thymus
Erythroid	Cortex	Marginal zone	Cortex
Fat	Cords	Red pulp	Medulla
Lymphoid	Germinal centres	White pulp	Stroma
Megakaryocytes	High endothelial venules (HEV)	Periarteriolar lymphoid sheath (PALS)	Hassal's corpuscles
Stroma	Lymphoid pollicles	Lymphoid follicles	
	Medulla		
	Paracortex		
	Sinuses		

Adapted with permission from (Haley, 2008) Copyright (2008) John Wiley & Sons.

2006). Conceptually, the approach considers that each lymphoid organ has distinct compartments that might be involved in specific immune functions (Table 17.4) and that the terminology used to describe the histomorphologic changes in these organs should be descriptive rather than interpretive (Haley, 2008). When performed in conjunction with an evaluation of gross anatomic changes, organ weights, haematologic measurements, and clinical chemistry, it does have the potential to determine whether or not exposure to a specific compound could cause modulation of the immune system. It should be noted, however, that drug-induced alterations in immune function can be found in the absence of any histologic change in the immune organs.

Haley (2008) has described several histologic changes and their potential implications. In the spleen, alterations in the periarteriolar lymphoid sheath (PALS) could be suggestive of an immunomodulatory effect. Alterations in red pulp could reflect changes in the circulating lymphoid populations, making the evaluation in conjunction with clinical pathology important. Additionally, alterations in marginal zones (B cells) are associated with effects on antibody responses to T-independent antigens. As usual, there are species-specific differences in tissue architecture that must be factored into the weight of evidence review. For example, the spleen of the rat functions predominantly as a lymphoid organ and so has extensive PALS, follicles, and germinal centres. The nonhuman primate is somewhat similar. On the other hand, the spleen in the dog functions more as a storage and filtering organ for blood and has fewer and smaller PALS and follicles. In the thymus, the most often reported change is cortical atrophy/lymphoid depletion. This may be a direct effect of a drug or can be an indirect effect associated with stress or even a significantly diminished nutritional status associated with decreased food consumption or direct GI toxicity. In addition to stress, reduced food consumption has also been associated with altered bone marrow histology.

An evaluation of the bone marrow can often detect an immunotoxic event, either direct or indirect. Additionally, haematologic findings can indicate that bone marrow should be evaluated. The bone marrow is evaluated to provide information on general cellularity, architecture and morphologic infrastructure. Direct bone marrow toxicity is usually determined by cytologic examination, which can provide a semi-quantitative evaluation of the hematopoietic lineages, including maturation status. Detailed quantification of myeloid and erythroid lineages can aid in the determination of the bone marrow response to a significant peripheral alteration in neutrophils and erythrocytes. For example, an increase in the myeloid:erythroid (M:E) ratio with decreased red cells and normal neutrophils is suggestive of a decrease in red cell production rather than an increase in neutrophil production. This assessment can be made histologically or by flow cytometry (Figure 17.2; see colour section). Finally, disorderly maturation of immature to mature cells can suggest immune-related effects. Disorderly maturation of either myeloid or erythroid precursors can be seen with neoplasias, myelodysplasia, cell- or lineage-specific arrest or toxicity including immune-mediated destruction, chronic inflammation, or recovery from viral infection.

17.2.1.6 Final Evaluation of Immunomodulation from STS

According to ICH S8, the weight of evidence review of STS should include: (1) statistical vs. biological relevance of the findings; (2) severity; (3) dose response relationship (particularly in relation to other drug-related toxicity and the projected clinical/pharmacodynamic exposure); (4) margin of exposure relative to the anticipated clinical exposure or pharmacologic activity; (5) treatment duration; (6) number of species affected; (7) potential for secondary effects mediated by stress or an acute phase response; (8) potential mechanism of action; and (9) reversibility. This approach is no different than that taken for evaluating the toxicity of any other organ system, though it may be somewhat more complicated. Statistically-significant effects do not necessarily indicate biologically-meaningful effects. For example, decreases in circulating leucocyte counts might be statistically signficant without biological consequence: reductions of more than 40% in circulating lymphocytes or of more than 75% in neutrophils could be necessary to produce clinically-significant effects (Hannet *et al.*, 2008; Johansen, 1983; Luster *et al.*, 1993). Typically, when neutrophils numbers drop below 1000/mm^3, patients are at risk for infections.

It is recognized that conditions such as crowding, altered environmental conditions, deprivation of food or water, transportation, isolation, and procedures including immobilization, handling, and some dosing procedures, can have an impact on the immune system (Ader and Cohen, 1993). However, regulatory authorities have made it clear that effects such as thymic atrophy in the presence of decreased body weight or physical activity should not be attributed to stress without adequate additional supporting data. While these effects can in fact be the result of stress, the evidence should be compelling. Such evidence could include the "stress leucogram" (increased circulating neutrophils with decreased lymphocytes) or alterations in thymus, spleen, and/or lymph node cellularity associated with adrenal weight increases and adrenal cortical hyperplasia. Measurement of cotisol in urine (dog, monkey) or serum corticosterone (rat) could also be useful in assessing potential stress effects.

17.2.1.7 Additional Factors to Consider

In addition to findings in STS, other factors to consider include: (1) pharmacologic properties of the test article (e.g., does it have the potential to target the immune system); (2) the intended patient population (e.g., patients immunocompromised due to disease state or other medications, pregnant women, infants or children); (3) structural similarities to known immunomodulators; (4) disposition of the drug (e.g., accumulation in immune tissues): and (5) any available clinical information (Table 17.5). Once all the information is available and all factors have been considered, a determination is made regarding whether a *cause for concern* exists. A finding of sufficient magnitude in any area could trigger additional testing. Multiple findings which may be insufficient alone to be a cause

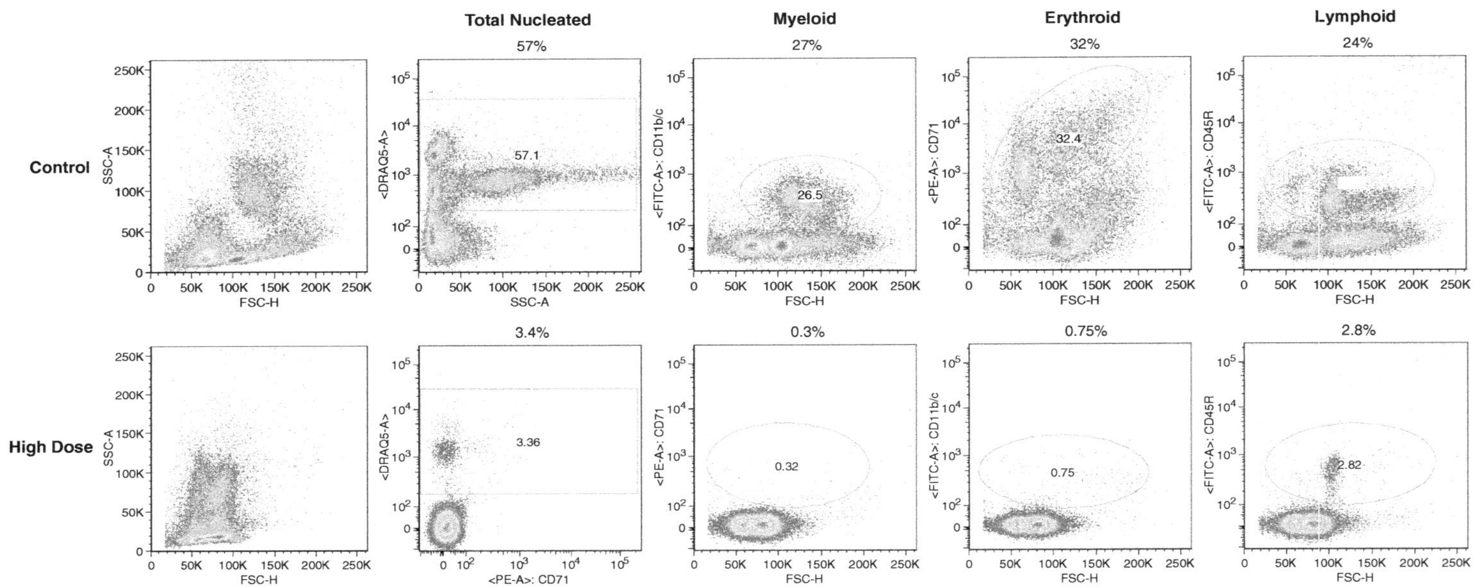

Figure 17.2 *Flow cytometric evaluation of bone marrow. Rats were dosed with the vehicle (control) or a high dose of a cell cycle inhibitor agent. At the end of the study, bone marrow was harvested from the femur and the various lineages in the bone marrow evaluated by flow cytometry. Data provided with the compliments of the Biomarkers Group, Drug Safety Research and Development, Pfizer (San Diego). (Full colour version in plate section.)*

Table 17.5 *Considerations in determining the need for specific immunotoxicity testing.*

Factor	Consideration	Possible methods
Topical administration	Dermal sensitization	LLNA, GPMT, BA
Inhalation administration	Respiratory sensitization	Weight of evidence including LLNA, pulmonary histology
Immunocompromised patients	Immunosuppression	TDAR, phenotyping, CMI, NK
Pregnancy	Developmental immunotoxicity	TDAR and/or CMI with DART evaluation
Accumulation in immune tissue	Immunomodulation	TDAR, phenotyping, CMI, NK
Structural similarity	Immunosuppression	TDAR, phenotyping, CMI, NK
Observations in clinical trials	Immunomodulation	TDAR, phenotyping, CMI, NK

Derived from ICH S8 (ICH, 2006) and FDA (2002). DART = developmental and reproductive toxicity.

for concern could be sufficient when considered together to trigger additional studies. Any decision to not perform additional studies should be scientifically justified.

17.2.1.8 What Assay(s) Should Be Conducted?

There are numerous methods to evaluate test article effects on the immune system (e.g., see Herzyk and Bussiere, 2008). ICH S8 recommends that the immune tests selected should be widely used and demonstrated to be adequately sensitive and specific for known immunosuppressive agents. Assays not fully validated should be scientifically justified and positive controls included, wherever feasible. Immunotoxicology studies should be conducted in compliance with Good Laboratory Practice (GLP) regulations.

When considering how to assess effects on the immune system, methods should be selected based on findings in STS and what is known about the biology/pharmacology of the test article. The T-dependent antibody response (TDAR) assay is most often recommended since it covers the functionality of multiple cell types (antigen presentation, T cells, B cells). If specific cell types are known to be affected, functional evaluation of these cells should be conducted if possible. If the cell type is known to participate in the TDAR, then this assay should be sufficient. Sheep erythrocytes (sRBC), keyhole limpet haemocyanin (KLH), and tetanus toxoid (TT) are the most commonly used and accepted antigens for the TDAR assay. Regardless of how standardized the antigen is, the assay should be optimized in each laboratory in terms of dose, route, and time-course of response. Study designs for stand-alone TDARs in rodents are shown in Figure 17.3a and b. Additionally, modifications to the plaque assay can be made to evaluate the effect of a drug on the T-independent antibody response (TIAR), an assay that might be considered when a drug specifically targets B cells.

To assess test article effects on cell-mediated immunity (CMI), the cytotoxic T cell response (CTL) or a delayed hypersensitivity response (DTH) assays would be appropriate. The CTL assay measures the ability of splenic T cells to recognize and lyse allogeneic target cells (e.g., tumour cells). The DTH assay evaluates test article effects on the ability of memory T cells to recognize foreign antigen with influx of radiolabelled inflammatory cells into the sensitization site as the experimental endpoint.

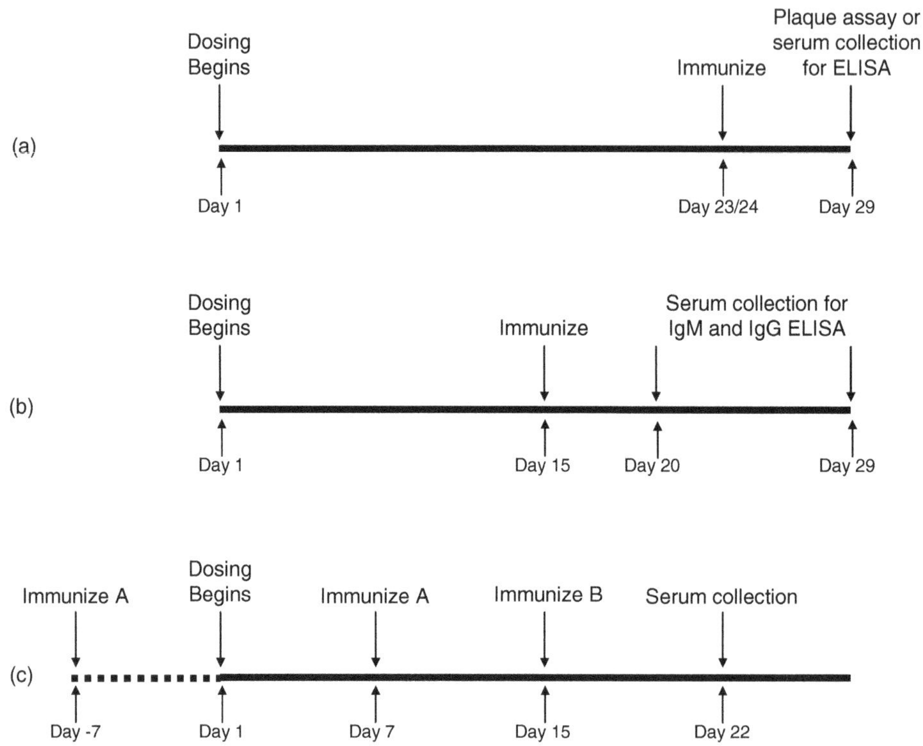

Figure 17.3 *Representative study designs for evaluation of the T-dependent antibody response (TDAR). (a) Rats are immunized on Day 23 or 24 of study with either sRBC or KLH by the intravenous route. For the sRBC antigen, spleens are harvested and the plaque assay performed on the day of study termination. For either sRBC or KLH, serum is taken at the end of the study for evaluation of the anti-antigen antibody response. Note that the time to peak response may be different for an ELISA vs. the plaque assay so simultaneous measurement of these end-points may necessarily require that one be performed at a slightly sub-optimal time and often it is the ELISA. These timelines are representative of the experience of one individual. Immunization conditions (concentration, route, day of evaluation) should be optimized in the laboratory. (b) In this scenario, antigen challenge occurs mid-study and animals are bled twice (approximately Days 20 and 29) for evaluation of the primary IgM (Day 20) and IgG (Day 29) antibody response. (c) A comprehensive TDAR evaluation in nonhuman primates involves immunization pre-study and two weeks later with one antigen (e.g., KLH) to evaluate impact of the drug on the anti-antigen 1 secondary (IgG) response, and immunization with a second antigen (e.g., TT) during the second week of dosing to evaluate the impact of the drug on the anti-antigen 2 primary (IgM, primary IgG) immune response.*

Innate immunity encompasses immunologic responses that do not require prior exposure to an antigen. These responses include recognition of virus or intracellular bacteria-infected cells and tumour cells by NK cells, phagocytosis of pathogens by macrophages, and the activity of neutrophils. This arm of the immune system can be evaluated using the natural killer (NK) cell assay or by evaluating macrophage or neutrophil function. An evaluation of NK cell function could be warranted if there is an increase in viral infection rates or if immunophenotyping shows a significant drop in NK cell numbers. NK cell assays are typically *ex vivo* evaluations of tumour cell lysis.

Test article effects on macrophage and neutrophil function can be evaluated by determining ability to phagocytose particulates *in vitro* (drug exposure *in vitro*) or *ex vivo* (drug exposure *in vivo*). Effects on macrophage and neutrophil function can also be evaluated *in vivo* with the reticuloendothelial system assay for clearance of intravenously-injected radiolabelled antigen (e.g., ^{51}Cr-sRBCs). Finally, oxidative burst, chemotaxis, or cytolytic activity can be measured *in vitro* or *ex vivo* for additional functional evaluation of both macrophages and neutrophils. Flow cytometry methods can also be used to assess these functions.

Although functional evaluation of the immune system is generally considered to be a more sensitive predictor of immunotoxicity than non-functional evaluation, when performed in conjunction with at least two functional tests, non-functional evaluations such as the enumeration of lymphocyte subsets (immunophenotyping) can greatly enhance the detection of immunotoxic chemicals (Iciek, 2008). In the absence of specific functional tests, test article effects on specific immune cells by flow cytometry (either in STS or in a stand-alone study) can provide useful information that could be directly adapted for use in clinical trials (see Figure 17.4; see colour section). Immunophenotyping also can be performed by immunohistochemical staining (IHC): an advantage to this method is that tissues from STS can be evaluated retrospectively. An important challenge with IHC is the need to develop methods that reverse changes produced during tissue fixation, particularly when using cross-linking fixatives such as formalin (Ward *et al.*, 2006). Approximately 85% of antigens fixed in formalin require some type of antigen retrieval for proper ICH. Immunochemical reagents are becoming available for nonrodent animals commonly used in drug development (see Figure 17.5; see colour section). ICH can look at cell types in specific organs so results can be interpreted in close conjunction with histologic effects, while flow cytometric methods offer the potential to better enumerate the cell types compared to IHC and can do this in a temporal manner rather than taking a snapshot at the end of the study. One disadvantage of flow cytometry is that immune cells in circulation represent a small percentage of total lymphocytes and might not indicate effects in lymphoid organs.

Host resistance assays are recommended in ICH S8 as a potential follow-on assay if a cause for concern is identified. Few laboratories have the capability to adequately perform these studies, however, and they are technically challenging and costly. In host resistance studies, it is important to consider the following: (1) strain, route of administration, and challenge size of the pathogen; (2) strain, age, and sex of the host; (3) physiological state of the host and the pathogen; (4) time of challenge with the pathogen (prior to, during, or after drug exposure); and (5) the potential for a direct effect of the drug on the pathogen. As with other immune function tests, no single host resistance model can predict overall immunocompetence of the host, primarily because each model uses different mechanisms for elimination of various pathogens. However, when the affected cells or the altered immune functions are known, the choice of the host resistance model can be made accordingly.

17.2.1.9 General Aspects of Study Design

In general, immunotoxicology studies should be conducted in compliance with Good Laboratory Practice (GLP) regulations, recognizing that this is not always feasible for some

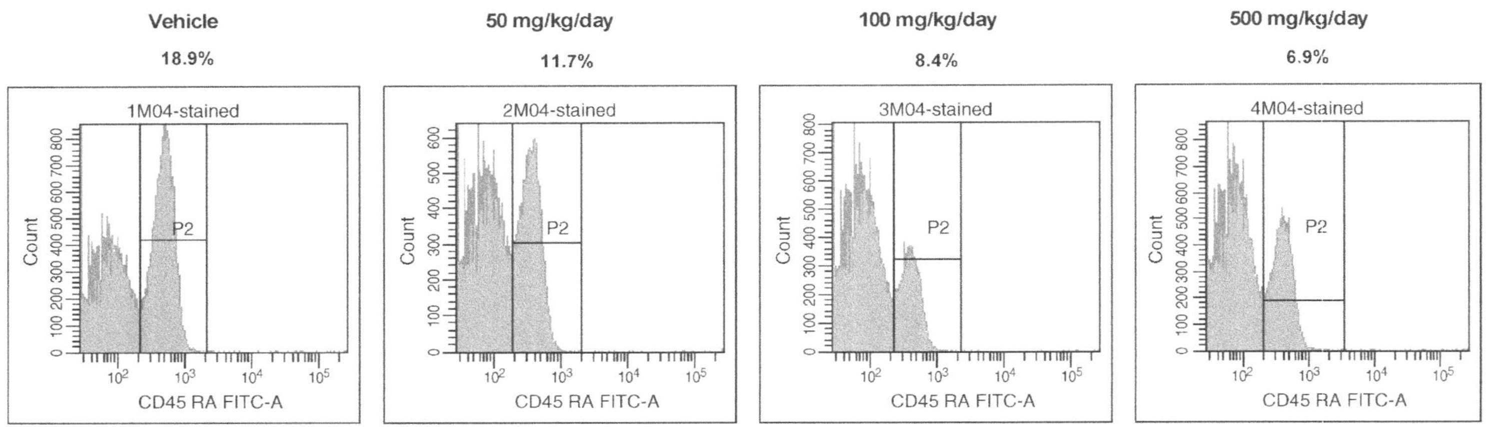

Figure 17.4 *Immunophenotyping evaluation of drug-induced alteration in circulating B cells. Rats were treated for two weeks with increasing concentrations of a drug which demonstrated altered splenic histology in the marginal zone region in a standard toxicology study. Data provided with the compliments of the Biomarkers Group, Drug Safety Research and Development, Pfizer (San Diego). (Full colour version in plate section.)*

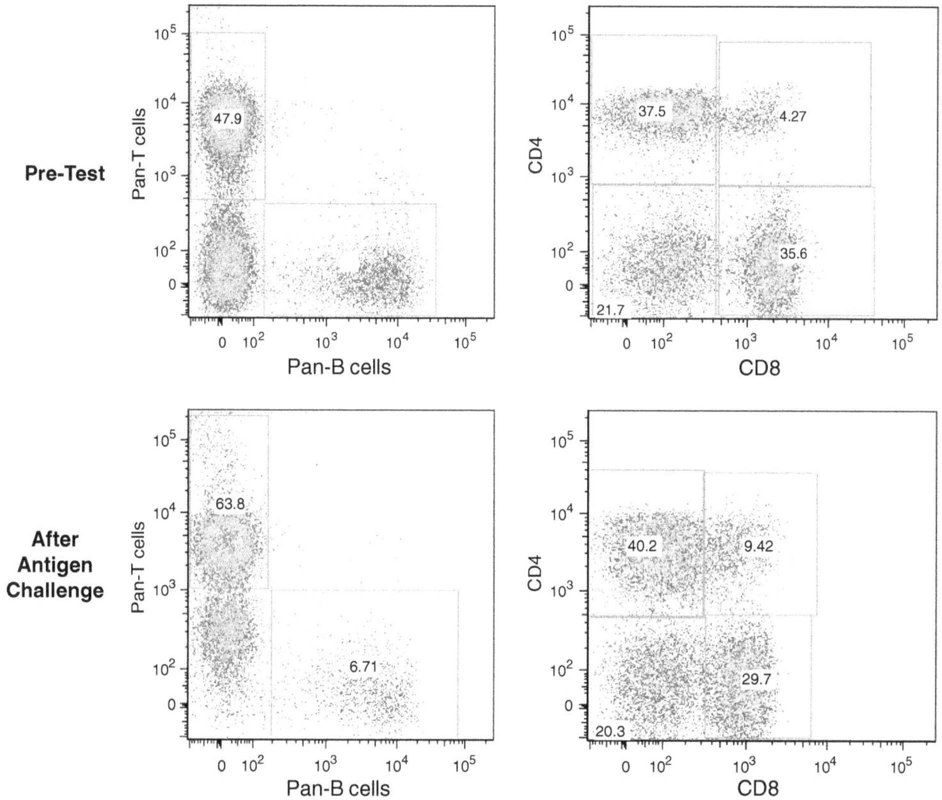

Figure 17.5 Evaluation of hypersensitivity response in dogs. Dogs which were determined to be hypersensitive to a specific allergen were challenged with the allergen and the changes in peripheral T and B cell populations were evaluated in an effort to develop potential biomarkers for future therapeutic intervention studies. Data provided with the compliments of the Biomarkers Group, Drug Safety Research and Development, Pfizer (San Diego). (Full colour version in plate section.)

specialized assays. In general, the conditions of the immunotoxicology study (dose, duration, route of administration, species) should be consistent with, to the extent possible, the nonclinical study in which the potential adverse immune effect was observed. If the STS did not include a period of non-exposure (e.g., recovery phase), then this should be included in an immunotoxicity assessment. For rodents, a sufficient number of animals should be used to allow for an appropriate evaluation of the end-points, typically 8–10 per sex. For nonhuman primates this is often 3–4 per sex but could be more depending on the nature of the end-point needing evaluation. Both sexes should be evaluated unless scientifically justified. Testing to an MTD is not recommended due to the potential to induce secondary immunologic effects as a result of stress. ICH S8 notes that the high dose should, however, be above the no observed adverse effect level (NOAEL) and below a level that would potentially cause secondary toxicity. Ideally, a last one dose level should provide a significant margin of exposure above the projected clinically-efficacious concentration. Thus, it is recommended to obtain pharmacokinetic data from stand-alone immunotoxicity studies.

Sponsors may wish to incorporate immune end-points into subchronic or chronic studies. This is acceptable with the understanding that some of the doses could induce secondary toxicity. When adding immunotoxicity end-points in rodent studies, it may be advisable that these be performed in a satellite group of animals. This recommendation is driven primarily by the potential of immune manipulation to impact and possibly confound pathology end-points. The ability to "read around" the immune manipulation is still somewhat controversial and therefore the satellite groups are generally preferred.

Finally, if a cause for concern is identified after the weight of evidence review, the question remains regarding when to conduct any additional studies, should they be warranted (Figure 17.6). Typically, these studies should be completed prior to the initiation of large-scale clinical trials, generally considered to be before the start of Phase 3. Earlier initiation of this testing might be considered based on the nature of the effects observed during the weight of evidence review and the type of testing that could be required clinically should positive effects be observed in the immunotoxicity evaluation. For example, if clinical methods need to be developed or validated prior to initiation of Phase 3, an earlier investigation could help prevent discontinuous clinical development.

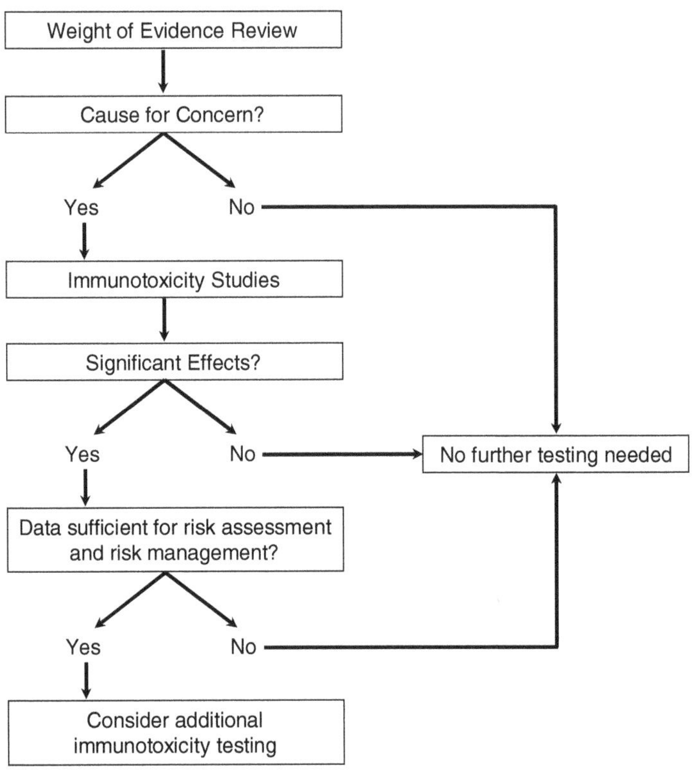

Figure 17.6 *Steps in the evaluation of unintended adverse immunomodulation. Derived from ICH S8 (ICH, 2006).*

17.2.2 Hypersensitivity

ICH S8 focuses on unintended adverse immunomodulation of the immune system, primarily immunosuppression and inflammation. Other aspects of immunotoxicity are not specifically covered (e.g., hypersensitivity, autoimmunity). However, the FDA (2002) does retain guidance on the immunotoxicological evaluation of investigational new drugs which considers both of these possible drug-related effects in addition to several other factors that may require special consideration in assessing a potential cause for concern.

Hypersensitivity refers to antigen-specific immunological reactions that have adverse effects. Small molecular weight drugs can become allergenic if they or their metabolite(s) covalently bind to proteins. Clinically, adverse drug responses are classified as Type A (predictable; 80% of all reactions) or Type B, which are unpredictable, non-immune or immune-mediated, and generally occur in predisposed individuals. For Type B reactions which appear to be immune-mediated, the Gel and Coombs classification system can be used to consider the potential mechanism. Type 1 reactions (immediate hypersensitivity) are mediated by IgE in humans, and for drug development can be subdivided into respiratory (asthma and asthma-like) and systemic responses (anaphylaxis, urticaria). Type 2 reactions are mediated by IgM and/or IgG with the pathologic result being antibody-mediated cellular cytotoxicity (ADCC) and/or complement activation and complement-dependent cytolysis. Type 3 reactions are mediated by IgG with immune complex deposition, and complement activation leading to tissue destruction. Finally, Type 4 reactions are mediated by T cells and are usually associated with delayed hypersensitivity responses.

17.2.2.1 Type 1, Immediate Hypersensitivity (Systemic, Respiratory)

To date, there are no accepted definitive, validated animal models to predict Type 1 hypersensitivity. Passive cutaneous anaphylaxis (PCA), active cutaneous anaphylaxis (ACA), and active systemic anaphylaxis (ASA) assays have been used to detect allergenic proteins but have not proven to be useful in the identification of small molecular weight drugs capable of causing drug allergy. These assays are not recommended for drug development (FDA, 2002).

Maybe the most common hypersensitivity reaction in humans is pseudoallergy, possibly comprising up to 77% of so-called hypersensitivity reactions (Demoly *et al.*, 1999). Pseudoallergic (anaphylactoid) reactions are occasionally observed in nonclinical studies and may result from activation of inflammatory mechanisms independent of the drug or antigen-dependent immune response (FDA, 2002). These reactions can be dose-related and are often associated with facial swelling, rapid or laboured breathing, rash/flushing, and/or drop in blood pressure (much like Type 1 hypersensitivity), and can be treated with antihistamines. For intravenous drugs, pseudoallergic responses can occasionally be elicited simply based on the rate of infusion of the drug. Pseudoallergy can generally be distinguished from Type 1 (IgE-mediated) allergy by demonstrating direct histamine-releasing potential using a basophil activation test or by measuring complement split products in the serum.

Immune-mediated systemic drug allergy is not common (estimated incidence of 0.01 to 0.1%) though some drugs do cause immune-related reactions in 5–10% of treated patients (Alvestad, *et al.*, 2007; Demoly and Bousquet, 2001; Pieters, 2008). Clinical manifestations include anaphylaxis, fever, cutaneous reactions, difficulty breathing, and blood dyscrasias. The aetiology of systemic hypersensitivity is considered to be very complex, which has led to its description as idiopathic immune-mediated drug-related hypersensitivity (IDRH). Most FIH-enabling nonclinical studies will not provide obvious signs of potential IDRH, though evidence of immune activation, inflammation, or altered haematologic profiles might need to be considered (FDA, 2002). Pieters (2008) describes a tiered strategy to evaluate test article potential for IDHR. The sponsor sequentially evaluates structural alerts, covalent binding potential, formation of reactive metabolites, potential to induce apoptosis, outcome of an *in vitro* basophil activation test, and signs from toxicology studies. Additionally, an *in vitro* screen in a panel of human T cell clones to identify potential for cross-reactivity could be used.

To date, there are no standardized, validated methods to evaluate the ability of drugs to cause respiratory hypersensitivity. Traditionally, guinea pigs have been used to assess respiratory hypersensitivity (Karol *et al.*, 1981; Karol *et al.*, 1985). While much has been learned about pulmonary hypersensitivity using the guinea pig model, it is not useful for routine drug safety assessment.

Assessment of respiratory sensitizing potential can be made in a tiered manner using standard toxicology studies and a sensitization test with the goal of using a weight of evidence approach to identify a cause for concern (Burns-Naas *et al.*, 2005; Maier, 2008). Adaptations of assays used to evaluate contact sensitization have been evaluated for their ability to predict respiratory sensitization. For example, the murine local lymph node assay (LLNA) and the mouse IgE test (MIGET) have been used to detect respiratory sensitizers. The MIGET has not been shown to reproducibly detect IgE production when relatively non-reactive drugs have been tested (FDA, 2002) and cytokine profiling to distinguish respiratory from contact allergens still remains somewhat controversial (Lebrec *et al.*, 2001; Ulrich *et al.*, 2001). The LLNA is currently considered to have the greatest potential as an adjunct test to predict respiratory hypersensitivity potential. A positive in the LLNA should only be considered suggestive of respiratory sensitizing potential since the route of exposure in the LLNA is dermal, the vehicle is generally different, and the inhalation dose in humans could fall well below the dermal sensitization threshold. Additional data are needed to support any conclusion based on results obtained with the LLNA.

Histomorphologic evaluation of the respiratory tract in STS can provide insights into test article sensitizing potential. Pathologic changes suggestive of sensitization that occur in the respiratory tract include accumulation of mononuclear cells or eosinophils and/or T cells, excessive mucus associated with goblet cell hyperplasia, as well as smooth muscle hypertrophy and hyperplasia indicative of airway remodelling. These structural changes have been observed in animals exposed to known respiratory allergens (Arts *et al.*, 1998; Pauluhn, 2003; Pauluhn *et al*,, 1995; Pauluhn *et al.*, 2000; Pauluhn and Mohr, 2005; Pauluhn *et al.*, 2005; Zhang *et al.*, 2004). Additional information that would be considered useful include test article protein reactivity, thiol-redox potential, dermal irritation, and/or quantitative whole body autoradiography (QWBA). A similar tiered approach has previously been proposed by Sarlo and Clark (1992) though that specific method was more useful for highly-reactive molecules and not for drug safety evaluation (FDA, 2002). If, after a weight of evidence review, there is a cause for concern and additional testing is deemed necessary, modifications of the inhalation induction and challenge methods described by Karol *et al.* (1985) could be used.

17.2.2.2 Types 2 and 3, Antibody-Mediated Cytotoxicity and Immune Complex-Mediated Hypersensitivity

As described in the FDA guidance (FDA, 2002), both Type 2 and Type 3 hypersensitivity responses can have similar presentations in both animals and humans, including anaemia, thrombocytopenia, vasculitis, glomerulonephritis, and pneumonitis. Additionally, some drugs can also generate multiple types of hypersensitivity response. Penicillin, for example, can induce all four types of hypersensitivity. Penicillin-induced blood dyscrasias can occur due to the production of IgG against penicillin metabolites bound to the surface of red blood cells (Type 2) and has also been implicated in Type 3 reactions leading to serum-sickness-like symptoms.

Type 2 reactions result when drug and/or metabolites bind to the target cells and produce hapten–protein complexes from which an immune response is generated. Tissue damage can result from the direct action of cytotoxic cells or by antibody activation of complement.

The distinquishing feature of Type 3 reactions is that immunoglobulin production is against soluble circulating antigen (Burns-Naas *et al.*, 2001). Schnyder and Pichler (2009) note that the formation of immune complexes usually occurs without symptoms. However, on rare occasions, complexes can bind to endothelial cells, resulting in immune complex deposition with complement activation. This could result in tissue damage in areas where immune complexes are deposited, most commonly the vascular endothelium in the lung, joints, and kidneys. The skin and circulatory systems might also be involved. In STS, signs of Type 3 hypersensitivity include immune complex disease (ICD), serum sickness, drug-induced lupus, and vasculitis (Schnyder and Pichler, 2009).

Type 2 and Type 3 reactions are rarely modelled in nonclinical species and signs from STS suggestive of these responses are more likely to be the result of a direct, non-immune mediated drug toxicity (FDA, 2002). Additionally, there are no nonclinical methods that are considered to be predictive of either Type 2 or Type 3 hypersensitivity reactions in humans. Anaemia in nonclinical studies with no other potential explanation (e.g., haemorrhage) can be the result of an immune-mediated mechanism (e.g., immune-mediated haemolytic anaemia, IMHA). IMHA might present with moderate to severe anaemia, marked reticulocytosis, increased numbers of spherocytes, autoagglutination, Heinz bodies, red cells in macrophages, and possibly leukocytosis (Krishnaraj, 2008). A diagnostic test for IMHA is the direct Coomb's test which measures the presence of polyclonal anti-RBC antibodies or complement on the surface of RBC. Immune-related vasculitis can be diagnosed by examining affected tissues immunohistologically for the presence of IgM and/or IgG and complement. Immune complex deposition could be further confirmed with electron microscopy.

17.2.2.3 Type 4, Delayed-Type Hypersensitivity

All drugs administered by the dermal route should be assessed for their potential to produce delayed-type hypersensitivity (allergic contact dermatitis, ACD). This assessment is generally not dependent on results obtained in STS, though redness at the site of application or histology suggestive of inflammation at the site should be taken as a potential indicator. Unlike the other forms of hypersensitivity, methods available to assess Type 4 potential are validated and well-accepted internationally, and utilize either guinea pigs or mice. The Buehler Assay (BA) and the guinea pig maximization test (GPMT) are highly reliable and have demonstrated high correlation with known human dermal sensitizers. The split-adjuvant and Draize tests are also acceptable, though generally used less often. Within the past decade, the LLNA has found broad acceptance as an alternative to the guinea pig tests and it is now used as a stand-alone test. It has a key advantage over the guinea pigs studies in that it can be used without adjuvants, coloured materials do not interfere with the assessment and, most importantly, it provides quantitative (rather than subjective) results that can be used to compare across compounds (e.g., across studies). A positive control should always be included and individual animal data should be reported. Notably, for development of dermal drugs some regulatory agencies require separate testing of the drug substance (active pharmaceutical ingredient, API), excipient(s), and final formulation (FDA, 2002).

17.2.2.4 Special Types of Drug Hypersensitivity

Other types of drug hypersensitivity reactions that do not belong clearly to the Gell and Coombs classification have also to be considered. These are immune mediated drug-induced hepatitis and severe cutaneous reactions including Steven-Johnson syndrome (SJS) and toxic epidermal necrolysis (TEN). In the case of drug-induced hepatitis, the effectors of cytotoxicity are antibodies directed to the drug but also drug-specific cytotoxic T-lymphoctes although only the former have been identified in patients. SJS and TEN are clearly mediated by CD8+ cytotoxic T-lymphocytes directed to drug expressed on keratinocytes.

17.2.2.5 Photosensitization

Photoallergic reactions with drugs are very rare. Only a few drugs administered systemically have been well documented to be photoallergenic, and include carprofen, chlorpromazine, fluoroquinolones, ketoprofen, promethazine, sulfanilamide, and tiaprofenic acid. Notably, these compounds are also known to be photoirritants. Photoactivation of a drug results in a covalent binding metabolite (e.g., the hapten) which binds to proteins and acts as a sensitizer. After a period of approximately 1–2 weeks after beginning a drug, a patient gets exposed to sunlight and subsequently experiences a hypersensitivity response that can vary from mild redness to bulbous or macropappular rash with itching.

The formation of a photoallergen occurs by the same mechanisms that induce phototoxicity. Thus, photoallergy is simply a special form of phototoxicity. Photoallergens would be expected to also be phototoxicants and this conclusion is supported by studies with known photoallergens (Bec *et al.*, 1986; de Vries *et al.*, 1990; Pendlington and Barratt, 1990; Tokura, 1998; Miranda *et al.*, 1999; Lovell and Jones, 2000; Tokura, 2000). There are no nonclinical models available that can be recommended to determine test article photoallergic potential.

17.2.3 Autoimmunity

In Gell and Coombs Types 2 and 3 hypersensitivity reactions, host tissues are damaged by their own immune system, creating autoimmune-like disease. In those situations, unaltered self antigens are not the target of the immune mechanisms but damage occurs to cells bearing hapten on membranes or to cells in close proximity to antigen–antibody complexes. Although the resulting pathology may be the same for autoimmune reactions and hypersensitivity, mechanisms of true autoimmune disease are different from hypersensitivity. In cases of autoimmunity, self antigens are the target, and in the case of chemical-induced autoimmunity, it is a modification of host tissues or immune cells by the chemical and not the chemical acting as an antigen/hapten that induces the disease state (Burns-Naas *et al.*, 2001). Often the pathologies observed can have similar presentations to Types 2 and 3 hypersensitivities, including haemolytic anaemia, vasculitis, and glomerulonephritis. At present, there are no standardized methods available that are predictive of the ability of the test article to cause autoimmunity in humans (FDA, 2002). Both the popliteal lymph node assay (PLNA) and the lymphocyte transformation test (LTT) have been proposed as potential screening tools for autoimmunity, but as yet no data are available to support the usefulness of either assay. Similarly, screening for autoantibody production in a nonclinical study can be performed but this has not been shown to be predictive.

17.3 Special Considerations

17.3.1 Immunomodulatory Drugs

ICH S8 was conceived to address "unintended" adverse immunomodulation. In addition to specifying the exclusion of hypersensitivity and autoimmunity, ICH S8 excludes consideration of *intentional* immunomodulators. Additional testing to evaluate off-target or unexpected immunological effects should be made on a case-by-case basis (Piccotti *et al.*, 2009). While some information to make this assessment can come from STS, additional information is likely to be available from discovery pharmacology studies, exploratory studies, and an evaluation of the available literature. In the case of an unprecedented mechanism where little may be known, sponsors might decide to conduct additional evaluations which could be done prior to or in conjunction with FIH-enabling studies. Additional causes for concern with immunomodulators include non-reversibility of effects (all studies with immunomodulators should evaluate the reversibility of effects), potential patient populations (e.g., children, elderly, those predisposed to infection), unacceptably low margin of exposure for the unexpected effects and, possibly, immunostimulators (e.g., for cytokine release).

To date, there is no consensus regarding which studies provide the most value in assessing potential clinical risk from immunomodulators, including lack of agreement on the value of host resistance assays (Piccotti *et al.*, 2009). However, if there is clear cause of concern, these studies should be considered.

17.3.2 Biopharmaceuticals

Many biopharmaceuticals act directly on the immune system or have secondary effects that alter immune function. For biotherapeutics, evaluation of immunotoxicity using a classical tiered approach or routine testing batteries more commonly employed for small molecule therapeutics and environmental chemicals is not generally recommended (ICH, 2011). Similarly, a standard approach such as that described in ICH S8, where immunologic assessment is driven by a weight of evidence review, identification of causes for concern, and an evaluation of data for human risk evaluation/management, is also not recommended to be generally employed for routine evaluation of protein therapeutics. Rather, an immunotoxic evaluation is likely to be conducted as an integral part of the overall pharmacologic assessment of the agent (Brennan *et al.*, 2010; Hastings, 2008).

Of interest though, as drug developers exploit more and more novel targets, the likelihood is lower that the biology of those targets is fully understood such that early pharmacology studies could have adequately explored potential immune modulation. So while biopharmaceuticals are specifically excluded from the scope of ICH S8 and immunotoxicity testing of biopharmaceuticals should continue to be considered on a case-by-case basis, the general approach described in ICH S8 does provide an initial assessment of the potential of the test article to cause unintended or unexpected immunomodulation. Flow cytometry, for example, can be used to evaluate functional competency of the immune system by evaluating NK cell activity, apoptosis, oxidative burst, cellular activation, cytokine secretion, and phagocytosis.

More often, though, functional immunological evaluation for biotherapeutics is performed using the TDAR in nonhuman primates (NHPs). This typically involves immunizing with KLH or tetanus toxoid (TT) and measuring the antigen-specific antibody response in serum using an enzyme-linked immunosorbant assay (ELISA). As described by Bussiere (2008) and represented in Figure 17.3c, the most comprehensive evaluation of the TDAR in NHPs utilizes both antigens over the course of treatment. The difficulty with immunomodulatory assessment in NHPs is that numbers of animals in each group are limited (often 3–4/sex/group), there are no consistent protocols for evaluation of the immune response (in particular the TDAR) in NHPs, the timing of incorporation of endpoints into GLP studies varies, the assays in NHPs are less well-characterized than in rodents, and the variability is greater. The geographical source of animals has also been shown to have significant impact on the variability of immune assessments; therefore, it is important to maintain the same source (e.g., Chinese, Mauritius) throughout the drug development programme.

17.3.2.1 Cytokine Release Syndrome (CRS)

CRS is a potential adverse effect attributed to cellular release of pro-inflammatory cytokines (e.g., TNF-α, IL-6, IFNγ, IL-8, IFNα) that might occur following intravenous infusion of protein biotherapeutics. CRS can be the result of: (1) direct stimulation of immune cells (e.g., OKT3; TGN1412); (2) NK cell activation as a result of antibody-dependent cellular cytotoxicity (ADCC) (e.g., Campath); (3) complement activation resulting from complement-dependent cytotoxicity (CDC) (e.g., rituximab); (4) tumour lysis syndrome (e.g., rituximab); or (5) protein load (e.g., IVIG) (Bugelski *et al.*, 2009; Brennan *et al.*, 2010; Vidal *et al.*, 2010). The potential of immunostimulatory biotherapeutics to induce CRS is highlighted with the unfortunate events associated with the first-in-human (FIH) clinical trial with TGN1412, a CD28 agonist IgG4 monocloncal antibody, when six healthy male volunteers suffered the most severe and life-threatening form of CRS (known as "cytokine storm"), and became critically ill (Suntharalingam *et al.*, 2006). Although CRS can be observed in appropriately-designed nonclinical toxicology studies, "cytokine storm" related to therapeutic protein administration has been primarily observed in humans. To date, no nonclinical method has been shown to predict CRS. Therefore, there are no regulatory guidelines or requirements for evaluation of CRS potential for therapeutics known to stimulate the immune system.

Table 17.6 *Possible risk factors associated with cytokine release by protein therapeutics.*

Attribute	Risk factor
Functional	Ligand on cytokine-producing cell Mimics or elicits "danger signal" to active innate immune system Activity mediated (all/part) by ADCC
Structural	Potential to bind and/or crosslink target(s), including multifunctional therapeutics Human IgG1 > rat IgG2b > human IgG4 Murine IgG2a Affinity for Fcγ receptors
Patient population	High target expression, high tumour burden

References used to derive considerations in this table include: Wing *et al.*, 1996; Lazar *et al.*, 2006; Gribble *et al.*, 2007; Kiewe and Thiel, 2008; Lordick *et al.*, 2008; and Brennan *et al.*, 2010.

Table 17.6 contains a list of risk factors which might suggest a potential for a biotherapeutic to produce CRS (Vidal *et al.*, 2010). *In vivo* evaluation of CRS can be difficult since cytokine release is temporal, not all cytokines necessarily follow the same temporal profile, some cytokine modulation may be normal for target modulation, and there could be species-restriction for the protein therapeutic. This is particularly true for the prediction of cytokine storm, and it is generally accepted that there are no good nonclinical models to predict this most severe form of CRS. If the intended therapeutic target is related to the immune system, careful evaluation of interspecies differences in relation to the biological effects of the target is mandatory in Europe before clinical studies (CHMP, 2007).

17.3.2.2 Immunogenicity, Anti-Drug Antibodies, and Generalized Systemic Immune Complex Disease (ICD)

The immunogenicity of protein therapeutics is generally considered to be most importantly associated with alterations in pharmacokinetics and pharmacodynamics. However, development of anti-drug antibodies (ADA) and formation of immune complexes that deposit in tissues can lead to specific pathologies in animal studies. In STS, immune complex deposition in the vascular endothelium in the lungs, joints, kidneys, and/or skin could result in inflammatory responses due to activation of complement, and recruitment of macrophages and neutrophils, producing tissue damage (Kumar *et al.*, 2010).

In animals with systemic ICD, lethargy, fever, rash, vomiting, hypoactivity, ataxia, and changes in food consumption can be observed. Clinical signs can include one, all, or a combination of the following: lethargy, fever, rash, vomiting, hypoactivity, ataxia, and changes in food consumption, and can occur as early as 7–10 days after an initial dose, or more acutely within minutes to a few hours after the administration of subsequent doses in an animal that has been sensitized by the initial dose. Clinical pathology signs suggestive of ICD include increased or decreased white cells, increased fibrinogen, reduced serum albumin, increased serum globulin, and proteinuria. In more severe cases of ICD, animals may have signs of disseminated intravascular coagulopathy (DIC) with reduced peripheral blood platelet counts and increased coagulation times (PT, APTT). DIC can be confirmed with an evaluation of fibrin split products, d-dimers, C-reactive protein and complement split products, end-points which can be included in clinical trials. Correlation of these data with ADA data can add to the weight of evidence for DIC.

Histologically, the renal glomerulus is a primary location for complex deposition, though lesions may be present in other tissues. If light microscopic inflammatory lesions consistent with ICD are present, other methods can confirm the presence of immune complexes. These include immunohistochemical (IHC) demonstration of the drug co-localized with IgM and/or IgG and complement (Figure 17.7a; see colour section). Positive findings in IHC can be further confirmed with electron microscopy (Figure 17.7b; see colour section). Immune complex formation in animals has not been proved to predict immune complex formation in humans (Kang and Saif, 2007). Nevertheless, test article-related ICD observed in animals should be considered carefully when dosing humans (FDA, 2002).

17.3.3 Drugs in Pregnancy and Children – Developmental Immunotoxicology

17.3.3.1 Regulatory Considerations

The interest in developmental immunotoxicology (DIT) is predicated around the possibility that the immune system may exhibit greater susceptibility (qualitative, quantitative, or temporal) to chemical perturbation during ontological development compared to adults (Burns-Naas *et al.*, 2008). Regulatory agencies have not routinely required assessment of DIT during the development of therapeutic agents. Rather, these assessments are driven by a cause for concern from STS in adult animals, similar to other known immunomodulators, or the potential for neonatal exposure. If a drug can be used in pregnant or lactating women and the drug can cross either the placenta or into breast milk (or when this information is unknown) then a DIT study should be considered (FDA, 2002).

In its guidance on nonclinical testing to support paediatric drug development (CHMP, 2008), the European Committee for Human Medicinal Products (CHMP) recognizes that major developmental differences exist between the immune systems of human neonates/infants and adults, and considers that these developmental differences are generally apparent until age 12. FDAs juvenile testing guidance (FDA, 2006) also recognizes the immune system as one that continues to mature after birth (until approximately 5–12 years of age) and may well be a novel target for drug-induced toxicity.

17.3.3.2 Methods to Assess DIT

Pathology evaluations have been a major end-point of standard nonclinical toxicology tests, and are an appropriate starting point for evaluation of DIT. The type of pathology evaluations used in standard nonclinical toxicology studies can be applied in developmental immunotoxicology studies, but some modifications will probably be required due to the size and age of the animals. For example, haematology evaluations should be given a priority when sample size is limited (Burns-Naas *et al.*, 2008). As with a study in adult animals, a similar list of immunologically-important organs (thymus, spleen, adrenal, liver) should be collected for a DIT assessment.

The histologic features of immune system organs in adult laboratory animals are well known (Dunn, 1954; Haley, 2003), but those features are not as well defined in neonatal animals. As described in Burns-Naas *et al.* (2008), preliminary studies suggest there is a remarkable progression in the histologic appearance of foetal immune system organs in the rat between GD 15 and GD 20. The immune system of the developing rat is

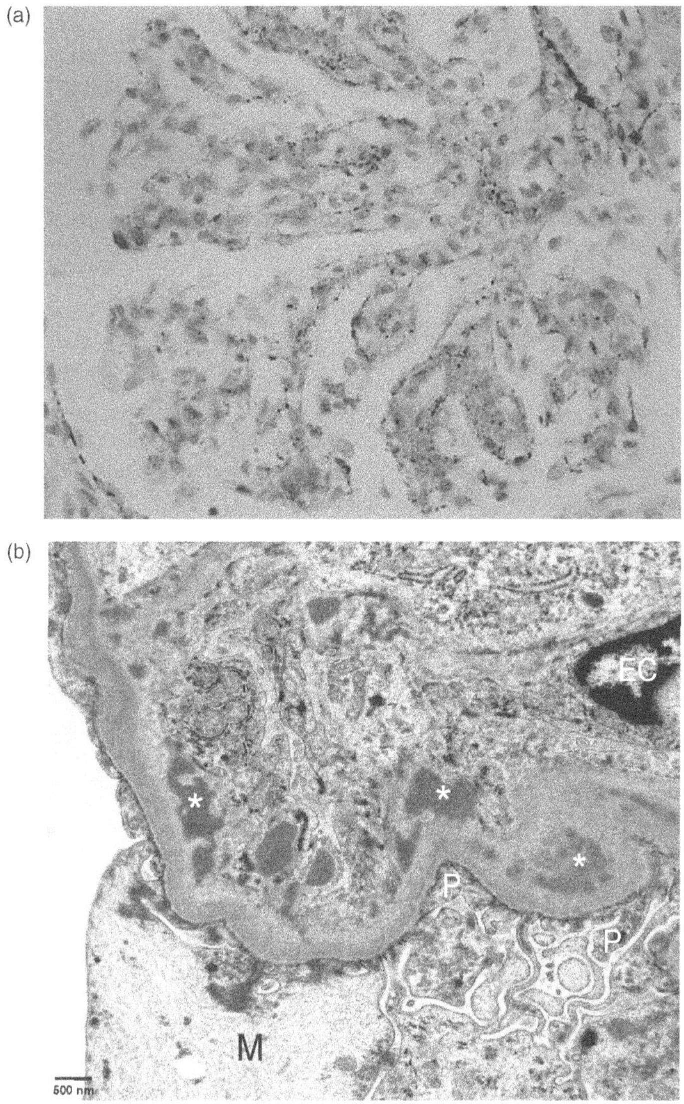

Figure 17.7 *Evaluation of Systemic Immune Complex Disease. (a) Renal glomerulus of Cynomolgus Monkey. Brown-staining granular pigment consistent with immune complex deposits is evident along the contours of the glomerular capillary network (immunohistochemical staining for SC5b-9; 600X). (b) Electron micrograph of renal glomerulus. Many electron-dense, immune-type deposits (*) of variable morphology and sizes are present in the subendothelial region of the glomerular capillary wall. An endothelial cell (EC) is evident projecting into the capillary lumen that is filled with undulating folds of endothelial cellular processes. Mesangial matrix (M) and foot processes (P) of podocytes are evident (5000X). Data with the compliments of Charles River Laboratories and the Pathology Group, Drug Safety Research and Development, Pfizer. (Full colour version in plate section.)*

anatomically intact by PND 22, but histologic features at this stage suggest relative inactivity (lack of stimulation by exogenous antigens). Therefore, histology must be combined with other end-points (e.g., organ weights, haematology, functional evaluation) for a complete evaluation of immune status in juvenile rodents. The developing immune system in nonhuman primates is similar to humans and histology might play a greater role in DIT in the nonhuman primate. However, functional impairment of the developing immune system in the absence of histologic alteration has been reported (Hussain *et al.*, 2005). The TDAR assay probably represents the single best functional test of immunocompetence in the developing immune system. There are several caveats to its use, however. First, the ability to measure a TDAR in non-adult rodents is limited as virtually no response is detectable at PND 10 and a measurable, but a suboptimal, response is detectable at weaning (PND 21) (Kimura *et al.*, 1985; Ladics *et al.*, 2000). The maximal response appears to occur at the point in which rodents reach young adulthood (PND 42–49). This observation is consistent with the differences in immune system development between mammalian species (Burns-Naas *et al.*, 2008; Dietert and Burns-Naas, 2008). Therefore, while it *can* be performed at PND 21, it isn't recommended for use in rodents until PND 42, unless justified scientifically. Because of a different developmental timeline between nonhuman primates and rodents (Burns-Naas *et al.*, 2008; Buse *et al.*, 2003) the TDAR can be used in the nonhuman primate shortly after birth, though a maximum response may take up to three months after birth to fully develop.

An assay for cellular immunity (CTL, CTH, NK) is generally agreed to be important in the overall assessment of DIT, particularly in the rodent because the developmental progression has the cellular response developing earlier postnatally than the humoral. Additionally, there are examples of developmental immunotoxicants which failed to alter the TDAR while significantly altering cellular immunity (Bunn *et al.*, 2001a, 2001b; Gehrs *et al.*, 1997; Karrow *et al.*, 2004; Miller *et al.*, 1998).

17.3.3.3 Study Design and Interpretation

There is consensus that, wherever possible, methods to evaluate the developing immune system be incorporated into existing developmental and reproductive toxicology (DART) protocols (Burns-Naas *et al.*, 2008; Holsapple *et al.*, 2003; Ladics *et al.*, 2005; Burns-Naas, 2012). For drugs in development, this generally means incorporation into either ICH S5 C-F DART or juvenile toxicology studies in rodents (Figure 17.8a), or in the newly-proposed expanded peri- and postnatal development study (PPND) for nonhuman primates (Figure 17.8b).

One key consideration that has been a foundational premise of DIT is that, in order to truly assess the hazard, animals must be exposed throughout all developmental windows. However, for drug development, exposure to the developing system is likely to occur only in two general scenarios: inadvertent exposure *in utero* via dosing the mother, or direct dosing of children to treat a childhood disease. In either case, the goal is to assess developmental effects resulting from these scenarios and not to generally assess a hazard, such as might be the desire when considering unintentional exposure to environmental chemicals. In the rodent, mothers are exposed beginning on GD 6 and continuing through weaning on PND 21 (Figure 17.8a, lower exposure bars). At this point, the pups can be evaluated for immunopathology end-points and a cellular functional assay. Evaluation on PND 21 may be important to understand whether the offspring is potentially

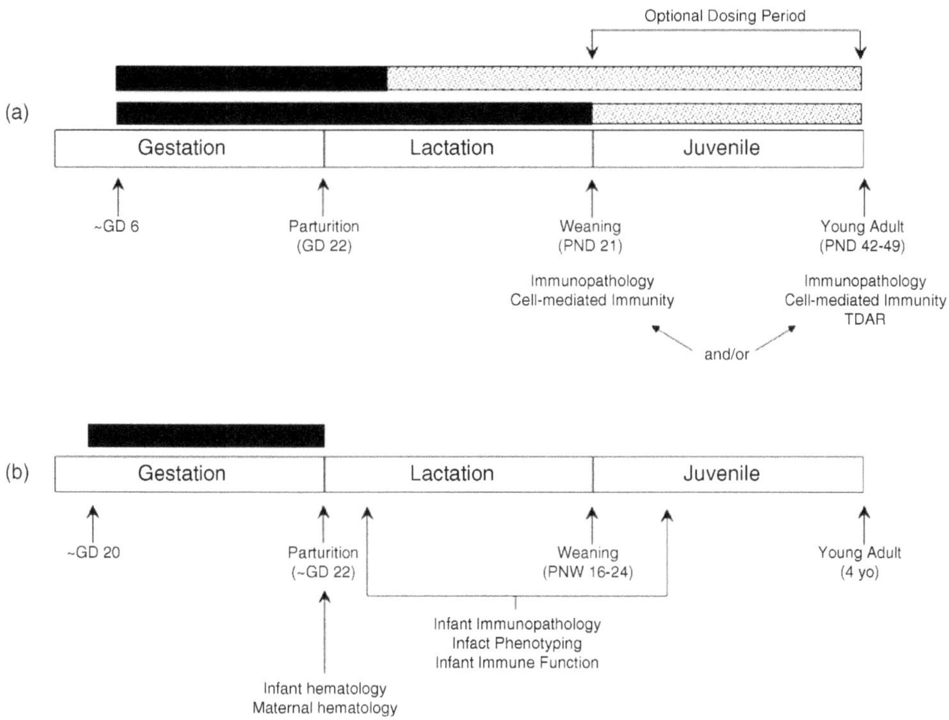

Figure 17.8 *Evaluation of developmental immunotoxicology in rats (A) and nonhuman primates (B). Black bars = maternal dosing; grey bars = direct dosing of rat pups. Derived with permission from (Burns-Naas* et al.*, 2008).*

immunocompromised since children often get their first set of vaccines within the first few weeks after birth. Figure 17.8a also shows an optional period of exposure by direct dosing of pups which might be needed to mimic longer-term exposure to the drug (e.g., to account for possible differences in human and rodent rearing of offspring). In this case, DIT evaluation at PND 42–49 allows full evaluation of immunopathology, a maximal TDAR, and a cellular response (the most rigorous assessment of DIT). Figure 17.8a (top bars) also shows the potential to begin direct dosing of pups on approximately PND 7. This scenario could be used if drug exposure via lactation were unknown, but would need to be considered possible. If the drug is intended for use in children from 0–12 years of age, direct dosing of pups from nontreated dams should begin on PND 7 and continue through PND 42–49 with full DIT assessment at that time. If the drug is intended for children over the age of 12, no DIT assessment is considered necessary as the immune system is considered fully developed at that time.

If DIT needs to be assessed in the nonhuman primate, as would be the case for biopharmaceuticals, mothers are exposed to the drug beginning during the period of organogenesis (approximately GD 20) and through either birth or the first month after birth. At birth, both maternal and infant haematological parameters can be evaluated, if desired.

Beginning at approximately one month after birth, infants can be assessed for immunopathology and immune function. It is important to remember that a negative DIT study (no adverse effects) in the absence of confirming exposure to the offspring is not sufficient, and overexposure resulting from poor high dose selection confounds the ability to determine whether effects are direct or secondary to overt toxicity.

17.4 Summary

Immunotoxicity testing has come a long way since the first Gordon Conference where the potential for drugs to produce toxic effects on the immune system was discussed. For pharmaceuticals in development, there is global agreement that all should be evaluated for potential to produce adverse immunomodulation. For small molecular weight drugs this is generally done through a weight of evidence review and specific studies as needed. For biotherapeutics, potential adverse effects on the immune system are typically evaluated in early pharmacology studies in addition to nonclinical toxicology studies.

Drugs that are developed to intentionally modulate the immune system (e.g., anti-inflammatory agents) should be evaluated on a case-by-case basis. A weight of evidence approach that includes early pharmacologic evaluation can be used to help identify potential off-target toxicity from exaggerated pharmacology. Both the TDAR and flow cytometry have found some utility in this evaluation, but there is significant disagreement in the scientific community over the usefulness of host resistance models.

Pharmaceuticals that are intended to treat children or pregnant women and which are also immunosuppressive should be considered for developmental immunotoxicology testing. With the appropriate design, this could be incorporated into an expanded peri-and postnatal study which could be performed in either rodents or nonhuman primates. Finally, where possible, test article effects on immune system parameters should be assessed as part of general nonclinical toxicology studies. Signs of adverse effects on the immune system should be appropriately addressed consistent with existing science and the 3Rs principles: refinement, reduction, and replacement.

References

Ader, R. and Cohen, N. (1993) Psychoneuroimmunology: conditioning and stress. *Ann. Rev. Psychol.*, **44**, 53–85.

Alvestad, S., Ludersen, S., and Brodtkorb, E. (2007) Rash from anti-epileptic drugs: influence by gender, age, and learning disability. *Epilepsia*, **48**, 1360–1365.

Arts, J.H.E., Kuper, C.F., Spoor, S.M., and Bloksma, N. (1998) Airway morphology and function in rats following dermal sensitization and respiratory challenge with low molecular weight chemicals. *Toxicol. Appl. Pharmacol.*, **152**, 66–76.

Bec, J.L., Lelrieu, P., Abravanel, G., and Paillous, N. (1986) Drug sensitization: photobinding of sulfanilamide to bovine serum albumin. *Photochemistry and Photobiology*, **4**(1), 41–45.

Brennan, F.R., Morton, L.D., Spindeldreher, S. *et al.* (2010) Safety and immunotoxicity assessment of immunomodulatory monocloncal antibodies. *MAbs*, **2**(3), 233–255.

Bugelski, P.J., Achuthanandam, R., Capocasale, R.J. *et al.* (2009) Monoclonal antibody-induced cytokine release syndrome. *Expert Rev. Clin. Immunol.*, **5**(5), 499–521.

Bunn, T.L., Parsons, P.J., Kao, E., and Dietert, R.R. (2001a) Gender-based profiles of developmental immunotoxicity to lead in the rat: assessment in juveniles and adults. *J. Toxicol. Environ. Health A*, **64**(3), 223–240.

Bunn, T.L., Parsons, P.J., Kao, E., and Dietert, R.R. (2001b) Exposure to lead during critical windows of embryonic development: differential immunotoxic outcome based on stage of exposure and gender. *Toxicol. Sci.*, **64**(1), 57–66.

Burns-Naas, L.A., Meade, B.J., and Munson, A.E. (2001) Toxic responses of the immune system, in *Casarett & Doull's Toxicology: The Basic Science of Poisons* (ed. C.D. Klaassen), McGraw-Hill, New York.

Burns-Naas, L.A., Lee, C., Evering, W. *et al.* (2005) Lack of respiratory and contact sensitizing potential of the intranasal antiviral drug candidate rupintrivir (AG7088): a weight-of-the-evidence evaluation. *J. Immunotox.*, **2**, 123–139.

Burns-Naas, L.A., Hastings, K.L., Ladics, G.S. *et al.* (2008) What's so special about the developing immune system? *Int. J. Toxicol.*, **27**, 223–254.

Burns-Naas, L.A. (2012) Developmental immunotoxicity testing, in *Developmental and Reproductive Toxicology: A Practical Approach, 3rd Edition* (ed. R.D. Hood), Informa Healthcare, London.

Buse, J.E., Habermann, G., Osterburg, I. *et al.* (2003) Reproductive/developmental toxicity and immunotoxicity assessment in the nonhuman primate. *Toxicol.*, **221**, 221–227.

Bussiere, J.L. (2008) Relevant immune tests across different species and surrogate molecules, in *Immunotoxicology Strategies for Pharmaceutical Safety Assessment* (eds D.J. Herzyk and J.L. Bussiere), John Wiley & Sons, Inc., Hoboken, NJ.

CHMP (Committee on Medicinal Products for Human Use) (2007) Guideline on strategies to identify and to mitigate risks for first-in human clinical trials with investigational medicinal products, EMA/CHMP/SWP/28367/07

CHMP (Committee on Medicinal Products for Human Use) (2008) Guideline on the need for nonclinical testing in juvenile animals of pharmaceuticals for paediatric indications, EMA/CHMP/SWP/169215/2005

Demoly, P., Leel, B., Messaad, D. *et al.* (1999) Predictive capacity of histamine release for the diagnosis of drug allergy. *Allergy*, **54**, 500–506.

Demoly, P. and Bousquet, J. (2001) Epidemiology of drug allergy. *Curr. Opin. Allergy Clin. Immunol.*, **1**, 302–310.

de Vries, H., Bojarski, J., Donker, A.A. *et al.* (1990) Photochemical reactions of quindoxin, olaquindox, carbadox and cyadox with protein, indicating photoallergic properties. *Toxicology*, **63**, 85–95.

Dietert, R.R. and Burns-Naas, L.A. (2008) Developmental immunotoxicity in rodents, in *Immunotoxicology Strategies for Pharmaceutical Safety Assessment* (eds D.J. Herzyk and J.L. Bussiere), John Wiley & Sons, Inc., Hoboken, NJ.

Dunn, T. (1954) Normal and pathologic anatomy of the reticular tissue in laboratory mice. *Journal of the National Cancer Institute*, **14**, 1281–1433.

Evans, E. (2008) Clinical pathology as crucial insight into immunotoxicity testing, in *Immunotoxicology Strategies for Pharmaceutical Safety Assessment* (eds D.J. Herzyk and J.L. Bussiere), John Wiley & Sons, Inc., Hoboken, NJ.

FDA (2002) Guidance for Industry, Immunotoxicological evaluation of investigational new drugs, Office of New Drugs, Center for Drug Evaluation Research, Food and Drug Administration, U.S. Department of Health and Human Services.

FDA (2006) Guidance for Industry, Nonclinical safety evaluation of pediatric drug products, Office of New Drugs, Center for Drug Evaluation Research, Food and Drug Administration, U.S. Department of Health and Human Services.

Gehrs, B.C., Riddle, M.M., Williams, W.C., and Smialowicz, R.J. (1997) Alterations in the developing immune system of the F344 rat after perinatal exposure to 2,3,7,8-tetrachlorodibenzo-p-dioxin: II.

Effects on the pup and the adult. *Toxicology.*, **122**(3), 229–240. Erratum in: *Toxicology* 130(1), 71 (1998).

Gribble, E.J., Sivakumar, P.V., Ponce, R.A., and Hughes, S.D. (2007) Toxicity as a result of immunostimulation by biologics. *Expert Opinion Drug Metab. Tox.*, **3**, 209–234.

Haley, P.J. (2003) Species differences in the structure and function of the immune system. *Toxicology*, **188**(1), 49–71.

Haley, P. (2008) Histomorphology of the immune system: a basic step in assessing immunotoxicity, in *Immunotoxicology Strategies for Pharmaceutical Safety Assessment* (eds D.J. Herzyk and J.L. Bussiere), John Wiley & Sons, Inc., Hoboken, NJ.

Haley, P., Perry, R., Ennulat, D. *et al.* (2005) STP position paper: best practice guideline for the routine pathology evaluation of the immune system. *Toxicol. Pathol.*, **33**, 404–408.

Hannet, I., Erkeller-Yuksel, F., Lydyard, P. *et al.* (1992) Developmental and maturational changes in human blood lymphocyte subpopulations. *Immunol. Today*, **13**, 215–218.

Hastings, K.L. (2008) Current regulatory expectations for immunotoxicology evaluation of pharmaceuticals, in *Immunotoxicology Strategies for Pharmaceutical Safety Assessment*, (eds. D.J. Herzyk and J.L. Bussiere), John Wiley & Sons, Inc., Hoboken, NJ.

Herzyk, D.J. and Bussiere, J.L. (2008) *Immunotoxicology Strategies for Pharmaceutical Safety Assessment*, John Wiley & Sons, Inc., Hoboken, NJ.

Holsapple, M.P., West, L.J., and Landreth, K.S. (2003) Species comparison of anatomical and functional immune system development. *Birth Defect Research (Part B)*, **68**, 321–334.

House, R.V. and Hastings, K. (2004) Multidimensional immunomodulation. *J. Immunotoxicol.*, **1**, 123–129.

Hussain, I., Piepenbrink, M.S., and Dietert, R.R. (2005) Impact of in ovo-administered lead and testosterone on developing female thymocytes. *J. Toxicol. Environ. Health A.*, **68**(15), 1309–1319.

ICH (2006) Harmonized Tripartite Guideline (S8), Immunotoxicity studies for human pharmaceuticals.

ICH (2011) Harmonized Tripartite Guideline (S6)(R1), Preclinical safety evaluation of biotechnology-derived pharmaceuticals.

Iciek, L. (2008) Evaluation of drug effects on immune cell phenotypes, in *Immunotoxicology Strategies for Pharmaceutical Safety Assessment* (eds D.J. Herzyk and J.L. Bussiere), John Wiley & Sons, Inc., Hoboken, NJ.

Johansen, K.S. (1983) Nitroblue tetrazolium slide test: use of the phorbol-myristateacetate-stimulated NBT-reduction slide test for routine and prenatal detection of chronic granulomatous disease and diagnosis of heterozygous carriers. *Acta Pathol. Microbiol. Immunol. Scand. C*, **91**, 349–354.

Kang, S.P. and Saif, M.W. (2007) Infusion related and hypersensitivity reactions of monoclonal antibodies used to treat colorectal cancer – identification, prevention, and management. *J. Support. Oncol.*, **5**(9), 451–457.

Karol, M.H., Hauth, B.A., Riley, E.J., and Magreni, C.M. (1981) Dermal contact with toluene diisocyanate (TDI) produces respiratory tract sensitization in guinea pigs. *Toxicol. Appl. Pharmacol.*, **58**, 221–230.

Karol, M.H., Stadler, J., and Magreni, C.M. (1985) Immunotoxicological evaluation of the respiratory system: animal models for immediate and delayed-onset hypersensitivity. *Fund. Appl. Toxicol.*, **5**, 459–472.

Karrow, N.A., Guo, T.L., Delclos, K.B. *et al.* (2004) Nonylphenol alters the activity of splenic NK cells and the numbers of leukocyte subpopulations in Sprague-Dawley rats: a two-generation feeding study. *Toxicology*, **196**(3), 237–245.

Kiewe, P. and Thiel, E. (2008) Ertumaxomab: a trifunctional antibody for breast cancer treatment. *Expert Opin. Invest. Drugs*, **17**, 1553–1558.

Kimura, S., Eldridge, J.H., Michalek, S.M. *et al.* (1985) Immunoregulation in the rat: ontogeny of B cell responses to types 1, 2, and T-dependent antigens. *J. Immunol.*, **134**, 2839–2852.

Krishnaraj, R. (2008) Specific drug-induced immunotoxicity: immune-mediated hemolytic anemia, in *Immunotoxicology Strategies for Pharmaceutical Safety Assessment* (eds D.J. Herzyk and J.L. Bussiere), John Wiley & Sons, Inc., Hoboken, NJ.

Kumar, V., Abbas, A.K., Fausto, N., and Aster, J. (2010) Diseases of the immune system, in *Robbins and Cotran Pathologic Basis of Disease, 8th Edition* (eds V. Kumar, A.K. Abbas, N. Fausto, and J. Aster), Saunders Elsevier, Philadelphia, PA.

Kuper, C.F., Herleman, J.H., Richeter-Reichelm, H.B., and Vos, J.G. (2000) Histopathologic approaches to detect changes indicative of immunotoxicity. *Toxicol. Pathol.*, **28**, 454–466.

Ladics, G.S., Smith, C., Bunn, T.L. *et al.* (2000) Characterization of an approach to developmental immunotoxicology assessment in the rat using SRBC as the antigen. *Toxicol. Methods*, **10**, 283–311.

Ladics, G.S., Chapin, R.E., Hastings, K.L. *et al.* (2005) Developmental toxicology evaluations: issues with including neurotoxicology and immunotoxicology assessments in reproductive toxicology studies. *Toxicol. Sci.*, **88**(1), 24–29.

Lazar, G.A., Dang, W., Karki, S. *et al.* (2006) Engineered antibody Fc variants with enhanced effector function. *Proc. Natl. Acad. Sci.*, **103**, 4005–4010.

Lebrec, H., Kerdine, S., Gaspard, I., and Pallardy, M. (2001) Th_1/Th_2 responses to drugs. *Toxicology*, **158**, 25–29.

Lordick, F., Ott, K., Weitz, J., and Jager, D. (2008) The evolving role of catumaxomab in gastric cancer. *Expert Opin. Biol. Ther.*, **8**, 1407–1415.

Lovell, W.W. and Jones, P.A. (2000) An evaluation of mechanistic in vitro tests for the discrimination of photoallergenic and photoirritant potential. *ATLA*, **28**, 707–724.

Luster, M.I., Portier, C., Pait, D.G. *et al.* (1993). Risk assessment in immunotoxicology II: relationships between immune and host resistance tests. *Fundam. Appl. Toxicol.*, **21**, 71–82.

Maier, C.C. (2008) Nonclinical models to assess respiratory hypersensitivity potential, in *Immunotoxicology Strategies for Pharmaceutical Safety Assessment* (eds D.J. Herzyk and J.L. Bussiere), John Wiley & Sons, Inc., Hoboken, NJ.

Maronpot, R.R. (2006) Enhanced histopathology of lymphoid tissues. *Toxicol. Pathol.*, **34**, 631–633.

Miller, T.E., Golemboski, K.A., Ha, R.S. *et al.* (1998) Developmental exposure to lead causes persistent immunotoxicity in Fischer 344 rats. *Toxicol. Sci.*, **42**(2), 129–135.

Miranda, M.A., Sarabia, Z., Hernandez, D. *et al.* (1999) An in vitro approach to drug photoallergy: use of drug-directed antibodies to assess photobinding of non-steroidal anti-inflammatories to skin cells. *Toxic. in vitro*, **13**, 701–705.

Pauluhn, J. (2003) Respiratory hypersensitivity to trimellitic anhydride in Brown Norway rats: analysis of dose-response following topical induction and time course following repeated inhalation challenge. *Toxicology.*, **194**(1–2), 1–17.

Pauluhn, J., Rungeler, W., and Mohr, U. (1995) Phenyl isocyanate-induced asthma in rats following a 2-week exposure period. *Fundam. Appl. Toxicol.*, **24**(2), 217–228.

Pauluhn, J., Thiel, A., Emura, M., and Mohr, U. (2000) Respiratory sensitization to diphenylmethane-4,4′-diisocyanate (MDI) in guinea pigs: impact of particle size on induction and elicitation of response. *Toxicol. Sci.*, **56**(1), 105–113.

Pauluhn, J., Woolhiser, M.R., and Bloemen, L. (2005) Repeated inhalation challenge with diphenylmethane-4,4′-diisocyanate in brown Norway rats leads to a time-related increase of neutrophils in bronchoalveolar lavage after topical induction. *Inhal. Toxicol.*, **17**(2), 67–78.

Pauluhn, J. and Mohr, U. (2005) Experimental approaches to evaluate respiratory allergy in animal models. *Exp. Toxicol. Pathol.*, **56**(4–5), 203–234.

Pendlington, R.U. and Barratt, M.D. (1990) Molecular basis of photocontact allergy. *Inter. J. Cosmetic Sci.*, **12**, 91–103.

Piccotti, J.R., Lebrec, H.N., Evans, E. *et al.* (2009) Summary of a workshop on nonclinica.l and clinical immunotoxicity assessment of immunomodulatory drugs. *J. Immunotoxicol.*, **6**, 1–10.

Pieters, R. (2008) Systemic hypersensitivity, in *Immunotoxicology Strategies for Pharmaceutical Safety Assessment* (eds D.J. Herzyk and J.L. Bussiere), John Wiley & Sons, Inc., Hoboken, NJ.

Sarlo, K. and Clark, E.D. (1992) A tier approach for evaluating the respiratory allergenicity of low molecular weight chemicals. *Fund. Appl. Toxicol.*, **18**, 107–114.

Schnyder, B. and Pichler, W.J. (2009) Mechanisms of drug allergy. *Mayo Clin Proc.*, **84**(3), 268–272.

Stockholm, S.L. and Scott, M.A. (2008) *Fundamentals of Veterinary Clinical Pathology, 2nd Edition* (eds S.L. Stockholm and M.A. Scott), Blackwell Publishing, Ames, Iowa.

Suntharalingam, G., Perry, M.R., Ward, S. *et al.* (2006) Cytokine storm in a phase 1 trial of the anti-CD28 monoclonal antibody TGN1412. *N. Engl. J. Med.*, **355**(10), 1018–1028.

Tokura, Y. (1998) Quinolone photoallergy: photosensitivity dermatitis induced by systemic administration of photohaptenic drugs. *J. Dermatological. Sci*, **18**, 1–10.

Tokura, Y. (2000) Immune responses to photohaptens: implications for the mechanisms of photosensitivity to exogenous agents. *J. Dermatological Sci.*, **23**, S6–S9.

Ulrich, P., Grenet, O., Bluemel, J. *et al.* (2001) Cytokine expression profiles during murine contact allergy: T helper 2 cytokines are expressed irrespective of the type of contact allergen. *Arch. Toxicol.*, **75**, 470–479.

Vidal, J.-M., Kawabata, T.T., Thorpe, R. *et al.* (2010) In vitro cytokine release assays for predicting cytokine release syndrome: the current state of the science, Report of a European Medicines Agency workshop. *Cytokine*, **51**(2), 213–215.

Ward, J.M., Erexson, C.R., Faucette, L.J., Foley, J.F., Dijkstra, C., and Cattoretti, G. (2006) Immunohistochemical markers for the rodent immune system. *Toxicol Pathol.*, **34**(5), 616–630.

Weiser, G. (2006) Interpretation of leukocyte responses in disease, in *Veterinary Hematology and Clinical Chemistry* (eds M.A. Thrall, D.C. Baker, T.W. Campbell, D. DeNicola, M.J. Fettman, E.D. Lassen, A. Rebar, and G. Weiser), Blackwell Publishing, Ames, Iowa.

Wing, M.G., Moreau, T., Greenwood, J. *et al.* (1996) Mechanism of first-dose cytokine release syndrome by CAMPATH 1-H: involvement of CD16 (FcYRIII) and CD11a/CD18 (LFA-1) on NK cells. *J. Clin. Invest.*, **98**, 2819–2826.

Zhang, X.-D., Fedan, J.S., Lewis, D.M., and Siegel, P.D. (2004) Asthma-like biphasic airway responses in Brown Norway rats sensitized by dermal exposure to dry trimellitic anhydride powder. *J. Allergy Clin. Immunol.*, **113**(2), 320–326.

18

Nonclinical Safety Assessment: Biotechnology-Derived Pharmaceuticals

Christopher E. Ellis[1*], *Melanie T. Hartsough*[2], *Martin D. Green*[3*], *and Hanan Ghantous*[1*]

[1]*CDER, Office of New Drugs, FDA, Silver Spring, USA*

[2]*Biologics Consulting Group Inc., Derwood, USA*

[3]*DVRPA/OVRR/CBER/FDA, WOC2, Rockville, MD, USA*

18.1 Introduction

Although the specific definition of a "biologic drug" differs with the particular health authority, in general the term refers to protein products as opposed to a small molecular weight (SMW) chemical drug. In this chapter, nonclinical approaches to support clinical trials and marketing applications for biologic drugs (which will be referred to as "biopharmaceuticals") are presented and discussed. The most important document for reference is ICH S6(R1) (ICH, 2011), and the scope of products covered is the same as outlined in this guidance document. These products include monoclonal antibodies, cytokines, growth factors, recombinant plasma factors, enzymes and hormones. Specific to the US, "biopharmaceuticals" applies to protein therapeutic, diagnostic and prophylactic productsderived from expression systems such as bacteria, yeast, insect, plant and mammalian cells and produced by cells in culture or by recombinant DNA technology, including transgenic plants and animals. The expected timing and framework for conducting nonclinical studies for biopharmaceuticals have been described in ICH M3(R2) (ICH, 2010a), S6(R1) (ICH, 2011) and S9 (ICH, 2010b). In addition, other relevant documents have been published by the EMA, WHO, and OECD and can be consulted as needed. This

Nonclinical Safety Assessment: A Guide to International Pharmaceutical Regulations, First Edition.
Edited by William J. Brock, Kenneth L. Hastings and Kathy M. McGown.

chapter is intended to provide the details, rationale and explanation of the framework for nonclinical safety assessments of biopharmaceuticals, which are set out in these guidance documents. Despite significant progress achieved in attaining harmonization of regulatory requirements for biopharmaceuticals, many differences persist, due in part to unique considerations related to risk assessment. These include severity and seriousness of disease indications, availability and/or features of existing therapies, and the intended patient populations. The authors anticipate continued evolution of specific nonclinical safety expectations, so this chapter focuses on general strategies and considerations and not on providing specific, proscriptive recommendations. As stated explicitly in ICH S6(R1) (ICH, 2011), biopharmaceutical safety assessments must be made using a case-by-case approach. For this reason, it is customary for those developing biopharmaceuticals to work more closely with regulatory authorities early in preclinical development as compared to sponsors of more traditional SMW drugs. The opinions expressed in this chapter are those of the authors and should be viewed accordingly, unless specific regulatory or statutory requirements are cited.

18.2 Unique Characteristics of Biopharmaceuticals

Biopharmaceuticals differ significantly from SMW drugs with respect to composition; absorption, distribution, metabolism and excretion (ADME) characteristics; inherent immunogenicity; species specificity, and likely mechanism of toxicity. These unique aspects of biopharmaceuticals necessitate special considerations when designing nonclinical pharmacology, pharmacokinetic (PK) and safety studies, determining specific types of studies appropriate for product development, and interpreting nonclinical study results.

Unlike SMW drugs (usually defined as <1 kD), biopharmaceuticals are heterogeneous mixtures of high molecular weight molecules (often 10 to >160 kD) defined by process-specific attributes, and so are probably not single defined molecular entities. Heterogeneity of protein products is due not only to the presence of host cell impurities but also to varying amounts of specific post-translational modifications (e.g., glycosylation, acylation, acetylation, deamidation, oxidation, phosphorylation), truncations, amino acid substitutions, degree of multimerization, and so on. Thus, biopharmaceutical products will probably contain many types of protein modifications that determine overall tertiary structure and function. These product-specific attributes have safety and functional implications by influencing the ADME characteristics, particularly with respect to distribution and elimination (refer to Section 18.6).

The goal of PK analysis for biopharmaceuticals is the same as for SMW drugs: to define the ADME characteristics of the product and the relationship of systemic/local exposure to the pharmacodynamic (PD) and toxicity observations. Whereas SMW drugs can undergo diffusion and active transport processes to arrive at their site of action, the size, composition and structural characteristics of biopharmaceuticals typically limit them to processes such as bulk flow. Therefore, biopharmaceuticals usually have limited absorption and distribution characteristics and are administered either by intravenous, subcutaneous or intramuscular routes or directly to the site of action. Additionally, there are significant differences in biotransformation and elimination mechanisms between SMW drugs and biopharmaceuticals. SMW drugs can undergo enzymatic metabolism, while biopharmaceuticals are ultimately catabolized to amino acids. Biopharmaceutical clearance, although often limited by molecular size, can be quite similar to SMW drug clearance in that it can occur by renal filtration mechanisms.

Biopharmaceuticals are usually foreign proteins that, when administered to animals, can elicit an immune response (i.e., are immunogenic). The resulting immune response can alter the PD, PK and/or toxicity profiles of biopharmaceuticals. Immune responses to SMW drugs are apparently rare, not typically observed in animals, and usually associated with hypersensitivity reactions. Thus, immunogenicity is an important consideration for nonclinical study design and interpretation (refer to "Section 18.4 for details).

Another unique aspect of biopharmaceuticals is that they are often species specific. Thus, pharmacologic and toxicological consequences of biopharmaceutical exposure can only be observed in animals sharing a close phylogenetic relationship with humans. This aspect is important because adverse effects of biopharmaceuticals are more often due to exaggerated pharmacology compared to SMW drugs. These unique aspects of biopharmaceuticals must be considered when selecting a species for pharmacology, PK and toxicology studies.

18.3 Species Selection

A pharmacologically relevant animal species is one in which the biopharmaceutical elicits a biological response similar to that expected in humans. The basis of this relevance is usually expression of a responsive orthologous biopharmaceutical target (receptor/antigen). Since the specificity of a biopharmaceutical often limits its binding affinity to orthologous targets in test species, it is important to identify a pharmacologically responsive animal species to avoid misleading study results. For example, an appropriate species to test a recombinant human hematopoietic colony stimulating factor (rhCSF) is one in which binding to the corresponding animal receptor initiates the desired pharmacologic response (haematopoiesis). In this scenario, where the PD response in the test species is similar to humans, nonclinical safety studies should be predictive of adverse effects in humans. Similarly, since biopharmaceutical clearance may depend on target-specific binding (often referred to as an "antigen sink"), PK studies should be conducted in a pharmacologically relevant species. Clearance mechanisms other than those mediated by biopharmaceutical targets might also be important. For example, glycosylated proteins containing mannose-type oligosaccharides, such as tissue-type plasminogen activator, could be cleared by the liver through the mannose-specific uptake system (Otter *et al.*, 1991; Opanasopit *et al.*, 2001).

When a test species does not express the orthologous target or the biopharmaceutical does not bind to the target in a manner similar to humans, nonclinical safety studies could result in a false assurance of safety. As an example, toxicity studies of a monoclonal antibody (mAb) directed against the human epidermal growth factor (EGF) receptor conducted in mice and rats demonstrated no adverse effects at systemic exposures approximately three to fourfold greater thanthose attained in humans (http://www.accessdata.fda.gov/drugsatfda . . . FDA, 2004a). However, clinical studies revealed moderate-to-severe gastrointestinal, pulmonary and dermatologic adverse events that were related directly to pharmacologic activity of the antibody. Data from a toxicology study in cynomolgus monkeys revealed dose- and duration-dependent increases in dermatologic and gastrointestinal lesions that were similar to those observed in clinical studies, effects that progressed with continued treatment. Further study confirmed that the mAb bound cynomolgus monkey but not rat, mouse, rabbit or dog EGF receptor. The initial toxicology studies in rodents did not demonstrate clinically-relevant adverse effects since they were not conducted in a pharmacologically relevant species.

18.3.1 Defining a Pharmacologically Relevant Species

In selecting a species for nonclinical safety studies, it is important to compare the animal to humans with respect to biopharmaceutical target (receptor/antigen) number, affinity of the biopharmaceutical for the target, and cellular response (e.g., effects on signal transduction pathways, translation, transcription, etc.) to biopharmaceutical binding. Although the properties of the orthologous target (receptor/antigen) in the animal species should be similar to those in humans, absolute equivalence of target density or affinity for the biopharmaceutical is not necessary. A decision tree for determining a relevant species is provided in Figure 18.1.

Identification of a pharmacologically relevant species often begins by searching publicly-available literature and genetic sequence databases such as NCBI's PubMed and GenBank®, respectively. It is often useful to determine information already known about the expression, cellular localization, tissue distribution, and physiological function of the orthologous target in candidate test species and relative concordance to the corresponding human target. The proposed mechanism of action (MOA) of the biopharmaceutical, such as inhibition or enhancement of target function, should also be considered. For example, data obtained from gene "knock-out" mice, resulting in loss of target expression and function, would be relevant where an mAb product binds and inhibits the interaction between the target with its receptor. Data obtained from phenotypic analysis of mice lacking the orthologous target gene should demonstrate similarities with that of mice administered the mAb product. Thus, these data would provide a reasonably good initial assessment of hazards associated with target inhibition.

Information obtained from literature searches not only helps in choosing a relevant species but also (1) helps define limitations of each species, (2) identifies potential safety risks of the biopharmaceutical, and (3) informs the design of nonclinical studies including end-points to be evaluated. Since adverse effects associated with biopharmaceuticals are often exaggerated pharmacology, understanding the fundamental biology of target activity can be useful in anticipating potential adverse effects in humans. The pharmacology of some biopharmaceuticals, and thereby hazards associated with them, might be well understood. Where little information is available for either the biopharmaceutical or the intended biologic target, one should anticipate providing more extensive safety information. A weight-of-evidence approach for safety evaluation of biopharmaceuticals includes collection and integration of all available information into overall safety assessment, thereby facilitating both biopharmaceutical development and the reduce/refine/replace (3Rs) principles without compromising patient safety.

Confirmation of an animal ortholog to a human biopharmaceutical target is determined by comparing the respective amino acid sequences. The higher the degree of protein similarity (or percent identity) between an animal ortholog and a human target, the more

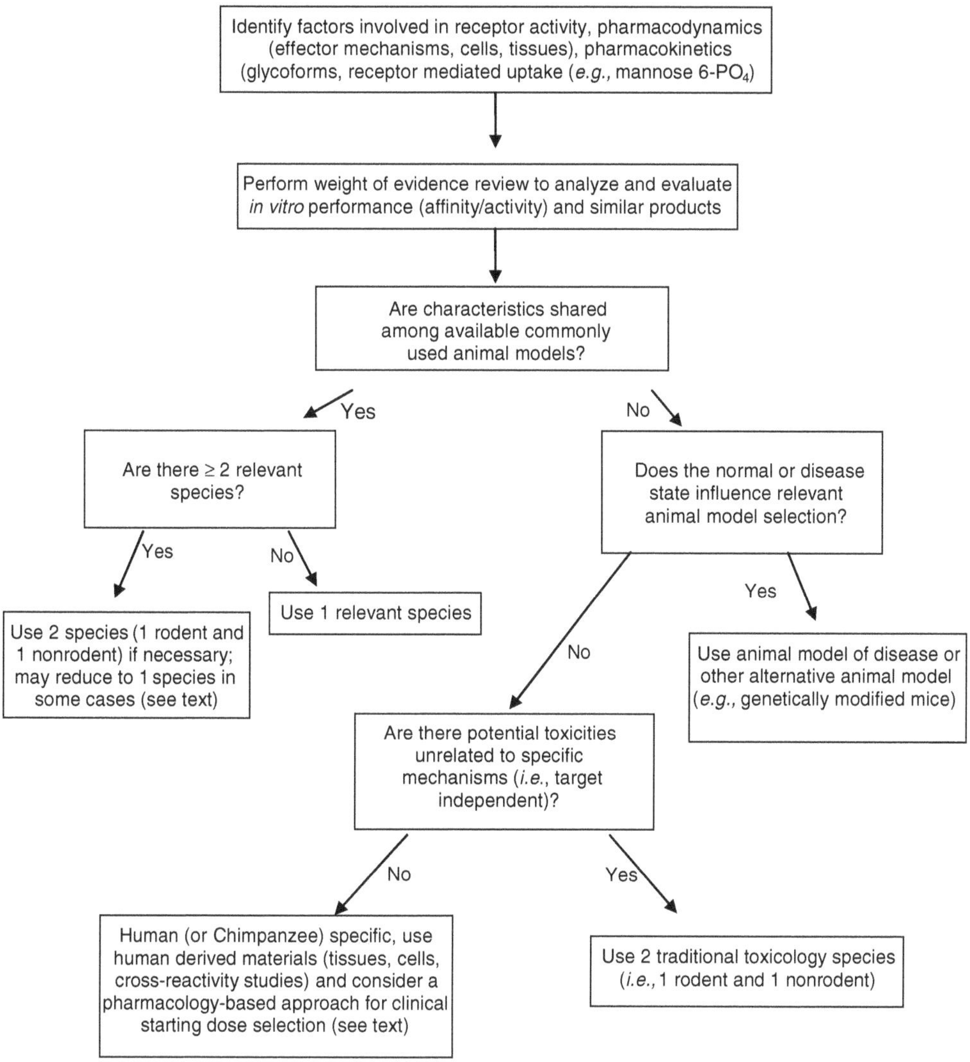

Figure 18.1 *Flowchart outlining considerations for selecting an appropriate animal model.*

likely the animal species will be pharmacologically relevant. Although the presence of an animal protein that is highly similar to the human target is important, data should be obtained to characterize the biopharmaceutical–target interaction in the candidate test species. This is most often accomplished by determining the binding affinity of the clinical candidate to the orthologous target (receptor/antigen) and/or its activity on cells of various species.

Methods used in binding studies include flow cytometry, surface plasmon resonance (SPR), or other quantitative assessment using purified recombinant proteins or cells, tissues or transfected cells expressing the orthologous targets. Functional assays are often performed to assess the capability of the biopharmaceutical to induce a known biological response (e.g., modulation of cellular proliferation or migration, antiviral activity) or change a PD marker (e.g., secretion of cytokines, induction of an enzyme, phosphorylation of a signalling component, transcriptional activation) associated with a biological response. The functional (PD) effect should be relevant to the desired biological effect. When feasible, a quantitative comparison of the PD effect should be made between human and animal cells. It is also desirable, when possible, to identify a PD marker that can be used to evaluate functional effects of the biopharmaceutical throughout nonclinical studies, which is particularly important for assessing the impact of immunogenicity.

When a difference in binding affinity or activity of the biopharmaceutical to animal and human target is evident, it is preferable to further characterize the nature of the difference to understand its overall significance. For example, some growth factors, such as neurotrophins, bind several receptor types with different affinities (e.g., high, medium and low affinity receptors) (Barbacid, 1995). Since these receptor types may have different levels of functional significance, larger affinity variations in those receptor types of lesser concern (often the low affinity receptors) could be acceptable. Additionally, some biopharmaceuticals (e.g., insulin and leutinizing hormone (Frank *et al.*, 1981; Mendelson *et al.*, 1975)) have spare receptors (i.e., receptors which exist in excess of those required to produce a maximal PD effect (Bourne and von Zastrow, 2004). Binding affinity differences for these products may pose less of a concern if biopharmaceutical target occupancy is suitable to induce a comparable pharmacological response.

For a biopharmaceutical, it is not unusual to observe dissimilar affinity/activity profilesbetween animals and humans. Pharmacological relevance of a given species, based on the type and degree of observed dissimilarity in affinity/activity profiles, depends on factors such as the degree of affinity difference and the relative importance of the functional end-point measured. Under these circumstances, further characterization of the nature of the difference should be considered. Differences between animal and human *in vitro* affinity/activity profile or PK parameters (such as faster relative biopharmaceutical clearance in the animal species) could result in altered PD effects. Therefore, compensation for these differences by altering the dose level and/or dosing frequency in a nonclinical study could be considered for more accurate risk assessment. Affinity and PD properties of a biopharmaceutical should be considered in determining species relevancy and in calculating FIH clinical starting doses.

18.3.2 Alternative Approaches

Sometimes no relevant species for nonclinical safety studies can be identified. Absence of target binding may occur due to either natural variation in target structure or lack of target expression in animal models (e.g., an orthologous target does not exist or the target is disease specific). Under circumstances where no relevant animal species can be identified, alternative approaches, such as use of surrogate molecules, genetically modified animal models, and/or animal models of disease, should be considered to evaluate product safety. Alternative approaches are not employed routinely, but are considered when there is scientific need. Although important PD and PK data might be obtained in alternative models, under most circumstances these are developed for nonclinical safety studies. A review by

Bussiere *et al.* (2009) discussing these alternative approaches, can be referred to for additional details and examples.

18.3.2.1 Surrogate Molecules

Surrogate (also known as analogous or homologous) molecules are generally either developed against the orthologous antigen of another species (e.g., mAb recognizing the animal ortholog of the human biopharmaceutical target) or are orthologous to the clinical candidate of the species to be utilized for nonclinical assessment. Orthologous proteins/antigens are identified typically by determining the percent similarity of the entire amino acid sequence and/or the sequence containing important binding or functional domains of the putative surrogate protein/target compared to those of the corresponding human biopharmaceutical/target. Where a test species lacks the corresponding ortholog of the human biopharmaceutical/target, the most suitable surrogate could be a paralog. The suitability of any surrogate protein/target is not only determined by comparison of the amino acid sequence with the clinical candidate/target but also by similarity in biologically meaningful attributes. The surrogate molecule should demonstrate similar binding affinity for its target and specific functional properties compared to the clinical candidate. While this approach allows for conducting nonclinical studies to obtain safety data relevant for the biopharmaceutical's clinical use, there are disadvantages. Manufacturing the surrogate molecule will likely differ from that of the clinical candidate. As a result, the surrogate molecule might exhibit variations in process-specific impurity and contaminant profiles and/or protein modifications, possibly resulting in disparate potency and/or pharmacology. An example of this approach is described for infliximab, which only binds to chimpanzee and human TNFα. Potential reproductive and chronic toxicities were evaluated using a surrogate anti-TNFα mAb that inhibits mouse TNFα activity (Treacy, 2000). Although efforts could be made to identify a NOAEL, safety data obtained using surrogates are generally used for hazard identification and not risk assessment.

18.3.2.2 Genetically Modified Models

Unlike surrogate molecules, genetically modified animal models allow for study of the clinical candidate directly. These models are most often transgenic or "knock-in" mouse models that express the human biopharmaceutical receptor/antigen (i.e., human target of the clinical candidate). The process of creating transgenic mice begins by microinjecting DNA constructs into fertilized mouse eggs. Most often, these DNA constructs are small plasmids containing the protein coding region of the human gene to be expressed along with heterologous regulatory elements necessary for protein expression. These constructs can also be large artificial chromosomes (e.g., bacterial, phage) that contain the entire human gene including regulatory elements. DNA constructs insert randomly (with preference for euchromatin regions) into the mouse genome. Due in part to multiple genomic copies of the DNA construct, transgenic models tend to express non-physiologically high levels of human protein. In addition, the heterologous DNA regulatory elements contained within plasmid DNA constructs, not only contribute to this non-physiological level of expression but also result in non-physiological regulation of expression, both temporal (e.g., developmental, cell cycle dependent etc.) and spatial (i.e., tissue distribution), since these regulatory elements do not originate from the human gene. In contrast, mice containing artificial chromosome DNA constructs, containing the entire human gene including regulatory elements, tend to demonstrate physiological regulation of protein expression, resulting in tissue distribution and temporal expression patterns that are similar to humans. An example of this approach is the nonclinical development of keliximab, in which human CD4 was expressed transgenically in murine CD4 knock-out mice (Brugelski *et al.*, 2000).

As opposed to transgenic mice created by random genomic insertion, gene "knock-in" (and "knock-out") mice are generated by targeting a specific locus within the mouse genome using homologous recombination techniques. The process of creating "knock-in" mice begins by transfecting DNA constructs into mouse embryonic stem (ES) cells. The genomic locus targeted is the mouse gene orthologous to the human biopharmaceutical target, therefore expression of the human protein is regulated by mouse DNA regulatory elements orthologous to those of the human gene. Unlike transgenics that may contain many copies of the inserted human gene, only two copies of the gene are present in somatic cells of "knock-in" mice (if targeting autosomes), so these mice tend to have physiological levels of the human protein. Additionally, "knock-in" mice tend to have more physiological regulation of expression of the human protein, as compared to transgenic mice containing plasmid DNA constructs, allowing mouse-like tissue specific and regulatory control of human protein expression.

While genetically modified models can be used to generate safety data with the clinical candidate, interaction of the biopharmaceutical with the human target in mice could result in different physiological effects compared to humans, since these models only introduce a single human protein and not an entire physiological pathway. Therefore, to the extent possible, it is useful to determine the functional similarity of protein pathways and interactions with important regulatory proteins between species. Important questions to address when considering genetically modified models include:

- Are functional pathway and important accessory proteins present in the mouse that will allow the human protein to demonstrate normal function?
- What information do you hope to obtain from the model?
- What types of toxicology studies will you perform?
- Is this the best or only way to obtain the desired information?

Phenotypic characterization of genetically modified models is critically important to establish baseline control values and identify important parameters for observation. For example, characterizing human protein expression, including the amount, tissue distribution and cell localization, may be considered. This can be important since high human protein expression in tissues that are not relevant, particularly with plasmid DNA construct containing transgenic mice, may result in toxicities that are not of clinical concern. These models have limitations, such as lack of historical data, which may hinder interpretation of findings. In addition, some genetically modified mouse models have shortened lifespans, thereby limiting study duration. These limitations are exacerbated by the technical challenges of producing mice with consistent, physiological expression and tissue distribution of the human target protein. Due to non-physiological regulation of protein expression, findings in transgenic models, particularly those containing plasmid DNA constructs, tend to be more difficult to interpret than "knock-in" models. Careful phenotypic characterization and understanding the limitations of any particular model are critical for study interpretation.

18.3.2.3 Disease Models

Although not commonly used in toxicology due to the underlying disease complicating study interpretation, animal models of disease are often used to obtain clinical trial enabling "proof-of-concept" PD data. If a diseased animal model is selected, it may be useful to incorporate safety end-points into pharmacology studies. Diseased animals in these "proof-of-concept" studies can be a source of safety data, but these models are usually not well characterized and often share little similarity with the human disease or condition. Given the caveats and limitations of these models, a cautious approach to interpreting safety results should be used. When feasible, attributes of the model should share significant similarities to the human disease or condition. However, absolute consistency of disease manifestations is not necessary for a model to be useful. Therefore, the potential value of nonclinical safety studies in diseased animals is dependent on the clinical relevance of the model itself.

Disease models that could be used for safety evaluation of biopharmaceuticals include those that target disease-specific proteins, such as tumour-associated or microbial antigens. Under these circumstances, to support clinical development in infected patients or those with an epitope specific for the pathological condition, nonclinical studies in diseased animals can provide important PD, PK and safety information, given that the biopharmaceutical target might only be present in these models. Due to the scientific complexity of studies in diseased animals, full GLP compliance may not always be feasible.

18.3.3 Utilizing Non-Pharmacologically Relevant Species

There are unique circumstances in which valuable safety information for a biopharmaceutical can be obtained in a species that may not be pharmacologically relevant. For example, safety of fusion or conjugate proteins can be evaluated in an otherwise non-relevant species. Observed toxicity could be due to instability of the linker region, resulting in systemic exposure to the "payload" (a conjugated toxin or radioisotope). In this case, toxicity could be due to blood flow and localization rather than target-binding. Where product instability may be an issue, further assessments of *in vivo* product stability could be important.

18.3.4 Additional Alternatives

It is uncommon that there are no available *in vivo* tools for safety evaluation of biopharmaceuticals. An example of this situation is an unconjugated mAb, directed against a nonhuman target (often of microbial origin) or one that is only expressed under certain pathological conditions (such as a cancer-specific epitope) and there is no animal model that expresses the therapeutic target. In situations such as this, toxicology studies in animal species lacking the target may be unnecessary. However, a short duration (i.e., up to one month) nonclinical safety study in a single "non-relevant" species should be considered to support a FIH clinical trial in healthy (uninfected or disease-free) individuals. Although additional *in vivo* nonclinical safety studies might not be necessary, development of disease models capable of providing clinically relevant safety information should be considered early in product development. It should be noted that there are situations in which a disease-"specific" epitope is not actually absent in non-diseased animals (and humans) but is up-regulated significantly in disease. Studies in animals may be useful since the biopharmaceutical target is expressed, albeit at a much lower amount. In these situations, non-diseased animals could identify a hazard, but could under-predict toxicities associated with target binding.

When a biopharmaceutical is human specific and/or no appropriate nonclinical model for safety evaluation can be found, a weight-of-evidence approach can be used to determine if additional biopharmaceutical-specific safety information is needed. This approach could include target-specific biological information from published literature and clinical safety information of approved products that target the same receptor/antigen, if available. This information may identify potential hazard(s) associated with the biopharmaceutical and/or its target and, along with clinical indication and patient population considerations, can then be used to inform risk-benefit assessments. Under these circumstances, an *in vitro* pharmacology-based approach, utilizing human-derived materials such as tissues and cells, could be useful for FIH dose selection.

18.4 Immunogenicity

Many biopharmaceuticals induce an immune response in laboratory animals that can alter the pharmacologic activity, PK and/or toxicity of the biopharmaceutical. Therefore, the potential for an immune response to the biopharmaceutical should be considered in nonclinical study design and interpretation. There are two basic considerations relevant to these anti-biopharmaceutical immune responses. First, is systemic exposure to active biopharmaceutical in nonclinical studies sufficient for adequate safety evaluation? Second, can nonclinical findings be adequately extrapolated to the clinical situation? A review by Ponce *et al.* (2009) can be referred to for additional details and examples.

Anti-drug antibodies (ADA), also known as anti-product antibodies, could affect animal exposure to active biopharmaceutical by altering its rate of clearance or neutralizing its function. Development of antibodies that increase the clearance rate and thereby reduce biopharmaceutical exposure appears to be common in nonclinical studies, while development of antibodies that increase biopharmaceutical exposure by inhibiting clearance is not observed commonly. Significant changes in blood levels of a biopharmaceutical in nonclinical studies are often indicative of "clearing" or "enhancing" antibody development even before the antibodies themselves are detected. In these cases, the presence of ADA that affect systemic exposure to the biopharmaceutical is likely. Determining the presence, type, and titre of ADA might not be useful; however, careful consideration should be given to collecting and storing serum for future measurement of ADA, which is sometimes needed. In general, TK assessments are particularly important to interpret nonclinical studies for immunogenic biopharmaceuticals.

Independent of PK effects, neutralization can occur when ADA bind to the biopharmaceutical and inhibit pharmacological activity. Additionally, if a biopharmaceutical contains regions that are highly similar to an endogenous protein, ADA may cross-react and neutralize critical physiological activity. The presence of neutralizing antibodies in nonclinical studies might not need to be determined if a PD marker is included to confirm biopharmaceutical activity. However, it may be important to determine if toxicities observed in nonclinical safety studies were due to neutralization of endogenous proteins rather than biopharmaceutical-specific effects. Therefore, if this distinction cannot be established otherwise, the presence of neutralizing antibodies to the biopharmaceutical and/or endogenous protein may need to be determined.

ADA could also produce toxicities that are not attributable directly to the biopharmaceutical. For example, ADA formation can lead to immune complex disease (or serum sickness). Deposition of ADA:biopharmaceutical complexes in the vasculature, perhaps the most common manifestation of immune complex disease, can result in complement fixation, inflammation, and tissue destruction. This does not appear to predict human toxicity.

Immunogenicity *per se* should not be considered an adverse effect since ADA often appear to have no observable effects. Thus, the presence of ADA, in the absence of reduced product exposure and/or activity, loss of endogenous protein function or immune-related toxicities, could be irrelevant to safety assessment. Even when observable effects due to ADA exist, nonclinical safety studies should often proceed since these effects do not necessarily invalidate these studies. Data interpretation can be complicated due to immunogenicity, which is common for biological products. However, data obtained from well-designed studies can be informative and important for proper safety assessment, even in the presence of a significant immune response to the biopharmaceutical. Nonclinical study design modifications may be considered due to the formation of ADA and could include modifying the dose level and/or frequency of biopharmaceutical administration and the number of time points to evaluate PK and PD. If TK and/or ADA assessments are either not adequate or indicate lack of sufficient systemic exposure to active biopharmaceutical the study is often uninterpretable.

Determining whether systemic exposure to the biopharmaceutical was adequate despite immunogenicity can be difficult. The most important determination is whether systemic biopharmaceutical exposure in animals was clinically relevant. If biopharmaceutical exposure and/or activity level in animals provides an appropriate safety margin over clinical exposure levels, then the safety data collected should be informative. If ADA affect a significant number of animals within a study group, summarizing PK and toxicity data from those animals that maintain adequate biopharmaceutical exposure could be useful. For example, in nonrodent studies when biopharmaceutical exposure is maintained in at least two animals in a group, then data from those could be analyzed separately from animals in which systemic exposure might not have been adequate.

Alternative approaches can be considered where significant ADA are observed in a pharmacologically relevant species. ADA formation can result in loss of biopharmaceutical exposure and/or PD activity, possibly limiting the usefulness of chronic toxicology studies. When chronic toxicity studies are needed and immunogenicity issues cannot be overcome, then development of a surrogate molecule can be considered. However, it should be noted that immunogenicity to the surrogate molecule can be observed in the intended species, potentially negating any expected utility. Developing a surrogate molecule exclusively to enable chronic toxicity evaluation is uncommon.

If adverse effects observed in nonclinical toxicology studies might be due to immunogenicity (e.g., loss of endogenous protein function, immune-related toxicities, etc.), characterizing the ADA response might be useful to elucidate the mechanism. Additionally, ADA characterization could be necessary for studies in which there is no useful PD marker. Appropriate characterization of the ADA response could include determination of specific antibody titre, number of animals affected, functional characteristics of the immune response (usually whether neutralizing or non-neutralizing), and correlation with any pharmacological and/or toxicological changes in the animals.

ADA formation can be assessed in conjunction with TK assessments. Immunogenicity assessments are typically performed prior to study initiation, at scheduled necropsy following the final dose of the biopharmaceutical and from surviving animals if a treatment-free period is included. Immunogenicity should be evaluated using sensitive, specific and reliable detection methods (Mire-Sluis *et al.*, 2004). Additionally, the potential effect of test article on assay performance should be determined. The FDA draft guidance "Assay development for immunogenicity testing of therapeutic proteins (FDA, 2009) can be referred to for specific details.

Immune responses in animals usually do not reliably predict similar responses in humans. Human mAbs induce ADA responses in animals but not necessarily in humans because the antibody is a foreign protein to the former but not the latter. Unlike exaggerated pharmacology related adverse effects, toxicity in animals occurring as a result of immune-mediated endogenous protein inhibition may not predict adverse immune responses in humans. However, since it is important to determine the clinical risk potential for an ADA response inhibiting endogenous protein function, findings in animals may nevertheless indirectly inform clinical safety (refer to Shankar *et al.* (2007) for further discussion). For example, serious immune-mediated toxicities in animals that result from inhibition of an endogenous protein could indicate a critical non-redundant function. In this case, the nonclinical study may identify an important non-redundant functional pathway that, if irreversibly inhibited due to an induced immune response, could lead to severe clinical adverse events.

18.5 Biological Activity/Pharmacodynamics

Establishing the biological activity of a biopharmaceutical is critical, not only in determining potential efficacy but also as an early indication of potential hazards due to exaggerated PD effects. Initially, the pharmacologic activity of a biopharmaceutical can be evaluated by *in vitro* and/or *in vivo* techniques. These include, but are not limited to, *in vitro* binding assays to demonstrate the affinity of the biopharmaceutical for the human target and *in vivo* studies to establish biological activity in pharmacologically relevant animal models.

Biopharmaceutical targets should be identified and characterized to the extent possible to understand the biologic consequences of target interaction. Since biopharmaceuticals are selected based on target specificity, general screening for binding to unrelated targets usually are not needed. However, valuable information can be obtained by examining binding of the biopharmaceutical to potentially related targets, such as paralogs of the intended clinical target, in order to confirm specificity. If binding to a paralogous or other highly similar target is observed, the biological implications should be explored. Important PD related questions to address include:

- Is there more than one receptor/target for the clinical candidate? If so, how does binding to each contribute to its biological effect?

- Do species chosen for *in vivo* studies express all relevant targets (i.e., orthologs of the human targets)?
- What similarities (and differences) are anticipated between the biological activity of the clinical candidate in nonclinical models compared to the clinical situation?

The dose-response characteristics of the biopharmaceutical should be determined early in development. Dynamic physiological processes can affect target expression and/or activity over the time course of biopharmaceutical treatment, resulting in nonlinear dose-response relationships. Nonlinear dose-responses include plateau effects, bell-shaped curves, and other unusual patterns. These nonlinear PD effects may be due to biopharmaceutical interaction with multiple targets with different affinities/functions acting in concert. Plateau effects are often due to either target binding saturation or interactions with spare targets (receptors/antigens). Bell-shaped curves can result from alterations in target activity, expression, turnover or other normal physiological adjustments to continuous biopharmaceutical exposure. Bell-shaped curves have been observed for some biopharmaceuticals where maximal PD and/or toxic effects were observed at doses other than the high-dose. Alterations in the amount of target, due to changes in expression and/or turnover, often can be determined experimentally.

Animal models of human disease can be used for "proof of concept" studies to demonstrate that the biopharmaceutical can bind to the target, ameliorate or slow progression of disease, or alleviate disease-associated signs. When the pharmacologic activity of a biopharmaceutical is dependent upon specific receptor/antigen binding to a target not present in available animal models, a number of nonclinical approaches to obtain valuable PD data can be considered. For example, if the orthologous target is absent in the animal species, xenograft or genetically modified models, expressing the human biopharmaceutical receptor/antigen, could be used to assess PD parameters in a normal physiological milieu. If the orthologous target is present in an animal model but the biopharmaceutical does not bind to it, studies with an appropriate surrogate molecule could be useful in demonstrating PD effect(s).

18.6 Pharmacokinetics/Toxicokinetics

The primary goal of studying PK and TK of biopharmaceuticals is to understand the relationship of systemic exposure to the biopharmaceutical and its therapeutic action and toxicity (refer to ICH S3A; ICH, 1995). When administered by the intravenous route, biopharmaceuticals, due to their high molecular weight and tertiary structure, usually do not undergo significant diffusion as would be expected for SMW drugs. Systemic exposure of biopharmaceuticals is initially confined to the circulating vasculature, but can eventually distribute to extravascular space by various factors, including bulk flow and convection. Catabolism of biopharmaceuticals occurs by the same processes that break down endogenous proteins and usually involves receptor-mediated endocytosis followed by intracellular proteolysis in lysosomes. Catabolism can also occur at extravascular sites. The route of absorption from these extravascular sites is influenced by molecular size and is partitioned between direct absorption into the bloodstream and lymphatic system. Similarly, elimination of a biopharmaceutical from the vascular compartment is also influenced by molecular size. Biopharmaceuticals of greater than 70 kD do not undergo renal glomerular filtration and degradation; instead, the liver plays a predominant role in their catabolism and PK/TK behaviour. In contrast, the smaller the molecular size of the biopharmaceutical, the more likely it is that the kidney and not the liver will play the major role in elimination. Those biopharmaceuticals that undergo renal filtration are often reabsorbed and/or degraded by various renal structures, including cells of the brush border and tubules. While disposition mechanisms are similar across species, it is important to realize that certain aspects will vary due to sheer physical differences, such as relative muscle mass when the intramuscular route of injection is used.

Glycosylation patterns of a biopharmaceutical could also play an important role in PK/TK. Terminal glycoforms, such as sialic acid and mannose residues, play significant roles in regulating catabolism and influence several PK/TK parameters, including systemic exposure, as measured by area under curve (AUC) and half-life. The effects of glycosylation on clearance (Cl) may vary across species, which could result in different product clearance rates due to the different rates of uptake as exhibited by asialoglycoprotein or mannose/GlcNAc receptor-mediated pathways (Park *et al.*, 2005).

Basic parameters that are used in characterizing systemic exposure are AUC and C_{max}. Half-life, total plasma Cl and volume of distribution (V_d) are also calculated and are basic parameters used in the analysis of PK/TK data. Because PK/TK assessments are essential for accurate interpretation of toxicity data and these assessments may vary between studies, PK/TK parameters should be included in general toxicology studies, regardless of whether independent studies are performed. This approach not only validates doses in the toxicology study but also provides a means of extrapolating systemic exposure data across various species. Hence it can be used as a means of supporting the selection of an initial, safe starting dose for clinical use in conjunction with determining therapeutic end-points that may be based on plasma levels associated with pharmacological effects. Additionally, establishing an association between dose and systemic exposure provides an upper limit to clinical dosing based on PK/TK parameters.

Unlike smaller, synthetically-produced SMW drugs, proteins are not metabolized by hepatic cytochrome P_{450} mechanisms. Instead, they are catabolized into individual amino acids that may then be excreted or reused for protein synthesis or energy production. This poses a problem for studies that rely on radiolabelling, such as mass balance assessments and tissue distribution studies typically performed for SMW drugs. Frequently, the radiolabelled amino acid of the biopharmaceutical will be released through catabolism and possibly incorporated into other proteins through normal endogenous protein synthesis (Wills and Ferraiolo, 1992). Subsequently, measurements of this type when applied to biopharmaceuticals will typically reflect normal protein turnover patterns. Therefore, studies assessing metabolism and excretion of biopharmaceuticals are not generally warranted, nor are they normally useful in providing information on the disposition of biopharmaceuticals relative to toxicity. Nevertheless, tissue distribution studies could provide insight into the localization of an administered biopharmaceutical. For example, tissue distribution studies for imaging agents could be informative since the interest is in identifying organ systems at risk from the radiolabel moiety aside from the targeted tissue or organ. Distribution studies of the radiolabelled biopharmaceutical are important because they provide information on the localization and potential for PD and toxicological activity, regardless of whether the biopharmaceutical is maintained as an intact molecule or the radiolabel is released as a consequence of protein degradation.

PK/TK profiles of biopharmaceuticals can be influenced by a variety of factors. These include, but are not limited to, immunogenicity to the biopharmaceutical, post-translational processing such as glycosylation during manufacture, pharmaceutical factors in the administered dose, antibody isotype, specific biopharmaceutical constituents (e.g., fusion proteins, pegylation, fragments), biopharmaceutical receptor/antigen density, and route of administration. As previously discussed, a major factor in extrapolating PK across species can be the development of ADA that could confound interpretation of the PK/TK data.

The route of administration in conjunction with molecular weight could influence the extent and time dependency of systemic exposure. For example, after subcutaneous administration, adsorption into the circulating blood volume is dependent on two parallel pathways. One pathway is direct absorption into the circulation via the blood capillaries, while the other occurs via the lymphatic system (Supersaxo *et al.*, 1990). The latter is associated with a delayed, systemic appearance and, in some cases, loss of systemic exposure due to uptake into lymphatic tissues. Biopharmaceuticals with higher molecular weights are more likely to be absorbed by the lymphatic system. T_{max} (time to reach maximum concentration) via the lymphatic pathway could be much longer than that via blood capillaries. Thus it is important to maintain consistency in comparing various routes of administration between nonclinical and clinical study designs. The route of administration and dosing regimen ideally should mimic the projected clinical trial. PK sampling should also be sufficient to describe the profile for a minimum of 3–5 half-lives and include predose and C_{max} estimates.

PK parameters are most often determined in studies conducted after administration of the biopharmaceutical to healthy animals. However, in some instances, the use of an animal model of disease that shares similarly mediated pathophysiology to the clinical disease could yield a pharmacological setting similar to that in humans and may better reflect PD properties associated with clinical outcomes. Additionally, it could provide a more clinically representative PK/TK profile. For example, if an mAb is directed towards an antigen that is over-expressed in tumour tissue, presence of the tumour antigen could alter the biodistribution of the biopharmaceutical, thereby influencing its blood concentration. If the tumour burden diminishes due to treatment efficacy, more antibody will be available systemically, ultimately affecting overall exposure to the biopharmaceutical.

Assessing the PK/TK profile in an animal species that does not express the therapeutic biopharmaceutical target should be considered carefully, because the major mechanisms of elimination of the biopharmaceutical could be at low levels or absent. For example, continuous exposure of biopharmaceuticals that target transmembrane receptors, which can decouple from downstream signalling processes (i.e., desensitization) or undergo internalization and/or down regulation (e.g., G-protein coupled receptors, receptor tyrosine kinases, etc.) (Moore *et al.*, 2007; Hupfeld and Olefsky, 2007), reduce receptor-mediated clearance mechanisms and could result in nonlinear biopharmaceutical elimination that would not be evident in non-pharmacologically relevant species. Paradoxically, this increased biopharmaceutical exposure could actually be associated with reduced PD and toxicologic effects due to target desensitization/down regulation. In addition, other protein-mediated mechanisms exist, which can be species dependent, that can affect the PK of biopharmaceuticals, such as Fc receptor-mediated mechanisms for mAbs (Qiao *et al.*, 2008).

In some cases, the underlying disposition factors for a biopharmaceutical could be reflected in a non-relevant animal species. For instance, when comparing nonclinical studies to the clinical setting, greater fidelity exists with small molecular weight biopharmaceuticals (<10 kD), which undergo extensive renal elimination. Saturation of various active processes often result in nonlinearity between PK/TK end-points and dose, thus complicating extrapolation and interpretation.

18.7 Nonclinical Safety Assessment

18.7.1 General Principles

Prior to FIH clinical trials, the basis for estimating clinical safety was nonclinical safety testing. The goals of nonclinical safety evaluation for biopharmaceuticals are identical to those for SMW drugs and include identifying a toxic dose (when feasible), target organs of toxicity (and reversibility) and a no observable adverse effect level (NOAEL), as well as determining adequate safety margins (human dose multiples), a safe clinical starting dose, and safety end-points for clinical monitoring. It is important to emphasize that multiples of the human dose necessary to establish adequate safety margins vary with each class of biopharmaceutical and clinical indication (refer to ICH S6(R1; ICH, 2011)). While some data regarding biopharmaceutical safety may be obtained from well-designed nonclinical pharmacology studies, toxicology testing is intended to answer specific questions regarding the acceptable risk to the patient and to provide an indication of toxicities that could be anticipated to occur upon clinical introduction of the product.

For biopharmaceuticals, specific toxicities are usually related to exaggerated pharmacological action, regardless of whether they are associated with the desired biological effect being sought in the clinic. In contrast, nonspecific toxicities, such as hypotension or acute immune-related events, can occur with any protein due to general aspects of protein chemistry and not to specific toxicities of a particular biopharmaceutical. In general, these latter properties are observed frequently after administration of biopharmaceuticals and are anticipated clinically and readily corrected by modifying the rate of infusion and/or pretreatment of subjects in the clinical study with antihistamine, for example. Therefore, since these hazards are well-characterized, it is unnecessary to perform animal studies to assess the potential for these nonspecific effects. In fact, nonclinical studies should be designed to avoid inducing these types of nonspecific toxicities (e.g., by altering infusion rates) since they could interfere with the identification of more clinically relevant biopharmaceutical-specific toxicities. Additionally, a cautious approach is warranted for nonclinical safety study interpretation because specific biopharmaceutical-related effects may not always appear to be dose-dependent, because of nonlinear dose response curves. For example, many hypersensitivity reactions demonstrate a bell-shaped dose-response curve, such that these reactions are not generated if administering a dose that is too low or too high (Descotes, 2004).

In general, toxicology studies should be performed according to Good Laboratory Practices (GLP, 21CFR, part 58). The timing of nonclinical studies relative to the conduct of clinical trials is addressed in ICH M3(R2) (ICH, 2010a). While this document was written specifically for SMW drugs and addresses the timing of nonclinical studies necessary for their development, many of the principles outlined are relevant to biopharmaceuticals. ICH M3(R2) (ICH, 2010a) and S6(R1) (ICH, 2011) allow flexibility in the design of supporting nonclinical toxicology programmes for biopharmaceuticals based upon the nature of the biopharmaceutical, the indication and patient population to be treated. As a general principle, sufficient nonclinical data of adequate dose and duration should be performed in advance of the proposed clinical studies.

18.7.2 Study Design Considerations

When choosing an appropriate test species, preference should be given to those that share an active cross-reactive or identical target with humans. Under most circumstances, two pharmacologically relevant species (one rodent and one nonrodent) can be used for toxicology studies. However, if the biopharmaceutical is well-understood, the target poses minimal safety concern and/or results of initial shorter duration studies in two species are concordant, then one species could be acceptable for longer duration safety testing.

In many cases, interaction of a biopharmaceutical with its specific target occurs only in humans, NHPs, and sometimes other nonrodent species, but not in rodents (i.e., situations where rodents are not pharmacologically relevant). In these situations, additional toxicology testing in rodents will not provide additional useful information, but instead could provide irrelevant data. Additionally, development of alternative models or assessment of a second pharmacologically relevant nonrodent species to fulfil the two species expectation is not appropriate.

In order to assess potential toxicities of a biopharmaceutical adequately, the design of toxicology studies should consider the animal species, age and physiologic state most relevant for the clinical indication and product class, as well as the intended doses, route of administration and treatment regimens planned for the clinical trial. Moreover, the number of animals used per dose group should be large enough to detect clinically relevant toxicities, both male and female animals should be used or justification provided for specific omissions, and stability of the product under the conditions of use and the comparability of critical product attributes (e.g., degree of pegylation) to those intended for the clinical study need to be considered. With many biopharmaceuticals, these considerations are interdependent, as the route of administration or the maximal feasible dose (MFD) for the nonclinical study could be influenced by the species selected for testing, and vice versa. For studies utilizing NHPs, five animals per sex for each dose group may be considered if a treatment-free period is included (i.e., three per sex for terminal sacrifice and two per sex for recovery sacrifice). Clinical observations, body weight, food consumption, clinical chemistry, haematology, coagulation indices, gross pathology, organ weights, histopathology, TK, ophthalmologic evaluation, cardiovascular assessments and sometimes immunogenicity assessments are often included for all dose groups in pivotal studies. Other end-points may be incorporated as necessary to address safety concerns unique to specific biopharmaceuticals based on expected effects related to exaggerated pharmacology. For example, if the biopharmaceutical is intended to activate or suppress the immune system, then evaluation of the PD effects (i.e., immune effects) would help define the potential hazards associated with the biopharmaceutical.

For repeat-dose toxicology studies, terminal sacrifice occurs typically within 1–3 days following the last dose. A treatment-free period (recovery group) is often included, primarily to determine reversibility of pharmacological and toxicological effects. Although complete recovery is not necessary, one should consider the time it will take for the biopharmaceutical to be eliminated (e.g., 3–5 half-lives), the biopharmaceutical level that may interfere with analytical assays (e.g., ADA assays), the duration of PD effects and reversibility of toxicities when defining the duration of the treatment-free period. In the case of mAbs with long half-lives, treatment-free periods could be 8–10 weeks in duration.

It is important to understand all aspects of biopharmaceutical safety over the course of nonclinical development that have the potential for adverse clinical consequences. This is particularly important for studies performed to support FIH trials. Therefore, the importance of including a treatment-free group should be considered carefully prior to removal of some or all of these animals from a study design. The more that is understood about the safety of a biopharmaceutical, particularly from biopharmaceutical-specific data obtained from shorter duration studies, the more likely that treatment-free period groups might not be necessary for all dose levels or all additional studies, since recovery may be predictable. However, one assumes significant risks by not including treatment-free groups for all or any dose level for any particular study because there may be unanticipated or unusual toxicities (i.e., new findings in longer duration studies) that are not well understood and of potential clinical concern and/or the dose-response curve and therefore toxicities related to exaggerated pharmacology might not be linear. With a nonlinear dose-response curve, the mid-dose may actually be more toxic than the high-dose; thus if a treatment-free group was only included for the high-dose and toxicities are observed in the mid-dose animals, reversibility of the toxicities will not be able to be assessed. An additional study might be necessary to adequately address safety concerns. The risk of not including treatment-free period groups at low- and/or mid-dose levels in longer-term toxicology studies can be mitigated to some extent by establishing the dose-response relationship in PD studies. For example, if longer-term studies are conducted for a biopharmaceutical where the dose-response curve in the dose range examined is known to be linear, then including a treatment-free period group at high-dose levels only may be sufficient.

There are many occasions when modified study designs, based on immunogenicity-related complications or differences in relative affinity/activity of the biopharmaceutical between species, should be considered. These modifications often include dose level and/or frequency adjustments to overcome loss of exposure to the active biopharmaceutical or reduced affinity/activity of the biopharmaceutical in the test species.

18.7.2.1 Dose Selection

Dose selection in a toxicology study for biopharmaceuticals is based primarily on binding affinity and activity data from both *in vitro* and *in vivo* studies and estimation of the efficacious or highest anticipated clinical dose. The importance of defining the shape and steepness of the dose-response curve, in all test species, to understand the relationship between dose level, frequency and duration of dosing with the degree of target occupancy compared to PD and toxicological effects of a given biopharmaceutical cannot be overemphasized. In order to ensure adequate safety assessment, the dose levels used should be biologically active in the species selected for study and it is often appropriate to include three dose levels of the biopharmaceutical along with an appropriate negative control group. Ideally, the doses selected will encompass the projected clinical dose equivalent, identify an overtly toxic dose and a NOAEL.

Allometric scaling of doses of a biopharmaceutical facilitates comparisons across species and allows retrospective determination of whether an animal model was predictive of toxicities observed in the clinic. Thus, selection of doses for toxicity testing may also consider any known PK parameters that could impact the distribution, elimination and/or toxicity of the biopharmaceutical. Following intravenous administration, biopharmaceuticals with high molecular weights (>70 kD) are largely confined initially to the vascular space. Distribution of these products is therefore limited, and toxicities are usually observed in tissues that either express the target (receptor/antigen) or have a high blood flow and subsequent high exposure. Since plasma volume is related to total body weight in both humans and test animal species, it is appropriate to scale doses of the biopharmaceutical on a body weight (mg/kg) basis. In contrast, smaller molecular weight biopharmaceuticals (<70 kD) that undergo first order elimination by renal or hepatic mechanisms scaling by surface area (mg/m^2) may be more appropriate. However, various factors, such as receptor-mediated uptake and disposition, could alter allometric scaling significantly.

A rationale for dose selection, particularly for the high-dose level, should be contemplated carefully. Establishment of a maximal tolerated dose (MTD) for biopharmaceuticals with inherently low toxicity is often not feasible. In some instances, an MFD in lieu of an MTD could be used as a high-dose. However, an MFD can be difficult to define, can result in non-specific "protein overload" effects that are not relevant clinically and, most importantly, can be a dose in gross excess of the amount necessary for proper safety evaluation (i.e., orders of magnitude greater than the maximal PD effect). Utilizing dose levels that far exceed the amount required for target saturation and maximal PD effect(s), which is often the case for MTDs and MFDs, in order to search for potential additional toxicities at these high-doses can be self-defeating, as they can result in nonlinear dose-response relationships leading to reduced biopharmaceutical-specific toxicities in the high-dose group. Therefore, nonclinical doses that provide an adequate dose or exposure multiple relative to the anticipated clinical dose or exposure should be selected. For most biopharmaceuticals, an adequate high-dose can often be the greater of either the dose necessary to achieve systemic exposures ~10-fold greater than those attained at the highest proposed clinical dose (i.e., 10-fold multiple) or the dose required for nonclinical target saturation (i.e., maximal PD effect). There are cases, however, when an MFD approach to select the highest dose level might be most appropriate. For example, a biopharmaceutical may not be soluble or the pharmaceutical quality may be altered at high protein concentrations in the desired test vehicle (i.e., protein aggregate formation). Determining an MTD may be considered for those biopharmaceuticals, such as immuno- and protein-conjugates, toxin containing fusion proteins and thrombolytics, that elicit frank toxicity.

An important consideration when defining nonclinical dose levels is species differences in target affinity/activity of the biopharmaceutical. The doses or exposure multiples selected (especially the high-dose) should be adjusted for these differences. For example, if the clinical candidate binds the animal target with threefold lower affinity than the human target, the nonclinical dose levels could be adjusted threefold higher to account for this affinity difference. This is an important concept when determining a pharmacologically relevant species since lower affinity/activity of a biopharmaceutical can be compensated for, at least to some extent, by increasing the dose level. If the affinity/activity difference is so great that this limitation cannot be overcome adequately, the species is not generally considered pharmacologically relevant.

When using a receptor saturating dose (i.e., maximal PD effect) as the high dose for a toxicology study, one should consider the presence of lower affinity targets and issues related to biopharmaceutical distribution peculiarities. It is important to consider the safety concerns related to PD effects of lower affinity targets, when they exist in conjunction with higher affinity targets, early in development. When lower affinity targets contribute to the maximal PD effect, it is beneficial to consider the biopharmaceutical dose level that is required to achieve saturation of these targets when determining the high dose level in the toxicology study. An exception to this approach is when the affinity/activity of the lower affinity target differs substantially in the test species compared to humans. One then needs to determine whether the pharmacological relevance of the test species remains valid, rather than adjusting for these differences. In cases like this, the toxicological evaluation of the biopharmaceutical in this test species may over- or under-predict safety concerns depending on the relative affinity/activity differences and the overall contribution of these lower affinity targets to the PD effect.

A second unique consideration, when establishing the high-dose level based on the maximal PD effect, relates to issues regarding both the limited distribution of the biopharmaceutical with the intended route of administration, and the biopharmaceutical target distribution, particularly when the target is located at multiple sites that may be more or less available for biopharmaceutical interaction. This is an important consideration, especially with large biopharmaceuticals that are administered systemically. To illustrate this point, consider the scenario in which an mAb product is administered intravenously with the intention of binding to a single protein target on cells located intravascularly but also has target expression in unintended extravascular tissues. Distribution of the mAb is initially limited to intravascular sites due to the size, composition and structure of the product and to the presence of high affinity intravascular binding sites. However, once systemic exposure levels exceed those necessary for intravascular target saturation, the mAb product is available to distribute to these unintended extravascular sites. So shortly after administration the PD effects and, thereby, safety issues are limited to intravascular sites but, later on, after intravascular target saturation, clinically-relevant toxicities of the biopharmaceutical might be evident at extravascular sites. Thus, if the high-dose chosen is based on the maximal desired PD response for intravascular target saturation, it may not actually equate to the maximal systemic PD response, which includes both intravascular and extravascular target saturation and extravascular toxicities could be missed. Therefore, potential limitations of PD end-points, used to establish a high-dose level based on a maximal PD effect, must be considered.

Although not as critical as high-dose selection, proper dose selection for low- and mid-dose group animals is still important. For most biopharmaceuticals, it might be appropriate to select a low- or mid-dose that approximates the estimated adjusted clinical efficacious dose (i.e., ~1 to threefold greater exposure for biopharmaceuticals with similar inter-species affinity/activity profiles). The low dose should not only be biologically active but should also achieve exposure levels expected to be less than the amount necessary for target saturation (i.e., below the maximal PD response). It is preferable in many circumstances not only to observe dose-dependent PD effects in the toxicology study, by using low- and sometimes mid-doses in the linear part of the dose-response curve, but also to use a dose where substantial biopharmaceutical-mediated desensitization/down-regulation of the target is unlikely to occur. Target down-regulation can occur as part of receptor-mediated biopharmaceutical clearance mechanisms that reduce active cell surface receptors, whereby receptor saturating doses can result in diminished biological activity. This mechanism is one of several by which biopharmaceuticals may not have a linear relationship of biological activity with dose. Thus, utilizing at least one non-saturating dose level in these studies is often appropriate.

18.7.2.2 Schedule and Duration of Dosing

The duration of dosing of a biopharmaceutical in nonclinical safety studies is dependent upon the proposed clinical use (i.e., acute versus chronic exposure). ICH S6(R1) (ICH, 2011) recommends a maximum dosing duration for biopharmaceuticals of six months in animal studies to support products that are to be administered chronically in humans. Initially, many biopharmaceutical products could enter clinical trials based on safety profiles obtained in single- and repeat-dose toxicology studies of limited duration (e.g., 14–28 days), with an appropriate treatment-free period included as part of the study design. The duration and frequency of biopharmaceutical administration (e.g., daily versus intermittent administration) should be as close as possible to or exceed that planned for the clinical trial(s). There are caveats to this basic principle, however. For example, human mAb products often have half-lives of 1–2 weeks in cynomolgus monkeys, compared to over three weeks in humans, resulting in weekly versus monthly dosing frequencies in nonclinical versus clinical situations. So in the case of mAbs, it is preferable that toxicology study designs cover the duration of dosing in the clinical trial. Appropriate data from *in vitro* and/or *in vivo* nonclinical pharmacology and PK studies can help define an appropriate dosing frequency. Therefore, dosing frequency differences between nonclinical and clinical situations can be acceptable. The most important consideration is that the duration of exposure in pivotal nonclinical safety studies is adequate to support the safety of exposure for the proposed clinical trial.

18.7.2.3 Route of Administration

Most often, the route of administration in toxicology studies should mimic that intended for clinical use. In contrast to SMW drugs, biopharmaceuticals are not often administered orally due to rapid degradation by gastrointestinal proteases and peptidases. Thus, on the rare occasion when a biopharmaceutical is administered orally, it should be demonstrated that an active biopharmaceutical can distribute to and/or have activity at its site of action, which is usually within the gastrointestinal tract. As opposed to orally (and dermally) administered biopharmaceuticals, systemic absorption of inhalation biopharmaceuticals, intended to act locally in the respiratory tract, can occur frequently based on physiochemical characteristics and particle size. So, systemic toxicities will often need to be monitored for these biopharmaceuticals. Although other routes are used occasionally to produce locally-confined therapeutic effects, the most common routes used for systemic administration are intravenous infusion or subcutaneous injection. Infusion rates of biopharmaceuticals might need to be adjusted if anaphylaxis/hypersensitivity reactions occur as a response to foreign protein infusion; however, when feasible, the rate should be consistent with the clinical situation.

In some cases, larger systemic doses are too toxic for intravenous or subcutaneous administration, whereas a smaller dose administered directly into the target region can be tolerated. Therefore, in order to gain access to targets located in protected body regions (e.g., central nervous system, eye), alternative and more invasive routes of administration can be employed for biopharmaceuticals. If such a system is necessary, devices such as reservoirs, pumps, catheters or other components can be used in the toxicology studies. In some cases, the size of the device could be a critical factor in the choice of the animal model for use in nonclinical studies. If the route of administration cannot be duplicated in any animal system, alternative routes could be justified, providing that they result in similar target organ exposure. Lastly, one may need to consider the route of administration, particularly when immunogenicity is a problem, since some routes are thought to be more immunogenic than others (Ponce *et al.*, 2009).

18.7.3 Specialized Studies

18.7.3.1 Safety Pharmacology

Nonclinical studies for most SMW drugs include a core battery of safety pharmacology studies that evaluate the effects of a compound on specific critical physiological functions, such as those of the cardiovascular, respiratory and central nervous systems (refer to ICH S7A; ICH, 2001). The objectives of these studies are threefold: to identify potential undesirable PD effects of a drug that may be relevant for safe human use, to help evaluate adverse effects observed in the PD or toxicology studies, and to provide information regarding the mechanism of any adverse PD effects. For biopharmaceuticals, standalone safety pharmacology studies are normally not needed. Instead, the battery of nonclinical toxicology studies should meet the objectives intended for traditional safety pharmacology evaluation. To accomplish this, safety pharmacology end-points are typically incorporated into toxicology studies. However, a more detailed assessment of a cardiovascular, respiratory, neurological or other safety pharmacology parameter may be needed due to the MOA of the biopharmaceutical, the indication, the patient population, or results of initial toxicology studies. Moreover, biopharmaceuticals could possess nonspecific properties that influence end-points normally investigated through safety pharmacology studies. For example, cardiovascular function and/or blood pressure could be influenced by the rate of infusion of biopharmaceuticals. These effects are common to biopharmaceuticals and well recognized. Adjustments are made routinely during clinical trials to avoid such effects. Some *in vitro* methods, such as the hERG assay for potassium channel blockade, are not designed for biopharmaceuticals and are not used to assess potential to produce QT prolongation.

18.7.3.2 Genotoxicity

The standard battery of assays recommended for SMW drugs as defined by the ICH S2B (ICH, 1997) guidance is designed primarily to detect substances that interact with DNA and induce gene mutations, chromosomal aberrations and/or DNA damage directly. Biopharmaceuticals are not expected to pass through the cellular and nuclear membranes of an intact cell and interact with DNA or other chromosomal material. Additionally, the standard assays (e.g., Ames test, *in vitro* mammalian chromosomal aberration assay and rodent *in vivo* micronucleus assay) may not provide informative data because the test cells might not contain active receptors (i.e., not relevant species) or because the biopharmaceutical has an indirect mechanism that is not present in isolated systems. Moreover, these assays rely on cytotoxicity to ensure assay validity, which is not applicable to most biopharmaceuticals. Thus, it is very important to carefully consider if and/or when such assays might be useful for safety assessment of any particular biopharmaceutical.

In determining whether genotoxicity testing is appropriate and necessary for any particular product, the properties of the biopharmaceutical should be considered. Causes for concern can include: (1) a manufacturing process that results in residual organic chemicals; (2) a construct that contains transporter sequences that will localize the biopharmaceutical to the nucleus of an intact cell; or (3) "free" organic linker or SMW drug released from the biopharmaceutical (e.g., from a protein- or immuno-conjugate) due to instability of the conjugation upon storage or upon dilution in serum. In general, it is very important to take into account the pharmacology, MOA and the final content of the biopharmaceutical to determine whether the standard genotoxicity assays will be informative. For example, if the biopharmaceutical is able to alter DNA or RNA integrity, (e.g., DNAses and ribozymes), one should contemplate the feasibility of the biopharmaceutical and byproducts to interact with nuclear material in intact cells under normal physiological conditions (i.e., in the absence of cell permeability enhancing agents and techniques) prior to performing standard genotoxicity tests. Similarly, general screening of a product for genotoxic contaminants is not a revealing tool, as the impurities and contaminants of a biopharmaceutical typically consist of residual host cell proteins and nucleic material, fermentation components, manufacturing process components such as column leachables and detergents, bacteria and viral particles and not organic chemicals typically found in SMW drug manufacturing.

18.7.3.3 Carcinogenicity/Tumour Promotion

The need for carcinogenicity testing of a biopharmaceutical that is administered chronically is made on an individual basis, taking into consideration the product characteristics and MOA, as well as the indication, patient population and intended clinical use. Therefore, it is important to understand how the carcinogenic risk will be addressed, both experimentally and for product labelling purposes. As discussed previously, a weight-of-evidence type approach utilizing all data sources should inform the development strategy for each biopharmaceutical. Rodent bioassays usually are not useful for biopharmaceuticals (refer to ICH S6(R1); ICH, 2011), since they are designed to identify complete carcinogens (i.e., chemicals involved in cancer initiation). In general, biopharmaceuticals are not initiators. However, biologic activities of certain biopharmaceuticals could raise concern regarding the potential for tumour promotion and progression. For example, growth factors may promote tumour progression directly through activation of their receptor or indirectly through production and/or activation of other molecules involved in growth regulation. Immune suppressants could increase tumour promotion by impairing endogenous tumour surveillance mechanisms.

Alternative approaches can be considered on a case-by-case basis to evaluate the tumourigenic potential of a biopharmaceutical in order to address specific mechanism-based concerns or on occasions when insufficient knowledge exists regarding the relationship of the MOA of the biopharmaceutical to carcinogenic potential. If standard rodent carcinogenicity studies are considered, one must take into account the species specificity of a biopharmaceutical and immunogenicity profile prior to committing to such studies. Use of NHPs are not appropriate since their relatively long life-span, background incidence of tumours and low numbers per group (inadequate for statistical analysis) make carcinogenicity studies impractical (Knight *et al.*, 2006; Gold *et al.*, 1999). Rosenblum and Dayan (2002) describe the decision process used to assess the need and feasibility of carcinogenicity studies for IL-10, which highlights important points that could be considered for other biopharmaceuticals.

18.7.3.4 Reproductive/Developmental Toxicology

If reproductive toxicology studies are needed, they should be conducted in compliance with ICH S5(R2) (ICH, 2000). However, inherent characteristics of biopharmaceuticals frequently require innovative approaches. Specific study design, dosing schedule, and/or species selection are related to immunogenicity, biological activity, PK characteristics and/or extent of embryo–foetal exposure. ICH S6(R1) (ICH, 2011) should be referred to for detailed considerations regarding these studies.

Reproductive toxicology studies with SMW drugs are generally performed in rodents and rabbits for which ample historical control data are available and that produce litters with sufficient progeny for adequate statistical analysis. If the biopharmaceutical demonstrates clinically-relevant activity in rodents and rabbits, then conducting embryo–foetal development (EFD) studies in both species is often appropriate. Although the short dosing duration (11 to 13 days in rodents) of these studies often limits the impact of immunogenicity, ADA formation may nonetheless limit the feasibility of a particular species for EFD studies.

In many instances, the NHP is the only pharmacologically relevant species in which to perform reproductive toxicology studies. The use of monkeys poses many challenges. NHPs are heterogeneous compared to in-bred laboratory animals, the availability of sexually mature animals is limited, NHPs produce one offspring per pregnancy, gestation periods are approximately 5–7 times that of rats and rabbits, and spontaneous abortion rates can be high. When it is necessary to assess risks to the conceptus of the NHP, an enhanced pre- and postnatal development (ePPND) study may be considered. Effects on female and male fertility can be addressed by incorporating standard end-points into repeat-dose toxicology studies. If the biopharmaceutical is an immune modulator, relevant end-points can also be included in an ePPND study.

When no relevant animal species is available, a genetically modified mouse model or use of surrogate molecules could be appropriate alternatives. Pharmacology experiments to characterize the genetically modified models or PD properties of the surrogate molecules are essential to ensure these approaches are suitable for toxicology studies. Examples of a surrogate molecule and a transgenic mouse model used for reproductive toxicology testing have been published (Treacy, 2000; Brugelski *et al.*, 2000).

18.7.3.5 Toxicities Involving the Immune System

The potential for a biopharmaceutical to produce adverse effects on immune function is generally recognized. Many biopharmaceuticals are intended to either stimulate or suppress the immune system directly. Others, such as mAbs, directed against growth factors, may indirectly interfere with immune function. For example, antibodies directed against the insulin-like growth factor (IGF-1) receptor could inhibit IGF-1 effects on T cell maturation (Timsit *et al.*, 1992). It is therefore important to ascertain potential adverse effects of the biopharmaceutical on immune system function. Factors to consider in selecting appropriate immune system end-points for a biopharmaceutical include its composition and structure, MOA, interaction with receptor/antigen targets, dose-response relationship, the specific type and nature of toxicity, species specificity and relevancy of any immune findings in the test species to the intended human population.

Although ICH S8 (ICH, 2008) specifically excludes biopharmaceuticals from consideration, the fundamental approach to immunotoxicity evaluation is the same. An initial evaluation of potential immunotoxicity can be obtained from clinical chemistry, haematology, and gross and histologic pathology findings obtained in standard repeat-dose toxicology studies. Immunotoxicity studies should address specific issues related to the biopharmaceutical and its target.

As with other physiological systems, there can be marked species differences in the immune system that could limit feasibility of testing and/or interpretation of data (Haley, 2003). For example, although lymphocyte subset analyses can be performed easily in rodents, NHPs and humans, specific phenotypic markers may not be expressed identically by all species. Additionally, appropriate reagents might not be available to measure these cell surface markers in a pharmacologically relevant animal species. Currently-available lymphocyte subset markers might not adequately assess immunotoxicity (refer to ICH S8; ICH, 2008). Animals treated with an immunomodulatory biopharmaceutic may exhibit clinically relevant immunotoxicity, but may not adequately model risk. For example, treatment of chimpanzees with an anti-CD3 monoclonal antibody HuM291 resulted in increased cytokine serum levels without eliciting signs of cytokine release syndrome. Humans treated with HuM291 demonstrated signs of mild to moderate cytokine release syndrome at doses 667–6667-fold lower than the highest dose tested in the chimpanzee, when compared on a mg/kg basis (Hsu *et al.*, 1999; Norman *et al.*, 2000). Clinical relevance of findings in immunotoxicity studies can be assessed *in vitro* using human leukocytes, depending on the availability of useful biomarkers in this setting.

The mammalian immune system exhibits a great deal of redundancy and compensatory mechanisms. If an adverse effect on a relatively discrete immune system end-point is observed, this might not be biologically meaningful. In general, a global evaluation of immunotoxicity is preferred where possible.

18.7.3.6 Local Tolerance

Adverse reactions at the site of application (local reactivity) could be caused by hypersensitivity or irritation to a biopharmaceutical and/or formulation components. Although it is difficult to distinguish between various mechanisms for local intolerance, it is important to evaluate local tolerance in a pharmacologically relevant animal species and to identify target-specific effects, using the same dosing regimen and route of administration as that intended for the clinical trial. A histological evaluation of the injection sites within a repeat-dose toxicology study is useful for assessing local tolerance without having to perform an independent study. Caution should be taken when interpreting results, however, since repeated injection of human proteins into animals could cause local intolerance that will not occur in humans.

18.8 Tissue Cross-Reactivity (TCR)

A human TCR study is an important part of the safety assessment of mAbs and imaging agents and is usually conducted utilizing a representative panel of human tissues prior to FIH trials (refer to ICH S6(R1); ICH, 2011). FDA guidances "Points to consider in the manufacture and testing of monoclonal antibody products for human use" (FDA, 1997) and "Developing medical imaging drug and biological products, part 1: conducting safety assessments" (FDA, 2004a) can be referred to for additional details. These studies are intended to identify, in a qualitative manner, all tissues that express the biopharmaceutical target(s). TCR studies could reveal unintended target binding to non-targeted tissues, with potentially important safety implications. When these studies are performed using fixed tissues, antigen structure might not be fully retained (i.e., antigens are denatured and cells are not intact) and therefore observed tissue binding may not be representative of *in vivo* binding.

Adverse effects of most biopharmaceuticals are related to exaggerated pharmacology, due to high target affinity and specificity, and so are not usually considered "off target". However, these effects can occur in tissues that were not targeted intentionally. For example, if the intended therapeutic target is that expressed on lung tissue but the target is also expressed on gastrointestinal tissue, then any gastrointestinal-related adverse effects would be unintentional but still target-specific. When the intended biopharmaceutical target, or perhaps an unintended cross-reacting paralogous target, is expressed on human tissues other than the intended tissue, binding could have inadvertent and potentially adverse consequences.

Data obtained from TCR studies using animal tissues have been used to identify pharmacologically relevant species. However, other methods may provide better comparisons across species. Since this method does not necessarily correlate with pharmacological activity, TCR studies are not generally recommended as a standalone method for determining relevant species. Cross-species data comparisons from a select number of tissues may be useful to follow up adverse findings in a toxicology study.

The general utility of TCR study data for any particular mAb can be determined by using positive control samples. In situations where mAb binding to target epitopes is predominantly tertiary structure-dependent, positive control samples may reveal little or no specific staining because fixation conditions might not be compatible with these antibodies (i.e., antibodies not binding a denatured epitope). In this situation, TCR studies do not provide valuable information. TCR studies with mAbs that recognize membrane-bound targets are thought to provide valuable target expression and binding information. This contrasts with mAbs that recognize cytosolically-expressed targets, thought to be inaccessible *in vivo* because of limited tissue penetration. However, tissue expression of these cytosolic targets can be revealed by these studies. The sensitivity and qualitative nature of the method limits its utility in many circumstances and therefore other methods to evaluate human tissue distribution of biopharmaceutical targets should be considered.

Although general TCR recommendations are available (refer to FDA "Points to consider . . . ", (FDA, 1997)), certain key design aspects of these studies are discussed below. Human TCR studies are usually performed according to Good Laboratory Practices (GLP, 21CFR, part 58). In general, the biopharmaceutical intended for use in the clinic is evaluated in these studies. In the case of immuno-conjugates, it might be better to utilize the parent antibody as long as additional data indicate that the conjugation does not affect mAb binding to, or affinity for, the target. For bi-functional antibodies, performing separate binding studies for each target is not normally necessary, although the tissue distribution and cellular expression of each target should be understood.

Paraffin-embedded tissues are not usually utilized for these studies due to inconsistent or poor antigen retrieval. However, these types of tissues might be useful if consistent and adequate antigen retrieval is demonstrated. Most often, cryopreserved tissues from at least three unrelated human donors are evaluated as a minimum effort to control for genetic polymorphism of antigen expression. If there is a reason to suspect genetic polymorphism of the antigen, it may be wise to include samples from additional donors to better characterize these findings.

Since the ability to detect cross-reactivity of the biopharmaceutical with non-targeted tissues could depend on product concentration, several concentrations are used. While biopharmaceutical affinity for the target as well as expected achievable peak plasma concentrations may be considered when choosing concentrations for TCR studies, concentrations should be optimized to produce strong, specific binding with limited background staining.

Inclusion of positive and negative controls is essential for interpreting study results. For example, staining with anti-human β2 microglobulin or anti-CD31 antibodies that detect protein expressed on endothelial cells and counterstaining with hematoxylin allow evaluation of tissue quality and morphology, thereby confirming that the tissues are suitable for immunohistochemistry. Moreover, positive and negative control material (tissues, cells or soluble target affixed to a solid matrix) with known antigen expression status (i.e., presence or lack of antigen), are appropriate to confirm binding capability of the mAb under the optimized test conditions utilized in the definitive study.

18.9 Clinical Starting Dose Selection for Biopharmaceuticals

The most common method for calculating a maximum recommended starting dose (MRSD) is based on allometric scaling with a NOAEL in the most relevant (usually assumed to be the most sensitive) species (refer to FDA guidance "Estimating the maximum safe starting dose in initial clinical trials for therapeutics in adult healthy volunteers" (FDA, 2005)). However, there are situations where no relevant species or alternative model is available for *in vivo* studies to determine a NOAEL, or where quantitative risk assessment is limited or not feasible (e.g., surrogate biopharmaceuticals were used). Where these issues cannot be addressed with *in vivo* methods, an *in vitro* pharmacology-based approach, such as a minimally anticipated biological effect level (MABEL) (refer to draft EMA CHMP "Guideline on strategies to identify and mitigate risks for first-in-human clinical trials with investigational medicinal products" (2007)), may be used to determine a safe clinical starting dose. Clear exceptions to using a MABEL include circumstances where the FIH trial occurs in a patient population that has an expectation of therapeutic benefit (e.g., oncology patients). Utilizing multiple approaches for selecting a safe clinical starting dose are often appropriate, since the best approach at the outset of nonclinical development could be uncertain. A flowchart outlining considerations for estimating a safe clinical starting dose for biopharmaceuticals in healthy volunteers is provided in Figure 18.2.

A pharmacology-based approach, such as a MABEL, can allow estimation of a safe clinical starting dose; however, no standardized and validated method for estimating a MABEL is available and the approach is considered case-by-case. For example, a MABEL could be defined as the dose where biopharmaceutical exposure levels are estimated to result in 10% of the maximal anticipated clinical effect. A

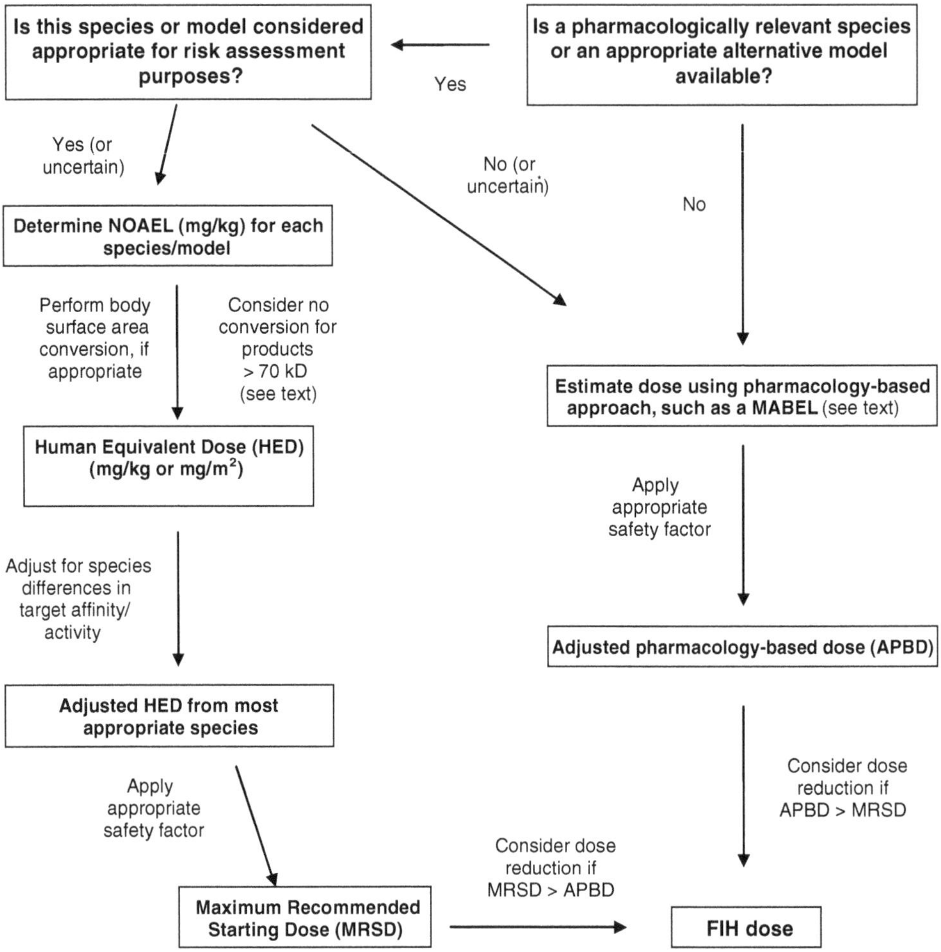

Figure 18.2 *Flowchart outlining considerations for estimating a safe clinical starting dose in healthy volunteers.*

manuscript by Muller and Brennan (2009) can be referred to for additional details including a retrospective discussion concerning the value of a MABEL in the case of TGN1412.

Calculating a safe starting dose using a pharmacology-based approach could be performed using PK/PD modelling information obtained from human cells expressing the biopharmaceutical target. This information can sometimes come from existing data obtained from discovery pharmacology studies. Larger safety factors can also be applied to doses determined using pharmacology-based approaches where there is a higher degree of clinical concern or uncertainty. The most appropriate FIH dose, as determined using NOAEL or pharmacology-based approaches, is often the lower of the two calculated doses.

Even when a pharmacologically relevant species and/or an alternative model are available, an *in vitro* pharmacology-based approach could be considered in situations where nonclinical studies are of limited utility for risk assessment or where significant uncertainty as to the quantitative predictability of *in vivo* nonclinical models exists. The importance of considering this approach varies proportionally with the amount of uncertainty as to the clinical predictability of safety data obtained from pivotal nonclinical safety studies. The amount of uncertainty is dependent, in part, on the overall similarity of the target pathway to be manipulated in the species or model selected compared to that of humans. Some pharmacologically relevant animal species and alternative models can underestimate the potential human risks associated with a biopharmaceutical class based on known species-specific biological differences. For example, a pharmacology-based approach may be appropriate for FIH dose selection of biopharmaceuticals targeting the immune system. Additionally, the maximal PD effect(s) in animals may be non-adverse but may nonetheless be of clinical concern depending on the uncertainty associated with a particular biopharmaceutical. In these cases, a FIH dose determined based on a NOAEL could far exceed the level necessary for maximal PD effects. Even for biopharmaceuticals not thought to pose significant clinical safety concerns based on the MOA and so on, it is prudent that a FIH dose not approach an estimated maximal clinical effect level.

18.10 Comparability

This section applies only to biopharmaceutical manufacturing changes occurring during the course of clinical development or post-approval and not to "biosimilars". Due to the heterogeneous nature of biopharmaceuticals and the common occurrence of changes in manufacturing, the biopharmaceutical used in nonclinical studies does not have to be identical to that used in clinical trials, but does have to be sufficiently comparable. Comparability assessments consist of rigorous physicochemical characterization and *in vitro* functional comparison of the pre- and post-change products (biopharmaceuticals) designed to determine the similarity of structural folding, post-translational processing, carbohydrate content, impurity profile, potency and other end-points as appropriate (refer to ICH Q5E (ICH, 2005) and "FDA guidance concerning demonstration of comparability of human biological products, including therapeutic biotechnology-derived products" (FDA, 1996)). These assays are performed to determine whether manufacturing changes might affect the safety, identity, purity or efficacy of the biopharmaceutical. In order for pre- and post-change products to be comparable, the physicochemical properties, biological activity and immunochemical properties must be highly similar, and when physicochemical differences are detected, these changes should have no adverse affect upon the safety or efficacy of the biopharmaceutical.

In most cases, comparison of the *in vitro* quality attributes of pre- and post-change products is enough to establish comparability, and additional *in vivo* or *in vitro* nonclinical studies are not necessary. However, sometimes quality data are insufficient and bridging nonclinical studies in an appropriate animal model may be needed. Considerations that could suggest the need for further nonclinical studies to establish comparability include: (1) obvious quality alteration; (2) biochemical alterations in the active moiety known to affect biopharmaceutical exposure *in vivo* (e.g., glycosylation, charge) or influence other *in vivo* characteristics; or (3) analytical testing is insufficient for comparison of safety and/or efficacy with the reference (pre-change) biopharmaceutical. Additionally, comparability studies may be needed if the final biopharmaceutical formulation is changed to include a new excipient.

Nonclinical determinations that could be needed to establish comparability include PK, PD, toxicology, and/or immunogenicity. PK bridging studies are the most commonly performed to assess comparability since manufacturing changes can result in alterations of the active moiety that can affect biopharmaceutical exposure *in vivo*. For example, glycosylation changes can influence the PK of a protein due to changes in clearance rates through the asioaloglycoprotein or mannose/GlcNAc receptor-mediated pathways. A direct comparison of PK parameters of the pre- and post-change products in a pharmacologically relevant animal species is preferable. PK comparisons made between two independent studies, one with the post-change product and one with the pre-change product, are difficult to interpret and are not usually considered adequate. A reasonable number of animals for a PK study would demonstrate statistically a 20% difference with 80% power. Comparability assessments are not intended to be the same as PK bioequivalence for SMW drugs. Moreover, when the only relevant animal model is a NHP and/or the animal species chosen is known to develop ADA that could limit the usefulness of the study, flexibility in the study design may be appropriate. In the majority of cases, these PK comparisons provide sufficient information for clinical dose adjustment and additional bridging studies are usually not necessary.

In some instances, additional nonclinical studies may be needed to establish comparability. The need for these studies is dependent upon the safety profile of the reference (pre-change) biopharmaceutical, the magnitude of the manufacturing change(s), and any identified differences in product purity, structure, or *in vitro* activity. PD comparisons can include *in vitro* assays such as receptor binding or *in vivo* studies in an animal model of disease. For example, it may be useful to perform a PD comparison when a major alteration in the active moiety occurs and *in vitro* potency is altered. It is not expected or necessary to apply the 20% difference/80% power rule for PD comparability studies. Bridging nonclinical safety studies are usually not needed for a typical comparability assessment. Alterations of the biopharmaceutical that could potentially result in a significant shift in the risk:benefit ratio that cannot be solved by altering the clinical trial (e.g., altering the clinical dose to account for potency or PK differences) could warrant a bridging toxicology study. This might be particularly important if there is a steep dose-response curve for a severe or unmonitorable clinical toxicity or if a small safety margin was established with the pre-change product in initial toxicology studies. If a bridging toxicology study is needed, it could consist of a single 1–3 month study with the post-change product in a pharmacologically relevant species.

Immunogenicity comparability assessment is usually not informative because: (1) these studies are insensitive due to the low number of animals used and inter-animal variability (e.g., differences in time of onset, persistence, type of antibody, incidence); and (2) immunogenicity in animals is not predictive of clinical immunogenicity. Considerations for including comparative immunogenicity end-points in a comparability study can include changes in the post-change product that are known to increase immunogenicity, such as the presence of certain leachables and increase in bacterial protein contaminants (i.e., endotoxin) or high order biopharmaceutical aggregates. Greater clinical concern exists for induction of ADA that have the potential to neutralize non-redundant endogenous protein function. Prior to performing an immunogenicity comparability study, the likelihood of the study informing clinical decision making, the utility of the study compared to a clinical assessment, the type of data to be collected and evaluated, the animal model and the predictive potential of the results should all be considered. Although these assessments are of limited utility in most cases, if immunogenicity comparative end-points are included in a nonclinical comparability study, then antibody titre along with the number of animals affected for pre- and post-change products should be compared side-by-side.

Disclaimer

The views expressed are those of the authors. No official support or endorsement is provided by the US Food and Drug Administration to those authors indicated with an asterisk*.

References

Barbacid, M. (1995) Structural and functional properties of the TRK family of neurotrophin receptors. *Ann. N. Y. Acad. Sci.*, **766**, 442–458.

Bourne, H.R. and von Zastrow, M. (2004) Drug receptors and pharmacodynamics, in *Basic and Clinical Pharmacology* (ed. B.G. Katzung), The McGraw-Hill Companies, Inc., pp. 13–14.

Brugelski, F.P.J., Rehm, S., Harmensen, A.G. *et al.* (2000) Preclinical development of keliximab, a Primitized™ anti-CD4 monoclonal antibody in human CD4 transgenic mice: characterization of the model and safety studies. *Human Exp. Tox.*, **19**, 230–243.

Bussiere, J.L., Martin, P., Horner, M. *et al.* (2009) Alternative strategies for toxicity testing of species-specific biopharmaceuticals. *Int. J. Toxicol.*, **28**(3), 230–253.

Descotes, J. (2004) Importance of immunotoxicity in safety assessment: a medical toxicologist's perspective. *Toxicol. Lett.*, **149**, 103–108.

EMA Committee of Medicinal Products for Human Use (CHMP) (2007) Guideline on Strategies to Identify and Mitigate Risks for First-in-Human Clinical Trials with Investigational Medicinal Products.

FDA (1996) Guidance Concerning Demonstration of Comparability of Human Biological Products, Including Therapeutic Biotechnology-Derived Products.

FDA (1997) Points to Consider in the Manufacture and Testing of Monoclonal Antibody Products for Human Use.

FDA (2004a) Pharmacology reviews for Erbitux® (BLA-125,084) (http://www.accessdata.fda.gov/drugsatfda_docs/bla/2004/125084_erbitux_toc.cfm) FDA 2011.

FDA (2004b) Guidance to Industry Developing Medical Imaging Drug and Biological Products, Part 1: Conducting Safety Assessments.

FDA (2005) Guidance for Industry Estimating the Maximum Safe Starting Dose in Initial Clinical Trials for Therapeutics in Adult Healthy Volunteers.

FDA (2009) Guidance for Industry (draft) Assay Development for Immunogenicity Testing of Therapeutic Proteins, Dec.

Frank, H.J., Davidson, M.B., and Serbin, P.A. (1981) Insulin binding and action in isolated rat hepatocytes: evidence for spare receptors. *Metabolism*, **30**, 1159–1164

Gold, L.S., Manley, N.B., Slone, T.H., and Rohrbach, L. (1999) Supplement to the carcinogenic potency database (CPDB): result of animal bioassays published in the general literature from 1993 to 1994 and by the national toxicology program in 1995 to 1996. *Environ. Health Perspect.*, **107**(Suppl. 4), 527–600.

Haley, P.J. (2003) Species differences in the structure and the function of the immune system. *Toxicology*, **188**, 49–71.

Hsu, D.-H., Shi, J.D., Homola, M. *et al.* (1999) A humanized Anti-CD3 Antibody, HuM291, with low mitogenic activity, mediates complete and reversible T-cell depletion in chimpanzees. *Transplantation*, **68**, 545–554.

Hupfeld, C.J. and Olefsky, J.M. (2007) Regulation of receptor tyrosine kinase signaling by GRKs and Beta-Arrestins. *Annu. Rev. Physiol.*, **69**, 561–577.

ICH S3A: (1995) Toxicokinetics: A Guidance for Assessing Systemic Exposure in Toxicology Studies.

ICH S2B: (1997) A Standard Battery for Genotoxicity Testing of Pharmaceuticals.

ICH S5(R2): (2000) Detection of Toxicity of Reproduction for Medicinal Products and Toxicity to Male Fertility.

ICH S7A: (2001) Safety Pharmacology Studies for Human Pharmaceuticals.

ICH Q5E: (2005) Comparability of Biotechnological/Biological Products Subject to Changes in their Manufacturing Process.

ICH S8: (2006) Immunotoxicity Studies for Human Pharmaceuticals.

ICH M3(R2): (2010a) Guidance on Nonclinical Safety Studies for the Conduct of Human Clinical Trials and Marketing Authorization for Pharmaceuticals.

ICH S9: (2010b) Nonclinical Evaluation of Anticancer Pharmaceuticals.

ICH S6(R1): (2011) Preclinical Safety Evaluation of Biotechnology-Derived Pharmaceuticals.

Knight, A., Bailey, J., and Balcombe, J. (2006) Animal carcinogenicity studies 2. Obstacles to extrapolation of data to humans. *ATLA*, **34**, 29–38.

Mendelson, C., Dufau, M.L., and Catt, K.J. (1975) Gonadotropin binding and stimulation of cyclic adenosine 3′-5′-Monophosphate and testosterone production in isolated leydig cells. *J. Biol. Chem.*, **250**, 8818–8823.

Mire-Sluis, A.R., Barrett, Y.C., Devanarayan, V. *et al.* (2004) Recommendations for the design and optimization of immunoassays used in the detection of host antibodies against biotechnology products. *J. Immunol. Methods*, **289**, 1–16.

Moore, C.A.C., Milano, S.K., and Benovic, J.L. (2007) Regulation of receptor trafficking by GRKs and arrestins. *Annu. Rev. Physiol.*, **69**, 451–482.

Muller, P.Y. and Brennan, F.R. (2009) Safety assessment and dose selection for first-in-human clinical trials with immunomodulatory monoclonal antibodies. *Clin. Pharmacol. Ther.*, **85**(3), 247–258.

Norman, D.J., Vincenti, F., de Mattos, A.M. *et al.* (2000) Phase I Trial of HuM291, a humanized Anti-CD3 antibody, in patients receiving renal allografts from living donors. *Transplantation*, **70**, 1707–1712.

Opanasopit, P., Shirashi, K., Nishikawa, M. *et al.* (2001) In vivo recognition of mannosylated protein by hepatic mannose receptors and mannan-binding proteins. *Am. J. Physiol. Gastrointest. Liver Physio.*, **280**, G879–G889

Otter, M., Barrett-Bergshoeff, M.M., and Rijken, D.C. (1991) Binding of tissue-type plasminogen activator by the mannose receptor. *J. Biol. Chem.*, **266**, 13931–13935.

Park, E.I., Yiling, M., Unverzagt, C. *et al.* (2005) The asialoglycoprotein receptor clears glycoconjugates terminating with sialic Acidα2, 6GalNAc. *Proc. Natl. Acad. Sci.*, **102**, 17125–17129.

Ponce, R., Abad, L., Amaravadi, L. *et al.* (2009) Immunogenicity of biologically-derived therapeutics: assessment and interpretation of nonclinical safety studies. *Regul. Toxicol. Pharmacol.*, **54**, 154–182.

Qiao, S.W., Kobayashi, K., Johansen, F.E. *et al.* (2008) Dependence of antibody-mediated presentation of antigen on FcRn. *Proc. Natl. Acad. Sci.*, **106**(27), 9337–9342.

Rosenblum, I.Y. and Dayan, A.D. (2002) Carcinogenicity testing of IL-10: principles and practicalities. *Hum Exp Toxicol.*, **21**, 347–358.

Shankar, G., Pendley, C., and Stein, K.E. (2007) A risk-based bioanalytical strategy for the assessment of antibody immune responses against biological drugs. *Nat. Biotechnol.*, **25**(5), 555–561.

Supersaxo, A., Hein, W.R., and Steffen, H. (1990) Effect of molecular weight on the lymphatic absorption of water soluble compounds following subcutaneous administration. *Pharm. Res.*, **7**, 167–169.

Timsit, J., Savino, W., Safieh, B. *et al.* (1992) Growth hormone and insulin-like growth Factor-I stimulate hormonal function and proliferation of thymic epithelial cells. *J. Clin. Endocrinol. Metab.*, **75**, 183–188.

Treacy, G. (2000) Using an analogous monoclonal antibody to evaluate the reproductive and chronic toxicity potential for a humanized Anti-TNFα monoclonal antibody. *Human Exp. Tox.*, **19**, 226–228.

Wills, R.J. and Ferraiolo, B.L. (1992) The role of pharmacokinetics in the development of biotechnologically derived agents. *Clin. Pharmacokinetic*, **23**, 406–414.

19

International Safety Regulations for Vaccine Development

Robert V. House
DynPort Vaccine Company LLC, Frederick, USA

19.1 Introduction

The introduction of vaccines in 1796 arguably resulted in one of the greatest increases in survival and quality of life for humanity of any medical intervention in history. The routine use of immunization has spared the lives of countless individuals who would otherwise have died of communicable disease. Unfortunately, this has resulted in an increasing state of complacency, or worse. Vaccines are blamed for maladies without strong scientific evidence, and usually with no evidence at all (Halsey, 2001; Offit, 2011). An anti-vaccine lobby is gaining strength on these specious accusations, with the tragic result that parents are being encouraged to limit or even reject vaccination of their children. Played to its logical conclusion, this trend would almost certainly result in an increase in preventable disease.

19.2 What "Toxicities" have been Attributed to Vaccination?

A variety of maladies have been attributed to the use of vaccination. Before we discuss how toxicity is assessed and how this assessment is regulated, it is useful to examine a few of these attributions.

Nonclinical Safety Assessment: A Guide to International Pharmaceutical Regulations, First Edition.
Edited by William J. Brock, Kenneth L. Hastings and Kathy M. McGown.

19.2.1 Immune System "Overload"

Some have opined that administration of multiple vaccines to children is somehow overloading their immune system, leading to an inability to resist naturally-acquired infections. But can the immune system in fact be quantitatively overloaded? Based on the work of Offit *et al.* (2002), we must consider a few facts. The potential immune repertoire of a neonate is approximately 10^9 to 10^{11} antigens, and the B-cell capability of neonates is approximately 10^7 B-cells per mL of circulating blood. The total "load capacity" of a neonate is therefore approximately 10^4 vaccines simultaneously, assuming 100 antigens/vaccine and 10 epitopes per antigen (10^3 epitopes). However, based on a standard vaccination regimen, children are now exposed to approximately 125 vaccine antigens (although not simultaneously). By contrast, in 1960, there were over 3200 antigens per five vaccines total. In the intervening 50 years there has been no evidence of massive immune dysfunction related to vaccine exposure.

19.2.2 Increase in Allergy/Atopy

Another dubious idea is that vaccination disrupts the immune response in such as way to increase the incidence of allergic disease. Much of the basis for this is the so-called "hygiene hypothesis", which states that preventing childhood infections (which are generally Th1-type immune responses) results in an immune response more strongly biased toward a Th2 (allergic) response. However, this is an immunological fallacy for a variety of reasons (Offit and Hackett, 2003). First, other strong Th2-biased responses (such as immune changes seen in pregnancy) do not predispose toward allergies. Secondly, helminth infections decrease, rather than increase, allergies. Finally, the increased prevalence of Th1 and Th2 conditions are not geographically exclusive. In fact, several major, well-controlled clinical trials have failed to detect a correlation between allergy and vaccination.

This is not to say that allergic reactions to vaccines don't occur; while such reactions are rare (few cases per every 10 000 vaccinations), they can occur to various vaccine components such as animal proteins (ovalbumin, chicken proteins, gelatine, calf lymph); yeast proteins (recombinant products); preservatives (thimerosal); adjuvants (aluminium); and antibiotics. Reactions can also occur to packaging (latex in stoppers). It is important to understand that allergy *to* a vaccine component is not synonymous with allergy caused *by* vaccination.

19.2.3 Autism

Perhaps the most contentious issue regarding vaccination is a supposed association with autism. This association was originally based on a now-notorious paper (Wakefield *et al.*, 1998) which attributed the development of autism to immunization with the Measles-Mumps-Rubella (MMR) vaccine. From this inauspicious beginning, a considerable number of studies on this alleged association have been published, with the great majority clearly discounting any causal association. The issue reached its zenith in 2010 when *The Lancet* published a retraction of the original paper (Anonymous, 2010). Sadly, although the weight of scientific evidence has now refuted any association between vaccination and autism, this is likely not to be the end of the public controversy given the special interests involved, not the least of which are distraught parents seeking a cause for their children's disorder(s).

19.3 How Vaccines are (Slightly) Different from Other Biopharmaceuticals

Most of the subsequent discussion in this chapter will deal with regulations covering preventive vaccines; that is, vaccines that are developed specifically to prevent infection. Where appropriate, any differences that are specific to therapeutic vaccines will be noted.

Unlike almost all other medicines, preventive vaccines are routinely administered to large numbers of otherwise healthy individuals. Most vaccine recipients are also very young, so consideration must be given to the status of the recipient's developing immune system. Thus, the risk–benefit ratio for vaccines must be weighted even more heavily in the direction of safety. Does this imply that vaccines should be completely safe? Not at all; as with any other medical intervention, vaccines have inherent risks that should be anticipated, tested for and controlled. As with other medical products, it is necessary to establish standardized regulations that provide a clear process for assessing safety, with sufficient flexibility to accommodate the complex biology and immunology that is the basis of immunization.

In the past, safety testing for vaccines was not quite as thorough compared to other medical products since vaccines were generally perceived as safe and were administered at most only a few times over the course of an individual's lifetime. This concept has changed with proliferating technologies that have resulted in a diversity of vaccine candidate formats. Modern vaccines include recombinant proteins and peptides, conjugated molecules, genetic constructs (such as DNA vaccines), and recombinant cells, as well as traditional live and attenuated whole organisms (which are becoming increasingly rare). In addition, recent advances in immunology have demonstrated the importance of innate immunity and have led to an explosion of new adjuvant technologies, which must be evaluated in combination with specific antigens, further increasing the complexity of studies required to assess overall safety.

19.4 Regulatory Framework for Assessing Safety of Vaccines

Vaccine development in the US follows an essentially three-tiered regulatory structure. At the highest level are legal statutes written by Congress and promulgated by the Executive branch. Examples of such statues include the Public Health Service Act (42 USC 262-63) Section 351, the Federal Food, Drug and Cosmetic Act (21 USC 301-392) and the Food and Drug Administration Amendments Act. Beneath this general framework are more specific FDA rules published in the Code of Federal Regulations (CFR). Examples that are pertinent vaccines include Protection of Human Subjects (21 CFR 50), Institutional Review Boards (21 CFR 56); and Good Laboratory Practices (21 CFR 58). These regulations should be familiar to anyone engaged in developing medical products. The most specific understanding of vaccine development comes at the most proximate level, published as FDA guidance documents. The specifics of guidance documents related to safety will be discussed below.

Vaccines are subject to specific regulations enforced by the FDA, and licensure is based on successful submission of a Biologics License Application (BLA). Section 351 of the Public Health Service Act, 42 USC 262 states that "the Secretary shall approve a biologics license application on the basis of a demonstration that the biological product that is the subject of the application is *safe, pure and potent* and the facility in which the biological product is manufactured, processed, packed or held meets standards designed to assure that the product continues to be safe, pure and potent (emphasis added).

For vaccines, the manufacturing and testing necessary to ensure the characteristics of the product remain unchanged and are paramount. In terms of safety assessment for vaccines, toxicological testing in animals forms only a part of the overall continuum of testing, and one must be cognizant of myriad regulations that cover many aspects of the development lifecycle. Testing thus should be developed early in the lifecycle and be robust enough to ensure that product characteristics of safety, purity and potency meet all appropriate standards, not only at the time of licensure, but also continue to meet these standards post-licensure.

What do these terms mean in practice? As defined in the Code of Federal Regulations (21 CFR 600.3(p)), safety is "the relative freedom from harmful effect to persons affected directly or indirectly by a product when prudently administered, taking into consideration the character of the product in relation to the condition of the recipient at the time". Purity is defined in CFR 21 CFR 600.3(r) as "relative freedom from extraneous matter in the finished product, whether or not harmful to the recipient or deleterious to the product. Purity includes but is not limited to relative freedom from residual moisture or other volatile substances and pyrogenic substances". Finally, potency is defined (21 CFR 600.3(s)) as "the specific ability or capacity of the product, as indicated by appropriate laboratory test or by adequately controlled clinical data obtained through administration of the product in the manner intended, to effect a given result". [Note that this "given result" does not necessarily imply the efficacy of the vaccine.] It is appropriate therefore to discuss these preliminary issues of quality before covering more traditional concepts of safety (toxicity) testing.

19.4.1 Quality Testing

A commonly-used expression in vaccine development is "the process is the product". Perhaps more than any other type of medicinal product, including even other biopharmaceutical products, the production process (and consequently the various quality checks to ensure consistent production) of vaccines is intimately associated with the regulatory process and, indeed, the ability to license the product. As stated above, it is crucial that manufacturers are able to demonstrate that a vaccine is safe, pure and potent. The term "safety" in this case subtends a number of different things, all of them covered by various regulations and guidelines. The key concept is "product characterization"; for vaccines, it is crucial that the product's biochemical/biophysical characteristics are well understood and documented, and that the manufacturing process is likewise well characterized to facilitate consistency in product over time. Special considerations should be given to adventitious agent testing, examination for unwanted (extraneous) materials, and evaluation of stability under various storage conditions.

Product characterization is assessed by designing and implementing lot release testing. While the exact list of required lot release assays is dependent on the vaccine itself, some examples include the following:

- *Sterility tests* to detect microbial contamination, whether bacterial or fungal;
- *General safety tests*, to detect extraneous toxic contaminants (a "blunt force" assay generally performed in guinea pigs and mice);
- *Identity tests* to confirm identity of the product. The type of test used is usually dependent on the vaccine characteristics but can include amino acid analysis (AAA), Western blots, SDS-PAGE, or immunologic assays;
- *Potency* measurements (*in vivo* or *in vitro*) to evaluate chemical composition of the vaccine product, its antigen content, and its immunogenicity. These three characteristics are, not surprisingly, closely related.
- *Purity* determinations including percent moisture, presence of endotoxin, and biochemical tests such as SDS-PAGE. Tests should also be included to determine the efficacy of removing process contaminants.

Whereas many vaccines are now based on recombinant proteins or peptides, many still are based on inactivated or attenuated live organisms. Such vaccines represent a difficult challenge; as described earlier, the acceptable risk–benefit ratio for vaccines, while historically high, is now much more conservative. As a consequence, it is crucial that strong demonstration of attenuation and lack of reversion be demonstrated. Various approaches are available to accomplish attenuation with a high degree of confidence (Kimman, 1992; Frey, 2007), and animal models are being developed to assess safety (Levenbook, 2011).

FDA Guidelines that cover various aspects of vaccine manufacture and testing include: Points to Consider in the Production and Testing of New Drugs and Biologicals Produced by Recombinant DNA Technology (FDA, 1985); Guidance for Industry, Content and Format of Chemistry, Manufacturing and Controls Information and Establishment Description Information for a Vaccine or Related Product (FDA, 1999); Draft Guidance for Industry, Characterization and Qualification of Cell Substrates and Other Biological Starting Materials Used in the Production of Viral Vaccines for the Prevention and Treatment of Infectious Diseases (FDA, 2006a) and Guidance for Industry Process Validation: General Principles and Practices (FDA, 2011). In Europe, guidance is found in: Quality of Biotechnological Products: Stability Testing of Biotechnological/Biological Products. CPMP/ICH/138/95 (CPMP, 1995); Note for Guidance on Pharmaceutical and Biological Aspects of Combined Vaccines CPMP/BWP/477/97 (CPMP, 1998) and Guideline on Quality, Non-clinical and Clinical Aspects of Live Recombinant Viral Vectored Vaccines EMA/CHMP/VWP/141697/2009 (EMA, 2010). Additional guidance is found in Guideline of Pharmaceutical Aspects of the Product Information for Human Vaccines. EMA/CMP/BWP/2758/02 (EMA, 2003).

19.4.2 Toxicology Testing

Following the initial safety assessment provided by the battery of tests required to demonstrate purity and characterization, nonclinical safety studies must be performed prior to initiation of human clinical trials. As with any other medicinal product, vaccines must be tested for safety in well-controlled studies. In the US, Federal regulations are quite specific: 21 CFR 312.23(a)(8) states that " . . . adequate information about the pharmacological and toxicological studies . . . *in vivo* or *in vitro studies* should be conducted on the basis of which the sponsor has concluded that it is reasonably safe to conduct the proposed clinical investigations. The kind, duration, and scope of animal and other tests required vary with the duration and nature of the proposed clinical investigations".

While regulations require that safety testing be performed, regulators have routinely recognized that the complex characteristics of vaccines would preclude the implementation of regimented requirements; thus, vaccines tend to be covered by guidance documents. This flexibility acknowledges that the study design for safety assessment should be case-by-case and driven by not only the unique character of the vaccine candidate, but the body of existing literature to devise a coherent and comprehensive plan.

With this in mind, there are a number of things that should be considered when designing preclinical safety assessments for vaccines. One should bear in mind that preclinical safety studies should help determine a safe and immunogenic dose for human clinical trials and to enable entry into those trials. Carefully-designed preclinical studies will inform what types of safety parameters should be included in clinical studies, as well as identify any potential target organ toxicities. In addition, study designs should incorporate as many clinical parameter considerations as are practical, such as the intended target population (and any existing clinical data or literature that would inform potential toxicities), how the route of administration might affect anticipated toxicity, and any novel or unique features of the vaccine candidate. As an example, a proposed vaccine against botulinum neurotoxin would likely include evaluation for potential neurotoxicity of the vaccine itself.

The balance of this chapter will focus on FDA, EMA, and WHO regulations. These regulations are generally congruent, and in most cases regulatory agencies will default to WHO guidelines where applicable. While regions other than the US and Europe have their own internal regulations governing the development of vaccines, compliance with the three entities listed above is generally necessary to facilitate international trade in vaccines.

19.4.3 General Toxicology Study Design Considerations

Regulatory guidelines for vaccines are relatively harmonized between the US and Europe. In Europe, the Note for Guidance on preclinical pharmacological and toxicological testing of vaccines (CHMP, 1997) provides a fairly comprehensive description of preclinical safety testing for vaccines; however, this guidance has increasingly been superseded by the WHO guidelines on nonclinical evaluation of vaccines, WHO Technical Report Series No. 927, Annex 1 (2005), which is very similar although slightly more detailed. For US regulations, the WHO guidance is the default regulation. The following sections are based on this guidance.

The obvious first issue in study design is the selection of which animal model to use. The issue of what constitutes a relevant animal species is one that deserves careful consideration prior to any safety assessment. A primary consideration should be that the species chosen should be "responsive" to the vaccine; that is, the animal should develop an immune response following vaccination. Ideally, the animal should be sensitive to the pathogenic organism or toxin against which the vaccine is being developed. In general, the FDA has required only one relevant animal species, although exceptions might be necessary on a case-by-case basis. The majority of times the relevant model tends to be a small animal (rodents or rabbits); nonhuman primates are generally not used unless the vaccine candidate characteristics dictate this model.

The route of administration, dose and dosing frequency chosen for toxicity studies should duplicate the intended route of clinical administration as closely as possible. This can be difficult when using small animal models, particularly if novel administration devices are employed. Generally, a full human-equivalent dose is preferred by regulators. However, many vaccines are administered in a dose of 500 μL; while this volume can be given intramuscularly in humans, it is impractical for rodents. Dividing this volume into multiple dose sites is one strategy, although admittedly less than ideal. Route of administration can also become a problem with mucosal administration, particularly with nasal vaccines where the human nasal environment is not easily replicated in animals. Finally, dose frequency (for vaccines which require multiple vaccinations, such as recombinant vaccines) might not be practical in animals with a short life span such as rodents. In these cases, an abbreviated or compressed schedule is usually acceptable. Although dose is an important concept in toxicology, it is probably less important for safety assessment of vaccines as long as the amount administered to animals is demonstrably immunogenic.

Vaccine toxicology studies can be conducted using either single-dose or repeated-dose paradigms, depending on existing knowledge about the vaccine candidate. For repeated-dose studies the number of doses should generally be $N+1$ ($N=$ number of doses to be given to humans) in an effort to gain a margin of safety, and it is preferable to utilize a range of dose concentrations. Each study should include a concurrent control group (the formulation matrix lacking only the relevant antigen is generally used), and if an adjuvant is employed an adjuvant-only formulation can be used.

Reversibility of any adverse effects should be evaluated in repeated-dose studies. This is generally accomplished using a staged post-mortem design in which toxicologic evaluations are performed shortly (within days) after cessation of exposure, as well as following a recovery period (two weeks is often used). To economize in use of animals and other resources, this recovery group might include only a control and high-dose group.

19.5 Parameters Monitored

End-point assessment for vaccine studies is very similar to any other biopharmaceutical product, with some minor exceptions. First, immunogenicity of the vaccine should always be assessed concurrent with toxicologic end-points; this serves to demonstrate that the vaccine is having its intended effect in conjunction with assessment of any adverse effects. Second, the local toxicity of vaccines should be assessed; this local reaction is generally termed "reactogenicity" and can routinely be measured using a standard or modified Draize scoring system. Local reactogenicity must be determined following administration of a full human dose (same volume to be used clinically) so the animal model must be able to accommodate an injection of this volume.

Routine toxicological end-points are integral to vaccine safety assessment. These include clinical observations, serum chemistries, haematologic analysis, body and organ weights, and histopathology. Histopathology is generally done on the full standard battery of tissues, with particular emphasis on "pivotal" organs such as the liver, brain, kidneys and so forth. In addition, special emphasis should be placed on histopathology of immune system organs and tissues (spleen, thymus, bone marrow and lymph nodes, both distant and those draining the site of injection).

19.5.1 Safety Testing for Adjuvants

Another way in which vaccines differ from most other medicines is in the use of adjuvants, which act to improve or "boost" immunogenicity, possibly through engagement of the innate immune response (Leroux-Roels, 2010). In general, adjuvants have limited, if any, function exclusive of their role in improving vaccines and, as such, are not licensed separately; rather, adjuvants are licensed in conjunction with the vaccine to which they are added (Sesardic, 2006). In general, regulatory agencies will expect to see data substantiating the need for an adjuvant, particularly in clinical trials; if there is no compelling reason to include an adjuvant, it should not be included. Before a consideration is made to include an adjuvant in a new vaccine candidate, the adjuvant should be tested separately as a new chemical entity, and the toxicology studies employed should be appropriate to the class of compound that the adjuvant represents. Recommended testing approaches for adjuvants are given in Guideline on Adjuvants in Vaccines for Human Use, EMA/CHMP/VEG/134716/2004 (EMA, 2005). While not strictly mandated by regulations, immunotoxicology assessment is a good idea given that the function of an adjuvant is often to "prime" the immune response (Brennan and Dougan, 2005). An explanatory note for "Guideline on Adjuvants in Vaccines for Human Use" was issued by EMA (EMA, 2006).

19.5.2 Reproductive Toxicology

In the United States, reproductive toxicity testing is described in Draft Guidance for Industry: Considerations for Reproductive Toxicity Studies for Preventive Vaccines for Infectious Disease Indications (FDA, 2006b).

Reproductive toxicology has long been a requirement for drug development; however, it is only in the past decade or so that regulations have been promulgated for this type of testing for vaccines. Reproductive toxicology testing is necessary when a vaccine could be administered to females of child-bearing potential; at present (2013) no testing requirements have been established for males regarding vaccine development. Standard reproductive toxicology testing paradigms established for drugs may not be appropriate for vaccines. Rather, studies should use an appropriate animal model, usually a species being used for other safety and efficacy studies. In general, small animal models are employed for these studies, although recently approaches have been proposed using nonhuman primates (Martin and Weinbauer, 2010). Study design is expected to evaluate both embryo–foetal and postnatal/neonatal toxicity. An understanding of the kinetics of antibody formation (and vector clearance in the case of live/attenuated vaccines) is crucial, with peak kinetics of antibody expression occurring during the period of organogenesis. For this reason, selection of animal model becomes of particular importance since the vaccine candidate should be immunogenic in the model of choice. Reproductive toxicity testing for vaccines is generally conducted using Phase 3 human dose and schedule.

19.5.3 Immunotoxicity

While vaccines are clearly intended to produce benefits in humans and animals, paradoxically they could strictly be characterized as immunotoxicants, given that immunotoxicology can be defined as an agent that modulates a resting or nominal immune state in either a positive or negative manner (House and Hastings, 2004). In practical terms, vaccines are evaluated for immunomodulatory activity very early in development, limiting the possibility of adverse immune findings prior to human trials. This is not to say that the possibility of immunosuppression or hyper-stimulation of the immune system should not be considered; in fact, while not mandated by regulations, potential immunotoxicity should be considered. The current thinking on immunotoxicity assessment is covered by ICH S8, Note for Guidance on Immunotoxicity Studies for Human Pharmaceuticals (ICH, 2004). This guidance is applicable for both US and European regulatory agencies. ICH M3 (R2), Non-clinical Safety Studies for the Conduct of Human Clinical Trials and Marketing Authorization for Pharmaceuticals (ICH, 2009) also includes wording relevant to immunotoxicity testing, although not specifically in the context of vaccines.

19.5.4 Genotoxicity

In nearly all cases, genotoxicity assessment is not required for vaccines. One notable exception is for vaccines that contain DNA or other genetic elements, such as plasmid DNA. With these vaccines there could be a risk that the genetic elements may become incorporated into the host genome, may become persistent in the host, may cause adverse immunological or immunotoxicological reactions, and may even pose an environmental hazard (Schalk *et al.*, 2006). Multiple guidance documents cover this issue, including Draft Guidance for Industry: Considerations for Plasmid DNA Vaccines for Infectious Disease Indications (FDA, 2007), Guidelines for Assuring the Quality and Nonclinical Safety Evaluation of DNA Vaccines (WHO, 1998) and Note for Guidance on the Quality, Preclinical and Clinical Aspects of Gene Transfer Medicinal Products, CPMP/BWP/3088/99 (CPMP, 2001). In addition, some useful guidance can be found in ICH S6, Preclinical Safety Evaluation of Biotechnology-Derived Pharmaceuticals (ICH, 1998) and its addendum (ICH, 2011). Williams *et al.* (2009) have published a useful summary of approaches designed to address genotoxicity issues in vaccines.

19.6 Clinical Safety Assessment of Vaccines

Safety is always of primary importance since vaccines are most often given to healthy individuals. As a consequence, while the overall strategy for clinical trials with vaccines is similar to other medicinal products, there are a few differences. In particular, safety assessment is the principal end-point for both Phase 1 and Phase 2 trials, and remains a key end-point for Phase 3 and for post-licensure assessment. Likewise, immunogenicity is a key assessment factor for Phases 1–3, with efficacy testing usually taking place during Phase 3 trials. A recent review by Marshall and Baylor (2011) provides an excellent overview of the FDA's clinical development expectations for vaccines.

Vaccine safety continues to extend into the post-licensure period, and a variety of programmes are in place or under development to track the long-term consequences of immunization. Examples include the Vaccine Adverse Event Reporting System (VAERS) (Iskander *et al.*, 2006) and the Vaccine Safety Datalink (Baggs *et al.*, 2011).

19.7 Summary

Vaccines are one of mankind's greatest medical advances, preventing many of the infectious diseases that have ravaged the human population throughout history. However, since they are routinely given to large numbers of otherwise healthy individuals, society has decided that evaluation of these agents must consider a near-zero tolerance for risk. Alarmingly, a vocal and increasingly influential anti-vaccine movement has begun to influence popular perception and understanding of vaccines and vaccinations around the world, often using fear and disinformation in an attempt to reduce or eliminate childhood vaccination. Clearly, there is an urgent need for a rational discussion and efforts to reverse this disturbing trend. A number of individuals have provided reasoned discussions in the literature (c.f., François *et al.*, 2005; Jacobson *et al.*, 2007; Poland *et al.*, 2009); however, these academic treatises are written for other academics. What is desperately needed is a more "popular" defense of vaccines for the general public.

As it turns out, based upon clinical data, vaccines by and large appear to be some of the safest medicinal products. Still, to address the ongoing need to ensure safety, regulations have been promulgated by the world's primary regulatory bodies (FDA and EMA/EMA) and health organizations (WHO). Through years of collaboration, many of these guidance documents and points to consider have been harmonized, providing a corpus of directives to pharmaceutical and biotechnology companies engaged in vaccine development. It is certain that as new technologies for vaccine discovery and development are employed (such as those reported by Momose *et al.* (2010)), these regulatory considerations will have to co-evolve with them. Only by doing so will vaccines continue to provide protection against infectious diseases.

References

Anonymous (2010) Retraction–Ileal-lymphoid-nodular hyperplasia, non-specific colitis, and pervasive developmental disorder in children. *Lancet*, **375**(9713), 445.

Baggs, J., Gee, J., Lewis, E. *et al.* (2011) The Vaccine Safety Datalink: a model for monitoring immunization safety. *Pediatrics*, **127**(Suppl 1), S45–S53.

Brennan, F.R. and Dougan, G. (2005) Non-clinical safety evaluation of novel vaccines and adjuvants: new products, new strategies. *Vaccine*, **23**, 3210–3222.

CPMP (1995) Quality of Biotechnological Products: Stability Testing of Biotechnological/Biological Products. CPMP/ICH/138/95. http://bit.ly/mIaQvg. Accessed June 2, 2011.

CPMP (1997) Note for guidance of preclinical pharmacological and toxicological testing of vaccines. CPMP/SWP/465/95. http://bit.ly/mKUzXg. Accessed April 15, 2011.

CPMP (1998) Note for Guidance on Pharmaceutical and Biological Aspects of Combined Vaccines. CPMP/BWP/477/97. http://bit.ly/jTl8Rq. Accessed June 1, 2011.

CPMP (2001) Note for Guidance on the Quality, Preclinical and Clinical Aspects of Gene Transfer Medicinal Products. CPMP/BWP/3088/99. http://bit.ly/mx0sm2. Accessed May 2, 2011.

EMA (2003) Guideline of Pharmaceutical Aspects of the Product Information for Human Vaccines. EMA/CMP/BWP/2758/02. http://bit.ly/m4moBt. Accessed June 3, 2011.

EMA (2005) Guideline on Adjuvants in Vaccines for Human Use. EMA/CHMP/VEG/134716/2004. http://bit.ly/kGqquE. Accessed April 15, 2011.

EMA (2006) Explanatory Note on Immunomodulators for the Guideline on Adjuvants in Vaccines for Human Use. EMA/CHMP/VWP/244894/2006. http://bit.ly/jlNhUs. Accessed April 15, 2011.

EMA (2010) Guideline on quality, non-clinical and clinical aspects of live recombinant viral vectored vaccines. EMA/CHMP/VWP/141697/2009. http://bit.ly/9HrYJj. Accessed June 1, 2011.

FDA (1985) Points to Consider in the Production and Testing of New Drugs and Biologicals Produced by Recombinant DNA Technology. http://1.usa.gov/jsp3r8. Accessed April 2, 2011.

FDA (1999) Guidance for Industry: Content and Format of Chemistry, Manufacturing and Controls Information and Establishment Description Information for a Vaccine or Related Product. http://1.usa.gov/ivhkmE. Accessed April 15, 2011.

FDA (2006a) Draft Guidance for Industry: Characterization and Qualification of Cell Substrates and Other Biological Starting Materials used in the Production of Viral Vaccines for the Prevention and Treatment of Infectious Diseases. http://1.usa.gov/ii7Hqn. Accessed May 2, 2011.

FDA (2006b) Guidance for Industry: Considerations for Developmental Toxicity Studies for Preventive and Therapeutic Vaccines for Infectious Disease Indications. http://1.usa.gov/luu4Tw. Accessed May 2, 2011.

FDA (2007) Draft Guidance for Industry: Considerations for Plasmid DNA Vaccines for Infectious Disease Indications. http://1.usa.gov/mFk7nn. Accessed May 2, 2011.

FDA (2011) Guidance for Industry: Process Validation: General Principles and Practices. http://1.usa.gov/hkVV6m. Accessed May 10, 2011.

François, G., Duclos, P., Margolis, H. *et al.* (2005) Vaccine safety controversies and the future of vaccination programs. *Pediatr. Infect. Dis. J.*, **24**(11), 953–961.

Frey, J. (2007) Biological safety concepts of genetically modified live bacterial vaccines. *Vaccine*, **25**(30), 5598–5605.

Halsey, N.A. (2001) Combination vaccines: defining and addressing current safety concerns. *Clin. Infect. Dis.*, **15**(33 Suppl 4), S312–S318.

House, R.V. and Hastings, K.L. (2004) Multidimensional immunomodulation. *J. Immunotoxicol.*, **1**, 123–129.

ICH (1998) ICH Topic S 6. Preclinical Safety Evaluation of Biotechnology-Derived Pharmaceuticals. http://bit.ly/iTczr1. Accessed May 12, 2011.

ICH (2004) ICH Topic S8 Note for Guidance on Immunotoxicity Studies for Human Pharmaceuticals. CHMP/167235/2004. http://bit.ly/k5Hyao. Accessed May 3, 2011.

ICH (2009) Addendum to ICH S6: Preclinical Safety Evaluation of Biotechnology-Derived Pharmaceuticals. S6(R1). http://1.usa.gov/8iyC3h. Accessed May 12, 2011.

ICH Topic M 3 (R2) Non-clinical Safety Studies for the Conduct of Human Clinical Trials and Marketing Authorization for Pharmaceuticals. CPMP/ICH/286/95, 2009. http://bit.ly/jaOqis. Accessed May 15, 2011.

Iskander, J., Pool, V., Zhou, W. *et al.* The VAERS Team (2006) Data mining in the US using the Vaccine Adverse Event Reporting System. *Drug Safety*, **29**, 375–384.

Jacobson, R.M., Targonski, P.V., and Poland, G.A. (2007) A taxonomy of reasoning flaws in the anti-vaccine movement. *Vaccine*, **25**(16), 3146–3152.

Kimman, T.G. (1992) Risks connected with the use of conventional and genetically engineered vaccines. *Vet. Q.*, **14**(3), 110–118.

Leroux-Roels, G. (2010) Unmet needs in modern vaccinology: adjuvants to improve the immune response. *Vaccine*, **28**(Suppl 3), C25–C36.

Levenbook, I. (2011) The role of non-human primates in the neurological safety of live viral vaccines (review). *Biologicals.*, **39**(1), 1–8.

Marshall, V. and Baylor, N.W. (2011) Food and Drug Administration regulation and evaluation of vaccines. *Pediatrics*, **127**, S23–S30.

Martin, P.L. and Weinbauer, G.F. (2010) Developmental toxicity testing of biopharmaceuticals in nonhuman primates: previous experience and future directions. *Int. J. Toxicol.*, **29**, 552–568.

Momose, H., Mizukami, T., Ochiai, M. *et al.* (2010) A new method for the evaluation of vaccine safety based on comprehensive gene expression analysis. *J. Biomed. Biotechnol.*, **2010**, 361841.

Offit, P.A. (2011) Why are pharmaceutical companies gradually abandoning vaccines? *Health Affairs*, **24**, 622–630.

Offit, P.A. and Hackett, C.J. (2003) Addressing parents' concerns: do vaccines cause allergic or autoimmune diseases? *Pediatrics*, **111**, 653–659.

Offit, P.A., Quarels, J., Gerber, M.A. *et al.* (2002) Addressing parents' concerns: Do multiple vaccines overwhelm or weaken the infant's immune system? *Pediatrics*, **109**, 124–129.

Poland, G.A., Jacobson, R.M., and Ovsyannikova, I.G. (2009) Trends affecting the future of vaccine development and delivery: the role of demographics, regulatory science, the anti-vaccine movement, and vaccinomics. *Vaccine*, **27**(25–26), 3240–3244.

Schalk, J.A., Mooi, F.R., Berbers, G.A. *et al.* (2006) Preclinical and clinical safety studies on DNA vaccines. *Hum. Vaccin.*, **2**(2), 45–53.

Sesardic, D. (2006) Regulatory considerations on new adjuvants and delivery systems. *Vaccine*, **24S2**, S2/86-S2/87.

Wakefield, A.J., Murch, S.H., Linnell, A.J. *et al.* (1998) Ileal-lymphoid-nodular hyperplasia, non-specific colitis, and pervasive developmental disorder in children. *Lancet*, **351**, 637–641.

WHO guidelines on nonclinical evaluation of vaccines WHO Technical Report Series No. 927, Annex 1 (2005). http://bit.ly/ksVaWB. Accessed May 5, 2011.

WHO Guidelines for Assuring the Quality and Nonclinical Safety Evaluation of DNA Vaccines (1998). Geneva, Switzerland. http://bit.ly/m3Hz1H. Accessed May 10, 2011.

Williams, J.A., Carnew, A.E., and Hodgson, C.P. (2009) Plasmid DNA vaccine vector design: impact on efficacy, safety and upstream production. *Biotechnol. Adv.*, **27**, 353–370.

20

Phototoxicity and Photocarcinogenicity

Robert E. Osterberg,[1] *Christopher P. Sambuco*[2]*, and Paul Donald Forbes*[3]
[1]*Osterberg Pharm-Tox Consulting, Rockville, USA*
[2]*Downingtown, USA*
[3]*Toxarus Inc., Malvern, USA*

20.1 History of Phototoxicity, Photocarcinogenicity and Photogenotoxicity Testing at the US Food and Drug Administration (FDA)

Most, if not all, humans take the physical phenomenon called light for granted even thought its source, photons from the Sun, might exist for only another 5 billion years. Light is central to our interactions with both artificial and natural environments and is as essential for our existence as are air and water. All people, as well as most living organisms, are or have been exposed to the Sun or to equipment that emits ultraviolet radiation (UVR). These exposures can produce damaging (sunburn), cytotoxic, genotoxic and/or carcinogenic responses in living tissues. Light contains UVA, UVB, and visible wavelengths and many substances interact with one or more of these radiations. The Grotthaus-Draper law states that light must be absorbed for a photochemical event to occur. Chromophores in drug products and DNA in dermal tissue are targets for photochemical reactions (FDA, 2003; Megaw and Drake, 1986). It can be observed that the structural characteristics of many photoactive chemicals include either a planar, tricyclic or polycyclic configuration that can absorb light and generate an electronically excited species that could cause biological damage. Incorporation of halogens in the chemical structures may produce even more damage (Oppenlander, 1988).

Interestingly, UVR exposures to chemicals found in drugs, cosmetics and foods can demonstrate an interaction between light absorption, the product and the skin that can result in a toxicity called photosensitization or photoirritation. There are many drugs and

Nonclinical Safety Assessment: A Guide to International Pharmaceutical Regulations, First Edition.
Edited by William J. Brock, Kenneth L. Hastings and Kathy M. McGown.

chemicals that demonstrate this form of toxicity, that is, psoralens, several antibiotics, porphyrins, retinoids and nonsteroidal anti-inflammatory drugs, and so on (Osterberg and Szarfman, 1996; Derelanko and Hollinger, 2002). Historically, the majority of systemically administered drugs have not undergone photosafety testing while drugs applied topically have routinely been assessed for this toxicologic potential.

Phototoxicity testing has not always been of high concern for the regulatory agencies of the world, including those in the United States. There are stories and references about phototoxic substances in existence for a few thousand years and also in various reports up to the present century (Urbach, 1998). With this in mind, the human tragedy that resulted in the promulgation of the US Food, Drug and Cosmetic Act in 1938 (FD&C Act) did not marshal significant interest in this toxicity.

Concern for photocarcinogenic substances arose at the same time as phototoxicity was recognized for regulatory investigations, the former being the extension of excessive exposures to UVR. It was known that UV light by itself is a carcinogen in humans. Historically, Findlay (1928) demonstrated that skin tumours in animals could be induced by UVR. Urbach (2008) showed that UVR-induced photocarcinogenesis was enhanced by topical or parenterally administered photoactive drugs of several classes. Furthermore, Winkelman *et al.* (1960) discovered UV-induced squamous cell tumours in genetically hairless mice. About the same time, Epstein (1965) could have been the first scientist to report on drugs and chemicals and UV-induced dermal carcinogenesis using a standardized set of experimental procedures that involved repeated chemical administration. Later, he expanded the list of photocarcinogenic chemicals using several animal models (Epstein, 1975). Experiments of this type stimulated other scientists to investigate this emerging area of concern. As an example, Forbes and colleagues demonstrated enhanced carcinogenic ability of UVR by application of a drug used in psoriasis, 8-methoxypsoralen, to the skin of hairless mice (Forbes *et al.*, 1975, Forbes et al., 1990). This finding was subsequently confirmed by Stern *et al.* (1997) and then Morison *et al.* (1998) in large clinical trials.

Scientists in the FDA's Center for Drug Evaluation and Research (CDER) in the 1980s became more concerned about the impact of phototoxicity information on human safety, especially when topical retinoids were being tested for safety and efficacy for the eventual use in acne. Forbes et al. (1979) demonstrated that topical retinoids and UVR decreased the latency period for the emergence of skin papillomas in mice. As a result of this and other reports describing drugs administered parenterally or topically to humans and resultant phototoxic responses, CDER requested that sponsors provide data during preclinical development if they absorbed UVR in the range of 280 to 700 nm, the biologically important parts of the UV spectrum. This information was used to determine whether additional animal testing should be performed to determine the severity of the potential adverse responses in humans. Testing for photocarcinogenicity in humans is considered to be unethical; therefore, animal testing is used as a surrogate. In the case of photocarcinogenicity, the most widely-used animal model was the Skh1-hr hairless mouse although other hairless or shaved species could be and have been used for testing drugs and chemicals.

Numerous scientific meetings occurred within the FDA and at national and international toxicology meetings in which the subject of phototoxicity and photocarcinogenicity (photo co-carcinogenicity) were extensively discussed. In March 1993, a CDER advisory committee meeting was held after a report that some oral fluoroquinolone antibacterials and UVA produced skin tumours in hairless mice (Klecak *et al.*, 1997; Ferguson, 2003). It was a surprise to the investigators to find that the longer wave length UVA had this influence on drug- and light-induced phototoxicity. The papillomas that were produced in the mice had shorter latency periods than those seen with UVA alone. Interestingly, the latency periods differed depending upon the fluoroquinolone that was investigated. This experiment identified 8-MOP as the most photoactive chemical followed by lomefloxacin and other fluoroquinolones. Ciprofloxacin and ofloxacin were the least photoactive and resembled the UVA control latency period for tumour production. At an FDA/CDER advisory committee meeting where a potent fluoroquinolone antibacterial was being discussed, the committee recommended to the agency that a black box warning was not appropriate in the product label. However, the findings of the photocarcinogenicity study could be inserted in the appropriate sections of the label (Warnings and/or Precautions) and the optional animal pharmacology section of the label.

From 1995 through 1997, when the International Conference on Harmonization (ICH) genotoxicity guidance (S2A and S2B) was being discussed, members of the Expert Working Groups unanimously excluded photogenotoxicity testing from the recommendations because of the lack of broad-based data and confidence in its regulatory utility. Earlier meetings within the CDER Pharmacology-Toxicology Coordinating Committee (PTCC) and the Genetic Toxicology subcommittee discussed the regulatory utility of photogenotoxicity testing that was being published in scientific journals. These FDA committees agreed not to endorse these tests for use in drug regulation at that time because of a general lack of confidence in the methods and a lack of data corroboration. Furthermore, in a November 2007 meeting in Amsterdam (DIA/EMA, 2007), it was mentioned that FDA pharmacology-toxicology reviewers lacked confidence in the value of photogenotoxicity tests because test results had not been very predictive. The experiences of international pharmaceutical companies suggested that photogenotoxicity tests, specifically the 3T3 neutral red uptake photocytotoxicity test, were overly sensitive or simply difficult to interpret and that at that time they had little practical value in the regulatory environment. As a result, the EMA/CPMP (now the CHMP) (European Medicines Agency/Committee for Medicinal Products for Human Use) representatives announced their intent to undertake revisions to their guideline because of the apparent lack of value in the inclusion of a photogenotoxicity test and its test results in a photosafety testing strategy.

Following numerous scientific meetings and seminars in which the subjects of phototoxicity and photocarcinogenicity were discussed, toxicologists in FDA CDER established a subcommittee of the PTCC with the intent to write FDA guidance for industry regarding photosafety testing. However, prior to FDA/CDER action, the ECVAM Science Advisory Committee (ESAC) released a statement in November 1997 in which it declared that the 3T3 NRU PT is a scientifically validated test that could be considered for regulatory acceptance. In addition, the EMA's Committee for Proprietary Medicinal Products (CPMP) released for consultation a "Note For Guidance On Photosafety Testing" that was finalized in late 2002 (EMA/CPMP, 2002). This guideline discussed photosafety testing for phototoxicity (photoirritation), photoallergy, photogenotoxicity and photocarcinogenicity. This was the first formal notification that photogenotoxicity, a genotoxic response after exposure to a chemical photoactivated by UV or visible light, was discussed for regulatory evaluation. In addition, this guideline discussed the 3T3 NRU PT phototoxicity test that uses the mouse fibroblast cell line Balb/c. This test also allows other cell lines to be used if the culture conditions are adapted to the specific needs of the cells. In an effort to decrease the amount of whole animal testing, topically applied chemicals might eventually be subjected to future alternative assays such as 3-D Skin models. Test strategies are also proposed to give guidance on the decision-making process for testing.

The Japanese JaCVAM undertook a peer review of a test battery consisting of the yeast growth inhibition phototoxicity assay and the red blood cell photohemolysis assay. Acceptance by the JaCVAM Regulatory Acceptance Board was pending at the time of this writing (Yanga and Xiong, 2007).

China also started research and utilization of alternative methods to replace animal testing, especially in the area of cosmetics with successful results regarding the 3T3 NRU PT assay with fibroblast cells (Gad, 2002).

FDA/CDER published its final guidance, Guidance for Industry: Photosafety Testing (FDA, 2003). This guidance was intended to help sponsors to decide whether photoirritation studies are needed in their drug development programme and to assess the potential human risk for photocarcinogenesis for their systemic or topical drug products (Table 20.1). Unlike the EMA/CHMP guideline, the FDA/CDER

Table 20.1 *Some drugs in current use reported to cause photosensitivity reactions in humans*[a].

Drug class	Examples of drug substances
Antimalarials	Chloroquine, quinine, mefloquine
Antimicrobials	Fluoroquinolones, nalidixic acid, sulfonamides, tetracyclines, aminoglycosides, isoniazid, nitrofurantoin, griseofulvin
Antihistamines	Loratadine, cyproheptadine, diphenhydramine, triprolidine, brompheniramine, chlorpheniramine
Antidepressants	Nortriptyline, desipramine, doxepin, imipramine, amitriptyline
Anticonvulsants	Phenobarbital, phenytoin, perphenazine, carbamazepine, lamotrigine
Antipsychotics	Prochlorperazine, promethazine, haloperidol, chlorpromazine, thioridazine, trifluoperazine
Cardiovascular drugs	Quinidine, captopril, enalapril, nifedipine, amiodarone, hydralazine, clofibrate, simvastatin, disopyramide
Cytotoxic drugs	Procarbazine, methotrexate, vinblastine, fluorouracil, vincristine
Diuretics	Spironolactone, hydrochlorothiazide, furosemide, ethacrynic acid, amiloride, triamterene, acetazolamide, metolazone
Hormones	Corticosteroids, estrogens, progesterones
Hypoglycemics	Glyburide, glipizide, tolbutamide, acetohexamide, chlorpropamide
Nonsteroidal anti-inflammatory drugs (NSAIDS)	Piroxicam, ibuprofen, indomethacin, diclofenac, naproxen, ketoprofen, phenylbutazone, sulindac, diflunisal
Dermatologic agents	Topical/systemic retinoids, methoxsalen
Miscellaneous drugs/ chemicals	Azathioprine, hematoporphyrin, PABA, acridine dyes

[a]Additional drugs can be reviewed in Osterberg and Szarfman (1996).

guidance does not recommend specific tests. The EMA/CHMP document indicates its preference for *in vitro* tests with descriptions of those for photogenotoxicity and phototoxicity. The FDA guidance does, however, discuss product warnings and labelling and under what conditions they may be appropriate rather than having to perform the long-term and expensive testing for photocarcinogenesis. Interestingly, the FDA guidance does mention the *in vitro* test model, namely the 3T3 neutral red uptake photocytotoxicity test, and indicates its potential utility. There may be some circumstances that allow the avoidance of photo co-carcinogenicity testing. These considerations include:

1. Drugs having structures significantly similar to known photochemical carcinogens.
2. Drugs that are in a known pharmacological class of photochemical carcinogens where the pharmacology of the product is believed to be directly related to the carcinogenic potential.
3. Drugs for which several other tests for photoreactivity, such as *in vitro* photogenotoxicity, adduct formation, human photoirritation, or short-term *in vivo* nonclinical tests are positive.
4. Drugs that have been identified as carcinogens with potential human relevance in other assays that do not include UV sunlight, such as traditional two-year bioassays or transgenic assays.

Warning statements for phototoxicity include advising patients to avoid sun exposure or, if such exposure is unavoidable, to use protective clothing and sunscreens. It also mentions that phototoxicity testing could be conducted during Clinical Phase 4 (post-approval) of the drug development process with the prior approval of the appropriate CDER review division. Four decision trees are included in the guidance to assist sponsors on the decision-making process for testing potential drugs. The sponsor should be aware that they should contact the appropriate review division to seek agreement on their desired course of action.

Both the EMA guideline and the FDA guidance mention photogenotoxicity testing as a potentially useful short-term test to measure photoreactivity. However, the interpretation of such assays is not always clear and, thus, their role in the evaluation of human risk should be carefully assessed. Recently the EMA released for review a "Note for Guidance on Photosafety Testing" (EMA/CPMP, 2002). Regarding the use of photogenotoxicity testing, specifically photoclastogenicity tests, the CPMP no longer recommends photoclastogenicity tests for regulatory purposes because test results suggest that these tests are substantially oversensitive and even incidences of pseudophotoclastogenicity have been reported. Furthermore, the document recommends the exclusion of photogenotoxicity testing as a *routine* part of the standard photosafety testing program (Table 20.2). One of the challenges related to identifying phototoxic agents is a function of disparate chemical pathways and exhibited clinical symptoms. Table 20.2 provides a suggested categorical organization that summarizes such information.

20.2 FDA Photosafety Testing Guidance

This guidance (the FDA's preferred term) is intended to assist sponsors with their decision to test for photoirritation and assess the potential of their drug product to

Table 20.2 *Selected chemical agents and compounds grouped by photochemical and photobiological effects.*

Category	Description	Example, comment, reference
A	Compounds with no reported relevant photochemistry, photobiology	Water, aliphatic alcohols, ethers
B	Compounds with some reported evidence for enhanced effectiveness of UVR or enhanced synthesis, redistribution, or localization of a photosensitizing agent	
B1	Agents with evidence for enhanced effectiveness of UVR, including neoplastic progression	Retinoids, e.g., retinoic acid; TPA; certain skin moisturizers
B2	Agents with evidence for enhanced redistribution, concentration or localization of a primary photosensitizing agent	Hypericin (chlorophyll transport to UVR exposed skin); levulinic acid (in-situ synthesis of porphyrin)
C	Evidence for photochemistry, photobiochemistry, cellular photobiology; but lack of evidence for photobiology in intact vertebrates	
C1	Only when perfused or infused	FD&C Red Food Dye
C2	Natural substances with photosensitizing potential, but not normally at risk in (intact) vertebrates	Chlorophyll, hematoporphyrin
D	Chemical agents and drugs approved for use, although reported as photosensitizers (case reports, adverse event reports)	
D1	Under unique circumstances or as relatively infrequent events	Amiodorone, NSAIDs, antibiotics, most approved FQAs; chlorpromazine
D2	Relatively mild reactions, but with some regularity	None known
D3	Relatively frequent reports	Lomefloxacin
E	Photodynamic compounds and other drugs employed therapeutically as photosensitizers	
E1	Photodynamic drugs	Thalocyanines; Photofrin and other porphyrin derivatives;
E2	Phototoxic drugs (other than PDT drugs)	8-MOP and other Psoralens
F	Compounds associated with photoallergy	TCSA
G	Highly efficient photosensitizers; the most effective phototoxic agents for intact vertebrates orally, topically, IV, etc. Generally not used clinically	Bay 3118

enhance UV-associated skin carcinogenesis. The guidance describes a consistent, science-based approach for photosafety evaluation of topically and systemically administered drug products in which basic concepts of photobiology and phototesting are described. A regulatory process is also discussed that can be used to assist in scientific and regulatory decisions and risk communication. The document does not recommend specific tests but refers to available test methods that might be useful. Other scientifically sound methods can also be used by drug sponsors. Such testing is only recommended when it is felt that the results would provide important safety information or would inform the practitioner and the consumer about potential risks of sun exposure and exposure to a drug product.

The guidance indicates that UVR is the carcinogen and that chemicals can enhance dermal carcinogenicity by hastening the production of skin neoplasms by several mechanisms and factors. Factors (FDA, 2003; Gad, 2002) that are to be considered include:

- Percutaneous penetration and absorption of a photoactive chemical into normal skin or skin altered by irritation, sunburn, and so on;
- The amount and/or location of the photoactive chemical in or on the skin;
- The amount of UVR exposure;
- Thickness of the stratum corneum;
- The degree of melanin pigmentation in the skin;
- Atmospheric conditions to which the skin is exposed such as temperature and humidity;
- The inherent photoactivity of the chemical;
- The absorption spectrum of the chemical;
- The intensity of the UVR.

The guidance further recommends that drugs that are applied topically to the skin should be tested as the drug product because of the potential influences of components, for example, excipients, in the drug product. Careful selection of topical vehicles (creams, lotions, gels, ointments and/or solutions) is recommended because some of their properties might influence a phototoxic response. Vehicles may reflect or scatter light to decrease the amount of UVR received on the skin or increase skin thickness or affect drug stability. Drug products that can decrease skin thickness could increase the amount of UVR absorbed to enhance photoirritation.

The intent of the guidance is to determine the potential of drugs to induce a photoirritation reaction before widespread human exposure. The guidance recommends a decision tree approach to determine if additional testing should occur and what type of testing is appropriate. To determine if such testing is appropriate, information regarding the ultraviolet/visible radiation absorption spectrum is necessary. If a drug substance or product absorbs in the radiation spectrum of 290–700 nm and will be directly applied to the skin or eyes or will affect the condition of the skin or eyes or will partition to those areas following systemic absorption, the drug should be a candidate for phototoxicity testing.

The guidance also proposes the use of warnings that may be sufficient to advise patients about sun exposure. It is thought that long-term photosafety studies can be avoided when sufficient information has already been obtained for a drug or members of its class to appropriately inform users regarding the potential for phototoxicity reactions. Patients are already cautioned against excessive sunlight exposures while using phototoxic drug products. Rather than conducting expensive and time-consuming photo co-carcinogenicity tests, a drug sponsor could strengthen its phototoxicity warning statements. This option of enhancing the warnings without conducting the long-term tests would be appropriate in those instances where photo co-carcinogenicity would not affect the approvability or significantly reduce the therapeutic utility of the drug product. However, communication regarding the overall risk to the patient should be informative and specified in the informed consent for clinical trials and in the warning section of the product label. In a revision to the Guidance for Industry entitled M3 (R2) Nonclinical Safety Studies for the Conduct of Human Clinical Trials and Marketing Authorization for Pharmaceuticals (ICH, 2009) there is a specific statement regarding photocarcinogenicity. The guidance indicates that testing for photocarcinogenicity in rodents using currently available models (e.g., hairless rodent) is not considered useful in support of pharmaceutical development and generally is not recommended. Furthermore, the guidance indicates that if phototoxicity data suggest a photocarcinogenic risk and an appropriate assay becomes available, the study should be completed before marketing and the results should be considered in the human risk assessment. The FDA does recommend that, prior to any toxicity test conduct, the appropriate review division should be consulted.

The guidance provided for warning statements regarding phototoxicity includes advising patients to avoid sun exposure or, if such exposure is unavoidable, to use protective clothing and sunscreens. It also mentions that phototoxicity testing could be conducted during Phase 4 (post approval) of the drug development process with the prior approval of the appropriate CDER review division. Four decision trees are included to give guidance on the decision-making process for testing potential drugs.

20.2.1 Status of In Vitro and In Vivo Phototoxicity Testing

20.2.1.1 Phototoxicity Testing In Vitro

One of the earliest documented demonstrations of phototoxicity *in vitro* was that of O. Raab. In the late 1890s, Raab, working under the direction of H. Tappeiner, was studying the pharmacological effects of acridine in *Paramecia* and found that survival was reduced when the organisms were exposed to light while suspended in a medium containing acridine. Light alone was not sufficient to reduce survival and the *Paramecia* survived well in the acridine solution when maintained in the dark (described in Blum, 1959). This finding stimulated a great deal of investigation. Over the years, similar findings were demonstrated with many other organisms. The published literature on *in vitro* assays employed in phototoxicity testing is extensive. However, three assays account for a substantial part of the recorded history of *in vitro* phototoxicology: the yeast test, the red blood cell haemolysis test and the 3T3 Neutral Red Uptake test.

20.2.1.2 The Phototoxicity Yeast Test

Daniels (1965) was one of the earliest clinical investigators to study yeast cell growth inhibition as a measure of phototoxicity induced by the combination of compounds and light exposure. Daniels introduced a test using *Candida albicans* and a UVA light source, reporting that the assay was useful in detecting well-known phototoxicants, and was relatively inexpensive, simple and fairly fast. Because *Candida albicans* was a well-recognized pathogen, other investigators chose less problematic yeasts for their investigations, including *Saccharomyces cerevisiae* which is commonly used in baking. The technique for the yeast test often involves the following procedures.

1. Media preparation in which dextrose agar is dissolved in distilled water, autoclaving the mixture and dispensing appropriate aliquots of the medium into petri dishes or microplates.
2. Inoculation of the prepared dishes or plates with yeast suspended in sterilized distilled water and mixed with a 1% dextrose agar.
3. Application of circular discs treated with the test compound onto the seeded dishes or microplates. Typically, multiple discs are prepared using a series of test compound concentrations. Chemicals that are not soluble in water can be dissolved in solvents, such as ethanol, methanol and acetone. In fact, for compounds that are not soluble in standard solvents, the discs can be "dipped" into the compound before being put in place. The lack of the necessity for test compounds to be soluble in water or other common solvents can be useful since this is a shortcoming of other *in vitro* assays.
4. Irradiation of the prepared dishes or microplates with an appropriate light source. The light sources that have been used in conducting the yeast test have varied. In many instances, a UVA fluorescent light source has been used, but other sources can be easily used. Irradiance and light dose levels have varied amongst investigators. In most applications, using a UVA dose in the range of 5–10 J/cm^2 is reasonable. A corresponding non-irradiated control must be kept in the dark for each irradiated dish or plate.
5. After irradiation, all dishes or plates are incubated at 25 °C for 72 hours.
6. After incubation, the dishes or plates are inspected for evidence of inhibition of yeast growth around the compound-treated discs. Inhibition of growth is manifested as a circular zone surrounding the compound-treated disc that is devoid of yeast. Beyond the affected zone, unaffected yeast growth appears as a homogenous, milky area covering the growth medium.
7. Interpretation of results can take various forms. It is always important to compare the irradiated and non-irradiated dishes or plates. Zones of growth inhibition can simply be scored as positive, as compared with a negative result when no growth inhibition occurs in either dark or other (e.g., vehicle) controls. Alternatively, the diameter of the zone of growth inhibition can be measured, and compared with appropriate controls. Some investigators have classified the severity of the phototoxicity based on the magnitude of the zone of growth inhibition and it is not unusual to see statistical analysis employed to assess significance.

A schematic representation of a petri dish used in an *in vitro* phototoxicity yeast test is presented in Figure 20.1.

A number of compounds have been examined in yeast with a comparison of the phototoxic response in guinea pigs (Sugiyama *et al.*, 1994). The data included in Table 20.3 provide for comparison of *in vitro* versus *in vivo* outcomes.

Based on the data in Table 20.3 from Sugiyama *et al.* (1994), several salient conclusions can be made:

- For all tested compounds, with a single exception, positive cutaneous findings of phototoxicity in the *in vivo* guinea pig model elicited positive findings in the *in vitro* yeast

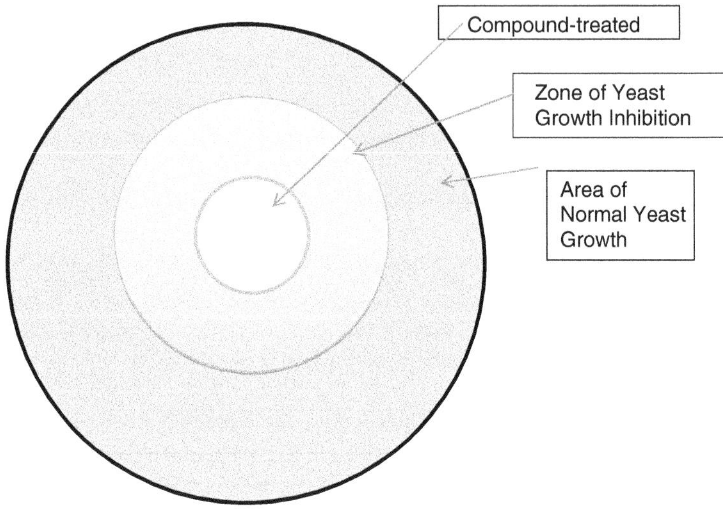

Figure 20.1 *Schematic representation of a petri dish used in an* in vitro *phototoxicity yeast test. Note the compound-treated disc, a zone of yeast growth inhibition and an area of normal yeast growth.*

assay. The exception was phantolid which was phototoxic in the guinea pig model, but not in the yeast assay based on the authors' criterion (i.e., a zone of yeast growth inhibition with a diameter ≥2 mm). However, there was a zone of yeast growth inhibition with phantolid (1.4 mm) which could be considered indicative of phototoxicity if the positive *in vitro* criterion was reduced.

- For three compounds (musk ambrette, Escalol 507 and rose Bengal) positive signs of phototoxicity occurred in the *in vitro* model with either negative or equivocal findings in the guinea pig model. Two other compounds could be included amongst these apparent "false positive" *in vitro* findings if the criterion for a positive response included the occurrence of yeast growth inhibition regardless of the magnitude of the diameter of inhibition. Bithionol and TBS had growth inhibition zone diameters of 0.3 mm and 1.6 mm, respectively.
- The results of four compounds appeared to represent "false positive" responses *in vitro*. Phototoxic compounds have been found to elicit photoallergic responses in man and animal models. TCSA, probably the most robust photoallergen amongst the tested compounds, was positive in both the *in vitro* and *in vivo* assays.
- Ten of the tested compounds elicited no inhibition of yeast growth (i.e., the diameter of the inhibition zone was 0) and were negative in the guinea pig model. The results of other *in vivo* phototoxicity investigations of these compounds were either negative or equivocal.

In summary, for compounds that are phototoxic *in vivo*, the *in vitro* yeast assay results reveal very good congruence. Surprisingly, this *in vitro* assay could also be useful in detecting photoallergens. However, the reality is that many photoallergens are also phototoxic. There are some indications that the *in vitro* assay results in some "false positive"

Table 20.3 In vitro *and* in vivo *comparison of phototoxicity results in the yeast assay and guinea pigs.*

Substance (solvent)	Test substance concentration (mg/mL)	Growth inhibition zone (mm)	Photoxic reaction	
			Yeast	Guinea Pig
Fragerances				
Musk ambrette (acetone)	20	2.0	+	−
Musk ketone (acetone)	300	0	−	−
Musk xylene (acetone)	300	0	−	−
Phantolid (acetone)	500	1.4	−	+
Galaxolide (acetone)	200	2.1	+	+
8-MOP (ethanol)	10	14.1	+	+
5-MOP (ethanol)	2	10.0	+	+
6-MC (ethanol)	100	6.4	+	−
UV Absorbers				
Parsol 1789 (ethanol)	100	0	−	−
Parsol MCX (ethanol)	Undiluted	0	−	−
ASL-24 (ethanol)	50	0	−	−
ASL-24S (distilled water)	50	0	−	−
Escalol 507 (ethanol)	Undiluted	3.0	+	±
Pharmacceuticals				
Sulfanilamide (methanol)	50	0	−	−
Indomethacine (ethanol)	10	0	−	−
Piroxicam (acetone)	20	0	−	−
Chlorpromazine (distilled water)	2	2.4	+	+
Antimicrobials				
TCC (acetone)	20	0	−	−
Bithionol (acetone)	200	0.3	−	−
TBS (acetone)	2	1.6	−	−
TCSA (acetone)	10	2.4	+	+
Dyes				
Rose Bengal (DMSO)	10	11.5	+	−
Acridine (acetone)	0.8	6.8	+	+
Antracene (acetone)	0.08	10.1	+	+

Adapted from Sugiyama *et al.* (1994).

Abbreviation key: 8-MOP – 8-methoxypsoralen; 5-MOP – 5-methoxypsoralen; 6-MC – 6 methyl coumarin; Parsol 1789 – 4-t-butyl-4-methoxydibenzoylmethane; Parsol MCX – 2- ethylhexyl-p-methoxycinnamate; ASL-24 – 2-hydroxy-4-methoxybenzophenone; ASL-24S - 2-hydroxy-4-methoxybenzophenone-5-sulfonic acid; Escalol 507 – 2-ethylhexyl-p-dimethyaminobenzoate; TCC – 3, 4, 4′-trichlorocarbanilide; TBS – 3, 4, 5-tribromosalicylanilide; TCSA – 3, 3′,4′,5-tetra-chlorosalicylanilide; DMSO – dimethyl sulfoxide.

occurrences (i.e., positive phototoxicity findings *in vitro* for compounds that are not phototoxic *in vivo*). This latter point is important because the occurrence of "false positive" phototoxicity findings in *in vitro* assays has been a recurring problem.

20.2.1.3 The Phototoxicity Red Blood Cell Haemolysis Test

Sacharoff and Sachs (1905) demonstrated that red blood cell haemolysis occurred with the combined action of sunlight and certain photoactive compounds. As in the yeast cell assay, sunlight alone did not induce haemolysis as long as the cells were suspended in glass which filtered out the shorter UVR wavelengths, and the test compound concentrations were diluted to levels that did not induce haemolysis in the dark. Interestingly, early investigations also demonstrated that certain compounds (e.g., eosin, fluorescein and erythrosine) elicited photohemolysis when the compound solutions were irradiated before addition of the RBCs (Ledoux-Lebard, 1902; Blum, 1930). Typically, the technique for the RBC haemolysis test involves the following procedures:

1. Fresh blood samples from humans or animals are obtained and the RBCs isolated by centrifugation.
2. RBCs are suspended in phosphate buffered saline to an appropriate volume.
3. Test compounds are diluted in an appropriate medium (e.g., PBS); this is typically done in the dark.
4. The mixture is exposed to light with corresponding samples being kept in the dark. In some instances this step is performed with incubation at 37 °C.
5. After light exposure, the mixtures are inspected for signs of haemolysis.
   - Haemolysis can be visualized by noting a change in the opacity of the mixtures. If little or no haemolysis occurs, the mixture appears translucent. With complete haemolysis, the mixture appears virtually transparent. If partial haemolysis occurs, the mixture appears more transparent compared with controls. Careful inspection of the mixtures is essential, particularly when the samples are coloured and assessments are often conducted at several time points after irradiation.
   - Opacity can also be measured spectrophotometrically, typically at 650 nm. With this technique, optical density (OD) at 650 nm (a wavelength at which RBC light absorbance occurs) is reduced when haemolysis occurs (Figure 20.2).
   - Some investigators have measured haemolysis by centrifuging the mixtures after irradiation and weighing any pellets that accumulate at the bottom of the vials. The magnitude of the pellet is smaller or nonexistent when haemolysis has occurred.

In the Vargas et al. (2008) investigation, all light exposures were performed with a UVA source, and mixtures of RBCs alone, RBCs and cinoxacin, and RBCs and both cinoxacin and allopurinol were assessed. Cinoxacin is a phototoxic fluoroquinolone antibiotic used here to elicit photohaemolysis. Allopurinol is a drug known to inhibit free radicals and reactive radical species. UVB was purposely avoided in this experiment because allopurinol phototoxicity can be elicited with UVB exposure. As shown in Figure 20.2, spectrophotometric measurements indicate the time course of the RBC haemolysis with little optical density reduction over time when RBCs alone were exposed to UVA, substantial optical density reduction with the combination of RBCs and

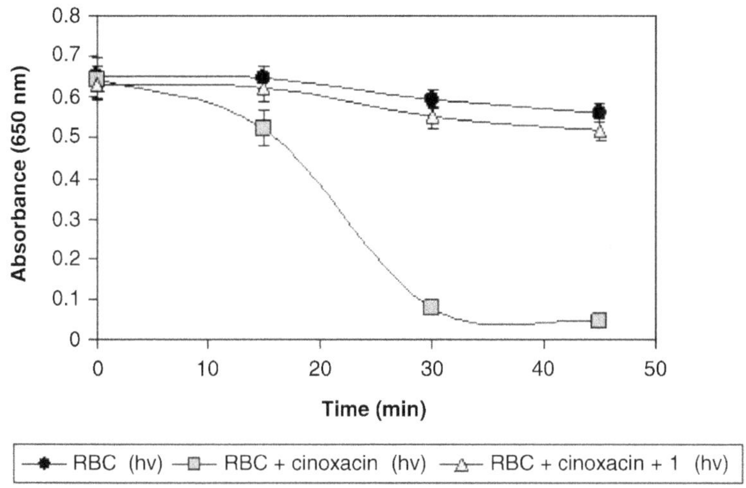

Figure 20.2 *Effects of allopurinol (1) on the photohaemolysis of RBC induced by cinoxacin under UVA light (hv). Dark controls for RBC, cinoxacin and 1, did not reveal any photohemolysis. Adapted from Vargas* et al. *(2008).*

a known phototoxic compound, cinoxacin, at 30 and 45 minutes after UVA exposure and a inhibition of that photohemolysis with the addition of allopurinol.

In validation studies of the photo-RBC test sponsored by the EU/COLIPA, Spielmann et al. (2000) used a protocol for measuring photohaemolysis at 520 nm and assessed photochemically-induced methemoglobinemia (met-Hb) at 625 nm as a second end-point (Table 20.4). met-Hb may be produced during extensive exposure to sunlight, especially as a result of type I photodynamic reactions. The salient results were summarized by the authors as follows:

- When both end-points in the Photo-RBC test in the final assessment were combined, a good overall fit with the *in vivo* evaluations was obtained.
- The three "false negative" results were explained in the following manner. Forfurosemide, a relevant phototoxic potency *in vivo* has not been proven, since the clinical data in humans were insufficient. Ofloxacin was tested as a clinical preparation at a very low concentration of the active ingredient, which may not have revealed its phototoxic potential. 5-MOP may have provided a negative result because of the lack of sensitive target molecules in erythrocytes.
- "False positive" results were obtained with PABA and hexachlorophene in the Photo-RBC test. PABA is easily oxidized by oxy-Hb in the dark in a pseudo-enzymatic reaction, which may be enhanced under light exposure (or increased temperature).
- The combined Photo-RBC test can be performed reproducibly, and it provides relevant mechanistic information on photodynamic reactions, which add important information for the evaluation of the photo-safety of test chemicals.

Table 20.4 *Results comparing phototoxicity in the RBC photohaemolysis assay and* in vivo *human patch test.*

Chemical	*In vivo*	Assessment		
		PHF	ΔOD_{max}	Final
2-Hydroxy-4-methoxybenzophenone	−	−	−	−
Chlorhexidine	−	−	−	−
Hexachlorphene	−	−	+	+
Sodium lauryl sulfate	−	−	−	−
p-Aminobenzoic acid	−	−	+	+
Penicillin G	−	−	−	−
Fuorsemide	+ (?)	−	−	−
Ofloxacin	+	−	−	−
5-MOP	+	−	−	−
6-Mehtylcoumarin	−	±	+	+
Acridine	+	±	+	+
Acridine (free base)	+	+	+	+
Amiodarone	+	±	+	±
Antracene	+	±	+	+
Bergamot oil	+	−	+	+
Bithionol	+	±	+	+
Chlorpromazine	+	±	+	+
Demelocycline	+	−	+	+
Fenofibrate	+	+	+	+
Ketoprofen	+	+	+	+
Musk ambrette	+	+	+	+
Nalidix acid sodium salt	+	±	+	+
Nalidixic acid free acid	+	−	+	+
Neutral red	+	+	+	+
Norfloxacin	+	−	+	+
Promethazine	+	−	+	+
Protoporphyrin IX free acid	+	+	+	+
Protoporphyrin IX disodium salt	+	+	−	+
Rose bengal	+	+	+	+
Tiaprofenic acid	+	+	+	+

PHF – photohemolysis factor (a photohemolysis value ≥3.0 and an optical density (OD) $\Delta OD_{max} \geq 0.05$ for met-Hb formation; ΔOD_{max} – optical density; + = positive results; − = negative results; ± = equivocal results. Adapted from Spielmann *et al.* (2000).

- An additional advantage of RBC cells is their resistance to the short-wave UVB part of sunlight, which enables RBC cells in the Photo-RBC test to be exposed to the entire solar spectrum.

In summary, for compounds that are phototoxic *in vivo*, the *in vitro* photohaemolysis assay results reveal fairly good congruence. As with the phototoxicity yeast assay, the photohaemolysis assay could also be useful in detecting photoallergens. Like the yeast assay, the RBC phototoxicity assay results in some “false positive” occurrences – a recurring problem with *in vitro* phototoxicity testing. The inability of the RBC photoassay to demonstrate phototoxicity with 5-MOP (and other psoralens) is particularly problematic. Clinically, psoralen-induced phototoxicity is unequivocal. Compounds in this chemical group are often used in the clinic in combination with light exposure to ameliorate disease and reports of phototoxicity in humans and animals are often the result of psoralen-contaminated entities (e.g., bergamot oil).

20.2.1.4 The 3T3 NRU Phototoxicity Test

The 3T3 Neutral Red Uptake Phototoxicity Test (3T3 NRU-PT) is the recommended tier-one screen of the EMA guidance on photosafety testing. This assay was validated by ECVAM in 2002 and showed high sensitivity and specificity using the test set of compounds selected for the validation study. The test set contained many known phototoxicants and relatively few known non-phototoxicants, but a follow-up study with 10 known phototoxicants and 10 known non-phototoxicants with topical use confirmed the Predictive Capacity obtained in the validation study (Spielmann et al., 1998).

The 3T3 NRU-PT was adopted by the OECD as Test Guideline (TG) 432 (OECD, 2004). Since the introduction of the EMA guidance in 2002, the 3T3 NRU-PT has been used quite extensively within the pharmaceutical industry. A number of companies found they were encountering an unexpectedly high percentage of positive results with this assay (about 50%), which led to a survey of European Federation of Pharmaceutical Industries and Associations (EFPIA) member companies to capture industry experience (Lynch and Wilcox, 2010). Phototoxicity data were provided by 10 EFPIA member companies on 361 pharmaceutical candidates covering a broad range of different drug classes. Of the 349 compounds tested in the 3T3 NRU-PT, 157 compounds (44%) produced a Photoirritancy Factor (PIF) value of >5 and were classified as positive, and 30 compounds (i.e., 8%) produced PIF values between 2 and 5 and were classed as equivocal. Of these 187, 26 were retested either on animals or humans and 85% of the retested substances were found to be negative in the animal model/human clinical tests. One of the conclusions of the survey was that the 3T3 NRU-PT appears to be over-sensitive and substantially over-predictive of *in vivo* photosafety hazards in animals and humans in the clinic. Figure 20.3 provides a schematic depiction of the 3T3 NRU-PT (OECD, 2004).

In this assay, Balb/c 3T3 cells are maintained in culture for 24 hours for formation of monolayers. Then 96-well plates are preincubated with different concentrations of the test chemical with some plates exposed to a dose of light (xenon arc solar simulator) while control plates are kept in the dark. The treatment medium is then replaced with fresh culture medium and, after 24 hours, cell viability is determined with the neutral red using a microplate reader to measure optical density. Cell viability at the tested chemical concentrations with and without light exposure is compared to assess the photoirritation potential. A dose of UVA equivalent to 5 J/cm^2 is delivered to the appropriate 96-well plates. An example of 96-well plates that have been processed and ready to be assessed by the microplate reader to measure optical density is shown in Figure 20.4.

The phototoxic potential of a test article is determined by comparing the IC_{50} (i.e., the concentration of the test chemical at which cell viability is reduced by 50%) without and with UVA exposure to determine the photoirritancy factor (PIF):

$$\mathrm{PIF} = \frac{\mathrm{IC}_{50}(-\mathrm{UVA})}{\mathrm{IC}_{50}(+\mathrm{UVA})}$$

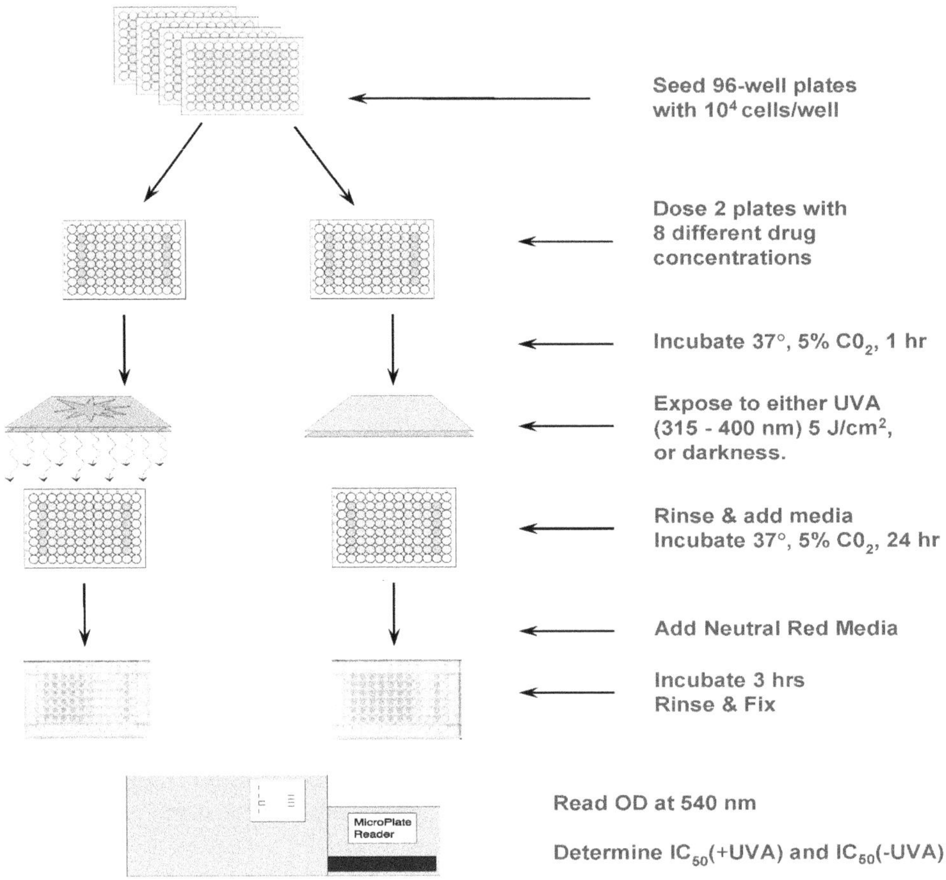

Figure 20.3 *Schematic depiction of the 3T3 NRU* in vitro *Photoirritation Test. Adapted from Spielmann* et al. *(1994).*

Additionally, the mean photo effect (MPE) is calculated. The MPE is a useful measure of phototoxic potential for cases in which two equally-effective concentrations (IC_{50}) in the dark (−UVA) and light (+UVA) cannot be determined. The MPE is based on comparison of the complete concentration response curves. It is defined as the weighted average across a representative set of photo effect values:

$$MPE = \frac{\sum_{i=1}^{n} W_i \, PE_{ci}}{\sum_{i=1}^{n} W_i}$$

where PEc is the photo effect at a concentration (C), and the weighting factors (w_i) are given by the highest response value (Peters and Holzhutter, 2002).

Based on the guideline, the phototoxicity potential of the test article is interpreted as follows:

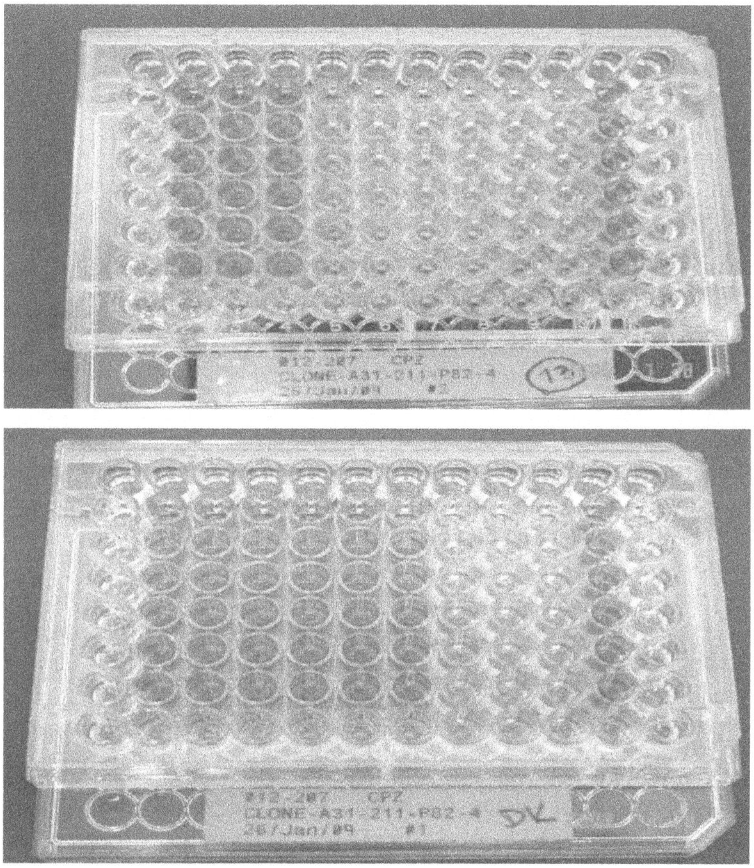

Figure 20.4 *The 3T3 NRU* in vitro *Photoirritation Test. Cells in the 96-well plates were exposed to test chemical dilutions and either exposed to light (top plate) or kept in the dark (bottom plate). Eight concentrations of the chemical were assessed (columns) in replicates of 6 (rows) along with the vehicle (2 bordering columns on each end of the chemical concentrations).*

Mean Photo Effect (MPE)	Photoirritancy Factor (PIF)	Phototoxic Potential
<0.1	<2	Non-phototoxic
>0.1 and <0.15	>2 and <5	Probably phototoxic
>0.15	>5	Phototoxic

Table 20.5 includes results of 3T3 NRU photoirritation tests for substances known to be clinically relevant.

From the data in Table 20.5, for most of these clinically-established phototoxicants the 3T3 NRU, MPE values indicate "phototoxic potential". However, the MPE values for

Table 20.5 *Results from the 3T3 NRU photoirritation test of selected phototoxicants.*

Substance	Concentration Range (mg/L)	MPE	PIF	IC_{50} (mg/L)	
				+UVA	−UVA
Chlorpromazine	0.1–120	0.51	39.6	1.02	40.4
Anthracene	0.0008–2.6	0.45	>32.7	0.08	NA
Doxycycline	0.0665–210	0.46	>132	1.55	NA
Amiodarone	0.024–75	0.06	3.6	3.03	10.8
Lomefloxacin	0.0045–13	0.14	>2.7	4.8	NA
8-MOP	0.01–30	0.28	1	NA	NA

Adapted from Spielmann *et al.* (1998); Lynch and Wilcox (2010) and Spielmann *et al.* (1994).

Amiodarone (0.058) and Lomefloxacin (0.135) indicate "no phototoxic potential" and only "probable phototoxic potential", respectively, although these two drugs are considered potent phototoxicants in man. The PIF values for these same respective drugs (3.6 and >2.7) indicate "probable phototoxic potential" or "phototoxic potential". Note that the ">" symbol assigned to the Lomefloxacin PIF value indicates that the IC_{50} value for cells kept in the dark (–UVA) was not achieved and that the highest concentration of the test article tested was included in the numerator of the PIF formula. Spielmann et al. (1994) also reported an IC_{50} (−UVA) concentration value of 24.3 mg/L and a PIF value of 6 for Amiodarone indicating a true "phototoxic" potential.

20.2.1.5 Difficulties Associated with the 3T3 NRU Phototoxicity Test

As indicated previously, there have been difficulties associated with this assay. The number of positive findings with this assay has been unexpectedly high. When *in vivo* studies in either animal models or man are conducted on test compounds found positive in the 3T3 NRU PT, the results often indicate a lack of phototoxicity (i.e., only 10% or 15% of compounds found to be positive in the *in vitro* test are also found to be positive in an *in vivo* model). In addition, there is some debate about whether the PIF value or the MPE value is the best predictor of clinical relevance.

Since test compounds can only be assessed in solutions, solubility in the recommended buffered salt solutions (e.g., Eagle's Balanced Salt Solution) can be very limited even when solvents (e.g., dimethylsulfoxide and ethanol) and mechanical mixing are employed. Related to solubility is the inability to assess finished clinical products, particularly topical formulations that may be formulated as a cream or ointment. Furthermore, it is not unusual to find that IC_{50} values are not achieved for the concentration series tested, particularly for cells not exposed to light (-UVA). The maximum concentration recommended in the OECD TG 432 is 1000 mg/L, 10 mmol/L or the solubility limit of the test substance in the treatment buffer. There is concern that, at least for some compounds, high concentrations may not be clinically relevant and that it might be more useful to compare concentrations in the 3T3 NRU PT that are representative of clinical distribution levels (e.g., C_{max} levels in the skin, blood and eyes).

The FDA and EMA guidances stipulate that the waveband of importance for considering phototoxic potential is 290–700 nm, and thus includes the UVB (280–315 nm) portion of the electromagnetic spectrum. Under normal conditions as specified in the

3T3 NRU PT guideline, the magnitude of UVB that is delivered to the cells is limited because the 96-wheel plate top in place during light exposure attenuates a substantial portion of the UVB.

Because any photoreaction requires sufficient absorption of light, the guideline stipulates that prior to conducting a 3T3 NRU PT for any test compound a UV/Vis absorption spectrum must be determined. Currently, the 3T3 NRU PT guideline stipulates that any chemical with a molar extinction/absorption coefficient of 10 litre/mol/cm or greater could require phototoxicity testing. This threshold has been questioned and there have been discussions of increasing the coefficient.

In vitro phototoxicity assays have been around for more than 100 years. The results of these assays have been an asset to the study of phototoxicology and have helped investigators learn a great deal about the interaction of light and chemicals. All of these assays are simple to perform, inexpensive and relatively quick, and they can be useful tools in helping investigators predict outcomes in more complicated organisms, for example, humans. One important finding that has been realized from these tests is that none of them can be used as unambiguous predictors of phototoxicity in the clinic. A huge advantage of the 3T3 NRU PT is the nearly non-existent occurrence of "false negative" results. As with all tests, including clinical trials, the 3T3 NRU PT has some problems and improvements can made, but its value as a screening tool is significant. It is unreasonable to consider that such a simple assay can resolve all of the needs for phototoxicity determinations.

20.2.1.6 Phototoxicity Testing In Vivo

The development of animal models for assessment of phototoxicity followed similar models in man (Marzulli and Maibach, 1970). In dermatology, patients presenting with skin reactions that appeared to be related to a combination of chemical and light exposure have often been subjected to testing to confirm the diagnosis. Eventually, standardized photo-patch tests were developed for use in the clinic, and human subjects were included in studies in order to screen chemicals for phototoxic liability (Magnus, 1976).

Animal models were initially developed to study the mechanisms of phototoxicity and to serve as surrogates for man in screening chemicals. The scope of animals used in phototoxicology has been very broad. For example, the literature includes studies in earthworms, rattlesnakes, insects and fish, but the most commonly-used animal models in phototoxicity testing have been mice, rats, guinea pigs, rabbits and pigs. Each of the commonly-used models has advantages and disadvantages. Unfortunately, regulatory guidance related to photosafety testing are not explicit about how to conduct testing for *in vivo* phototoxicity and, aside from the Japanese guideline for photosensitivity (photoallergy) testing (JMHLW, 1989), there are no guidelines comparable to that for the 3T3 NRU PT that give specific methods for testing. Therefore, the techniques used in the conduct of *in vivo* phototoxicity testing are highly variable.

20.2.1.7 Animal Models

There is no perfect animal model for phototoxicity testing. As with any animal model, important considerations would include sensitivity to the light source chosen for testing and relevance to humans.

In assessing the sensitivity to light exposure, the first step should always include determining the minimal dose of light alone that is required to elicit a response. Phototoxicity elicited by a combination of a drug or other chemical and light exposure represents an enhancement of the response by light exposure alone. Drug- or chemical-induced enhancement cannot be determined unless the response to light alone is carefully characterized. For example, when the intent is to assess cutaneous phototoxicity, the observed minimal erythema dose (MED), the observed light dose required to elicit a minimal cutaneous response, must be known. The MED_0 in hairless mice, rabbits, lightly pigmented miniature swine (e.g., Hanford miniature swine) and man tends to be quantitatively similar. The MED_0 in rats and guinea pigs is greater, as compared with these four species. Furthermore, the time courses of cutaneous responses vary amongst species and are dependent on light dose. Comparable characterization of light sensitivity must be established for other target organs and tissues prior to any phototoxicity testing.

20.2.1.8 Selection of a Light Source

The FDA and EMA guidances are consistent in that drugs that absorb light in the 290–700 nm waveband may require phototoxicity testing. A source that emits light that includes this entire waveband has advantages in phototoxicity testing. Figure 20.5 depicts an emission spectrum for a xenon arc lamp as commonly used for phototoxicity testing.

The emission spectrum covers the entire waveband of regulatory concern. With the xenon arc lamp a UVB dose equivalent to 0.5 MED (human) is commonly used in *in vivo* phototoxicity studies. In animal models, this light dose alone produces virtually no detectable adverse effects in the target tissues (e.g., skin and eyes), but is sufficient to elicit phototoxicity with most known phototoxicants. Of course, selection of the drug dose is always an important consideration in phototoxicity testing. Table 20.6 includes radiometric data captured with a meter commonly used in phototoxicology with definitions and terminology included in Table 20.7. These meters have multiple detectors, each of which has the ability to give a useful measurement of a portion of the electromagnetic spectrum.

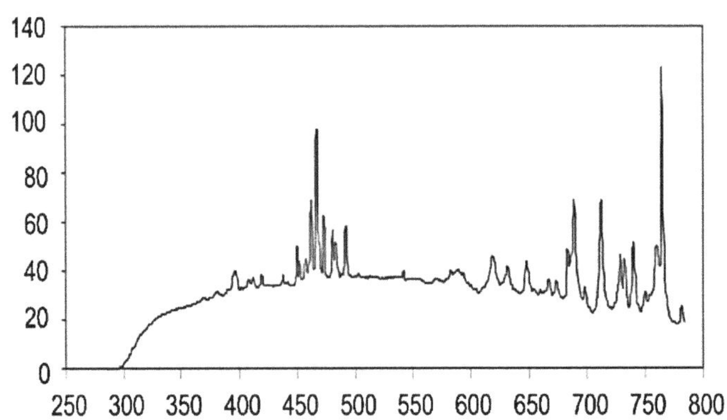

Figure 20.5 *An emission spectrum (intensity versus wavelength) of a xenon arc lamp as commonly used in phototoxicity testing.*

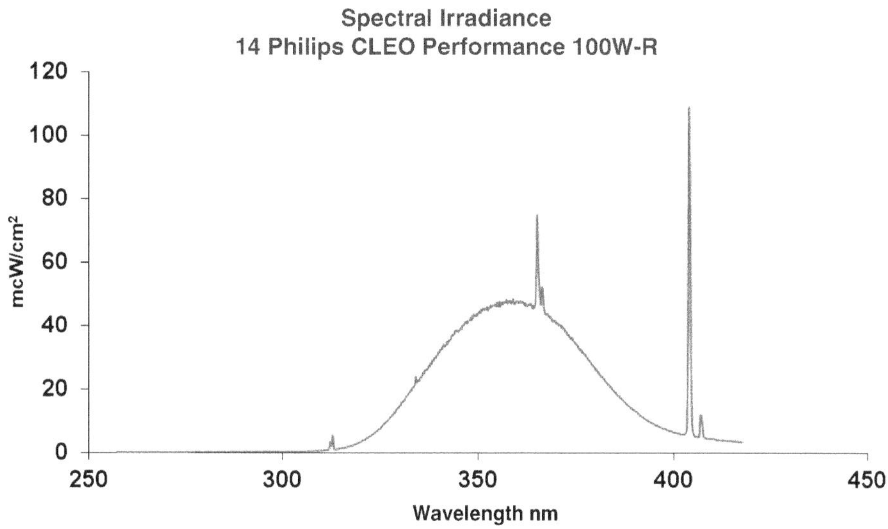

Figure 20.6 *Spectral emission of a fluorescent lamp that can be used in phototoxicology.*

The most problematic aspect of delivering a 0.5 MED to either animal models or humans with the xenon arc lamp is the paucity of UVA that is delivered to the target. With a 1.7 MED/hour UVB irradiance dose from a xenon arc lamp delivering a 0.5 MED to the target, the UVA dose is about 1.5 J/cm^2. This is a relatively low UVA dose and mighty not be sufficient to allow for detection of some phototoxicants. If the exposure duration is doubled, the delivered dose would be about 3.0 J/cm^2. At this dose, the MED would be about 1 MED of UVB. To deliver a more robust UVA dose without running into trouble with inducing the UVB responses would be to use UVA fluorescent lamps. An emission spectrum of a UVA fluorescent lamp is included in Figure 20.6.

Fluorescent lamps emit radiation nearly exclusively in the UVA portion of the electromagnetic spectrum. The spikes along the curve represent mercury lines that are inherent in these lamps. Based on the measurements in Table 20.6, one can deliver nearly 30 J/cm^2 of UVA with fluorescent lamps without having to worry about the UVB component of the emission spectrum. UVA alone does have some ability to elicit cutaneous erythema in human skin and blanching in hairless mouse skin, but the threshold dose for eliciting these responses is typically considered to be about 40 J/cm^2. Therefore, we can deliver high UVA doses to targets in the lab with fluorescent lamps without having to worry about the UVB component of the lamp output causing problematic skin reactions. A 20 J/cm^2 UVA dose is useful in conducting phototoxicity testing. It is important to keep in mind, however, that UVA exposure is responsible for driving phototoxicity for a very large portion of phototoxicants in the clinic. It might be necessary to implement unique light sources in evaluating phototoxicity based on the absorption characteristics of drug and intended use.

20.2.1.9 Formulation Administration and Light Exposure

The regimen for formulation administration and light exposure in phototoxicity testing is dependent on pharmacokinetic characteristics and the intended use of the formulation. Generally, the formulation is administered by an appropriate route, light exposure is

Table 20.6 *Radiometric measurements of sunlight, a xenon arc lamp and fluorescent UVA lamps.*

Light source	Waveband	Measurements
Sunlight [June, Horsham, PA (USA) @ 1100 – 1200 Hours]	UVB	2.7 MED/Hour
		5.8 SED/Hour
		16 mcW/cm^2
	UVA	5.3 mW/cm^2
	Photopic	110,000 Lux
		9700 ft-cd
		151 W/M^2
Xenon Arc Lamp	UVB	1.7 MED/Hour
		3.6 SED/Hour
		9.9 mcW/cm^2
	UVA	1.46 mW/cm^2
	Photopic	20,000 Lux
		32 W/M^2
Fluorescent UVA Lamps With Plate Glass Filtration	UVB	0.57 MED/Hour
		1.20 SED/Hour
		3.35 mcW/cm^2
	UVA	5.0 mW/cm^2
	Photopic	1886 Lux
		2.77 W/M^2

All measurements were made with a calibrated PMA2100 meter with separate detectors for UVB, UVA and visible (photopic) light [Solar Light Company, Philadelphia, PA (USA)]. This meter allows for measurements of multiple units in each waveband. Sunlight was evaluated on a clear mid-June day in Horsham, PA (USA) between 1100–1200 hours. The xenon arc measurements were made at a distance of 1.2 meters between the source and the detectors and a WG320 Schott filter was in place. The UVA source was a bank of 14 Philips Natural 62W/R fluorescent lamps with plate glass filtration at a distance of about 36 cm between the source and the detectors.

performed and the animals are maintained for observation. In earlier phototoxicity studies, test formulations tended to be administered topically, usually to the skin, followed by light exposure soon after administration (Scott et al., 1970; Forbes et al., 1977). Since the route of formulation administration was topical for these early evaluations, it was

Table 20.7 *Terminology and UVR quantities.*

Term	UVR quantity	Comment
Minimal Erythema Dose (MED, Instrumental MED_i)	200 J/M^2	This quantity is a common estimate of a UVR dose required to elicit minimal erythema in human skin after exposure to a broad band UVR source (e.g., sunlight). Many instruments are designed with this UVR quantity in mind in order to facilitate biological response predictability.
Standard Erythema Dose (SED)	100 J/M^2	Approximately 0.5 MED
Minimal Erythema Dose (MED, Observational MED_o)	Individually determined	Any measured UVR quantity that produces a minimal erythema (MED_o).
Robertson-Berger Unit (RBU)	0.5 J/M^2	400 RBU = 200 J/M^2 = 1 MED_i

assumed that light exposure should be done shortly after application. With advancement in technology, phototoxicity testing was conducted with systemic formulation administration. During the same time period, the field of pharmacokinetics (PK) made substantial advances so that PK data could be utilized in determining the appropriate timing for light exposure. PK data can also dictate the frequency of formulation administration required before light exposure. On rare occasions, multiple light exposures after one or more formulation administrations have been used in phototoxicity testing based on the characteristics and intended usage of the formulation. Positioning animals for light exposure has been variable. Light exposure can be done on either free-moving or restrained animals, and the restrained animals can also be anaesthetized. For haired animals depilation is necessary for light exposure to the skin. The utilization of a restraining method allows for delivery of a more accurate light dose. For light exposure to the skin, it is very useful to mask the restrained animal so that only a portion of the skin is exposed to light. Masking the animal has two important advantages: the skin surface area that can be affected by phototoxic responses is limited, and the light-exposed skin can be readily compared with surrounding, light-protected skin in the same animal.

20.2.1.10 Evaluation of Phototoxic Responses

Evaluations of phototoxic responses in the skin of animals are typically performed by visual inspection of the target sites, and are performed during and for several days after light exposure. The characteristics of the skin responses are variable amongst species. In the hairless mouse, typical cutaneous responses can include early occurrence of oedema (blanching) and/or erythema followed by flaking, erosion, ulceration and eschar formation. Blanching is seldom seen in other animals typically used in phototoxicity testing. In rats, guinea pigs, swine and rabbits, cutaneous erythema, oedema flaking, erosion/ulceration and eschar formation are common signs of phototoxicity. Fissuring is often seen in rabbit skin. Amongst the animals commonly used in phototoxicity, swine are probably the best models for assessing hyperpigmentation. The time course of skin reactions can be very different amongst species and can very much depend on the characteristics of the drug or chemical under investigation, drug/chemical dosage and light irradiance and dose. Figure 20.7 represents schematic depiction of the time courses of skin inflammatory responses in animals.

With light exposure alone (UVR, Figure 20.7), erythema typically occurs shortly after exposure and tends to maximize over the following few hours with the other responses characteristic of sunburn occurring over the next few days. An increase in light dose can easily modify the time course of skin responses, shortening onset and increasing severity. Most phototoxicants induce a time course of skin responses comparable to that seen for 8-methoxypsoralen (8-MOP) and light exposure (Figure 20.7). The 8-MOP time course is somewhat delayed, as compared with light exposure alone. The anthracene plus UVR time course depicted in Figure 20.7 is limited to only a few known phototoxicants, but is very important because the response is very different from responses seen with either light alone or most other phototoxicants and the response is typical of compounds used in photodynamic therapy. Topical administration of anthracene plus light exposure elicits very early signs of inflammation. The inflammatory response often begins during light exposure, is accompanied by a neurological component (i.e., the animals appear to be in discomfort), and begins to diminish soon after completion of light exposure.

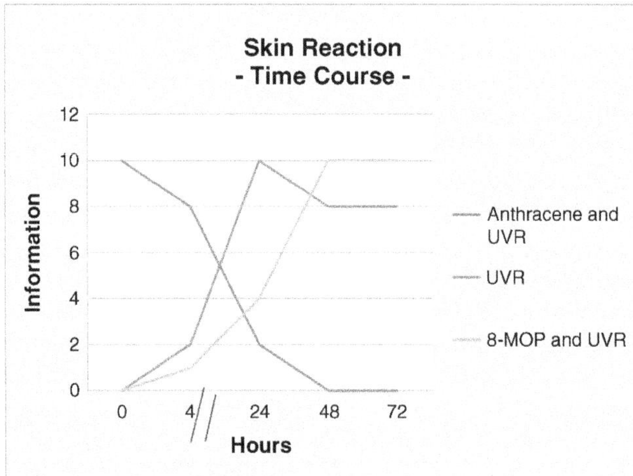

Figure 20.7 *Schematic representation of the time course of phototoxicological responses in the skin of animals. 8-MOP – 8-methoxypsoralen.*

Investigators have used changes in rodent ear thickness to assess phototoxicity (Scott *et al.*, 1970; Sambuco and Forbes, 1984). Measurements of ear thickness are recorded before and after formulation administration and light exposure. This method is objective, nondestructive and quantifiable. Repeated measurements have been found not to alter the response and allow for phototoxicity to be assessed over an extended period of time (Gabriel et al., 1986).

In order to assess ocular phototoxicity in animals, the eyes are examined before and after formulation administration and light exposure by an indirect ophthalmoscope in conjunction with a 28 dioptre and/or 20 dioptre hand-held lens to examine ocular structures (lens and fundus oculi) and slit lamp biomicroscopy is performed to evaluate the lids, adnexal structures, cornea, anterior chamber, lens and anterior vitreous for any abnormalities. At the time of sacrifice, the eyes are removed and subjected to extensive histopathological evaluation.

Like the *in vitro* phototoxicity tests, the animal models are not perfect. When some drugs (e.g., chlorpromazine and doxycycline) are administered to animals via the routes employed in the clinic, phototoxicity is difficult to demonstrate. At least some of these drugs can be demonstrated to elicit phototoxic responses with intracutaneous administration prior to light exposure.

Since the earliest demonstrations of phototoxicity, investigators have tried to use biomarkers as unequivocal predictors. In fact, cell death in the *in vitro* tests and erythema induction in animal models can be considered to be biomarkers. In recent years, more sophisticated biomarkers have been developed. These markers can be used to assess cell proliferation, cell damage and death, modification in DNA synthesis and repair, modification in cell metabolism and respiration, inflammatory processes, and so on. Biomarkers could be the future for phototoxicity testing, but at the current time there is no definitive biomarker test that addresses all of the needs for predicting clinical events.

Some drugs and chemicals increase sensitivity to light in man. In order to help predict clinical phototoxicity, *in vitro* and *in vivo* tests have been developed. Regulators have produced guidance and guidelines to aid in directing testing. However, there is no perfect preclinical test for phototoxicity. All of the preclinical tests have advantages and shortcomings. Appropriate preclinical phototoxicity screening with good predictive clinical value can be accomplished with good interaction amongst the shareholders (i.e., drug developers, regulators and testing facilities) and with the realization that there is no single, simple test to address all of the concerns for phototoxicity. Biomarkers could be useful in the future as predictors of clinical events.

20.3 Status of *In Vivo* Testing for Photocarcinogenesis

Ultraviolet (UV) radiation is a natural and variable component of our environment; its one unambiguous benefit is the vitamin D3 production that it initiates. UV radiation is better known for the several types of skin damage it causes, including the production of skin tumours. These factors are taken into account in developing programmes of safety studies for new pharmaceutical products.

Amongst laboratory mammals, rodents in general and mice in particular are well suited for toxicology studies. Mice and rats are thus the animals most widely used in experimental carcinogenesis. Their dense fur is, however, a disadvantage for photocarcinogenesis studies. The earliest laboratory studies on photocarcinogenesis depended on the exposure of repeatedly depilated mouse skin, or of the more sparsely haired areas such as ears and extremities (Blum, 1959; 1964). The tumours that were produced included many that exhibited malignant criteria, but few that were morphologically similar to those found in human skin damaged by UV radiation. Removing the hair in order to expose the underlying skin introduced an unmeasured stimulatory effect on cell turnover, along with other confounding effects. The discovery of UV-induced squamous cell tumours in genetically hairless mice was thus a pivotal laboratory finding (Winkelman *et al.*, 1960, 1963). Genetically hairless mice were described in detail in the 1920s (Grüneberg, 1952). By the 1950s, breeding studies had resulted in the availability of this allele in a diversity of mouse stocks and strains, housed in universities, government laboratories, and research foundations (Green, 1966). In general, the hairless stocks and strains were characterized by small litters and relatively inefficient output of the desired hairless phenotype. Typically, heterozygous haired dams were used because the homozygous hairless dams raised very few offspring successfully. Exceptions were the animals reported by Epstein (Epstein, 1965, 1975), and those from the Skh stocks developed at Temple University (Forbes *et al.*, 1981). Animals derived from the Skh lines have played a significant part in phototoxicology studies for the last two decades, and they have been identified under a variety of designations (IARC, 1992). One inbred variant is congenic for the "C" locus, and therefore produces both pigmented and albino offspring. This strain is designated HRA:HRII-C+/Skh.

For studies for regulatory submission, most of the historical data involve genetically hairless (*hr*/*hr*) mice. The original impetus for using this type of test system was that hair is a very effective UV blocker, and removing the hair from conventional mice or rats on a daily basis was not practical. Hairless mice of the stocks most commonly used are immunocompetent, exhibit DNA repair mechanisms, and produce squamous cell carcinomas (or their precursors) after repeated exposure to UV radiation. Such animals are maintained at dozens of academic and testing facilities. One commercial source provides barrier rederived hairless mice with the designation Crl:SKH1-Hr^{hr} (SKH1-Elite).

20.4 Photocarcinogenesis Study Designs

The published literature on photocarcinogenesis contains an array of basic research study designs, including the use of many species, radiation sources, the order, methods and rates of dose delivery, measure and interpretation of endpoints, and so on (IARC, 1992). Considerably more uniformity is likely when the results of a photocarcinogenesis study are intended to support a claim for efficacy or safety in a regulatory submission. For regulatory submission, photocarcinogenesis studies usually involve repeated intercurrent exposures to simulated sunlight and a chemical, a consumer product, or a candidate cosmetic or pharmaceutical ingredient. The test determines whether the selected material influences the time required for the known carcinogen (ultraviolet radiation; UVR) to produce skin cancer in a well-characterized animal model system (Forbes, 1996; Forbes et al., 2003; Sambuco et al., 2003).

20.5 Photo Co-Carcinogenesis

In their discussion of factors that influence photocarcinogenesis, Fry and Ley (1984) use the term *co-carcinogen* to cover exogenous and endogenous modifiers of the expression of cancer; they considered the beginning of experimental co-carcinogenesis of UVR and chemicals to be a study published by Findlay in 1928. Following that definition, virtually all photocarcinogenesis studies of concern to toxicologists would qualify as *photo co-carcinogenesis.*

For safety testing, the selection factors for candidate materials include the anticipated period of consumer or worker exposure to the product, the likelihood of cutaneous metabolic or mitogenic effects via topical or systemic route of exposure, and the probability of exposure of the product to sunlight, particularly if its photochemistry has not been fully characterized (Davies *et al.*, 1990; Osterberg and Szarfman, 1996). Many of the photocarcinogenesis studies designed for regulatory submission have contained "calibration" groups receiving only UVR, receiving "high" and "low" weekly doses, respectively. The two weekly radiation dose rates are defined to serve as internal UVR response calibrators. Radiation dose delivery occupies five consecutive days per week and differs by daily exposure duration. The specified doses (differing by a factor of about 2) provide an adequate response range while limiting the required study duration to one year in-life (Sambuco et al., 1991). There is a substantial body of information available on UVR dose-response relationships in this test system (Forbes *et al.*, 1981; De Gruijl *et al.*, 1983). The calibration groups provide a dynamic range of response, permitting accurate interpolation and reasonable extrapolation for data from the groups also receiving the test agents. Deviations from a "zero-effect" level in tumour response can be expressed in terms of an "amplification factor" (i.e., expressed as the mathematic equivalent of changing the UV dose by a specified fraction).

In carcinogenicity studies, statistical evaluations are far more robust for categorical animal-based measures (prevalence) than they are for continuous (mass or "burden") or quasi-continuous (tumour multiplicity or yield) measures based on numbers of lesions (IARC, 1992). Consequently, the photocarcinogenic study bases its determinations on prevalence, but all recognized tumours are documented, and tumour yield is summarized by treatment group and reported graphically as well. If tumours develop independently of each other, tumour prevalence and tumour yield should represent two expressions of the same process, at least until most animals in a group have developed several tumours (Burns et al., 1983; De Gruijl and van der Leun, 1994; De Gruijl and Forbes, 1995).

In most chemical carcinogenesis assays the proportion of individuals responding is relatively small, so the sensitivity of the test is critically dependent on group size. Similarly, the sensitivity of the test is often dependent on the duration of treatment and of observation, both of which may approach the natural life span of the animals. Comparisons to untreated "control" animals are generally made within organ-specific and type-specific categories of tumours and other lesions. In contrast, most or all of the animals in a photocarcinogenesis assay develop tumours, and effectiveness is judged in terms of the time to tumour appearance (or, less frequently, the multiplicity of the tumours produced). The tumour data are derived during the in-life phases of the study, and data collection is a function of visual inspection of the animal. The relationship between specific morphologic responses and the production of histologically confirmed cancers in chronically-irradiated hairless mice is established by an extensive body of literature. With occasional exceptions, the tumours produced by chronic UV exposure of hairless mice are squamous cell carcinomas or their precursors (Dunnick et al., 1991; Mark et al., 1989; Iversen, 1988). If histopathologic evaluation of tumours and other tissues is undertaken at the end of a study, it is understood that this is an evaluation of *what the lesions became*, and not necessarily *what they were* at the time of their first detection and measurement.

Intercurrent UVR and test article (TA) treatments are used in a photocarcinogenicity study. Topically applied TAs are delivered under both protected (post-irradiation) and exposed (pre-irradiation) conditions, by alternating treatment sequence on alternate days (within each week). TA applied *after* irradiation provides a test of influence by the unmodified test article. It also provides a situation in which the quantity of radiation delivered to the surface of the skin can be estimated directly without questions concerning optical attenuation or interaction by the TA. Test article applied *prior to* irradiation examines the influence of photoproducts as well as the possibility of photosensitized processes analogous to phototoxicity. It also introduces some uncertainty as to the amount of "effective" radiation actually delivered to the skin.

How chemical agents enhance photocarcinogenesis is not clearly defined, but several mechanisms have been postulated. The agent or its photoproducts could affect incoming radiation, or some optically significant aspect of cutaneous structure. Emollients, for example, might reduce random "light scatter" in the stratum corneum, resulting in greater transmission to the deeper target tissues. Alternatively, an agent could sensitize or participate in photobiological processes which themselves lead to carcinogenesis as is thought to occur with 8-MOP and other psoralens. The agent itself, or its photoproducts, or the consequences of photosensitized injury could contribute to the successful evolution of a presumptive photoinduced tumour. For example, croton oil enhances photocarcinogenesis, presumably as a consequence of its tumour-promoting potential. Agents that suppress immune response could enhance photocarcinogenesis by interfering with natural defence mechanisms (Davies et al., 1990; De Gruijl et al., 1993; Davies and Forbes, 1988a, 1988b; Forbes, 1981); Forbes and Davies, 1981.

A reliable safety test needs to respond to effects induced by the primary agent, or its photoproducts, or the consequences of photosensitized biological damage. It would not, and probably should not, differentiate between effects based on changes in the probability of carcinogenic events and those based on changes in subsequent tumour evolution. In this case, lack of specificity is a virtue; the safety testing protocol is designed to detect any adverse change in the effectiveness of an inevitable environmental hazard (i.e., UV photons). Ideally, a "guideline" test, with minor adaptations, would be broadly applicable to a diversity of products; it would not require knowledge of the mechanism by which the product might influence the photobiologic response (Davies et al., 1990; Forbes et al., 1989).

In a photocarcinogenesis safety test, selection of the test article dose must take into account not only the usual drug tolerance criteria, but also the possibility of interactions with the background UVR. One potentially limiting factor (in maintaining treatment over several months) is irritancy or induced inflammatory reactions in skin (Ichihashi et al., 2003). Even more problematic is the possibility that persistent inflammation might be a predisposing factor in photocarcinogenesis, as in other forms of carcinogenesis. A case in point is the family of chemical agents known as retinoids. Along with a number of other potential primary irritants, retinoids have been approved for treatment of a variety of dermatologic conditions. Several investigators have reported enhancement of photocarcinogenesis by all-*trans* retinoic acid and other retinoids (Forbes *et al.*, 1979; Davies and Forbes, 1988a). According to Powers *et al.* (1991) and Kligman and Kligman (1992) and Kligman (1993), a majority of studies on photocarcinogenesis in mice (using a diversity of research procedures and protocols) have not reported enhancement by retinoic acid (RA). Some of the factors involved with these differences in findings and interpretations are expanded upon below.

Reports that RA can promote tumour growth (or reduce tumour latency) are not limited to those involving UV radiation. In hairless mice, either RA or TPA (12-*O*-tetradecanoylphorbol-13-acetate) effectively promoted the growth of papillomas initiated by UVR or DMBA (Davies *et al.*, 1981). Furthermore, three retinoids (all-*trans* retinoic acid, 13-*cis* retinoic acid, and N-(4-hydroxyphenly) retinamide (4-HPR)), administered orally, all acted as tumour promoters when the initiator was 7,12 dimethylbenz(*a*)anthracene (DMBA). In the same study, the all-*trans* form and the 13-*cis* form also acted as tumour promoters when applied topically, but the 4-HPR did not do so (McCormick *et al.*, 1987).

Irritation, inflammation, hyperproliferation, and hyperplasia have been reported after application of RA to animal or human skin (Powers et al., 1991). One preclinical study of epidermal cellular kinetics suggested that topical retinoid application elicited a distinctive response. The study provided evidence of persistence of hyperproliferative activity (HPA) induced by repeated all-*trans* retinoic acid (RA) application, compared with earlier return to baseline after TPA application. Furthermore, if RA or TPA were applied in the form of a "promoter" after "initiation" of skin with 20 UV exposures (Monday to Friday for four weeks), there was additional epidermal activity initially; then, although TPA-treated epidermis returned to the control level of activity by week 21, no significant adaptation to RA treatment was seen (Sambuco and Forbes, 1983).

The skin reactions produced by RA are not necessarily identical with those of other skin irritants. The time course, dose response, components of inflammation, and involvement of putative mediators of inflammation in the irritant reaction induced by different chemicals was compared using a mouse ear swelling technique. Different chemicals do not act by a common inflammatory pathway (Patrick et al., 1987). Bason *et al.* (1991) indicate that irritation, or irritant dermatitis, is a complex biologic syndrome. Fujiki et al. (1989) report on differences in structural and biological activity amongst 23 newly-identified tumour promoters.

The role of inflammation and hyperplasia in tumourigenesis has been investigated and discussed by many clinical and preclinical researchers. Marks and Fürstenberger (1987) indicate that hyperplasia is a response of skin to chemical irritation and mechanical injury and that hyperplastic transformation provides an important physiological defence mechanism. Furthermore, these investigators suggest a possible link between hyperplasia and neoplasia in that tumour promotion is a process of hyperplastic transformation of skin that is over-activation of a normal physiological process. With respect to inflammation and the initiation-promotion model, Boutwell (1989) has pointed out that some carcinogens/initiators and, in general, skin promoters cause an inflammatory reaction in the skin leading to epidermal hyperplasia. This research model involves fairly distinctive morphological changes in the target tissues. Klein-Szanto (1989) in describing histopathology results from laboratory animal studies provides measurements of epidermal and dermal thickness, as well as the morphometric picture prior to the appearance of experimentally-induced skin tumours. Grasso *et al.* (1991) draw attention to indications that chronic lesions associated with repeated injury and repair of the skin can lead to cancer in humans. They also point out that prolonged injury to mouse skin can predispose to tumour production. Describing the reaction to painting with crude oil middle distillates, some of which were devoid of any recognized polycyclic aromatic hydrocarbon carcinogens, they point out that extremely high regenerative activity would provide a powerful hyperplastic stimulus to any cells within the epidermis, rendering them more vulnerable to transformation. The hyperplastic stimulus need not be in the form of chemical application. The interactive effects of dermal abrasion, in particular, have been investigated by Argyris (1989), who concludes that sequela to such damage can include very effective tumour promotion.

Clinical studies leave no doubt that UVR can strongly influence epidermal kinetics (Kligman, 1969; Lever and Schaumburg-Lever, 1975; Greaves et al., 1978). Clinically, the damage associated with chronic exposure to sunlight involves both dermal and epidermal changes. Bernstein and Uitto (1996) describe in detail how the process of chronologic ageing is distinct from ageing induced by sunlight, or photoageing. Hyperplasia is evident after exposure of animal skin including during the process of photocarcinogenesis (Sams et al., 1964; Stenbäck, 1975; Bissett et al., 1987). Sencar mice exhibit hypersusceptibility to single-dose UV-induced hyperplasia and tumourigenesis. Curiously enough, Sencar mice are not hypersusceptible to hyperplasia or tumourigenesis from chronic low dose UV (Strickland and Swartz, 1987).

An unresolved question has to do with the possible influence of inflammation-producing agents during the process of tumour induction by sunlight. One photocarcinogenesis study compared the effects of 8-MOP and anthracene as photosensitizers. In hairless mice exposed daily to a UV solar simulator, the exposed skin pretreated with 8-MOP or with anthracene became distinguishable from the surrounding skin after about five weeks of exposure (as judged by the degree of erythema, thickening and dry desquamation). This effect was not seen in areas treated with the vehicle only. Compared with the vehicle alone, the 8-MOP solution but not the anthracene solution markedly enhanced the photocarcinogenic response (Forbes et al., 1976). This indicates that a superimposed irritant response during the course of UV exposures will not necessarily enhance photocarcinogenesis. The authors also noted that the irritant response was transient, since the reactions on the 8-MOP and anthracene groups gradually resolved. By week 10 these two groups were indistinguishable from the vehicle-treated group. Similarly, Starcher et al. (1996) showed that the inhibition of neutrophil elastase effectively suppressed skin tumour development in UV-irradiated mice, even when the radiation dose was adequate to produce inflammatory infiltrates and cutaneous degenerative changes. Again, these data suggest that induced inflammation is not sufficient to enhance photocarcinogenesis. Kelfkens *et al.* (1991, 1999), noted differences in the inflammatory response relative to spectral and dose-rate influences during experimental photocarcinogenesis in mice. Perceptible inflammation associated with benzoyl peroxide did not appear to influence the rate of photocarcinogenesis (Epstein, 1988; Iversen, 1988) although Logani et al. (1984) previously noted UVR-induced skin tumour-promoting activity with methyl ethyl ketone peroxide.

Under certain circumstances, retinoids can have anti-neoplastic effects. The laboratory initiation-promotion model has been used to investigate the influence of RA on several stages of tumourigenesis (Yamasaki, 1989). Lippman et al. (1995) found that isotretinoin provided increased resistance to neoplastic conversion in oral tissues, apparently by modifying the expression of mutant p53 gene proteins.

In the overall scheme of tumourigenesis, the significance of hyperplasia induced by non-genotoxic agents has been debated for several very practical reasons. Grasso (1989) points out that exposure to substances that are well below the level of exposure used in the animal experiment, even for non-genotoxic photocarcinogens, the risk for man is negligible. In laboratory animals, modifications of urinary bladder epithelium have been extensively investigated and this field has provided a large body of data on the relationship of hyperplasia to tumourigenesis. Modelling analyses demonstrate that induced cell proliferation is sufficient to account for the increase in bladder tumour prevalence after exposure to sodium saccharin (NaS). If sufficient numbers of initiated cells are generated spontaneously, the increased and sustained proliferative activity induced by NaS generates tumors (Cohen and Ellwein, 1990). The authors conclude that, as the mechanisms of carcinogenesis become more thoroughly understood, a more rational approach can be taken for extrapolation from high-dose experimental data in animals to low-dose natural exposure and assessment of the risk faced by human populations exposed to chemical agents. The effects of toxicity and consequent cell proliferation are particularly critical for non-genotoxic agents because a threshold effect is likely. Powers *et al.* (1991) have commented on the diverse repertoire of retinoid effects on the biology of cells and tissues and on the relevance of animal toxicology tests and their value in calculating risks associated with retinoids as topical therapeutic agents in humans. They conclude that, considering all available toxicity information, the retinoids can be used safely and effectively. Griffiths and Voorhees (1995) point out the clinical attractiveness of retinoid therapy for photodamaged skin.

Thus, the published preclinical literature provides evidence that a few compounds, including some retinoids, can provoke cutaneous irritation, hyperproliferation, and persistent hyperplasia. To what extent these findings suggest the mechanism by which the test article acts as a promoter of chemically- or UV-induced tumourigenesis, or (when applied intercurrently) enhances photocarcinogenesis, is not yet known. Furthermore, until findings are available from prospective clinical trials, the influence of drugs (such as retinoids) on skin cancer development rates in susceptible humans will remain a matter of conjecture.

The photocarcinogenesis safety test is not designed to reveal mechanisms of effect, but it can estimate the amount of effect in one potentially useful way. An advantage of a study design containing UVR "calibration" doses is the immediate availability of an internal dose–response measure. Thus, when a test agent influences the effects (e.g., time-to-tumour) of a carcinogenic dose of radiation, it is possible to quantify that influence by equating it to the UV radiation dose which would have produced equivalent change. The tumour amplification or protection factor is measured by the apparent increase or reduction of the "carcinogenic effective" radiation caused by the presence of a test article. A dose–response calibration is provided in each study by a pair of groups receiving low and high doses of UV radiation. Results from these groups are used to estimate the parameters of the dose-response relationship:

$$Y = aX^b$$

where Y is the median latent period for 1 mm tumours and X is the cumulative weekly radiation dose. The observed latent period in a test group can then be used to estimate the "effective" weekly radiation dose. "Effective/Actual" provides the estimate of TA influence.

20.6 Future Testing Concepts, With Emphasis on Biomarkers

Photosafety testing comprises a relatively recent addition to the pharmaceutical regulatory scene. In November 2007, an international workshop was convened to discuss what were considered to be unclear and contradicting conclusions with respect to the photoreactive potential of a drug and its toxicological implications for human exposure. Primarily, the issue was the lack of sufficient consensus on interpreting the results of phototoxicity studies. The problem was compounded by the different testing strategies recommended in the guidance documents. "Photosafety" connotes toxicology safety testing involving interaction with light. Reports indicate that several categories of pharmaceutical products contain members that are associated with exaggerated responses to light (i.e., visible or ultraviolet radiation). One of the clinical end-points affected is the production of light-induced skin tumours (i.e., photocarcinogenesis). Several publications in the scientific literature provide information on the quantity and quality of light associated with tumour production, and on the pharmaceutical products that influence the rate of photocarcinogenesis. As a function of controlled environments and exposure factors, the animal studies provide the more reproducible quantitative data. International standards such as the CIE/ISO *Action Spectrum For Non-Melanoma Skin Cancer* are based largely on data from such "preclinical" studies.

Photocarcinogenesis studies conducted according to the CIE standardized protocol provide direct evidence useful for photocarcinogenesis risk identification and risk assessment. In preparation for full photocarcinogenesis tests, "tolerance" (dose range-finding) studies have been found to provide some predictive value, suggesting an approach to the evaluation of "abbreviated photocarcinogenesis studies".

Several investigators have been developing and evaluating abbreviated and alternative photocarcinogenesis tests. The principle aim has been to significantly shorten the time required for determining whether a substance has the potential to enhance photocarcinogenesis. Since 2003, regulatory guidance in Europe and the US strongly suggest the value of abbreviated and alternative tests, particularly those involving the use of "biomarkers" such as biochemical, histochemical and histological end-points associated with recognized early events in the process of carcinogenesis.

With the encouragement of regulatory reviewers, study sponsors have contracted for such studies and submitted the resulting data in support of their products. Several study designs (protocols) have received favourable reviews when submitted for FDA evaluation. Once the resulting data were submitted, however, the reviewers have asked that appropriate positive controls be included in order to demonstrate the validity of the model. The most direct response to this request is that, at this time, no adequate or definitive direct comparison of "positive control articles" in a photocarcinogenesis study with biomarker end-points has been performed, and therefore the relationship between these biomarkers and photocarcinogenesis cannot be assured. Given the lack of clarity of the relationships between the available biomarkers and photocarcinogenesis (and the enhancement of photocarcinogenesis by an exogenous agent other than UVR alone), the short-term safety test design cannot be considered as a proven concept. Consequently, at the time of writing, the abbreviated study designs based on evaluation of biomarkers cannot confidently be recommended as adequate for regulatory submission (i.e., for use as an adequate tool for risk identification and assessment).

Four points are offered in conclusion:

1. **Status of photocarcinogenesis testing:** The standardized protocol for photocarcinogenesis testing (i.e., irradiating hairless mice for 40 weeks) is the proven method for evaluating the effects of superimposed test agents.
2. **Observation:** Selected biomarkers provide evidence of influence by moderately large doses of UVR, but have not yet been shown to elicit graded responses to UVR levels adequate to initiate late-appearing tumours.
3. **Status:** The currently-available evidence does not lend sufficient confidence to the thesis that the biomarkers are adequate surrogates for modification (enhancement or inhibition) of photocarcinogenesis. For that reason, the use of this abbreviated photosafety design concept has not yet been recommended with confidence as an adequate substitute for a standard photocarcinogenesis study, and the results of other methodological studies are awaited.
4. **For the future:** The data base on abbreviated testing has not been widely available for peer review. Currently, the best hope for such development could be through the study nomination process supported by the US National Toxicology Program,

utilizing the phototoxicology capabilities of the National Center for Toxicological Research.

References

Argyris, T.S. (1989) Epidermal tumor promotion by damage in the skin of mice, in *Skin Carcinogenesis: Mechanisms and Human Relevance* (eds T.J. Slaga, A.J.P. Klein-Szanto, R.K. Boutwell, D.E. Stevenson, H.L. Spitzer, and B. D'Motto), Alan R. Liss, Inc., NY, pp. 63–80.

Bason, M., Lammintausts, K., and Maibach, H.I. (1991) Irritant dermatitis (irritation), in *Dermatotoxicology* (eds F.N. Marzulli and H.I. Maibach), Hemisphere Publishing Corp., NY, pp. 223–254.

Bernstein, E.F. and Uitto, J. (1996) The effect of photodamage on dermal extracellular matrix. *Clinics Dermatol.*, **14**, 143–151.

Bissett, D.L., Hannon, D.P., and Orr, T.V. (1987) An animal model of solar-aged skin: histological, physical, and visible changes in UV-irradiated hairless mouse skin. *Photochem. Photobiol.*, **46**, 367–378.

Blum, H. (1959) *Carcinogenesis by Ultraviolet Light*, Princeton University Press, Princeton, NJ.

Blum, H.F. (1930) Studies of photodynamic action: I. Hemolysis by previously irradiated fluorescein dyes. *Biol. Bull.*, **58**, 3.

Blum, H.F. (1964) *Photodynamic Action and Diseases Caused by Light*, Hafner Publishing Co., NY.

Boutwell, R.K. (1989) Model systems for defining initiation, promotion, and progression of skin neoplasms, in *Skin Carcinogenesis: Mechanisms and Human Relevance* (eds T.J. Slaga, A.J.P. Klein-Szanto, R.K. Boutwell, D.E. Stevenson, H.L. Spitzer, and B. D'Motto), Alan R. Liss, Inc., NY, pp. 3–15.

Burns, F., Albert, R., Altshuler, B., and Morris, E. (1983) Approach to risk assessment for genotoxic carcinogens based on data from the mouse skin initiation-promotion model. *Environ. Health Persp.*, **50**, 309–320.

Cohen, S.M. and Ellwein, L.B. (1990) Cell proliferation in carcinogenesis. *Science*, **249**, 1007–1011.

Daniels, F. (1965) A simple microbiological method for demonstrating phototoxic compounds. *J. Invest. Dermatol.*, **44**, 259–263.

Davies, R.E. and Forbes, P.D. (1988a) Retinoids and photocarcinogenesis: a review. *J. Toxicol. Cutan. Ocular Toxicol.*, **7**, 241–253.

Davies, R.E. and Forbes, P.D. (1988b) Effect of UV radiation on survival of non-haired mice. *Photochem. Photobiol.*, **43**, 267–274.

Davies, R.E., Forbes, P.D., and Urbach, F. (1981) Promotion of carcinogenesis by all-*trans* retinoic acid; effect of initiator. *Proc. Amer. Assoc. Cancer Res.*, **22**, 95.

Davies, R.E., Forbes, P.D., and Urbach, F. (1990) Effects of chemicals on photobiologic reactions of skin, in *DNA Damage and Repair in Human Tissue* (eds B.M. Sutherland and A.D. Woodhead), Springer, NY.

De Gruijl, F.R. and van der Leun, J.C. (1994) Estimate of the wavelength dependency of ultraviolet carcinogenesis in humans and its relevance to the risk assessment of a stratospheric ozone depletion. *Health Phys.*, **67**, 314–325.

De Gruijl, F.R. and Forbes, P.D. (1995) UV-induced skin cancer in a hairless mouse model. *BioEssays*, **17**, 651–660.

De Gruijl, F.R., Van der Meer, J.B., and Van der Leun, J.C. (1983) Dose-time dependency of tumor formation by chronic UV exposure. *Photochem. Photobiol.*, **37**, 53–62.

De Gruijl, F.R., Sterenborg, H.J.C.M., Forbes, P.D. et al. (1993) Wavelength dependence of skin cancer induction by ultraviolet irradiation of albino hairless mice. *Cancer Res.*, **53**, 53–60.

Derelanko, M.J. and Hollinger, M.A. (eds) (2002) *Handbook of Toxicology*, 2nd edn. CRC Press, Boca Raton, FL, pp. 129–201.

DIA/EMA (2007) Announcement: Photosafety Evaluation of Drugs: A Meeting and Workshop; NH Barbizon Palace Hotel, Amsterdam, Netherlands, 21–22 November 2007.

Dunnick, J.K., Forbes, P.D., Eustis, S.L. et al. (1991) Tumors of the skin in the HRA/Skh mouse after treatment with 8-methoxypsoralen and UVA radiation. *Fund. Appl. Toxicol.*, **16**, 92–102.

EMA/CPMP (2002) Note for Guidance on Photosafety Testing http://www.ema.europa.eu/pdfs/human/swp/039801.

Epstein, J.H. (1965) Comparison of the carcinogenic and cocarcinogenic effects of ultraviolet light on hairless mice. *J. National Cancer Inst.*, **34**, 741–745.

Epstein, J.H. (1975) Animal models for studying photocarcinogenesis, in *Models in Dermatology*, vol. 2 (eds H. Maibach and N. Lowe), Karger, Basel, Switzerland, pp. 303–312.

Epstein, J.H. (1988) Photocarcinogenesis promotion studies with benzyol peroxide (BPO) and croton oil. *J. Invest. Dermatol.*, **91**, 114–116.

Ferguson, J. (2003) Phototoxicity due to fluoroquinolones, in *Quinolone Antimicrobial Agents*, 3rd edn (eds D.C. Hooper and E. Rubenstein), ASM Press, Washington DC, pp. 449–458.

Findlay, G.M. (1928) Ultraviolet light and skin cancer. *Lancet*, **2**, 1070.

Food and Drug Administration (FDA) (2003) Guidance for Photosafety Testing www.fda.gov.

Forbes, P.D. (1981) Hairless mice for carcinogenesis studies, in *Proceedings of the Second NCI/EPA/NIOSH Collaborative Workshop: Progress on Joint Environmental and Occupational Cancer Studies* (eds H.F. Kraybill, I.C. Blackwood, and N.B. Freas), U.S. Government Printing Office, Washington, DC, pp. 131–153.

Forbes, P.D. (1996) Carcinogenesis and photocarcinogenesis test methods, in *Dermatotoxicology*, 5th edn (eds F.N. Marzulli and H.I. Maibach), Chapter 42, Hemisphere Publishing (Taylor & Francis), New York.

Forbes, P.D. and Davies, R.E. (1981) Enhancement of photocarcinogenesis by 8-MOP, in *Psoralens in Cosmetics and Dermatology, Proceedings of the International Symposium ("Proc. Int. Psoralens SIR")*, Pergamon Press, Paris, France, pp. 365–370.

Forbes, P.D., Davies, R.E., and Urbach, F. (1975) Phototoxicity and photocarcinogenesis: comparative effects of anthracene and 8-methoxypsoralen in the skin of mice. *Food Cosmet Toxicol.*, **14**, 303–306.

Forbes, P.D., Davies, R.E., and Urbach, F. (1976) Phototoxicity and photocarcinogenesis: Comparative effects of anthracene and 8-methoxypsorlen in the skin of mice. *Food Cosmet. Toxicol.*, **14**, 303–306.

Forbes, P.D., Urbach, F., and Davies, R.E. (1977) Phototoxicity testing of fragrance raw materials. *Fd. Cosmetic Toxicol.*, **15**, 55.

Forbes, P.D., Urbach, F., and Davies, R.E. (1979) Enhancement of experimental photocarcinogenesis by topical retinoic acid. *Cancer Lett.*, **7**, 85–90.

Forbes, P.D., Blum, H.F., and Davies, R.E. (1981) Photocarcinogenesis in hairless mice: dose-response and the influence of dose-delivery. *Photochem. Photobiol.*, **34**, 361–365.

Forbes, P.D., Davies, R.E., Sambuco, C.P., and Urbach, F. (1989) Inhibition of ultraviolet radiation-induced skin tumors in hairless mice by topical application of the sunscreen 2-ethyl hexyl-p-methoxycinnamate. *J. Toxicol. Cutan. Ocular Toxicol.*, **8**, 209–226.

Forbes, P.D., Davies, R.E., Urbach, F., and Dunnick, J. (1990) Long-term toxicity of oral 8-methoxypsoralen plus ultraviolet radiation in mice. *J. Toxicol. Cutaneous Ocular Toxicol.*, **9**, 237–250.

Forbes, P.D., Beer, J.Z., Black, H.S. et al. (2003) Standardized protocols for photocarcinogenesis safety testing. *Front. Biosci.*, **8**, 848–854.

Fry, R.J.M. and Ley, R.D. (1984) Ultraviolet radiation carcinogenesis, in *Mechanisms of Tumor Promotion and Skin Carcinogenesis*, vol. 2 (ed. T.J. Slaga), CRC Press, Boca Raton, FL, pp. 73–96.

Fujiki, H., Suganuma, H., Suguri, S. et al. (1989) Diversity in the chemical nature and mechanism of response to tumor promoters, in *Skin Carcinogenesis: Mechanisms and Human Relevance* (eds T. J. Slaga, A.J.P. Klein-Szanto, R.K. Boutwell, D.E. Stevenson, H.L. Spitzer, and B. D'Motto), Alan R. Liss, Inc., New York, pp. 281–291.

Gabriel, K.L., Forbes, P.D., and Davies, R.E. (1986) Phototoxicity, in *Photobiology of the Skin and Eye* (ed. E.M. Jackson), Marcel Dekker, Inc., New York.

Gad, S.C. (2002) Chapter 11, in *Drug Safety Evaluation*, John Wiley and Sons, Inc., New York, pp. 391–392.

Grasso, P. (1989) Relevance for man of skin carcinogenicity in experimental animals, in *Skin Carcinogenesis: Mechanisms and Human Relevance* (eds T.J. Slaga, A.J.P. Klein-Szanto, R.K. Boutwell, D.E. Stevenson, H.L. Spitzer, and B. D'Motto), Alan R. Liss, Inc., New York, pp. 17–24.

Grasso, P., Sharratt, M., and Cohen, A.J. (1991) Role of persistent, non-genotoxic tissue damage in rodent cancer and relevance to humans. *Ann. Rev. Pharmacol. Toxicol.*, **31**, 252–287.

Greaves, M.W., Hensby, C.N., Black, A.K. et al. (1978) Inflammatory reactions induced by ultraviolet irradiation. *Bull. du Cancer*, **65**, 299–303.

Green, G.L. (1966) *Biology of the Laboratory Mouse*, 2nd edn., McGraw-Hill Book Co., NY, New York.

Griffiths, C.E.M. and Voorhees, J.J. (1995) Effects of retinoids on photodamaged skin, in *Photodamage* (ed. B. Gilchrist), Blackwell Science, Inc., Cambridge, Massachusetts.

Grüneberg, H. (1952) *The Genetics of the Mouse*, Martinus Nijhoff Press, The Hague, The Netherlands.

IARC (1992) *Monographs on the Evaluation of Carcinogenic Risks to Humans. Solar and Ultraviolet Radiation*, vol. 55, IARC, Lyon, France.

Ichihashi, M., Ueda, M., and Budiyanto, A. (2003) UV-induced skin damage. *Toxicol.*, **189**, 21–39.

International Conference on Harmonization (ICH) (2009) Nonclinical safety studies for the conduct of human clinical trials and marketing authorization for pharmaceuticals, www.ich.org.

Iversen, O.H. (1988) Skin tumorigenesis and carcinogenesis studies with 7,12 dimethylbenz[a] anthracene, ultraviolet light, benzoyl peroxide (Panoxyl gel 5%) and ointment gel. *Carcinogen.*, **9**, 803–809.

Japanese Ministry of Health, Labour and Welfare (JMHLW) (1989) Guidelines for Toxicity Studies of Drugs. Notification 1 No. 24. Pharmaceutical Affairs Bureau.

Kelfkens, G., deGruijl, F.R., and van der Leun, J.C. (1991) Tumorigenesis by short-wave ultraviolet A: Papillomas versus squamous cell carcinomas. *Carcinogen.*, **12**, 1377–1382.

Kelfkens, G., deGruijl, F.R., and van der Leun, J.C. (1999) The influence of dose rate on ultraviolet tumorigenesis. *J. Photochem. Photobiol. (Part B. Biology)*, **10**, 41–50.

Klecak, G., Urbach, F., and Urwyler, H. (1997) Fluoroquinolone antibacterials enhance UVA-induced skin tumors. *J. Photochem. Photobiol. B*, **37**, 174–181.

Klein-Szanto, A.J.P. (1989) Morphological evaluation of the effects of carcinogens and promoters, in *Skin Carcinogenesis: Mechanisms and Human Relevance* (eds T.J. Slaga, A.J.P. Klein-Szanto, R.K. Boutwell, D.E. Stevenson, H.L. Spitzer, and B. D'Motto), Alan R. Liss, Inc., New York, pp. 45–62.

Kligman, A.M. (1969) Early destructive effect of sunlight on human skin. *J. Amer. Med. Assoc.*, **210**, 2377–2380.

Kligman, L.H. (1993) Tretinoin and photocarcinogenicity: an update. *J. Toxicol. Cutan. Ocular Toxicol.*, **12**, 205–220.

Kligman, L.H. and Kligman, A.M. (1992) Petrolatum and other hydrophobic emollients reduce UVB-induced damage. *J. Dermatol. Treatment*, **3**, 3–7.

Ledoux-Lebard, M. (1902) Action de la lumiere sur la toxicité de L'eosine. *Ann. Inst. Pasteur.*, **16**, 587.

Lever, W.F. and Schaumburg-Lever, G. (1975) *Histopathology of the Skin*, 5th edn, J.B. Lippincott Company, Philadelphia, PA.

Lippman, S.M., Shin, D.M., Lee, J.J. et al. (1995) p53 and retinoid chemoprevention of oral carcinogenesis. *Cancer Res.*, **55**, 16–19.

Logani, M.K., Sambuco, C.P., Forbes, P.D., and Davies, R.E. (1984) Skin-tumor promoting activity of methyl ethyl ketone peroxide: a potent lipid-peroxidizing agent. *Food Chem. Toxicol.*, **22**, 879–882.

Lynch, A.M. and Wilcox, P. (2010) Review of the performance of the 3T3 NRU in vitro phototoxicity assay in the pharmaceutical industry. *Exp. Toxicol. Pathol.* doi: 10.1016/j.etp.2009.12.001

Magnus, I.A. (1976) *Dermatological Photobiology: Clinical and Experimental Aspects*, Blackwell Scientific Publications, London, England.

Mark, R., Forbes, P.D., Sambuco, C.P. et al. (1989) Comparative histopathologic appearance of UV-induced skin tumors in hairless mice, cryptothrix mice, and Fuzzy rats. *J. Toxicol. Cut. Ocular Toxicol.*, **8**, 525–537.

Marks, F. and Fürstenberger, G. (1987) From the normal cell to cancer: the multistep process of experimental skin carcinogenesis, in *Concepts and Theories in Carcinogenesis* (eds A.P. Maskens, P. Ebbessent, and A. Burny), Elsevier Science Publishers B.V., NY.

Marzulli, F.N. and Maibach, H.I. (1970) Perfume phototoxicity. *J. Soc. Cosm. Chem.*, **21**, 685–715.

McCormick, D.L., Bagg, B.J., and Hultin, T.A. (1987) Comparative activity of dietary or topical exposure to three retinoids in the promotion of skin tumor induction in mice. *Cancer Res.*, **47**, 5989–5993.

Megaw, J. and Drake, L. (1986) An overview of photobiology, in *Photobiology of the Skin and Eye* (ed. E.M. Jackson), Marcel Dekker, Inc., NY.

Morison, W.I., Baughman, R.D., Day, R.M. et al. (1998) Consensus workshop on the toxic effects of long term PUVA therapy. *Arch. Dermatol.*, **134**, 595–598.

Organisation for Economic Cooperation and Development (OECD) (2004) In vitro 3T3 NRU phototoxicity test. Test Guideline No. 432.

Oppenlander, T.A. (1988) Comprehensive photochemical and photophysical assay exploring the photoreactivity of drugs. *Chimia*, **42**, 331–342.

Osterberg, R.E. and Szarfman, A. (1996) Assessment of risk for photocarcinogenesis: regulatory reviewer viewpoint. *Photochem. Photobiol.*, **63**, 362–365.

Patrick, E., Burkhalter, A., and Maibach, H.I. (1987) Recent investigations of mechanisms of chemically induced skin irritation in laboratory mice. *J. Investig. Dermatol.*, **88**, 24s–31s.

Peters, B. and Holzhutter, H.G. (2002) In vitro phototoxicity testing: development and validation of a new concentration response analysis software and a biostatistical analysis related to the use of various prediction methods. *Altern. Lab. Anim.*, **30**, 415–432.

Powers, W.J. Jr., Gendimenico, G.J., and McKenzie, B.E. (1991) Retinoids: a specific example in dermatotoxicology, in *Dermatotoxicology* (eds F.N. Marzulli and H.I. Maibach), Hemisphere Publishing Corp., New York, pp. 687–702.

Sacharoff, G. and Sachs, H. (1905) Ueber die hämolytische Wirkung der photodynamischen Stoffe. *Munch. Med. Woch.*, **52**, 297.

Sambuco, C.P. and Forbes, P.D. (1983) Interactions of ultraviolet radiation, 12-0-tetradecanoyl-phorbol-13-acetate and retinoic acid in the skin of hairless mice. *Food Chem. Toxicol.*, **21**, 595–600.

Sambuco, C.P. and Forbes, P.D. (1984) Quantitative assessment of phototoxicity in the skin of hairless mice. *Food Chem. Toxicol.*, **22**, 233–236.

Sambuco, C.P., Davies, R.E., Forbes, P.D., and Hoberman, A. (1991) Photocarcinogenesis and consumer product testing: technical aspects. *Toxicol. Methods*, **1**, 75–83.

Sambuco, C.P., Forbes, P.D., Davies, R.E. et al. (2003) Photocarcinogenesis: measuring the reproducibility of a biologic response to ultraviolet radiation exposure in mice. *Frontiers Biosci.*, **8**, a26–a33

Sams, W.M., Smith, J.G., and Burk, P.G. (1964) The experimental production of elastosis with ultraviolet light. *J. Invest. Dermatol.*, **43**, 467–471.

Scott, C.W., Stasse, J., Bonomo, R., and Campbell, A.H. (1970) Evaluation of the phototoxic potential of topically applied agents using longwave ultraviolet light. *J. Invest. Dermatol.*, **55**, 335–338.

Spielmann, H., Balls, M., Brand, M. et al. (1994) EEC/COLIPA project on in vitro phototoxicity testing: first results obtained with a Balb/c 3T3 cell phototoxicity assay. *Toxicol. In Vitro*, **8**, 793–796.

Spielmann, H., Balls, M., Dupuis, J. et al. (1998) The International EU/COLIPA in vitro phototoxicity validation study: Results of Phase II (Blind Trial). Part 1: The 3T3 NRU phototoxicity test. *Toxicol. In Vitro*, **12**, 305–327.

Spielmann, H., Müller, L., Averbeck, D. et al. (2000) The Second ECVAM Workshop on Phototoxicity Testing: The Report and Recommendations of ECVAM Workshop 42. ATLA **28**, 777–814.

Starcher, B., O'Neal, P., Granstein, R.D., and Beissert, S. (1996) Inhibition of neutrophil elastase suppresses the development of sklin tumors in hairless mice. *J. Invest. Dermatol.*, **107**, 159–163.

Stenbäck, F. (1975) Cellular injury and cell proliferation in skin carcinogenesis by UV light. *Oncology*, **31**, 61–75.

Stern, R.S., Nichols, K.T., and Vakeva, L.H. (1997) Malignant melanoma in patients treated for psoriasis with methoxsalen (psoralen) and ultraviolet radiation (PUVA): the PUVA follow up study. *New Engl. J. Med.*, **336**, 1041–1045.

Strickland, P.T. and Swartz, R.P. (1987) Inheritance of susceptibility to phototumorigenesis and persistent hyperplasia in F1 hybrids between SENCAR mice and BALB/c or C57BL/6 mice. *Cancer Res.*, **47**, 6294–6296.

Sugiyama, M., Itagaki, H., and Kato, S. (1994) In vitro assays to predict phototoxicity of chemicals: (II) Yeast growth inhibition assay and battery system with photohemolysis assay. *AATEX*, **2**, 193–202.

Urbach, F. (1959) Enhancement of photocarcinogenesis by photoactive agents. *J. Invest. Derm. (Suppl.)*, **32**, 373–378.

Urbach, F. (1998) Historical aspects of phototoxicology. *Int. J. Toxicol.*, **17**, 537–540.

Vargas, F., Rivas, C., Zoltan, T. et al. (2008) *In vitro* studies of the dual properties of Allopurinol anti- and photo-oxidants mechanisms. *Rev. Colomb. Cienc. Quím. Farm.* **37**, 69–83.

Winkelman, R.K., Baldes, E.J., and Zollman, P.E. (1960) Squamous cell tumors induced in hairless mice with ultraviolet light. *J. Invest. Dermatol.*, **34**, 131–138.

Winkelmann, R.K., Zollman, P.E., and Baldes, E.J. (1963) Squamous cell carcinoma produced by ultraviolet light in hairless mice. *J. Invest. Dermatol.*, **40**, 217–224.

Yamasaki, H. (1989) Short-term assays to detect tumor-promoting activity of environmental chemicals, in *Skin Carcinogenesis: Mechanisms and Human Relevance* (eds T.J. Slaga, A.J.P. Klein-Szanto, R.K. Boutwell, D.E. Stevenson, H.L. Spitzer, and B. D'Motto), Alan R. Liss, Inc., pp. 265–279.

Yanga, Y. and Xiong, X. (2007) Establishment and use of 3T3 NRU assay for assessment of phototoxic hazard of cosmetic products. AATEX, 14, Special Issue, 515–518, in Proc. 6th World Congress on Alternatives and Animal Use in the Life Sciences, Tokyo, Japan.

21

Degradants, Impurities, Excipients and Metabolites

Robert E. Osterberg[1] *and Mark W. Powley*[2*]
[1]*Osterberg Pharm-Tox Consulting, Rockville, USA*
[2]*CDER, Office of New Drugs, FDA, Silver Spring, USA*

21.1 Degradants, Impurities, and Excipients

21.1.1 Introduction and History

The United States Food and Drug Administration (FDA) has been charged with devising strict standards for the pharmaceutical and food industries to follow to ensure the cleanest, most effective and safest products that they can produce. Numerous federal and state laws and regulations mandate the quality of foods and drugs with consequences to those products and producers that do not meet the quality standards. The standard of quality refers to the physical, chemical, microbiological, biological, bioavailability and stability attributes that a drug product should maintain if it is to be deemed suitable for therapeutic or diagnostic use. Quality is also understood to convey the properties of safety, identity, strength, quality, and purity. However, attainment of this paradigm has not always been the case.

Adulteration of a product (to prepare for sale by replacing more valuable with less valuable or inert ingredients) and its lack of purity have been and is a problem in the United States as well as in other countries regarding imported drugs. In colonial times

[*] This author was responsible only for the sections addressing metabolites. The views expressed are those of the author. No official support or endorsement by the US Food and Drug Administration is provided.

Nonclinical Safety Assessment: A Guide to International Pharmaceutical Regulations, First Edition.
Edited by William J. Brock, Kenneth L. Hastings and Kathy M. McGown.

and the time after the American Revolution, the US imported most of its drugs from Europe. The drugs that entered into the US were often substandard regarding purity and many had been degraded due to the long journey by sea from Europe and the lack of refrigeration. Some drugs were not what they were reported to be since substitution with other drugs and/or substances of questionable quality often occurred and sufficient technology did not exist to discover any changes. As a result, many imported drugs were not effective for their intended therapeutic use or were unintentionally dangerous. This troubled medical and pharmaceutical professionals who observed an increasingly corrupt drug supply (Swann, 2008).

As a result, in January 1820, a group of 11 physicians, led by Dr Lyman Spaulding, met in Washington D.C. to establish a drug pharmacopeia and discuss what drugs would and would not be selected for inclusion. The publication of the United States Pharmacopeia (USP) was a milestone in the history of drug regulation because it was the first compendium of standard drugs in the United States. At this time, the USP contained 217 active drug substances (most were crude botanicals) that had an established utility which was best demonstrated and understood at the time. From these medicaments, drug products could be made that offered the greatest therapeutic advantages. The USP created a system of standards and quality control and a National Formulary (NF). This action effectively enhanced the reliability of the practice of medicine and pharmacy. The first revision of the US Pharmacopeia occurred in 1830.

Imported drugs continued to be of substandard quality. Around 1845, following a protest to a British drug manufacturer regarding the quality of the drugs received, the manufacturer reportedly responded that "the products are only as good as the Americans would pay for"! Indeed, the Americans were "over a barrel" then and for many more years.

The use of many of these substandard drugs by Americans usually did more harm than good. During the Mexican–American War (1846 to 1848), it was reported that many more American soldiers died from the consequences of treatment with these adulterated drugs than from actual battle wounds and diseases acquired during the war. It was Congress' understanding of pharmaceutical fraud during the Mexican–American War, the many reports of drug adulteration and degradation acquired over many years and developing anger amongst the general population that helped to craft a federal law that attempted to bring about quality pharmaceuticals. As a result, in 1848 President Polk signed into law the Drug Import Act that established US Custom Laboratories and required the US Customs Service to enforce the purity standards of the USP and stop the entry of adulterated drugs into the United States. The Act officially recognized the USP and the pharmacopeias and dispensatories of Edinburgh, London, France and Germany as the source of standards for drugs entering US ports.

The situation regarding the purity of drugs was still not satisfactory. Wives of congressmen protested the lack of efficacy with drugs being taken to fight diseases and also the poor quality of the food supply that was attributed to poor federal enforcement. By the turn of the twentieth century, several bills to improve federal regulation of foods and drugs had been introduced into Congress but failed to be passed for many reasons, including negative lobbying by interested parties. Specifically, the states of Connecticut, Georgia, Illinois, California and the Oklahoma Territory and most other states had outlawed drug adulteration and/or failure to label a medicine. Drugs especially of concern were morphine, cocaine, digitalis, nux vomica, chloroform, cantharides, strychnine and ergot. Violations were considered to be misdemeanours and penalties were assessed but more stringent federal laws were absent. Around this time, Samuel Adams wrote a series of articles in *Collier's* magazine that exposed patent medicine abuses. Shortly thereafter, the book *The Jungle* by Upton Sinclair appeared that told of the horrific happenings in the Chicago meat packing industry. As a result of these two events and others, numerous bills were introduced into Congress but passage was again thwarted. However, public reaction, State Food and Drug officials, the General Federation of Women's Clubs, the American Pharmaceutical Association, the American Medical Association and Dr Harvey Wiley successfully campaigned for passage of the Food and Drugs Act of 1906 that was signed into law by President Theodore Roosevelt.

In summary, the Food and Drugs Act forbade commerce in adulterated and misbranded drugs, required drug manufacturers to abide by the official standards in the USP/NF or meet the individual standards chosen by drug *manufacturers* as stated on the labels. The making of false or misleading label statements regarding a drug constituted misbranding. Interestingly, the Sherley Amendment to the Act (1911) prohibited labelling medicines with false therapeutic claims that were intended to defraud the purchaser, a difficult standard to prove. It also placed the burden of proof on the federal government to show fraud and misbranding. During this period, the Bureau of Chemistry was created and the "Poison Squad" led by Dr Wiley was charged to enforce the law. Sadly, very little, if any, federal legislation was introduced for two decades following the passage of the Sherley Amendment. In 1933, the FDA recommended a complete revision of the obsolete 1906 Food and Drugs Act. This legislation engendered heated discussions for five years until a human tragedy occurred that ended this particular and continuous legislative battle.

In 1937, the Massengill chemical company introduced the drug product Elixir of Sulfanilamide into commerce to treat bacterial infections. The company used a new and untested chemical (a.k.a. pharmaceutical necessity or excipient) called diethylene glycol to make the product tasty and attractive to children via its blue colour and to bring into solution the water insoluble sulfonamide. As a result of adding this assumed safe excipient, more than 100 children died from kidney failure and hundreds more were sick following the therapeutic use of the elixir. Public outrage led to the passage of the Food, Drug and Cosmetic Act of 1938 (FDCA) (a.k.a the Copeland-Lea Bill). Amongst other provisions of the Act, this legislation required that new drug substances and drug products had to be shown to be safe before marketing and this eventually started a new system of drug regulation. Furthermore, the Act eliminated the provisions of the Sherley amendment that required the government to prove fraud, and authorized standards of identity, quality and fill-of-container for foods. Interestingly, the Elixir of Sulfanilamide was removed from the market not because it caused great harm but because it was fraudulent. According to the USP, an elixir must contain at least 10% ethanol and Elixir of Sulfanilamide did not contain any ethanol. Interestingly, even today there have been numerous reports of poisonings due to diethylene glycol contamination in pharmaceuticals, especially in developing countries in Africa and the Carribean (History of the FDA).

To ensure the quality of foods and drugs and their components, the FDA currently enforces Good Manufacturing Practices (GMP) under Section 501(B) of the 1938 Food, Drug and Cosmetic Act and uses the phrase "current good manufacturing practices". This is to ensure that a drug product is manufactured according to good industry standards that can change with time as technology improves. In 1978, the FDA wrote its own GMP guideline that is presently in use in evaluating drug quality. As a result of the activities of the International Conference on Harmonization (ICH), the US, Japan and the EU, the main signatories, plus other countries that adopted the ICH guidelines (Canada, Australia, Singapore, and so on), follow this guidance to produce a quality drug product. The ICH activities have had a major effect on the world's drug development.

21.1.2 ICH Impact

The ICH is a joint regulatory industry initiative whose purpose is to rationalize and harmonize regulatory requirements for drug registration amongst the three major drug developing regions in the world: the EU, Japan and the USA. The World Health Organization (WHO) is involved in disseminating information and providing input beyond the ICH regions. The ICH's impetus is to control costs of health care, control the cost of research and development by reducing needless duplication of efforts and to bring safe and efficacious drugs to the market faster. In addition, a lack of research duplication leads to less use of research animals. To achieve these goals, the ICH has defined four areas of guideline development: Quality, Safety, Efficacy and Multidisciplinary (see ICH). These guidelines are discussed in Chapter 2 (ICH).

21.1.3 Impurities/Degradants in Drug/Biological Products

One of the missions of the FDA and its Centers for Drug Evaluation and Research (CDER) and Biological Evaluation and Research (CBER) is to determine if a drug/biological product contains impurities (contaminants that provide no therapeutic use and could be toxic) and impurities that are unavoidable during drug manufacture. Furthermore, to ensure a quality product, the identity and amount of each impurity must be ascertained. Impurities in a drug product must reside at FDA-determined safe levels to provide for a safe medicament. However, a degradant (also an impurity) is a chemical that has been changed into a less complex compound. Degradants could be responsible for additional therapeutic effects or could interfere with a drug and reduce its efficacy. The reduction of a drug's efficacy by a degradant could occur by blocking its activity at a receptor or by a reduction in the amount of non-degraded drug available for a therapeutic effect that was administered. Furthermore, degradants could expand the toxicity potential of the drug by introducing additional toxic effects not seen with the drug substance alone. Degradants must also be identified and quantified where possible. When dealing with the inherent complexity of many biological drugs (proteins, polypeptides, their derivatives and products of which they are components; they can be produced from recombinant or non-recombinant cell culture expression systems) there is no single stability-indicating assay or parameter that profiles the stability characteristics of the product. Therefore, the manufacturer should provide such a stability-indicating profile for their product based on data obtained from lots of the drug used in nonclinical and clinical studies and manufacturing consistency lots (see ICH Q6B). This ICH guidance does not cover antibiotics, synthetic peptides and polypeptides, heparins, vitamins, cell metabolites, DNA products, whole blood, cellular blood components, and so on, and manufacturers should refer to ICH Q6A.

Specifically, CDER has three offices that are responsible for determining the safety and quality of drug products. The Office of New Drugs, the Office of New Drug Chemistry and the Office of Generic Drugs embody review physicians, pharmacologists, toxicologists, pharmacists and chemists whose jobs require the evaluation of impurities found in drug and drug products. To facilitate the safety evaluation of impurities, the Office of New Drugs and its pharmacology and toxicology components formed an Inactive Ingredients subcommittee of the Pharmacology and Toxicology Coordinating Committee (PTCC) in 1988 to act as consultants to CDER drug review divisions. The subcommittee's focus involved evaluating the toxicities of impurities such as degradants, extractables, leachables, excipients, flavours, solvents and other contaminants in a consistent manner. Extractables, leachables and excipients are discussed below. If requested by a review division, the subcommittee reviews impurity data and recommends safe levels of exposure or request additional information that could engender a sponsor to conduct studies to obtain more toxicity data. On rare occasions, the subcommittee could act as an intermediary between a sponsor and a review division if requested. A few years later, the PTCC determined that the subcommittee had an additional and important use.

21.1.4 Impurities in New Drug Substances

When the ICH began its discussions and deliberations on quality issues, members of the subcommittee were invited to join certain quality expert working groups to bring a toxicology perspective since quality issues were primarily issues for chemistry discussions. The utility of the toxicology perspective involved determining which impurities were of concern and then determining their safe levels. Toxicology involvement in the Q3A, B and C expert working groups began sequentially and generated important considerations during the discussions.

For example, in Q3A discussions regarding impurity qualifications it was recognized that an impurity would be qualified if certain conditions were met. Qualification is the process of acquiring and evaluating data to establish the safety of an individual impurity or of a given impurity profile at the level(s) specified in the guideline. Initial discussions involved the determination of the safe level of an impurity. Some members of the expert working group recalled an *ad hoc* advisory committee meeting which took place in the early 1990s at the FDA that entertained discussions on safe levels of impurities. It was proposed by a Canadian representative that the value of 0.1% was a good starting point because of Canadian successes in regulating new drugs with impurities at or below this level. Furthermore, the Canadian representative stated that the pharmaceutical manufacturers involved in their discussions did not oppose that level because the level was reasonable and attainable. FDA representatives accepted that value also in their review activities and, as a result, proposed to the expert working group that 0.1% be accepted for the Q3A guideline. This value was acceptable also to the ICH Steering Committee and was adopted in the guideline.

The Q3A guideline states that an impurity is qualified if its specification limit is at or below the threshold concentration:

(a) 0.1% or 1 mg whichever is lower if the daily dose of a drug substance is 2000 mg or less; or,
(b) 0.05% if the daily dose is more than 2000 mg per day.

It should be understood that these numbers are not the rule of law because, based upon the identification of an impurity and its inherent toxicity, the acceptable limit in a drug product can be decreased. As an example, if the impurity is determined to be a nitrosamine and potentially carcinogenic to humans, carcinogenicity studies may be requested and a safe level determined from those data.

It was also understood that the level of an impurity in a drug substance that was *adequately* tested in nonclinical and/or clinical studies is considered to be qualified at that level. The term "adequately tested" involved anticipated exposure levels, duration of exposure and the route of exposure amongst other considerations. However, if the impurity data did not satisfy the toxicology reviewer, certain questions could be asked of the sponsor about the impurity that could lead to additional testing. For example:

1. Is the impurity level above threshold or is the threshold adequate?
2. Is the molecular structure known?
3. Is the toxicity documented or sufficient?
4. Is the impurity related to others of known toxicity?
5. Has the patient population and therapeutic use of the drug been considered?

If the impurity and its level in the drug substance are of concern, the sponsor of the drug can eliminate the impurity, reduce the level of the impurity to an acceptable level or conduct toxicology tests to qualify it at a higher level. The Q3A guideline suggests that qualification of the impurity at a higher level than accepted could occur by conducting two *in vitro* genotoxicity studies involving point mutations and chromosomal aberrations and conducting a general repeat-dose toxicology study in one species, usually the rat if applicable, for at least 14 to 90 days or more depending upon several considerations. Other tests could also be requested, if indicated. The guideline states that "the study duration should be based on available relevant information and performed on the species most likely to maximize the potential to detect the toxicity of an impurity. On a case-by-case basis, single-dose studies can be appropriate, especially for single-dose drugs". Initially, the expert working group recommended that the active drug including the impurity(ies) be tested in these studies. Years later, the FDA changed its collective mind and requested that the impurity itself be tested since this would increase the sensitivity of the assays to pick up toxicities that could be masked by the components of the active drug substance/-product. It is recommended that the impurity undergo a QSAR evaluation using any one of several modalities presently available to predict specific toxicities such as mutagenicity, teratogenicity and carcinogenicity. If no "red flag" is raised upon the analysis, the impurity could undergo further biological testing as suggested in the guidance. Tests recommended are a repeat-dose toxicity test in a rodent specie for up to 90 days using the intended therapeutic route of administration and two *in vitro* genotoxicity tests that are acceptable to the agency. Other tests could be requested by the agency (see below). If the impurity cannot be structurally identified or synthesized, the level of the impurity might have to be reduced to a lower concentration in the drug substance.

Impurities that are covered by the Q3A guideline are:

1. Organics that are usually a by-product of syntheses;
2. Extractables and leachables from containers and/or in manufacturing;

3. Residual solvents from the manufacturing process; and
4. Extraneous contaminants such as pesticides, other drugs, and so on that are GMP issues

Impurities that are not covered by the Q3A guideline are:

1. Biological and biotechnological impurities;
2. Peptides and oligonucleotides;
3. Radiopharmaceuticals, fermentation and semi-fermentation products such as antibiotics;
4. Botanicals and crude products of animal or plant origin.

Examples of impurities from INDs/NDAs that were discovered in drug substances that may produce known toxicities from drug exposures are:

Drug substance	Toxic impurity?	Observed toxicity
Tetracycline	4-epihydrotetracycline	Fanconi syndrome-kidney
Meperidine analogue	MPTP	Parkinson's disease
L-tryptophan	Approximately 61 impurities	Eosinophilia-Myalgia syndrome
Clidinium bromide	Ro 23333	Anticholinergic symptoms
Ibuprofen	Isobutyl acetophenone	Burning sensation-mouth/throat

21.1.5 Impurities in New Drug Products

However, considerations are different to some extent when a drug product is being evaluated in accordance with the ICH Q3B guidance. Impurity concerns involve:

1. Degradation products of the active drug substance;
2. Reaction products of the active drug substance with an excipient and/or the immediate container or closure system.

It should be noted that impurities from excipients or extracted or leached from a container closure system that are present in a drug product are excluded as well as those exclusions listed in the Q3A guidance. As stated in Q3A, the level of an impurity in a drug substance that was *adequately* tested in nonclinical and/or clinical studies is considered to be qualified at that level. This concept also applies to impurities in drug products.

The qualification thresholds for impurities in drug products are as follows:

Maximum daily dose of drug substance	Threshold (total daily intake)
$\leq$10 mg	1.0% or 50 μg (lowest value)
10 to 100 mg	0.5% or 200 μg (lowest value)
$\geq$100 to 2000 mg	0.2% or 2000 μg (lowest value)
$\geq$2000 mg	0.1%

If a drug impurity cannot meet the qualification thresholds, the toxicity test data that may allow for a higher level of impurity are the same as listed in the ICH Q3A guidance namely:

1. A repeat dose 14 to 90-day toxicity test in a rodent specie;
2. Two genotoxicity tests – an *in vitro* bacterial reversion test and an *in vitro* chromosomal aberration test;
3. Other tests as needed (i.e., *in vivo* genotoxicity, carcinogenicity, immunotoxicity tests, and so on).

21.1.6 Residual Solvents

This guidance pertains to organic volatile chemicals *not deliberately* used as excipients. The addition of ethyl alcohol to a drug product is an example of a deliberate excipient use although it is often used as a solvent. Residual solvents are residuals that were not completely removed by manufacturing processes. They may or may not be toxic at residual levels. Since there is no therapeutic benefit from residual solvents, they should be removed to the greatest extent possible to meet product specifications, good manufacturing practices or other quality-based requirements.

In order to avoid potential toxicities from these solvents, the ICH recommended:

1. Use of less toxic solvents identified in Class 3;
2. Acceptable levels of the more toxic solvents identified in Class 2;
3. Avoiding the unacceptably toxic solvents with *exceptions* in Class 1.

An example of an exception would be the unavoidable use of a very toxic solvent to produce a subpart H drug product (a drug product having a use that no other approved drug has for lifesaving or disease/disability preventing results, for example, cure for a cancer or prevention of blindness).

The following are some examples of residual solvents and their classes:

Class 1, solvents to be avoided such as known or highly suspected human carcinogens and environmental hazards: benzene, carbon tetrachloride, 1, 1, 1-trichloroethane, 1, 2-dichloroethane, 1, 1-dichloroethene.

Class 2, solvents to be limited such as non-genotoxic animal carcinogens or possible causative substances of other irreversible toxicities (teratogens): chloroform, dichloromethane, methanol, tetrahydrofuran, pyridine, toluene.

Class 3, solvents with a low toxic potential such as solvents with safe exposure levels of 50 mg or more per day: acetone, DMSO, ethanol, heptane, propyl acetate, formic acid, methylethyl ketone.

For identified solvents with a potential for use in some drug products for which no adequate toxicological information was available, *Table 4* was established in the hopes that a future maintenance activity could evaluate them at the appropriate time. Examples of these Table 4 solvents are: isopropyl ether, petroleum ether, methylisopropyl ketone, trichloroacetic acid. During a future maintenance activity, additional solvents could be evaluated and included in the residual solvent classes.

In the Q3C guidance, permissible daily exposures (PDEs) were calculated with the following formula:

$$\text{PDE} = \frac{\text{NOEL} \times \text{Weight Adjustment}}{\text{F1} \times \text{F2} \times \text{F3} \times \text{F4} \times \text{F5}}$$

Factors : F1 – extrapolate animal to human

F2 – 10 for human variability

F3 – duration of exposure

F4 – severity of toxicity

F5 – up to 10 for no NOEL in study

This equation can be used for residual solvent classes 2 and 3 and was obtained and used from the Pharmacopeial Forum, Nov–Dec 1989 and Environmental Health Criteria 170, WHO, 1994. These methods are similar to those used by the US EPA (IRIS) and the US FDA (Red Book). The residual solvent calculation assumes 100% systemic absorption by any route of exposure. For residual solvents in class 1, the Gaylor-Kodell method of risk assessment is appropriate (Gaylor and Kodell, 1980).

21.1.7 Extractables and Leachables

In the realm of drug product purity, the FDA has concerns about foreign substances that can migrate from containers which contain the medicament and might adulterate the product. Section 501 (a)(3) of the FDCA states that a drug is deemed to be adulterated "if its container is composed, in whole or in part, of any poisonous or deleterious substance which may render the contents injurious to health . . . ". Substances such as glass, high-density polyethylene resin, metal, and so on can be used to manufacture a packaging component. A packaging component can be any single part of a container closure system such as containers (e.g., ampules, vials, bottles), container liners (e.g., tube liners), closures (e.g., screw caps, stoppers), closure liners, stopper overseals, container inner seals, administration ports (e.g., on large-volume parenterals) overwraps, administration accessories, and container labels. Concern is also applicable to any component from which substances could migrate into the dosage form such as an ink or an adhesive (see DHSS, FDA, CDER, 1999). Interestingly, chemical and toxicological information regarding inks, adhesives, excipients, and so on are usually contained within Drug Master Files (DMFs). These DMFs are the sole property of the manufacturer of the product or container system and are proprietary. The owner of the DMF must give the FDA permission in writing to allow the FDA to review the DMF or allow another pharmaceutical manufacturer to utilize the information in support of their product. If the DMF is insufficient in its data content, the FDA alerts the owner of the DMF only regarding the nature of the deficiency. The other party is only told that there is a deficiency. It is the responsibility of the DMF holder to amend their DMF.

The foreign substances that could be obtained from a drug's packaging are called extractables and leachables. Extractables are chemical species that can be released from a container which has the potential to contaminate a drug product. An extractable could be produced through an interaction with a container under *stressed conditions* such as exposure to high temperatures for a specified length of time, exaggerated concentrations of solvents, irradiation and/or sterilization processes. The purpose of elevated temperatures is to increase the rate of impurity extraction so that a short exposure time could simulate a longer exposure time. High temperatures could also maximize the amount of extractables obtained from a sample and possibly release a chemical that normally would not be extracted. However, a leachable is a substance that has migrated from the container into a drug substance or drug product under *normal conditions* of use. This impurity may be what would usually be found in a drug product following migration from a container. Sources of extractables and leachables from containers include plastic components, adhesives, inks, vulcanizing agents, coatings, antioxidants, accelerants and elastomers (Osterberg 2005).

Identified extractables and leachables should be characterized for their toxicity potentials and their safe exposure levels should be determined. Exposures to these impurities can occur during transportation of the drug substance or a component of the drug product to a manufacturing unit while in its primary container or while the product is being transported and/or stored in its primary container. The Center for Veterinary Medicine has similar concerns for extractables and leachables that might migrate from drug and food container closures regarding animal drugs and medicated feeds. The Center for Food Safety and Applied Nutrition has similar concerns with respect to human foods.

There is a correlation between the degrees of concern regarding the routes of administration with the likelihood of packaging component–dosage form interactions for different classes of drug products. The highest concern level for packaging associated with the intended route of administration occurs with inhalation aerosols and injectable solutions and suspensions. A high level of concern exists for ophthalmic solutions and suspensions, transdermal ointments and patches and nasal aerosols and sprays. A low level of concern resides with topical solutions and suspensions, topical and lingual aerosols and oral solutions and suspensions. There is medium concern for sterile powders, powders for injection and inhalation and low concern for topical and oral powders, oral tablets and capsules.

The differences in concern levels reflect the degree of concern for the integrity and quality of the drug product. A packaging system found acceptable for one drug product is not automatically assumed to be appropriate for another product. The container should adequately protect the dosage form. It should be compatible with the dosage form and it should be composed of materials that are considered safe for use with the drug product and the route of administration. The drug container should protect the drug product from light, if it is light sensitive. It should also protect the drug product from temperature, oxygen, loss of solvent, water or microbial contamination or loss of potency by a reaction of the drug product with the container. There should be no harmful leachables bleeding into the drug product within the container (DHSS, FDA, CDER, 1999).

A standardized approach for making a determination that a packaging material is safe has not been established. Packaging materials can vary in type and chemical composition. There are many different types of plastic, glass, paper and metals, and so on that are components of packaging material. One standard approach would not fit all. The approach for the toxicological evaluation of the safety of extractables should be based on good scientific principles and take into consideration the specific container system, drug product formulation, dosage form, route of administration and a chronic or short-term dosage regimen. For a drug product such as an injection, inhalation, ophthalmic or transdermal, a comprehensive approach is suggested. A quantitative extraction study on the packaging component to determine which chemical species could migrate into the dosage form should be performed. This should be followed by the toxicological evaluation of the extractables to determine the safe level of exposure under the intended conditions of product use.

For many injectable and ophthalmic drug products, data from the conduct of the USP Biological Reactivity Tests (*In Vitro* and *In Vivo*) and USP Elastomeric Closures for Injections tests could be considered as sufficient evidence of material safety (see General Chapters below). In the current USP, General Chapter 87 discusses three *in vitro* tests, namely the Agar Diffusion Test, the Direct Contact Test and the Elution Test. Each test involves the use of cell cultures and the Chapter should be reviewed for specific descriptions, test methods and interpretations of test results. General Chapters 85, 88 and 151 describe animal-based standards and tests using mice, guinea pigs, rabbits and the Limulus Amoebocyte Lysate test (FDA recommended replacement test for the Rabbit Pyrogen test). These General Chapters should also be reviewed for specific test descriptions and result interpretations. Regarding elastomeric closures for injections, General Chapter 381 should also be reviewed for specific testing information and interpretation. The FDA could also request that certain toxicity studies be performed when concerns arise. Through the efforts of the USP's Council of Experts and its Expert Committees, chapters in the USP are reviewed and modified where considered necessary through a public review and comment process.

In a presentation made in 2005, the Product Quality Research Institute (PQRI) and its Toxicology Subgroup suggested that qualification of impurities should be performed only on leachables and only on those that occurred above data-supported thresholds. In general, regulators agree but want to know about extractables because they potentially could be released into the drug product as leachables. If some extractables are not detected at established thresholds in the leachable determination, they could be removed from regulatory consideration (PQRI, 2006). It was also stated that qualification of a product-related leachable composite mixture was sufficient to qualify those leachables for registration and that product samples should be qualitatively representative of the end-of-shelf-life leachable profiles. PQRI also indicated that the risk assessment of leachables could come from one or more data sources such as:

- *in silico*, structure activity relationships;
- literature;
- *in vitro* or *in vivo* testing.

PQRI also referred to the USP General Chapters 87 and 88 for additional information but indicated that the General Chapters were not necessary when a more comprehensive toxicological evaluation was available.

Through its activities in support of the ICH, the FDA has also helped to identify a decision tree for identification and qualification of impurities that can also apply to leachables and extractables. If a leachable is identified by chemical analyses, and considering the ICH guidances ICH Q3A and B, one could follow the Decision Tree for Identification and Qualification of impurities. Questions that should be answered via chemical analyses and toxicological tests are:

1. Is the leachable level above threshold as defined in the guidances?
2. Are the molecular structures known and are they similar to other chemicals with known toxicities?
3. Are the toxicity data documented and sufficient in quantity, quality and type?

In addition, one should also consider the patient population and potential therapeutic uses of the drug product containing the leachable(s). If toxicity data are lacking so questions cannot be answered, consider the relevant data that are needed, that is, genotoxicity tests, carcinogenicity tests, repeat-dose studies by the route and duration of drug therapy and special tests (teratology and reproduction toxicity tests, local tolerance tests, and so on). The ICH M3 guidance should be reviewed for the types of toxicological testing that might be necessary to determine the toxicity potentials of these leachables.

21.2 Metabolites

21.2.1 Metabolites and Nonclinical Evaluation

An assumption made during drug development is that nonclinical toxicology data are useful for predicting clinical outcome. The choice of nonclinical models is therefore vital to minimizing clinical trial subject and patient risk. While efforts are made to assure appropriate selection, the task is complicated by well-known species differences in drug metabolism. Substrate specificity, induction, as well as expression patterns of drug metabolizing enzymes and transporters are known to differ amongst nonclinical species. More importantly, these differences also exist between nonclinical species and human. The results of this metabolic variability are qualitative and quantitative differences in circulating levels of drug metabolites.

Interspecies differences in metabolism can lead to two metabolite-related scenarios in drug development. The first involves detection of a unique clinical metabolite (i.e., detected only in human) or a disproportionate clinical metabolite (i.e., present at higher plasma concentrations in human vs. nonclinical models). While unique and disproportionate human metabolites are considered to be historically infrequent (Davis-Bruno and Atrakchi, 2006; Robison and Jacobs, 2009), identified occurrences are likely to increase as a result of recent regulatory focus. Encountering a unique or disproportionate human metabolite is of particular concern because of clinical safety implications. For instance, a traditional nonclinical toxicology evaluation will provide no data to support the safety of a truly unique human metabolite and may provide inadequate data in regards to a disproportionate human metabolite.

An alternative scenario involves formation of a unique or disproportionate nonclinical metabolite. This situation does not impact clinical safety but might present problems to the development process. Determining whether a nonclinical toxicity has human relevance could require resource-intense investigations. While not included in recommendations by regulatory entities such as the FDA or ICH, identification of important nonclinical metabolites could assist with data interpretation (Baillie *et al.*, 2002).

21.2.2 The FDA and ICH

In 2002, a position paper addressing potential concerns with drug metabolite safety was published on behalf of the Pharmaceutical Research and Manufacturers of America (Baillie *et al.*, 2002). Additional perspectives were subsequently published on this topic leading to the issuance of a draft FDA guidance (FDA, 2006) and eventually a final FDA guidance (FDA, 2008). The International Conference for Harmonization's most recent guideline regarding nonclinical drug development, ICH M3(R2) (ICH, 2009), also includes discussion of metabolite safety. These regulatory documents cover the topic of metabolite safety in varying detail but there is overlap on a few key points (summarized below). Note that where there is inconsistency, the ICH guideline receives preference over the FDA guidance (Robison and Jacobs, 2009).

21.2.3 Systemic Exposure Threshold

Systemic exposure is a fundamental consideration for establishing toxic potential. Clinical metabolites with limited exposure are not generally a concern while those with substantial systemic exposure may merit further evaluation. Based on the FDA guidance document, a metabolite is of interest when steady-state systemic exposure is greater than 10% of parent drug exposure. The ICH definition differs slightly in that it is based on the fraction of systemic exposure to total drug-related material (e.g., metabolite systemic exposure greater than 10% of exposure to total drug-related material). This difference is important, for instance, when a drug is extensively metabolized and the parent drug accounts for only a small percentage of the total drug-related material. In this case, numerous metabolites could account for greater than 10% of exposure to the parent. These same metabolites may be considered minor if compared with exposure to total drug-related material. The ICH guideline also indicates that additional nonclinical characterization is needed only when clinical exposure to a metabolite is "significantly higher" than that observed in nonclinical species.

Another difference between the regulatory recommendations is that ICH does not consider the 10% threshold to be appropriate in all cases. For drugs administered in very low doses (for example, less than 10 mg/day) it may be acceptable to increase the threshold to a higher percentage of systemic exposure to drug-related material.

21.2.4 Safety Assessment Strategy

While the FDA guidance provides a general strategy for evaluation of metabolites, the ICH guideline does not address this topic. According to the FDA, an appropriate nonclinical assessment will provide coverage (defined below) for a clinical metabolite of concern in at least one species per relevant end-point. These relevant end-points include, but are not limited to, *in silico* assessment of genotoxic potential, *in vitro* genetic toxicology studies (e.g., assays that measure point mutations and chromosomal aberrations), general toxicology study of appropriate length per ICH M3(R2), embryo–foetal development study, and carcinogenicity study. Data from these studies are key to determining whether further nonclinical evaluation might be needed to support clinical safety.

21.2.5 Timing

The stage of development when nonclinical data should be available is an additional aspect of the regulatory recommendations. Early clinical trials usually involving limited number of subjects and duration are typically acceptable with little or no nonclinical data for a metabolite. However, the recommended data should be provided to support late-stage clinical trials (that is, prior to Phase 3 per ICH and prior to initiating large-scale clinical trials according to the FDA). Regardless of when the information is needed, early identification of metabolite issues is encouraged in order to minimize the potential for delays.

21.2.6 Exceptions

Drug metabolism involves Phase 1 (e.g., oxidation, reduction, etc.) and Phase 2 reactions (e.g., conjugation with glucuronide, sulfate, glutathione, etc.). Phase 2 metabolites are generally considered to be less toxic than the parent drug or Phase 1 metabolites and, therefore, a safety evaluation is not normally recommended. This might not be the case for pharmacologically active or chemically reactive Phase 2 metabolites. Acyl-glucuronides are one example of a Phase 2 metabolite considered to be chemically reactive and toxicologically significant (Faed, 1984). Overall, circulating metabolites with toxic potential should be considered for evaluation regardless of whether they are Phase 1 or Phase 2.

21.2.7 Data Collection

Metabolite-related data are collected and used to make decisions at all stages of drug development. According to ICH M3(R2), *in vitro* metabolite data should be provided prior to the first clinical trial. More definitive *in vivo* data in both nonclinical species and humans become available as needed. The types and utility of metabolite-related data are described below.

21.2.8 *In Vitro* Data

Tentative structural information for *in vitro* metabolites is typically available early in development. This information is derived from experiments conducted in hepatocytes or liver subcellular fractions (e.g., microsomes or S9) from multiple species, including human. The *in vitro* profiles are useful for determining which nonclinical species are qualitatively similar to the human and can provide early indication of whether unique metabolites could occur *in vivo*. Metabolites with genotoxic structural alerts are also identified at this stage.

It may be appropriate to determine the pharmacologic activity of significant *in vitro* metabolites early in development. Metabolites with activity at the target receptor (primary pharmacology) or off-target receptor (secondary pharmacology) are of concern, especially when activity approaches that of the parent drug. Because an unbound molecule is primarily responsible for *in vivo* pharmacologic activity (Trainor, 2007; Walker *et al.*, 2009), determining plasma protein binding for metabolites possessing pharmacologic activity can also be warranted (Walker *et al.*, 2009). These authors suggest that a decrease in protein binding of a pharmacologically active metabolite, relative to the parent compound, is an important consideration and could result in substantial pharmacologic activity compared to the parent compound.

There are obvious limitations to the use of *in vitro* data. However, the *in vitro* structural, pharmacologic, and disposition data can alert an investigator to metabolites that may justify *in vivo* measurement.

21.2.9 *In Vivo* Metabolite Data

In contrast to the useful qualitative and tentative structural information data provided by *in vitro* experiments, definitive clinical metabolite data is obtained from radiolabelled ADME studies. During the radiolabelled study, human volunteers are typically administered a single clinical dose of drug containing a radiolabel (for example, ^{3}H, ^{14}C, and so on). Plasma, urine, and faeces samples are processed and analyzed using the best available technology such as LC-MS, radiometric analysis and NMR. These analyses provide quantitative data as well as structural information for all detectable metabolites. From this information it is possible to definitively identify metabolites accounting for > 10% of drug-related material. However, due to the cost involved in synthesizing a radiolabelled compound, this type of study is typically conducted after proof of concept has been established for a molecule.

Based on the *in vitro* data, an investigator may choose to develop a fully-validated bioanalytical method prior to Phase 1 clinical study. A more likely scenario is that plasma concentrations of a metabolite will not be evaluated in nonclinical studies to support a Phase 1 clinical trial. Because of the desire to identify important clinical metabolites earlier in development, recent efforts have focused on establishing non-radiolabel-based methods to evaluate human metabolites (Tiller *et al.*, 2008; Vishwanathan *et al.*, 2009). When used to analyze samples from early repeat-dose nonclinical and clinical studies, the data can be used to determine if unique human metabolites exist and whether human exposures are expected to be similar in nonclinical species. Although exploratory methodologies have utility, a higher degree of confidence is associated with data collected using a more rigorously validated bioanalytical method. Data obtained from the validated methods can be used to directly compare clinical and nonclinical exposure and establish coverage (discussed below).

21.2.10 Regulatory Decision Making

After determining that a human metabolite is of significant concern (see Table 21.1) and requires follow-up, the next step is to determine whether coverage is provided in nonclinical species administered the parent drug. Coverage is dependent on both exposure and dose. To meet the exposure-based criteria, a nonclinical model must have equivalent steady-state systemic exposure (e.g., $AUC_{0\text{-}t}$ and/or C_{max} as appropriate) compared with human at the clinical dose. With regards to the dose criteria, it is most desirable to achieve equivalent exposure at a dose that is less than the nonclinical NOAEL; however, higher doses may be acceptable with adequate scientific justification (Atrakchi, 2009). Because of the potential need to provide metabolite coverage in embryo–foetal development and carcinogenicity studies, sufficient circulating concentrations are best found in a rodent model. If a metabolite is covered for all relevant end-points and lacks genotoxic potential (e.g., determined by SAR/QSAR or *in vitro* assessment), further evaluation is likely not needed.

Table 21.1 *Metabolite characteristics of significant concern.*

***In vitro* data**
- unique to human
- pharmacologically active
- decreased protein binding vs. parent drug
- structural alert(s) for genotoxicity

***In vivo* data**
- metabolites that are a significant fraction of drug-related material
- unique to human
- disproportionate human metabolite likely not covered by nonclinical model

In contrast, a human metabolite lacking nonclinical coverage in studies with the parent compound might require nonclinical testing following direct administration of the metabolite. One drawback to this approach is the potential for different pharmacokinetic profiles to be obtained for a metabolite formed *in vivo* vs. a synthesized metabolite directly administered. Well-described differences in PK characteristics such as absorption and clearance (Preuksaritanont *et al.*, 2006; Smith and Obach, 2006; Pang *et al.*, 2008) must be taken into account when choosing this strategy. Other negative aspects are the need to synthesize and characterize the metabolite, to develop a formulation for administration to a nonclinical model, and to conduct range-finding studies to confirm adequate systemic exposure (Powley *et al.*, 2009). In spite of these complications, a well-designed study could allow for collection of relevant data to support clinical safety.

Another important aspect of regulatory decision making is the consideration of additional relevant information. The toxicology profile of the parent drug from both nonclinical and clinical evaluations are of great importance. For instance, an embryo–foetal development study with a metabolite is not necessary for a teratogenic parent drug. A drug's indication, patient population, availability of alternative drugs, standard of care, and so on, will also factor into the final decision. It is worth noting that recommendations for a life-threatening indication are likely to be less extensive when compared to a non-life-threatening indication (FDA, 2008).

In summary, evaluating the nonclinical toxicity of an important clinical metabolite may be necessary to minimize risk to human trial participants. Although regulatory recommendations have been made by both the FDA and the ICH, it is important to note that decisions should be based on the totality of information available for each molecule.

References

Atrakchi, A.H. (2009) Interpretation and considerations on the safety evaluation of human drug metabolites. *Chem. Res. Toxicol.*, **22**, 1217–1220.

Baillie, T.A., Cayen, M.N., Fouda, H. *et al.* (2002) Drug metabolites in safety testing. *Toxicol. Appl. Pharmacol.*, **182**, 188–196.

Davis-Bruno, K. and Atrakchi, A. (2006) A regulatory perspective on issues and approaches in characterizing human metabolites. *Chem. Res. Toxicol.*, **19**, 1561–1563.

Faed, E.M. (1984) Properties of acyl glyucuronides: implications for studies of the pharmacokinetics and metabolism of acidic drugs. *Drug Met. Rev.*, **15**, 1213–1249.

FDA, CDER (2006) Draft Guidance for Industry: Safety Testing of Drug Metabolites.

FDA, CDER (2008) Guidance for Industry: Safety Testing of Drug Metabolites.

Gaylor, D.W. and Kodell, R.L. (1980) Linear interpolation algorithm for low dose assessment of toxic substances. *J. Environ. Pathology*, **4**, 305.

DHHS, FDA, CDER (1999) Guidance for Industry, Container Closure Systems for Packaging Human Drugs and Biologicals, Chemistry, Manufacturing and Controls Documentation, May 1999. http://www.fda.gov/Drugs/GuidanceComplianceRegulatoryInformation/Guidances/ucm064979.htm.

History of the FDA http://fda.gov/AboutFDA/WhatWeDo/History/default.htm.

ICH (2009) M3(R2) Guidance on nonclinical safety studies for the conduct of human clinical trials and marketing authorization for pharmaceuticals www.ich.org.

Osterberg, R.E. (2005) Potential toxicity of extractables and leachables in drug products. *Amer. Pharm. Rev.*, **8**(2), 64–67.

Product Quality Research Institute (PQRI) (2006) Safety thresholds and best practices for extractables and leachables in orally inhaled and nasal drug products http://www.pqri.org/publications/index.asp.

Pang, K.S., Morris, M.E., and Sun, H. (2008) Formed and preformed metabolites: facts and comparisons. *J. Pharm. Pharmacol.*, **60**, 1247–1275.

Powley, M.W., Frederick, C.B., Sistare, F.D., and DeGeorge, J.J. (2009) Safety assessment of drug metabolites: implications of regulatory guidance and potential application of genetically engineered mouse models that express human P450s. *Chem. Res. Toxicol.*, **22**, 257–262.

Preuksaritanont, T., Lin, J.H., and Baillie, T.A. (2006) Complicating factors in safety testing of drug kinetics: kinetic differences between generated and preformed metabolites. *Toxicol. Appl. Pharmacol.*, **217**, 143–152.

Robison, T. and Jacobs, A.C. (2009) Metabolites in safety testing. *Bioanalysis*, **1**, 1193–1200.

Smith, D.A. and Obach, R.S. (2006) Metabolites and safety: what are the concerns, and how should we address them. *Chem. Res. Toxicol.*, **19**, 1570–1579.

Swann, J.P. (2008) Pharmaceutical regulation before and after the FD&C Act, in *The Pharmaceutical Regulatory Process, Chapter One, 2nd Edition* (eds Berry, R. and Martin, R.P.), Informa Healthcare USA Inc., New York, NY.

Tiller, P.R., Yu, S., Bateman, K.P. *et al.* (2008) Fractional mass filtering as a means to assess circulating metabolites in early human clinical studies. *Rapid Commun. Mass Spectrom.*, **22**, 3510–3516.

Trainor, G.L. (2007) The importance of plasma protein binding in drug discovery. *Expert Opin. Drug Discov.*, **2**, 51–64.

Vishwanathan, K., Babalola, K., Wang, J. *et al.* (2009) Obtaining exposures of metabolites in preclinical species through plasma pooling and quantitative NMR: addressing metabolites in safety testing (MIST) guidance without using radiolabeled compounds and chemically synthesized metabolite standards. *Chem. Res. Toxicol.*, **22**, 311–322.

Walker, D., Brady, J., Dalvie, D. *et al.* (2009) A holistic strategy for characterizing the safety of metabolites through drug discovery and development. *Chem. Res. Toxicol.*, **22**, 1653–1662.

Index

Nonclinical Safety Assessment: A Guide to International Pharmaceutical Regulations, First Edition.
Edited by William J. Brock, Kenneth L. Hastings and Kathy M. McGown.

www.ingramcontent.com/pod-product-compliance
Ingram Content Group UK Ltd.
Pitfield, Milton Keynes, MK11 3LW, UK
UKHW050942290926
15470UKWH00005B/1594